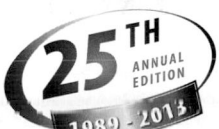

25TH ANNUAL EDITION 1989 - 2013

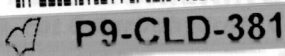

Calor... P9-CLD-381

Contents

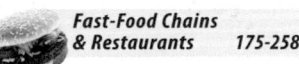

EXTRA DIET GUIDES & COUNTERS

Weight Control Tips

✅ Eat & Drink Sensibly

- Avoid fad diets. Eat 3 sensible portion-controlled meals.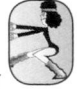
- Limit fats, high-fat foods/snacks and sugar. Eat adequate fresh fruit & vegetables.
- Limit soft drinks, energy drinks, fruit juice and alcohol. Quench your thirst on water. *(See Sample Meal Plan ~ Page 11)*

✅ Exercise Daily

- Aim for at least 30 minutes daily – even in 5-10 minute lots. For motivation, find an exercise buddy, personal trainer or join a gym. *(Extra Notes ~ Page 12)*

✅ Reshape Eating Behaviors

- Be aware of eating and shopping behaviors that lead to overeating.
- Also focus on social and emotional situations that may trigger compulsive eating. *(Extra Notes ~ Page 14)*

✅ Keep a Food & Exercise Journal

- A journal helps you see exactly what you eat and drink, and how much you exercise. *(Extra Notes ~ Page 15)*
- An excellent motivator and proven weight loss aid. Keeps you honest!

✅ Arrange Moral Support

- Gain the support of family and friends.
- Get extra professional help if required, from your doctor, dietitian, psychologist, exercise trainer, or slimming group.
- Beware of family saboteurs who discourage you from adopting a healthier lifestyle!

🩺 DOCTOR CHECK-UP

Ask your doctor to check your blood pressure, blood sugar and blood cholesterol levels.

HEALTHY WEIGHTS
~ MEN & WOMEN ~
(Over 18 Years)

Based on weights with least risk of disease or death from heart disease, diabetes, stroke and cancer.

Based on Body Mass Index of 20-25

BMI calculated as: $\dfrac{\text{Weight (kg)}}{\text{Height (m)}^2}$

Height (No Shoes) Ft Ins		Healthy Weight Range (Pounds)
4'7"	~	86-108
4'8"	~	88-110
4'9"	~	92-114
4'10"	~	97-121
4'11"	~	99-123
5'0"	~	101-127
5'1"	~	105-132
5'2"	~	110-136
5'3"	~	112-140
5'4"	~	114-145
5'5"	~	119-149
5'6"	~	123-156
5'7"	~	127-158
5'8"	~	129-162
5'9"	~	134-167
5'10"	~	138-173
5'11"	~	143-178
6'0"	~	145-182
6'1"	~	149-187
6'2"	~	156-193
6'3"	~	158-198
6'4"	~	162-202
6'5"	~	170-211
6'6"	~	172-215
6'7"	~	175-220

Body Fat Distribution & Health

Moderate amounts of body fat do not compromise health. However, excess fat above the hips carries a far greater health risk than fat on or below the hips - better to be a 'pear-shape' than an 'apple-shape'.

Abdominal obesity greatly increases the risk of developing diabetes, heart disease, high blood fats, hypertension, stroke, sleep apnea, arthritis and some cancers. So-called 'cellulite' carries no extra health risk.

Waist Circumference directly reflects the increased health risk of abdominal obesity. Waist size associated with a high health risk: **Men** ~ Over 40 inches
Women ~ Over 35 inches

Body Mass Index (BMI)

BMI is a general (but not specific) indicator of body fatness.
Although BMI alone is not diagnostic, the higher the BMI, the greater the health risk of developing diabetes, high blood pressure and heart disease. BMI does not apply to heavily muscled persons. BMI is used in a different way for children.

Abdominal obesity greatly increases the risk of ill-health and earlier death.

Check Your BMI: Find your height (no shoes) - look across the row to the weight nearest your own. Then track down to BMI.

Ht	WEIGHT (LBS) ~ ADULTS													
5'1"	100	106	111	116	122	127	132	137	143	148	153	158	185	211
5'2"	104	109	115	120	126	131	136	142	147	153	158	164	191	218
5'3"	107	113	118	124	130	135	141	146	152	158	163	169	197	225
5'4"	110	116	122	128	134	140	145	151	157	163	169	174	204	232
5'5"	114	120	126	132	138	144	150	156	162	168	174	180	210	240
5'6"	118	124	130	136	142	148	155	161	167	173	179	186	216	247
5'7"	121	127	134	140	146	153	159	166	172	178	185	191	223	255
5'8"	125	131	138	144	151	158	164	171	177	184	190	197	230	262
5'9"	128	135	142	149	155	162	169	176	182	189	196	206	236	270
5'10"	132	139	146	153	160	167	174	181	188	195	202	207	243	278
5'11"	136	143	150	157	165	172	179	186	193	200	208	215	250	286
6'0"	140	147	154	162	169	177	184	191	199	206	213	221	258	294
6'1"	144	151	159	166	174	182	189	197	204	212	219	227	265	302
6'2"	148	155	163	171	179	186	194	202	210	218	225	233	272	311
6'3"	152	160	168	176	184	192	200	208	216	224	232	240	279	319
6'4"	156	164	172	180	189	197	205	213	221	230	238	246	287	328
BMI	19	20	21	22	23	24	25	26	27	28	29	30	35	40

BMI Classification:

BMI Below 19
Underweight

BMI 19-24.9
Healthy Weight
(Low Health Risk)

BMI 25-29.9
Overweight
(Moderate Health Risk)

BMI 30-40
Obese (High Health Risk)

BMI Over 40
Morbid Obesity
(Very High Risk)

Interactive BMI Calculator
www.calorieking.com

Calories & Weight Loss

Calories in Food

Calories in food are derived from protein, fat and carbohydrate. Alcohol also provides calories. Vitamins, minerals and water provide no calories.

Calorie Values Per Gram	
Fat/Oil	~ 9 Calories
Carbohydrate	~ 4 Calories
Protein	~ 4 Calories
Alcohol	~ 7 Calories

Note that fats have over double the calories of protein and carbohydrate. The higher the fat content of food, the higher the calories.

Sample Calculation

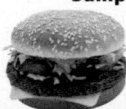

QUARTER POUNDER®
WITH CHEESE
has 510 calories
derived from:

26g Fat (x 9 cals/gram)	=	234
40g Carbohyd.(x 4 cals/gram)	=	160
29g Protein (x 4 cals/gram)	=	116
Total Calories	=	510

Calorie Levels for Weight Loss

Start with a calorie-controlled diet that allows a moderate weight loss of ½ - 1 pound per week. Weight loss is usually much greater in the first few weeks due to extra fluid losses.

Note: It is better to increase exercise rather than lessen food calories too drastically.

Suggested Calories for Weight Loss	
Women: Non-active	1000 - 1200
Active	1200 - 1500
Men: Non-active	1200 - 1500
Active	1500 - 1800
Teenagers:	1200 - 1800

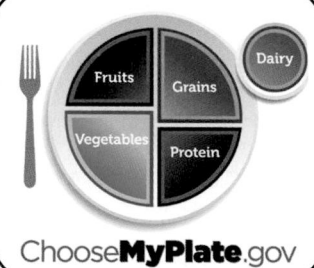
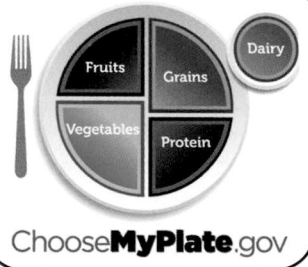

ChooseMyPlate.gov

The MyPlate symbol represents the recommended proportion of foods from each food group. It focuses on the importance of making smart food choices in every food group, every day. Daily physical activity is also important. *(More info: www.ChooseMyPlate.gov)*

Examples of Single Serving Sizes

Grains (Eat 6 servings per day):
- 1 slice wholegrain bread (1 oz)
- ½ bun, small bagel or English muffin
- 4 small crackers or 1 tortilla
- 1 oz ready-to-eat wholegrain cereal
- ½ cup cooked cereal, rice or pasta

Vegetables (Eat 3-5 servings per day):
- 1 cup raw leafy vegetables
- 1½ cups raw chopped vegetables
- ½ cup cooked vegetables
- ½ - ¾ cup vegetable juice

Fruit (Eat 3-5 servings per day):
- 1 medium apple, orange, banana
- ½ cup canned fruit (in own juice)
- ¼ cup dried fruit
- ½ cup fruit juice (unsweetened)
- ¼ medium avocado

Protein (2-3 servings per day):
- 2-3 oz (cooked) lean meat/poultry/fish
- 2 eggs or 6 oz tofu or ¼ cup nuts
- 1 cup (cooked) dried beans or chickpeas

Dairy (2-3 servings per day):
- 1 cup (8 fl.oz) milk/soy (enriched)/yogurt
- 1½ oz cheese or ½ cup cottage cheese

Portion Size Counts!

Food portion size is critical to controlling calorie intake for weight control.

Super-sized food servings have become more common when eating out and in the home. This can mean a day's worth of calories being consumed in one meal; or a snack being equivalent to a full meal.

It is easy to underestimate portion size of foods and drinks, and unwittingly consume excess calories – even if the fat content is low or even zero!

To more accurately estimate portion size of different foods, weigh and measure your food with food scales, measuring spoons and cups. Better control of calories will result.

For a visual idea of portion sizes, visit www.CalorieKing.com See examples (fries and cola) on this page.

Allow for Extra Calories in Packaged Food

The actual weight of packaged foods is usually 5-10% more than the label net weight (the minimum legal weight) – and in some cases up to 50% more. However, manufacturers calculate the calories based on the net weight. For actual calories, weigh the product and calculate the extra calories.

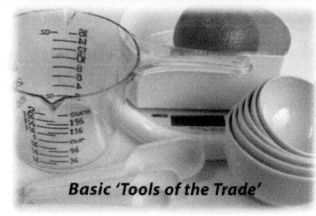

Basic 'Tools of the Trade'

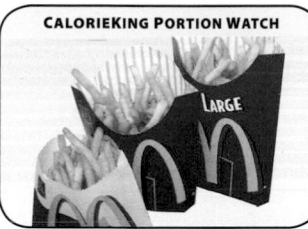

CALORIEKING PORTION WATCH

Fries	Cal	Fat	Carb
Small	230	11	29
Medium	380	19	48
Large	500	25	63

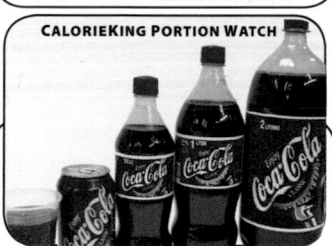

CALORIEKING PORTION WATCH

Cola	Cal	Fat	Carb
8 fl.oz Cup	100	0	25
12 fl.oz Can	150	0	37
20 fl.oz Bottle	250	0	63
1 Liter Bottle	400	0	100
2 Liter Bottle	800	0	200

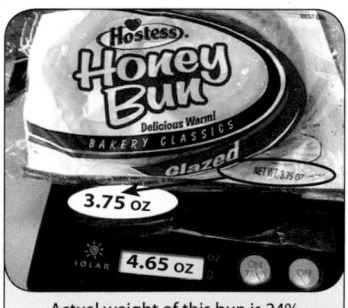

Actual weight of this bun is 24% more than the stated net weight.

▶ Fat in the Diet

Fats in the diet are essential for good health. However, too much fat can contribute to obesity and a higher risk of heart disease, high blood pressure, diabetes, gallstone and certain cancers.

Dietary fat and oils have over double the calories of carbohydrates and protein. (Example: Changing from whole-milk to non-fat milk halves the calories.)

MAXIMUM DESIRABLE FAT INTAKE (DAILY)

Calories	Fat
1200 cals	30g fat
1500 cals	40g fat
1800 cals	50g fat
2000 cals	60g fat
2200 cals	70g fat
2500 cals	80g fat
3000 cals	110g fat

ZERO GRAMS TRANS FAT

*Don't be fooled by **Zero Grams Trans Fat** boldly displayed on some high-fat snacks. They are still high in fat and calories.*

Examples: Cheetos 99c pkg ~ 24g fat, 380 cals
Lay's Chips (2¾ oz pkg) ~ 27g fat, 430 calories

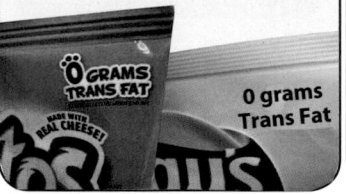

0 grams Trans Fat

▶ Beware low-fat foods

It is a mistake to think that eating low-fat or fat-free foods allows you to eat double the quantity. You can end up with even more calories than eating smaller amounts of regular-fat products.

Food products which are fat-free but high in calories include soda drinks, fruit juices, beer, alcoholic spirits, sugar and candy. Bread, rice and pasta also have negligible fat but need to be eaten in controlled amounts.

Ultimately, **it is food portion size as well as total calories that count** whether from fat, carbohydrate or protein. Remember, cows get fat on grass!

Reduced fat and fat-free foods are not necessarily low calorie. Portion size is still important.

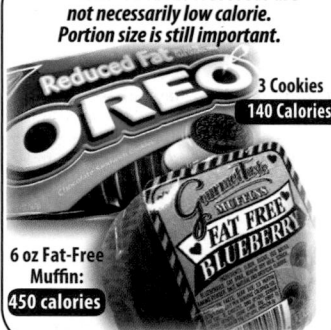

3 Cookies
140 Calories

6 oz Fat-Free Muffin:
450 calories

FOOD LABEL MEANINGS

FDA Nutrition Claim Definitions
(All are on a Per Serving Basis)

Low Calorie: 40 Calories or less
Light or Lite: One third fewer calories or, 50% or less fat than regular product
Fat-Free: Less than half a gram of fat
Low-Fat: 3 grams or less of fat
Reduced Fat: 25% less fat than regular product
Fewer or Less Calories: At least 25% fewer calories than regular product

▶ Meats, Poultry, Fish

- **Choose lean cuts** of meat with little marbling. **Trim all visible fat from meat** and remove the skin from poultry. Removal of fat after cooking, is okay (to prevent dryness). Choose 'extra lean' ground beef.
- **Avoid high-fat meat products** such as salami, bacon, sausage and franks.
- **Broil or bake. Avoid frying in oil.** Allow casseroles to cool and skim off surface fat.
- **Avoid fried fish,** frozen fish in batter and canned fish in oil.

▶ Fats & Oils

- **Use minimal amounts** of all types of fat and oil. All are high in calories.
- **Choose** 'light' and 'reduced fat' spreads but still use sparingly.
- Use minimal amounts of oil when stir-frying. Use no-stick sprays like Pam.

▶ Salad Dressings & Sauces

- **Avoid regular mayonnaise and oil dressings.** Choose 'light', 'reduced fat' or 'fat-free' brands.
- **Choose low-fat or fat-free sauces** (mainly tomato-based). Avoid 'pesto', 'alfredo', 'cheese' and 'creamy' sauces.

▶ Milk, Cheese

- **Choose low-fat or nonfat milks and yogurts.** Avoid full-cream milk, cream, Half & Half.
- **Cheese:** Choose fat-free, and low-fat cheese. Part-skim ricotta is still high in fat. Low-fat cottage cheese is a good choice. Cheese substitutes can still be high in fat.

▶ Snacks, Cookies, Candy

- **Avoid** high-fat snacks such as potato chips, corn/tortilla chips, cheese puffs, buttered popcorn, chocolate and carob bars.

▶ Desserts/Sweets

- **Avoid high-fat desserts,** such as cake, pie, pastries, cheesecake, full-fat puddings.
- **Choose** fresh fruits, fresh fruit salad, canned fruit in water pack, low-fat ice cream. Use low-fat yogurt in place of cream.

▶ Fast-Foods & Take-Out

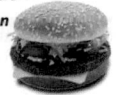

Check the Fast-Foods Section of this book for actual fat and calorie counts.

- **Avoid deep-fried foods such as** chicken, french fries and onion rings.
- **Pizzas:** Avoid sausage/pepperoni. Choose vegetarian topping and modest quantity of cheese. Eat a moderate serving. Eat extra salad and fresh fruit.
- **Hamburgers:** Choose medium size, lower fat burgers. Avoid bacon. Have a side salad (with fat-free dressing).
- **Delis:** Choose sandwiches/bread rolls, pitas with low-fat fillings and plain salad. Limit meat/cheese to small portions.
- **Coffees:** Avoid large sizes of latte and frappuccino. Request nonfat milk and no whipped cream. Avoid cookies and pastries.

Extra Information: www.CalorieKing.com

FRYING ADDS FAT!

The greater the surface area of potato exposed to fat or oil, the higher the fat content and calories.

	Whole Potato (3 oz) **0g Fat**	65 Cals
	Roasted Potato (3 oz) **5g Fat**	155 Cals
	Fries (Large cut, 3 oz) **12g Fat**	220 Cals
	Fries (Small, 3 oz) **15g Fat**	265 Cals
	Potato Chips (3 oz) **30g Fat**	450 Cals

Naturally-Friendly Carbs

- **Carbohydrate foods in their more natural forms** (not overly processed) are essential to good health. They are the main source of fuel for the body, and also provide important vitamins, minerals, antioxidants and fiber – all of which help protect against heart disease, diabetes, hypertension, constipation-related ailments and many other diseases.

- Carbohydrates even help the body produce serotonin, the 'feel good' brain chemical that helps control appetite and overeating. Too little serotonin can lead to mood swings and depression.

Carbohydrates are found in different forms in food as:

- Sugars in fruit, sugar cane, milk
- Starches in whole grains, legumes, nuts, seeds and vegetables
- Dietary fiber (See Fiber Guide ~ Page 264)

Glycemic Index & Diabetes ~ Page 21

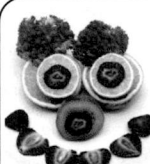

Carbohydrate foods (minimally processed) are essential to good health.

Be sure to eat adequate fruit (2 servings) and vegetables (5 servings) every day.

Low-Carbohydrate Diets

- Popular low-carbohydrate diets are extreme in their recommendations to initially cut carb intake to as little as 20 grams per day – the amount in 1 thick slice of bread, or 1 medium apple, or 1 small potato.

  This greatly increases the risk of nutritional deficiencies and compromises health, particularly if fat intake is excessive through fatty meats, high-fat dairy products, and fried foods.

- While overweight Americans do need to reduce carbohydrate intake, it should be done **sensibly as part of reducing portion size and total calories.**

- Simply eating 'low-carb' food products without regard to portion size, calories or fats, will do little to promote weight loss or good health.

- **Low-carb diets (and indeed any diet) only work if total calories are reduced.**

- Refined sugars should be one of the first targets in reducing carb intake.

Extra Info ~ www.CalorieKing.com

RECOMMENDED CARBOHYDRATE INTAKE		
Calories (Daily)	Carbohydrate (Grams)	Percent Carbohydrate Calories
1200 cals	120g	40%
1500 cals	170g	45%
1800 cals	210g	47%
2000 cals	250g	50%
2500 cals	345g	55%
3000 cals	450g	60%

How Much Do We Need?

- As shown in the chart, well-balanced diets above 2000 calories contain 50-60% of total calories from carbohydrates.

- At lower calorie levels used for weight control (1200-1500 calories), carbohydrates account for as little as 40% of total calories. This is because protein calories have nutritional priority.

- Carbohydrates & Diabetes ~ *See Page 21*

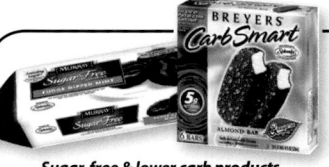

Sugar-free & lower carb products may still be high in calories and fat.

- Many overweight, inactive people consume over 500 calories of refined sugars per day, either self-added or as part of food products. This is equivalent to over 30 level teaspoons – a significant amount in weight control terms. Halving this amount would be reasonable and worthwhile.

Note: Naturally occurring sugars in fruits, vegetables and milk are fine when consumed in normal recommended amounts. These foods are also rich in other nutrients.

Refined sugar is referred to as having 'empty calories' because it supplies calories but negligible nutrients and no fiber.

- **Most sugar in our diet is 'hidden'** in processed foods such as soft drinks, fruit drinks, candy, cookies, cake, jam, sauces, ice cream, desserts, canned foods, and breakfast cereals.

Certainly enjoy moderate quantities of these foods, but for serious weight control, look for 'low calorie', 'diet' or 'sugar-free'.

However, be careful not to substitute sugar-rich foods with high-fat foods which might boost calories even more!

- Be aware that sugar comes in different forms such as sucrose, glucose, fructose, malt, high-fructose corn syrup, molasses, honey and maple syrup. Check the label.

- **Sugar alcohols such as sorbitol,** mannitol and maltitol are carb-based and have ½ - ¾ the calories of regular sugar. While not counted as sugar on food labels, they do add to the carb count. Excess amounts can cause bloating, gas and diarrhea.

- **Sugar-free sweeteners** such as *Equal, DiabetiSweet, NutraSweet, Splenda, Sweet'n Low* and *Stevia* make it easy to reduce sugar in drinks and recipes. Use only in moderation. Note: Most recipes can be adapted to contain less sugar with little effect on taste or quality.

Extra Info ~ www.CalorieKing.com

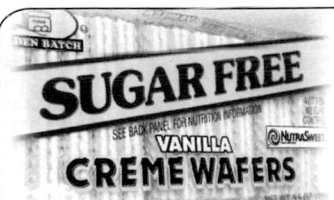

Sugar-free snacks and foods may be higher in fat and calories than the regular product.

Example	~ Creme Wafers (3):
Regular	~ 115 cals, 6g fat
Sugar-Free	~ 160 cals, 10g fat

SUGAR CONTENT OF SOME COMMON FOODS

	Teaspoons of Sugar
Coca Cola or *Pepsi*, 12 fl.oz	10
20 fl.oz size	17
Iced Tea, sweetened, 12 fl.oz	8
Chocolate Milk, 12 fl.oz	6
Honey Smacks Cereal, ¾ cup, 1 oz	4
Popcorn, caramel, 1 cup	3.5
Chocolate Bar, 1.5 oz	6
M&M's 1.7 oz pkg	7
Muffin, large, 4 oz	6
Choc Chip Cookie, 1 oz	2
Donut, iced	6
Apple Pie, 1 piece	7
Jell-O, ½ cup	4.5
Jam, 1 Tbsp, ¾ oz	2.5
Syrup, maple, 1 Tbsp	3

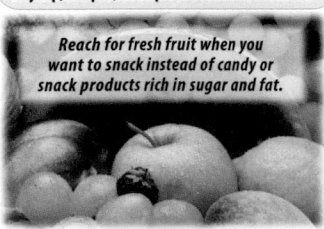

Reach for fresh fruit when you want to snack instead of candy or snack products rich in sugar and fat.

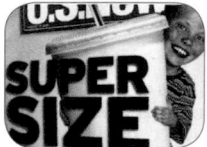

The XL Generation

Some 15% of American kids and adolescents are overweight; and childhood obesity has doubled over the last 20 years. Diabetes, high blood pressure and high cholesterol are major problem areas for overweight children and adolescents, as are depression, low self-esteem, sleep apnea and bone joint problems.

To address this problem, cooperation is required between kids, parents, schools and government. Weight control is a family and community affair.

Five Simple Tips To Get Started:

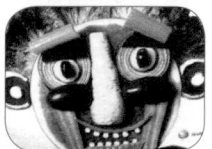

❶ Watch Soda Intake

Limit soda and sugary drinks to one serving on the weekends. Soda should not be an everyday beverage – water should be. When at restaurants or using a soda fountain, choose small servings with ice or choose diet soda instead. Schools should provide water and restrict access to soda as should parents when eating out or in the home!

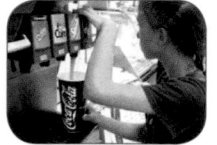

❷ Cut back on Fast-Foods and Eating Out

Many more calories are consumed when you eat out. Healthy meals prepared at home are best for the whole family.

❸ Say "No" to Super-Sizing

When meals are upsized, loads more calories are consumed. Choose sensible portion sizes when eating out and at home. Use smaller plates and choose smaller packages.

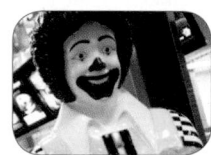

❹ Limit Between-Meal Snacking

Watch out for high-fat and high-calorie snacks – they can have more calories than a meal! Keep your eye on portion sizes and limit salty snack foods and candy to parties and special occasions. Choose fresh fruit, vegetables, nuts and low-fat milk instead.

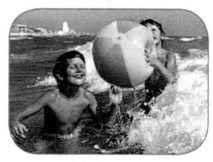

❺ Get Moving ~ Watch Less TV

Kids need at least 60 minutes of physical activity every day. It's critical for their fitness, and greatly lessens the risk of obesity.

Encourage kids to be active out of school hours. Wearing a pedometer can be highly motivational for kids to move more – as can playing dance video games such as *Dance Dance Revolution. Dance Central* (XBox360) and *Wii Fit (Nintendo)* are also excellent fitness motivators.

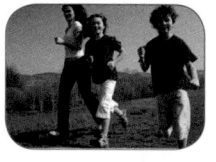

Limit TV and non-active computer games to just one hour per day. Also limit the accompanying snacks! Include exercise in family activities.

Extra information and tips ~ www.CalorieKing.com

**For Healthy, Overweight Persons ~ Not for Persons With Any Medical Condition
~ Please Check With Your Doctor & Dietitian ~**

 Breakfast (approx. 300 cal)

	1 Small Fruit or ½ oz Dried Fruit
Plus	Cereal: 1½ oz Dry (high fiber)
	or 1 cup cooked Oatmeal
Plus	½ oz Almonds/Seeds
Plus	Milk (from daily allowance) or Yogurt (low-fat)

Daily Milk Allowance (approx.160 calories)
2 cups Non-Fat Milk or 1½ cups Low-fat (1%) Milk
or equivalent Soy Drink, Yogurt, Cheese, Tofu

Fat Allowance (140 calories; 15g Fat)
4 tsp Fat or 6-8 tsp Diet Margarine or 3 tsp Oil
or 1½ Tbsp Mayonnaise or ½ medium Avocado
or 1½ Tbsp Peanut Butter or 30g Nuts/Seeds

 Lunch (approx. 440 calories)

	2 slices Wholegrain Bread (2 oz)
	or 4 Crispbreads/Crackers or 6" Pita
Plus	2 oz lean Meat, Chicken or Turkey
	or 3½oz Tuna (in water) or 2½ oz Salmon
	or 1 oz Cheese or ½ cup (4 oz) Cottage Cheese
	or ½ cup (4 oz) Ricotta Cheese (low-fat)
	or ½ cup (4 oz) Fruit Yogurt (low-fat)
	or ½ cup (4 oz) Bean Salad
Plus	Large Salad (Oil-free dressing)
Plus	1 small Fruit or ½ oz Dried Fruit

 Dinner (approx. 360 calories)

	Soup (fat-free)
Plus	3 oz lean Meat (cooked weight)
	or 4 oz Chicken Breast (no skin)
	or 3 oz Chicken Thigh/Leg (no skin)
	or 5 oz Fish (grilled, no fat)
	or ¾ cup (6 oz) Beans (Soy, Kidney, Pinto etc)/Lentils
	or Low-fat Entree (e.g. Lean Cuisine)
Plus	1 small Potato
	or ½ cup Rice/Pasta/Sweet Corn
	or 1 slice Wholegrain Bread
Plus	2-3 servings Vegetables/Salad
Plus	1 small Fruit + Diet Gelatin Dessert

 Breakfast ~ Choice 2

	1 Small Fruit
Plus	2 Eggs (no added fat)
	or 2 oz Cheese (low-fat)
	or 4 oz Cottage Cheese (low-fat)
	or 2 oz Lean/Canadian Bacon
Plus	1 Tomato
Plus	1 Slice Wholegrain Toast

 Between Meals

Water, Coffee, Tea, Diet drinks,
Fruit from main meals; Raw vegetable
pieces, Milk from Daily Allowance

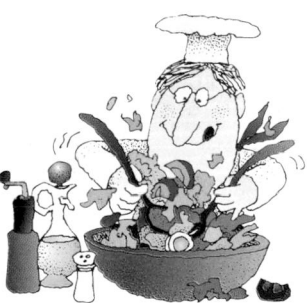

Exercise & Weight Control

- **Persons who exercise regularly lose more weight** and keep it off longer than non-exercisers.

- **Exercise also improves general health and well-being.** Mood, confidence and self-esteem are enhanced by a sense of control and accomplishment.

- **Exercise is a good way to 'wake up' a sluggish metabolism** and burn extra fat tissue.

- **Aerobic (huff and puff) exercise most days** is great for burning calories and for cardiovascular fitness. But, it is strength training that mainly builds the muscles that burn calories even while we sleep.

- **Strength training is the key to retaining or rebuilding muscles.** As we age, we lose some 6 pounds of muscle per decade. This results in a lower metabolism and fewer calories being burnt.

  Muscles are the furnaces that burn calories. The more muscle you have, the more calories you will burn.

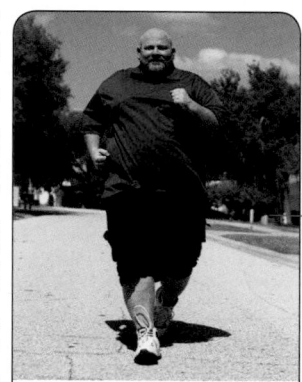

Brisk walking each day is a safe and effective way to burn calories and keep fit.
Try it – you'll like it!

- **Regular strength training (2-3 times weekly)** can increase our metabolic rate for several days following exercise – and an extra 100 calories per day being burnt. While 2-3 pounds of muscle may be gained in the first 8-10 weeks, weight from exercised muscles is okay. It is excess fat (particularly abdominal fat) that is a potential health hazard. Gaining muscle and losing fat also helps body reshaping – even if the scales don't show it.

- **Avoid injury** by beginning with walking, low impact aerobics, or weight-supported exercise (e.g. swimming, cycling). Avoid competitive sports. Allow 2-3 days of recovery between strength training sessions. Get professional advice ~ particularly if you have a medical condition.

- **How Much?** Start with 10-20 minutes per day and progress to 30-60 minutes per day.

  Also walk up stairs instead of using elevators. Take a brisk walk at lunch. Use an exercise bike, treadmill or stair machine while watching TV. Walk the dog.

- **How Often?** While aerobic fitness requires only 3-4 sessions weekly, **weight control is a daily event which requires daily exercise to burn calories.** Add in strength training 2-3 times weekly.

- **For motivation,** find an exercise buddy, personal trainer or join a gym.

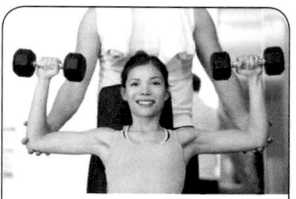

Strength training is the key to retain or rebuild muscles.
Muscles burn extra calories even while you sleep.
For extra guidance, seek a qualified trainer or join a gym.

Calories Used in Exercise

LIGHT	MODERATE	HEAVY
130 lbs ~ 3 Cals/Min	130 lbs ~ 5 Cals/Min	130 lbs ~ 8 Cals/Min
170 lbs ~ 4 Cals/Min	170 lbs ~ 6 Cals/Min	220 lbs ~ 12 Cals/Min
220 lbs ~ 5 Cals/Min	220 lbs ~ 7 Cals/Min	170 lbs ~ 10 Cals/Min

LIGHT	MODERATE	HEAVY
Walking, slow	Walking, brisk	Walking (power), Jogging
Cycling, light	Cycling, moderate	Cycling (vigorous), Spinning
Frisbee playing	Swimming, crawl	Swimming, strenuous
Gardening, light	Weight-training, light	Weight-training, heavy
Golf, social	Tennis, moderate	Wrestling/Judo, advanced
Tennis, doubles	Racquetball, beginners	Racquetball, advanced
Housework, cleaning	Aerobics, light	Tae Bo, Kick Boxing
Calisthenics, light	Football, touch	Football, training
Bowling	Basketball, Baseball	Basketball (Pro)
Ping-pong, social	Walking Downstairs	Climbing Stairs
Ice Skating, light	Snow Skiing (downhill)	Skipping Rope
Aquarobics, light	Shovelling snow	Skiing (cross country)
Skate Boarding	Dancing (ballroom)	Aquarobics, advanced
Line/Square Dancing	Rowing, moderate	Dancing (strenuous), Zumba
Tai Chi, Yoga	Volleyball, competitive	Rowing, vigorous
Volleyball		Martial Arts

Note: Only those sports or activities that are sustained over a period of time (e.g running) qualify for heavy exercise. Stop-start sports such as tennis are considered 'moderate'.

Interactive Calculations ~ www.CalorieKing.com/tools

WALKING PROGRAM

USE DISTANCE, STEPS OR TIME			
Weeks	Distance	Steps Pedometer	Time
1-2	1 mile	2000	20 mins
3-5	1.5 miles	3000	28 mins
6-8	2 miles	3500	35 mins
9-10	2.5 miles	4500	45 mins
11+	3.5 miles	6000	60 mins

10,000 STEPS PER DAY

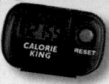

A pedometer can motivate you to be more active. It clips to your belt or waist band and registers each step.

Aim for 8,000 - 10,000 steps per day, instead of an average of only 3,000 - 4,000 steps.

For Extra Information:
www.CalorieKing.com

Reshaping Eating Behaviors

- Eating is a behavior that is largely controlled by people with whom we live or socialize, places in which we carry out our lives, and our emotions. Become aware of those situations that commonly lead to extra food being eaten.

- We may also be unaware of 'bad' eating habits that can lead to excess calorie intake; e.g. eating quickly, large mouthfuls, eating when tense or bored, finishing a large serving of food when not hungry.

Tips to help uncover and correct those 'bad' or problem eating habits:

- **Don't eat while engaged in other activities;** for example, watching TV, reading. Eat only at the table, not at the fridge or while standing.

- **Don't eat quickly.** Chewing slowly allows time to register a feeling of fullness. Don't use fingers, only utensils. Cut food into smaller pieces. Don't load your fork until the previous mouthful is finished.

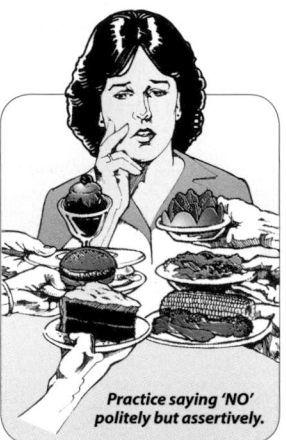

Practice saying 'NO' politely but assertively.

- **Don't purchase problem high calorie foods.** Shop from a set list to prevent impulse buying. Avoid shopping with children.

- **Buy snack foods** in the smallest package. The larger the serving size or package, the more you are likely to eat or drink.

- **Plan meals in advance. Stick to a set menu.**

- **Plan a strategy to avoid uncontrolled eating** and drinking at social events, or when your emotions urge you to binge.

  Rehearse repeatedly in your mind exactly what you will do in such situations. Remind yourself several times each day that you are in charge of your actions and that you can be strong-willed. Seek counseling or coaching on various strategies.

- **Distract yourself** when you feel the urge to snack impulsively. Engage in some activity that will distract you from thinking about food. Examples: go for a walk, brush your teeth, phone a friend.

  If you eat out of boredom, find some new hobby or interest that gets you out of the house. Even enrol in an adult education class.

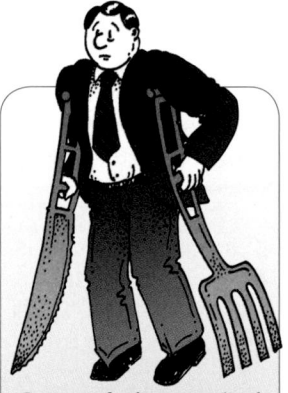

Do you use food as an emotional crutch? If so, professional counseling may be helpful.

The food journal is the most powerful proven aid for dieters. Persons who keep a food and exercise journal not only lose more weight, they also keep it off. Here are some of the reasons:

- **Recording your eating and exercise habits** jolts you into realizing just what you do eat and drink each day; and also whether you exercise sufficiently.

- **Helps you identify problem foods** and drinks with excessive calories and fat.

- **Helps identify moods,** situations and events that lead to excessive eating of unwanted calories. You can then plan to overcome or avoid them.

- **Prevents 'calorie amnesia',** the forgetfulness that leads to rebound weight gain after successful weight loss. Recording puts you back on the right track.

- **Helps you develop greater self-discipline.** You will think twice about overindulging if you have to record it - especially if someone checks your journal regularly. It certainly keeps you honest!

- **Motivates you** to carefully plan your meals and to exercise each day.

- **Serves as a check system** for your doctor, dietitian or counselor to assess your progress and make recommendations.

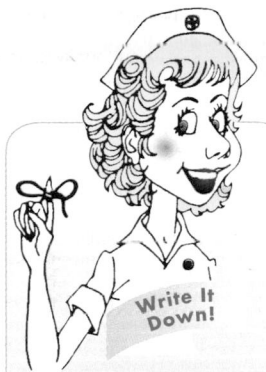

Write It Down!

"Keeping a journal gives me feedback on exactly what I eat and drink each day.

It helps prevent 'calorie amnesia' and reminds me to exercise each day.

It's a 'must' for successful weight control!"

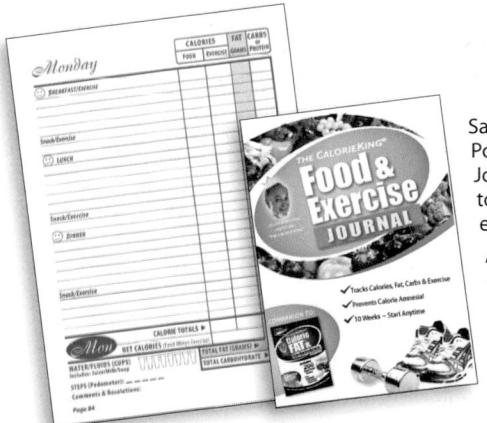

Sample Page from The Pocket Food & Exercise Journal, a 10-week journal to record food and exercise.

At day's end, exercise calories are deducted from food calories.

Includes Weekly Summary Page & Progress Checklist.

What is Diabetes?

Diabetes occurs when the body has difficulty processing glucose sugar in the blood.

- **After digestion,** sugar and starches are changed into **glucose** – the simplest form of sugar vital for body energy and growth.
- Insulin is the hormone which acts like a key that opens the door to body cells and allows glucose to enter.
- **Without enough insulin,** glucose builds up in the blood and passes into the urine. High blood glucose levels lead to frequent urination, extreme thirst, and tiredness.
- **Untreated diabetes increases the risk of damage to nerves and blood vessels.** This, in turn, increases the risk of heart disease, stroke, blindness, kidney damage, foot ulcers and gangrene (with amputation), impotence and other complications.

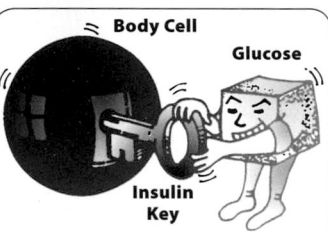

*Insulin acts like a key.
It opens the door to body cells
and allows glucose to enter.*

People with type 1 diabetes and some with type 2 have too few or no keys and require insulin injections.

Others (primarily type 2) make enough insulin but the body doesn't use it as well as it should – particularly if obese and inactive.

SYMPTOMS OF DIABETES

- Frequent urination
- Extreme thirst
- Unusual hunger
- Rapid weight loss
- Extreme fatigue
- Blurred vision
- Skin infections that are slow to heal
- Tingling/numbness in feet

Note: Diabetes can be present even with no symptoms.

DON'T IGNORE DIABETES

IT'S A SERIOUS DISEASE!

TYPE 2 DIABETES

- Occurs in 90% of diabetes cases
- Occurs mainly in adults - particularly in overweight and inactive persons
- Insulin is produced but body cells resist its action and glucose cannot enter cells
- Usually treated with meal planning and physical activity. Sometimes requires medication (pills or insulin)

TYPE 1 DIABETES

- Occurs in 10% of diabetes cases
- Usually in children and young adults
- Pancreas produces little or no insulin. Daily insulin injections (or use of an insulin pump) are necessary, as well as:
  - matching pre-meal insulin to the amount of carbohydrate eaten
  - weight control and regular physical activity

GESTATIONAL DIABETES

- Occurs in some women during pregnancy. It usually disappears after the baby's birth.
- Women who have had gestational diabetes still have a high risk of developing type 2 diabetes within 5 to 10 years.
- Requires weight control, a healthy lifestyle and regular medical checks

Are You At Risk for Diabetes?

Pre-Diabetes -- An Early Warning!

Pre-diabetes means that your blood glucose levels are higher than normal, but not high enough to be called diabetes.

If you have pre-diabetes, you have a higher risk for getting diabetes later on.

The good news is that you can start taking steps to prevent diabetes by making healthy lifestyle changes – such as losing weight if overweight, and being more physically active.

WHAT'S YOUR RISK?

Find out if you're at risk for diabetes by answering the following questions:

☐ I have been told I have pre-diabetes

☐ I have a family history of diabetes

☐ I am African American, Latino American, Asian American, Native American or a Pacific Islander

☐ I have had gestational diabetes (diabetes during pregnancy)

☐ I am over age 45

☐ I am overweight

☐ My waist is larger than: 35 inches (for a woman) or 40 inches (for a man)

☐ I get little or no physical activity

☐ My blood pressure is higher than 130 over 85

☐ My HDL (good cholesterol) is too low

☐ My triglycerides (blood fats) are too high

✓ CHECK YOUR RESULT

• If you've put a check mark in two or more of the boxes, you may be more likely to develop type 2 diabetes.

• Talk with your healthcare provider to see if you should have a blood test for diabetes.

BLOOD GLUCOSE CLASSIFICATION OF DIABETES

Normal:	**Below 100 mg/dl***
Pre-Diabetes:	**100-125 mg/dl***
Diabetes:	**Over 125 mg/dl***

(*Fasting Blood Glucose)

KNOW YOUR BGL
(Blood Glucose Level)
Everyone over the age of 45 should have a blood glucose test every three years

Importance of Weight Control

• **Type 2 diabetes** is more common in people who are overweight.

• **Being overweight** means that your insulin doesn't work as well to control blood glucose levels.

• **Losing just 10 to 20 pounds** can help you better manage your diabetes and lower your risk for heart disease.

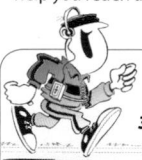

• **Keys to weight control include:**

• Following a healthy eating plan

• Controlling food portions

• Being physically active most days of the week

• Keeping food records

• Setting realistic goals

• **Work with a registered dietitian** who can help you reach a weight that's ideal for you.

KEEP MOVING!
Every day, do at least 30 minutes of moderate intensity exercise.
(even in 5-minute sets)

It's the key to improving insulin action.
Add muscle strength training 3-4 times a week to double the benefits.

Managing Diabetes

Don't battle diabetes alone. Establish a partnership with your doctor, dietitian, certified diabetes educator, and pharmacist.

Extra Support: • *Joslin Diabetes Center*
  • *American Diabetes Association*
  • *American Association of Diabetes Educators*
  • *Juvenile Diabetes Research Foundation*
  • *National Diabetes Education Program*

Hints to keep blood glucose within safe limits:

- **Control your food intake.** Know what and when you will eat. Seek referral to a dietitian for expert advice.

- **Exercise regularly.** It assists weight control and can improve sensitivity of body cells to insulin. Plan physical activity into your daily routine.

- **Monitor your blood glucose** at home and work with a blood glucose meter. It will help you become familiar with your blood glucose patterns, and the effects of food, activity and medication.

- **Take insulin or oral medication as prescribed.** If on insulin, know what action to take if hypoglycemia (low blood glucose) occurs. Also educate your family and friends. More Info: www.joslin.org

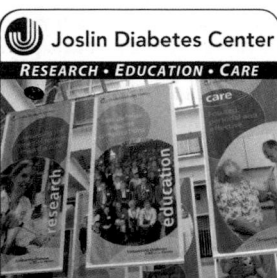

Joslin Diabetes Center, an affiliate of Harvard Medical School, is the world's largest diabetes research center, diabetes clinic and provider of diabetes education.

MORE INFORMATION
www.joslin.org or call 800-344-4501

Be Heart Smart ~ Know Your ABC's

If you have diabetes, you are at a higher risk for heart attack and stroke than someone without diabetes. But you can fight back!

Be smart about your heart!

Take control of the ABC's of diabetes and live a long and healthy life. Talk to your healthcare provider about your ABC targets.

Ⓐ is for A1C

The A1C (A-one-C) test – short for hemoglobin A1C. It reflects your average blood glucose (sugar) over the last 3 months.
Suggested Target: Below 7%

Ⓑ is for Blood Pressure

High blood pressure makes your heart work too hard.
Suggested Target: Below 130/80

Ⓒ is for Cholesterol

Bad cholesterol, or LDL, can build up and clog your arteries. **Suggested Target: Below 100**

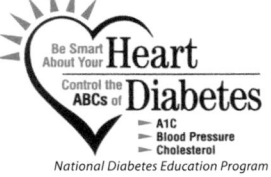

Be Smart About Your **Heart**
Control the ABCs of **Diabetes**
  ➤ A1C
  ➤ Blood Pressure
  ➤ Cholesterol
National Diabetes Education Program

Be smart about your heart!

Take control of the ABC's of diabetes and live a long and healthy life.

Talk to your healthcare provider about your ABC targets.

Take action now to lower your risk for heart attack, stroke and other diabetes problems.

* * *

◀ Note: These targets are suggested by the National Institutes for Health and the American Diabetes Association

Guidelines for choosing a healthy diet apply equally to people with or without diabetes. Eating a wide variety of foods that are mainly low in fat, low in refined sugars, and high in fiber, is recommended.

However, actual food quantities, as well as when you eat, will also influence control of blood glucose. Your dietitian will individualize a meal plan to suit your food preferences, lifestyle and medical status.

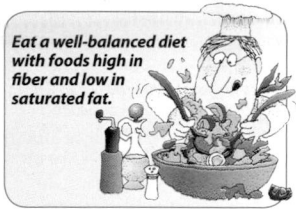

Eat a well-balanced diet with foods high in fiber and low in saturated fat.

Here are a few tips:

- **Maintain a healthy weight.** If overweight, even a modest weight loss plus daily physical activity can help manage blood glucose in type 2 diabetes.

- **Don't skip meals.** If you take insulin or an oral hypoglycemic agent, regular meals are important.

  If on insulin, eat meals at the same time each day. Eat a similar amount of food at each meal. Eating about the same amount of carbohydrate over the day will make best use of insulin and prevent wide variations in blood glucose levels.

- **Know which foods contain carbohydrate;** and learn how to check the *Nutrition Facts Label* on foods. Check the serving size, total fat and total carbohydrate – not just the sugar content. All carbohydrate breaks down to sugars after digestion.

- **Choose wholegrain breads, cereals and pasta.** Eat fresh fruits, vegetables and legumes. These foods contain more fiber and slow the release of glucose into your blood after a meal.

- **Limit foods high in saturated fat, trans fat and cholesterol.** Enjoy fish, soy foods, and other foods rich in omega-3 fats. *(Extra Notes: Page 259)*

- **Limit sugars and foods high in added sugar** particularly if overweight. Small amounts of sugar as part of a meal may occasionally be okay. Check with your dietitian. *(Extra Notes: Page 9)*

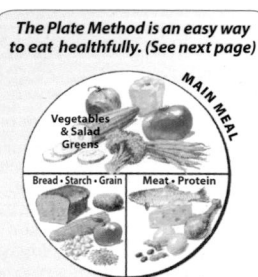

The Plate Method is an easy way to eat healthfully. (See next page)

MAIN MEAL

Vegetables & Salad Greens

Bread • Starch • Grain

Meat • Protein

ALCOHOL TIPS

- **If you drink alcohol, have only moderate amounts:**
  Men ~ 1-2 drinks/day
  Women ~ 1 drink/day
  For some people, safe drinking will mean no alcoholic drinks at all.

  (Also see Alcohol Guide ~ Page 23)

- **Drink along with your food** – especially if you use insulin or diabetes pills.

- **Do not omit any carb food** in exchange for an alcoholic drink. However, non-alcoholic beers (12 fl oz) count as one carb exchange.

- **Alcohol increases the risk of hypoglycemia** (low blood sugar) and drug interactions if you take insulin and certain types of diabetes pills.

- **Check with your doctor and dietitian.**
  Extra Info: www.joslin.org

The Plate Method – An Easy Way to Eat Healthfully

The plate method is a helpful tool to guide your food choices until you see a dietitian for your own meal plan.

For a healthy meal:

- Fill half of your plate with non-starchy vegetables (broccoli, green beans, carrots).
- Fill a quarter of your plate with carbohydrate (wholegrain bread, pasta, potato, brown rice).
- Fill the other quarter of your plate with 3-4 ounces of lean meat, poultry, or fish.
- Use 1-2 teaspoons of tub margarine or a heart-healthy vegetable oil.
- Add a small piece of fruit or 8 ounces of skim/low-fat milk or yogurt.

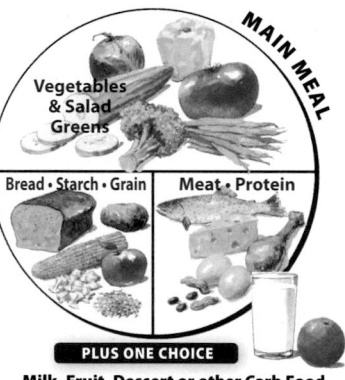

MAIN MEAL

Vegetables & Salad Greens

Bread · Starch · Grain

Meat · Protein

PLUS ONE CHOICE

Milk, Fruit, Dessert or other Carb Food

How Much Carbohydrate Should You Eat?

A dietitian can best determine how much carbohydrate you need at each of your meals, based on your lifestyle, food preferences, and overall diabetes control.

Until you see a dietitian, aim to keep the amount of carbohydrate you eat the same at each of your meals.

CARB CHOICES MEAL PLAN
One Carb Choice = 15 Grams of Carb

The amount in: 1 slice Bread **or** ¾ cup Cereal (unsweetened) **or** 1 small Potato **or** 1 small Fruit

Breakfast
- Eat 2-3 carb choices (30-45 grams)
- Include a low-fat protein source such as egg whites or skim milk.

Lunch and Dinner
- Eat 3-4 carb choices (45-60 grams carb)
- Include fruit and non-starchy vegetables. Choose small portions of low-fat protein foods.

Snacks: If needed, eat 1-2 carb choices (15-30 grams carb).

Note: Above plan is for adults. Carbohydrate amounts will vary with physical activity level.

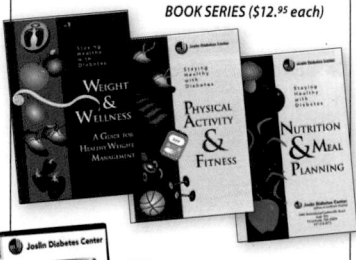
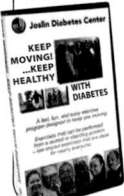

Carb Type Affects Blood Glucose

The various forms of carbohydrate affect blood glucose levels in different ways. It is difficult to predict the effect of particular foods, sugars, or meals, simply by their carbohydrate content.

Thus the same amount of carbohydrate from different foods may affect blood sugar levels very differently. Many factors affect the rate of digestion and absorption such as:

- the type of sugar, starch, and fiber
- the degree of processing and cooking (which increases digestion rate)
- the amount of protein and fat (which slow stomach emptying and digestion).

Glycemic Index (GI)

The GI is a method of ranking carbohydrate foods on a scale (0-100) according to how they affect blood glucose levels. (See next column).

The higher the GI value, the greater the food's ability to rapidly raise blood glucose levels, and the more insulin needed by the body (not desirable).

Eating low-GI foods may lead to better control of blood glucose and insulin levels (which in turn lowers the risk of damage to blood vessels and nerves). The slower digestion of low-GI foods may also help to delay hunger pangs and benefit weight control.

Cautionary Notes on GI

Choosing low-GI foods is not a license to eat unlimited amounts. Calorie restriction and portion control for weight control is of prime importance.

Also remember, Low-GI foods are carbohydrate foods and must still be counted as part of any dietetic carbohydrate plan.

GI is not meant to be used by itself without regard to portion size, and other dietary recommendations for healthy eating. Foods are not good or bad on the basis of their GI.

While GI may be a helpful tool for some people with diabetes, what is most important is to control the total amount of carbohydrate that you eat.

LOWER-GLYCEMIC FOODS

Slower-Acting Carbohydrates

These foods are more slowly digested and absorbed. They help maintain more even blood glucose levels, as long as excessive amounts are not eaten. Use these foods regularly but still limit portion size for weight control.

Examples:
- Dried beans, peas, lentils
- Nuts and seeds
- Wholegrain breads
- Bran cereals, oats
- Sweet corn, barley, buckwheat
- Wholegrain pasta, basmati rice
- Fresh fruit: apples, avocados, bananas (firm), cherries, grapefruit, grapes, olives, oranges, peaches, pears, plums. Fresh juices.
- Vegetables: broccoli, yam, sweet potatoes, salad greens
- Milk, yogurt, soy drinks
- Dark chocolate
- Sugar alcohols (sorbitol, maltitol)

HIGHER-GLYCEMIC FOODS

Quicker-Acting Carbohydrates

These foods more rapidly raise blood glucose levels. Eat only in moderation.

- White bread, rice cakes, bagels, croissants, doughnuts
- Low-fiber cereals: Cornflakes, *Rice Krispies, Froot Loops*
- White potatoes, white rice
- Watermelon, ripe bananas, cantaloupe, pineapple
- Soda, sugar-sweetened sports and energy drinks
- Sugar, candy, popcorn (plain)
- Ice cream (low-fat), frozen yogurt

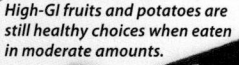

High-GI fruits and potatoes are still healthy choices when eaten in moderate amounts.

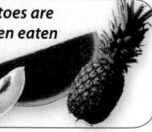

>> **Calorie and fat values have been rounded off.**
Calories ~ to the nearest 5 or 10 calories.
Fat ~ to nearest half gram. **Note:** Trace amounts of fat (less than 0.3 grams) have been treated as zero.

>> **Carbohydrate figures** in this book are for total carbohydrate, and not **Net Carbs** (which deducts fiber, polydextrose and sugar alcohols from total carbs).

>> Because manufacturers' figures on labels are rounded off, figures in this book may differ slightly from the label. Serving sizes may also vary.

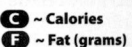

C ~ Calories
F ~ Fat (grams)
Cb ~ Carbohydrate (grams)

Abbreviations

tsp	= teaspoon
Tbsp or T	= Tablespoon
oz	= ounce(s)
c	= cup
fl.oz	= fluid ounce(s)
g	= gram(s)
avg	= average
pkg	= package

Volume Measures

(All measures are level)
3 tsp	= 1 Tbsp
2 Tbsp	= 1 fl.oz
½ cup	= 4 fl.oz
1 cup	= 8 fl.oz
2 cups	= 1 Pint
2 Pints	= 1 Quart

Note: 8 oz weight is not the same as 8 fl oz volume (space occupied). Dense foods weigh more per set volume. Examples:
1 cup popcorn weighs ½ oz
1 cup milk weighs 8½ oz
1 cup pudding weighs 10 oz

Metric Conversion

½ oz	= 14 grams
1 oz	= 28.4 grams
2 oz	= 57 grams
3½ oz	= 100 grams
1 fl.oz	= 30 mls
1 cup (8 fl.oz)	= 240 mls
33 fl.oz	= 1 liter (volume)

IMPORTANT DISCLAIMER

* The authors and publishers of this book are not physicians and are not licensed to give medical advice. This book is not a substitute for professional advice. Users should consult their medical professional before making any health, medical or other decisions based on the material contained herein.

* This book is a compilation of original material from other sources intended for educational purposes only. Because food manufacturers constantly change their products, only they are the authoritative source for food's most current nutritional information.

* Persons using the information herein for any medical purposes, such as matching insulin dosage to carbohydrate intake, should not rely solely on the accuracy of figures herein and should independently check food labels or contact the food manufacturer for the latest data.

* Because nutrition data for food products is subject to change, users should consult the most recent edition of this book, and the author's website www.calorieking.com for the most up-to-date information.

* WARRANTY DISCLAIMER:

THE AUTHOR AND PUBLISHER DISCLAIM ANY LIABILITY ARISING DIRECTLY OR INDIRECTLY FROM THE USE OF THIS BOOK. THE INFORMATION HEREIN IS PROVIDED "AS IS" AND WITHOUT ANY WARRANTY EXPRESSED OR IMPLIED. ALL DIRECT, INDIRECT, SPECIAL, INCIDENTAL, CONSEQUENTIAL OR PUNITIVE DAMAGES ARISING FROM ANY USE OF THIS INFORMATION IS DISCLAIMED AND EXCLUDED.

This information is also provided subject to Family Health Publications' Terms and Conditions found at the website, www.calorieking.com/terms and incorporated herein.

INFORMATION SOURCES
• U.S. Dept. of Agriculture
• Food Manufacturers
• Food Industry Boards & Councils
• Author extrapolations

FEEDBACK WELCOME!
Please contact the author with your queries and suggestions.
feedback@calorieking.com

Alcohol Guide (A)

- **Health Hazards: Excessive alcohol intake** contributes to obesity, high blood pressure, stroke, heart and liver disease, some cancers, and even impotence. **Concentration and short-term memory** are reduced as well as athletic performance.

  Other alcohol hazards include: Fetal Alcohol Syndrome, stomach upsets, menstrual problems, depression, snoring, sleep problems, work absenteeism, impaired judgement, and social/ family problems.

- **Alcohol contributes to obesity:** Through its high calories and by lessening the body's ability to burn fat. Fat storage is promoted, particularly in the belly – a health danger zone. Alcohol can also stimulate the appetite.

- **Alcohol is potentially more harmful while dieting:** Blood sugar levels may drop with resultant fatigue and further impairment of concentration, reflexes and driving skills – and maybe even the dieter's resolve!

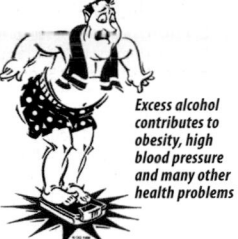

Excess alcohol contributes to obesity, high blood pressure and many other health problems

LOWER RISK ALCOHOL LIMITS

 WOMEN: No more than **1 drink** per day

 MEN: No more than **2 drinks** per day (Over 65 y.o. ~ 1 drink)

(At least 2 days a week should be alcohol-free)

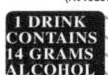 **1 DRINK CONTAINS 14 GRAMS ALCOHOL** →
- 12 fl.oz Regular Beer (5% Alc.)
- OR 14 fl.oz Light Beer (4.2% Alc.)
- OR 5 fl.oz Wine (12% Alc.)
- OR 1½ fl.oz Spirits (80 Proof)

Note: You cannot save daily drinks for one occasion.
Binge drinking is particularly harmful:
4 drinks for males or 3 drinks for females (within 2 hours).

For some people, safe drinking means no alcohol at all. Even one drink may impair driving skills, particularly if tired. For women who drink frequently, breast cancer risk is increased by 9% for each drink after the first drink.

It is advisable not to drink at all if you are:
- pregnant, trying to conceive or breastfeeding
- taking medication or have liver or heart disease (unless approved by your doctor or pharmacist)
- planning to drive, use machinery or play sports
- studying or needing to concentrate
- a child or adolescent

 Women and adolescents are more prone to alcohol's ill-effects due to their lower body weight, smaller livers and lesser capacity to metabolize alcohol. As we age, our ability to handle alcohol decreases.

HOW TO CALCULATE ALCOHOL CONTENT

Percent alcohol on label refers to alcohol volume (ml alcohol/100ml). Note: 100ml = 3½ fl.oz

To convert to grams (weight) of alcohol, multiply the percent volume by 0.8 – since 1 ml of alcohol weighs only 0.8 grams.

EXAMPLE:
12 fl.oz Can Beer (5% alcohol)
5% alc. volume
= 5% of 12 fl.oz = 0.6 fl.oz
= 18ml alcohol (Note: 1 fl.oz = 30ml)
Weight (18ml x 0.8) = 14.4g alcohol

GOVERNMENT WARNINGS!

(1) According to the Surgeon General, women should not drink alcoholic beverages during pregnancy because of the risk of birth defects.
(2) Consumption of alcoholic beverages impairs your ability to drive a car or operate machinery, and may cause health problems.

EXTRA INFORMATION
Alcohol & Diabetes ~ See Page 21
Alcohol & The Heart ~ See Page
Tips to Avoid Harmful Drinking ~ Page

23

Quick Guide

Alc ~ Alcohol (Grams)
Cb ~ Carbohydrate

Beer:
Beer Contains Zero Fat:

Regular Beer (5% Alc. Vol.):	C	Alc	Cb
7 fl.oz Glass	80	8.5	4
12 fl.oz Bottle/Can/Glass	140	14	10
16 fl.oz Bottle/Can	185	19	13
22 fl.oz Bottle	260	26	18
24 fl.oz Can	280	28	20
32 fl.oz Bottle	370	38	28
40 fl.oz Bottle	470	47	35
50 fl.oz Football	590	59	50

Light Beer (4.2% Alc. Vol.):	C	Alc	Cb
7 fl.oz Glass	65	7	4
12 fl.oz Bottle/Can/Glass	110	12	7
16 fl.oz Bottle/Can	145	16	9
22 fl.oz Bottle	200	22	13
24 fl.oz Can	220	24	14

Non-Alcoholic Brews:	C	Alc	Cb
(Less than 0.5% alcohol by volume)			
Average all Brands, 12 fl.oz	70	1	14

Beer Brands

Note: Figures shown are for the United States except for the states of Utah, Colorado, Kansas and Oklahoma who have certain restrictions limiting the alcohol content to not more than 4% by volume (3.2% by weight).

Per 12 fl.oz Serving
Percentage alcohol listed is by volume - not by weight.

Alc ~ Alcohol (Grams)

	C	Alc	Cb
Amstel, Light (3.5%)	95	10	5
Anchor: Porter (5.6%)	210	15	23
Steam (4.9%)	165	14	14
Asahi: Kuronama (5.3%)	165	14	14
Select (4.7%)	140	13	11
Super Dry (4.9%)	150	14	11
Bass, Pale Ale (5.1%)	155	14	12
Beck's: Original (5%)	145	14	12
Premier Light (2.3%)	65	7	4
Big Sky: Original IPA (6.2%)	195	18	17
Moose Drool (5.3%)	175	15	16
Scape Goat (4.7%)	155	14	14
Trout Slayer Ale (4.7%)	145	14	12
Blatz: Original (4.6%)	145	13	13
Light (3.9%)	110	11	8
Blue Moon: Belgian (5.4%)	165	15	13
Grand Cru Ale (8.2%)	230	21	19
Harvest Pumpkin Ale (5.8%)	180	17	14
Spring Ale (5.7%)	180	16	15
Summer Ale (5.2%)	150	15	13
Winter Abbey Ale (5.7%)	180	16	14
Bohemia (4.73%)	140	14	12

Brands (Cont)

Alc ~ Alcohol (Grams)

Per 12 fl.oz Serving

	C	Alc	Cb
Bud: Bud Light (4.2%)	110	12	7
Chelada Light (4.2%)	150	12	16
Dry (5%)	130	14	8
Ice (5.5%)	150	16	9
Ice Light (4.1%)	110	12	7
Light Lime (4.2%)	115	12	8
Light Platinum (6%)	140	17	5
Budweiser: Pale Lager (5%)	145	14	11
American Ale (5.3%)	180	15	18
Chelada (5%)	185	14	20
Select (4.3%)	100	12	3
Select 55 (2.4%)	55	7	2
Busch: Original (4.6%)	120	13	7
Ice (5.9%)	135	17	4
Light (4.1%)	95	12	3
Carlsberg, Pilsner (5%)	135	14	10
Carta Blanca (4.6%)	145	13	11
Castlemaine XXXX, Bitter (4.6%)	140	14	10
Cerveza, Aquila (4%)	125	11	11
Colt 45, Malt Liquor (5.6%)	155	16	11
Coors: Banquet (5%)	150	14	12
Extra Gold (5%)	150	14	13
Light (4.2%)	100	12	5
Corona: Extra (4.6%)	150	13	14
Light (4.1%)	100	12	5
Dos Equis XX: Amber (4.6%)	145	13	12
Lager (4.6%)	140	13	11
Fosters: Lager (5%)	145	14	11
Premium Ale (5.5%)	145	16	12
Genesee: Lager (4.5%)	150	13	14
Genny Light Lager (3.6%)	95	10	6
George Killian's, Irish Red (5%)	160	14	15
Grolsch: Blonde (2.8%)	120	18	16
Light (3.6%)	95	11	6
Premium (5%)	145	14	10
Guinness: Draught (4%)	125	12	10
Extra Stout (6%)	175	17	14
Hamm's: Original (4.7%)	145	13	12
Special Light (3.9%)	110	12	8
Harp, Pale Lager (5%)	150	13	12
Heineken: Lager (5%)	150	14	11
Special Dark (5%)	165	14	15
Premium Light (3.5%)	100	10	7
Hurricane: Malt Liquor (5.9%)	135	17	4
High Gravity (8.1%)	185	23	6
Icehouse: Original (5.5%)	150	16	10
Light (5%)	125	14	7
Keystone: Ice (5.9%)	140	17	6
Light (4.2%)	105	12	5
Killian's, Irish Red (5%)	165	14	14
King Cobra (6%)	135	17	5

Brands (Cont)   Alc ~ Alcohol (Grams)

Beer Contains Zero Fat:
Per 12 fl.oz Serving

	C	Alc	Cb
Kirin: Ichiban (5%)	145	14	10
Light (3.2%)	95	9	8
Labatt: Blue (4.7%)	135	14	10
Blue Light (4%)	110	11	8
Landshark, Lager (4.7%)	150	13	14
Leinenkugel's: Orig. (4.6%)	150	13	14
Summer Shandy (4.2%)	130	12	12
Lone Star: Pale Lager (4.7%)	135	13	12
Light (3.9%)	110	11	9
Lowenbrau, Original (5%)	140	14	12
Magic Hat, #9 (5.1% alc)	155	15	14
Magnum, Malt Liquor (5.6%)	160	16	11
Michelob: Original Lager (5%)	165	14	15
Golden Draft (4.7%)	125	13	8
Golden Draft Light (4.1%)	110	12	7
Honey Lager (4.9%)	175	14	16
Light (4.3%)	125	12	9
Pale Ale (5.6%)	185	16	5
Porter (5.9%)	185	17	16
Ultra (4.2%)	95	12	3
Ultra Amber (5%)	95	12	3
Mickey's, Malt Liquor (5.6%)	160	16	11
Miller: Chill, 100 Cal, (4.2%)	100	12	3
Genuine Draft /High Life, (4.7%)	145	13	13
High Life Light (4.2%)	110	12	7
Lite (4.2%)	95	12	3
MGD 64 (2.8%)	65	8	2.5
Milwaukee's Best:			
Premium (4.3%)	130	12	11
Ice (5.9%)	145	12	7
Light (4.2%)	100	12	4
Minnesota's Best, Original (4.9%)	140	14	10
Modelo, Especial (4.4%)	145	13	13
Molson: Canadian/Golden (5%)	135	14	11
Ice (5.9%)	160	16	12
Light (4%)	115	12	9
Molsons XXX (7.3%)	200	21	11
Moosehead, Lager (5%)	140	14	11
Natural: Ice (5.9%)	130	17	4
Light (4.2%)	95	12	3
Negra Modelo (5.4%)	170	15	15
Newcastle, Brown Ale (4.7%)	140	13	10
Old English "800", Malt (5.9%)	160	17	11
Old Milwaukee: Lager (4.5%)	150	13	13
Light (4.3%)	125	12	8
Ice (5.5%)	150	16	10
Old Style: Lager (4.7%)	145	13	12
Light (4.2%)	115	12	7
Olympia Gold, Light (2.1%)	70	6	6
Pabst: Blue Ribbon (4.7%)	145	13	12
Light (3.9%)	110	11	8

Cb ~ Carbohydrate

Per 12 fl.oz Serving Unless Indicated

	C	Alc	Cb
Pacifico, Clara (4.4%)	145	13	13
Peroni Nastro Azzurro, (5.1%)	150	14	12
Pete's, Wicked Ale (5.3%)	175	15	18
Piels, Lager (4.3%)	125	12	9
Pilsner Urquell, Lager (4.4%)	155	13	16
Point: Amber Classic (4.7%)	160	14	11
Special Lager (4.6%)	150	13	9
2012 Black Ale (4.6%)	150	13	9
Red Dog, Lager (5%)	150	14	14
Red Hook: ESB (5.8%)	185	16	16
India Pale Ale (4.7%)	190	13	19
Red Stripe, Jamaican Ale (5%)	155	14	10
Rolling Rock, Extra Pale Ale (4.5%)	130	13	10
Samuel Adams:			
Boston Lager (4.9%)	175	14	19
Sam Adams, Light Lager (4%)	125	13	9
Sapporo, Prem. Lager (4.9%)	140	14	10
Schaefer: Lager (4.6%)	145	13	12
Light (3.9%)	110	11	8
Schell's: Deer (4.8%)	135	14	8
Light (4%)	100	11	7
Schlitz: Lager (4.6%)	145	13	12
Light (3.8%)	110	11	8
Schmidt's: Pale Lager (4.6%)	145	13	13
Light (3.8%)	110	11	8
Sheaf, Stout (5.8%)	190	16	19
Shock Top, Belgian White (5.2%)	165	15	15
Sierra Nevada: Bigfoot (9.6%)	330	28	32
Pale Ale (5.6%)	175	16	14
Glissade Golden Bock (6.4%)	205	18	18
Porter (5.6%)	195	16	18
Sol, (4.2%)	130	12	11
Southpaw, Light (5%)	125	14	7
St Pauli Girl, Lager (5%)	135	14	9
Sparks: Lager (6%)	255	17	35
Flavors ~ see page 27			
Steel Reserve:			
High Gravity Malt Liquor (8.1%)	220	23	16
Steel 6 (6%)	160	17	11
Stella Artois, Pale Lager (5.2%)	155	15	12
Stroh's: Pale Lager (4.6%)	145	13	12
Light (3.9%)	115	11	7
Tecate: Pale Lager (4.6%)	140	13	11
Light (4%)	110	10	8
Trader Jose:			
Premium Lager (5%), 11.2 fl.oz	145	14	14
Prem. Lager Light (3.8%), 11.2 fl.oz	105	14	8
Victoria, (4%)	135	12	14
Warsteiners, Verum (4.8%), 11.2 fl.oz	140	13	12
Weinhard's: Priv. Reserve (4.8%)	150	14	13
Hefeweizen (4.86%)			
Widmer, Hefeweizen (4.9%)	165	14	13
Zeigenbock, Amber (4.9%)	145	14	11
Home Brewed Beer:			

Similar to regular beers, according to alcohol content.

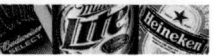
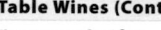

Alc ~ Alcohol (Grams) **Cb** ~ Carbohydrate

Non-Alcoholic Brews

Less Than 0.5% Alcohol
Average All Brands:
(Busch NA, Coors NA, Haake Beck, Kaliber, Kingsbury, O'Douls, Old Milwaukee NA, Pabst NA, Stroh's NA, Texas Select):

	C	Alc	Cb
12 fl.oz Can/Bottle	70	1	14
O'Doul's, Amber, 12 fl.oz	90	1	18
Sharp's, 12 fl.oz	60	1	12

Cider ~ Alcoholic

Per 12 fl.oz

	C	Alc	Cb
Ace: Cider (5%), av. all flavors	155	14	12
Joker (6.9%)	135	19	12
Hornsby's: Draft Cider (6%)	170	16	16
Hard Apple Cider (5.5%)	200	15	27
Woodchuck: Amber (5%)	200	14	21
Dark & Dry (5%)	180	14	16
Granny Smith (5%)	160	14	14
Pear (4%)	150	12	18
Raspberry (4%)	170	12	22
Wyder's: Apple (5%)	150	14	14
Pear (4%)	140	12	22
Raspberry (4%)	120	12	17

Quick Guide

Table Wines:
Average All Varieties (11.5% Alc.)
(Wine Contains Zero Fat)

	C	Alc	Cb
4 fl.oz, 1 small wine glass OR ½ large wine glass	100	12	3
6 fl.oz, (3/4 large wine glass)	145	18	5
8 fl.oz, (1 large wine glass)	195	25	7
½ Carafe/Bottle, 12 fl.oz	295	37	10
1 Bottle, 750ml, 25.4 fl.oz	620	78	20

Table Wines

	C	Alc	Cb
Red: Per 4 fl.oz			
Burgundy/Cabernet/Merlot, av.	100	11	4
White: Per 4 fl.oz			
Dry (Chenin; Fume Blanc; Chardonnay)	95	11	4
Sparkling, 4 fl.oz	95	11	4
Zinfandel Sweet (Moselle/Sauterne), 4 fl.oz	85	11	2

Table Wines (Cont)

	C	Alc	Cb
Champagne: Per 4 fl.oz			
Average 1 glass	85	11	2
with Orange Jce (3:1 orange)	75	8	4
with Orange Jce (1:1 orange)	65	5	7
Mulled Wine (Gluhwein), 4 fl.oz	180	14	20
Non-Alcoholic Wine: Less than 0.5% Alcohol			
Ariel: White varieties, av., 4 fl.oz	35	0.5	8
Red varieties, av., 4 fl.oz	25	0.5	5
Reduced Alcohol Wine (6%):			
Average all types, 4 fl.oz	80	6	10
Sake (Gekkeikan), (16%), 4 fl.oz	120	15	5

Flavored Wines

Average All Brands (6% alcohol)
(Examples: Arbor Mist, Wild Vines, Boone's Farm)

	C	Alc	Cb
1 small wine glass, 4 fl.oz	80	6	10
1 large wine glass, 8 fl.oz	160	11	20
1 bottle, 750 ml (25.4 fl.oz)	510	35	64

Dessert Wines

	C	Alc	Cb
Madeira (18%), 2 oz	85	9	5
Marsala (18%), 2 oz	110	9	11
Port, Muscatel (18%), 2 oz	85	9	5
Sherry (15%), 2 oz			
Dry, 1 Sherry glass	90	7	7
Sweet/Cream, average	90	7	8
Vermouth (Martini & Rossi):			
Extra Dry (18%), 2 oz	65	9	2
Martini Rosso (16%), 2 oz	90	8	8

Cooking Wines

Holland House:

	C	Alc	Cb
Marsala, (14%), 2 T., 1 fl.oz	45	4	4
Red/White, (10%): 2 T., 1 fl.oz	20	2	1
1 cup, 8 fl.oz	160	24	8
Sherry, (17%), 2 Tbsp, 1 fl.oz	45	5	2

Cooking with Wine:
For alcohol to evaporate, sufficient heat and cooking time (at least 30 minutes) is required.
Red and white table wines would then contain negligible residual calories.
Sweetened wines (marsala/sherry) would contain 10 calories per 1 fl.oz.
Flambé Desserts: Only surface alcohol is burned off, so negligible reduction in alcohol or calories.

Quick Guide

Alc ~ Alcohol (Grams)

Spirits/Liquors:
Includes Bourbon, Brandy, Gin, Rum, Scotch, Tequila, Vodka, Whiskey.
Note: All spirits with same alcohol proof have similar calories and zero fat.

Average All Brands	C	Alc	Cb
80 Proof (40% Alcohol by Volume):			
1 fl.oz	65	9.5	0
1½ fl.oz (1 shot)	100	14	0
3 fl.oz (Double shot)	195	28	0
½ Bottle, 350 ml (12 fl.oz)	770	113	0
1 Bottle, 700 ml (4 fl.oz)	1540	227	0
86 Proof (43% Alc): 1 fl.oz	70	10	0
1½ fl.oz (1 shot)	105	15	0
1 Bottle (24 fl.oz)	1670	244	0
100 Proof (50% Alc), 1½ fl.oz	125	18	0
Shochu (Soju) ~ Izakaya Lounges,			
Average all types (25% alc), 2 fl.oz	65	12	0

Flavored Spirits

Captain Morgan: Per 1½ fl.oz			
Original (35%)	85	12	0.5
Black Label (40%)	100	14	0
Parrot Bay (21%), average	95	7.5	11
Silver Spiced (35%)	95	12	2
Malibu Rum: Per 1½ fl.oz			
Original/Banana (21%)	80	7.5	30
Pineapple (21%)	75	7.5	22
Southern Comfort (35%), 1½ fl.oz	100	12	3

Hard Lemonade & Sodas

Margaritaville,			
Spiked Lemonade/Tea (5.5%), 12 fl.oz	225	15	30
Mike's: Per 11.2 fl.oz Unless Indicated			
Lemonade: Hard, Orig , (5%), av.	220	14	33
Light (4%)	110	11	14
Harder (8%) av., 16 fl.oz	395	22	22
Punch : Hard (5.5%)	230	15	34
Harder (8%): Fruit Punch, 23.5 fl.oz	730	0	96
Mango (8%), 23.5 fl.oz	690	0	87
Margarita (5.5%)	235	15	34
Sparks: Per 12 fl.oz (Half of 24 oz Can)			
Blackberry; Iced Tea (8%), av.	295	23	34
Lemonade (8%)	275	23	29
Original (6%)	260	17	35
Tilt: Per 16 fl.oz Can			
Blue/Green/Purple (6%), av.	340	23	45
Pink (6%)	320	23	41
Red/Yellow (6%)	280	23	30
Twisted Tea: Light (4%), 12 fl.oz	115	11	9
Original (5%) av., all flavors, 12 fl.oz	210	14	31

Coolers & Premix Cocktails

Ready-To-Drink:
Zero Fat Unless Indicated

	C	Alc	Cb
Bacardi Silver: Per 12 fl.oz			
Lemonade/Sangria (6%), av.	270	17	41
Raz/Strawberry (5%)	240	14	36
Mojito, (5%)	230	14	34
Bacardi: Per 4 fl.oz			
Party Drinks (Ready To Pour):			
Bahama Mama; Mai Tai (10%)	130	9	16
Mojito (15%)	160	14	16
Rum Island Ice Tea (12.5%)	150	12	16
Bartles & Jaymes: Per 11.2 fl.oz			
Malt Based Coolers (3.2%):			
Exotic Berry	190	9	31
Margarita	235	9	43
Mojito	240	9	43
Pina Colada	245	9	45
Pomegr. Rasp./Strawb. Daiquiri	200	9	35
Sangria	230	9	25
Captain Morgan's,			
Parrot Bay (4.1%), av. all flavor, 11.2 fl.oz	210	10	35
Chi Chi's: Long Is. Iced Tea, 4 fl.oz	145	12	17
Mexican Mudslide, 4 fl.oz (8g fat)	240	1.5	42
Mojito, 4 fl.oz	160	11	21
Pina Colada 4 fl.oz (6g fat)	240	4	42
White Russian 4 fl.oz (7g fat)	245	1.5	43
Daily's (6.9%):			
Bag-In-Box Cocktails, 4 fl.oz	110	6	15
Single Serve Bottles, all flav., 8 fl.oz	220	12	30
Jack Daniels, Country Cocktails (5%),			
average all flavors, 10 fl.oz	245	12	40
Jose Cuervo:			
Margaritas:			
Classic Lime (10%), 6 fl.oz	210	14	29
Golden (12.7%), 4·7 fl.oz	170	14	19
Seagram's:			
Escapes Coolers (3.2%):			
Bahama Mama, 12 fl.oz	150	9	39
Strawberry Daiquiri, 12 fl.oz	170	9	44
Skinnygirl:			
Vodka with flavors (30%), 1½ fl.oz	75	11	0
Cocktails (10%), av., 3 oz	70	8	4
Smirnoff: Per 11.2 fl.oz			
Ice (4.5%): Original/Grape, av.	205	12	37
Apple/Stawberry Acai, av.	235	12	36
Mango	225	12	33
Pomeg./Raspb./Triple Black	225	12	37
TGI Friday's: Per 6 fl.oz			
On The Rocks:			
Margarita (7.5%)	180	6	28
Long Island Ice Tea (15%)	245	12	27
Mudslide (10%)	355	8	30
Blenders (12.5% alc), av.	435	10	51

Coolers & Premix Cocktails (Cont)

Ready-To-Drink:

The Club Premix Cocktails: Per 3.4 oz Serving (½ can)

	C	Alc	Cb
Censored on Beach; Margarita (7.5%)	105	6	17
Gin/Vodka Martini (21%), average	155	17	0.2
Long Island Ice Tea (15%)	145	12	17
Manhattan (17%)	115	13	5
Mudslide/Pina Colada (10%), average	200	8	16
Screwdriver (7.5%)	95	6	14
Whiskey Sour (10%)	95	8	11

Shooters
Alc ~ Alcohol (Grams)

	C	Alc	Cb
Alabama Slammer	110	14	2
Amaretto Sour	120	6	19
B52	145	14	11
Beam Me Up Scotty	145	13	13
Blue Tequila	160	18	6
Jager Bomb	205	8	30
Jager Bomb, w/ Sugar-Free Red Bull	155	8	18
Jell-O Shot, 3 oz: With 1½ oz Vodka	180	14	14
With Diet Jell-O	110	14	0
Kamikaze	75	8	3
Kool-Aid	160	15	14
Orgasm	100	12	6
Peppermint Patty	195	8	11
Stinger	170	18	12
Surfer on Acid	90	7	11

Cocktail Mixers ~ Non-Alcoholic

Bacardi: Per 8 fl.oz, Prepared from 2 fl.oz concentrate

	C	Alc	Cb
Daiquiris; Rum Runner	120	0	32
Margarita	90	0	25
Mojito	110	0	30
Pina Colada	170	0	36
Baja Bob's (Sugar Free): Per 4 fl.oz			
Cranberry Cosmo Martini	10	0	2
Pina Colada	30	0	4
Jose Cuervo,			
Margaritas: av. all flav, 4 fl.oz	85	0	21
Light (Sugar Free), Lime, 4 fl.oz	5	0	1
Mr & Mrs T:			
Bloody Mary: Original, 5 oz	30	0	7
Bold & Spicy, 4 oz	35	0	7
Mai Tai	130	0	32
Margarita	100	0	26
Pina Colada	170	0	44
Strawberry Daiquiri	180	0	46
TGI Friday's:			
Mudslide, 2.3 fl.oz	110	0	3
Cosmo; Berrytini, 2 fl.oz	80	0	20
Strawb. Daiquiri; Marg., 4 fl.oz	190	0	46

Cocktails
Alc ~ Alcohol (Grams)

Made to Standard Recipes (Standard Size):

(Main Reference: The New American Bartender's Guide)

Zero Fat Unless Indicated	C	Alc	Cb
Adios Mother F.	260	23	23
Bacardi & Coke (w/ 1½ oz Bacardi)	160	14	17
Bellini, 4.5 fl.oz	95	11	7
Bloody Mary (w/ 1½ oz Vodka)	125	10	7
Blushin' Russian (20g fat)	405	14	23
Bourbon & Soda (w. 2 oz Bourbon)	130	19	0
Brandy Alexander (10g fat)	300	20	15
Chupa Naranjas (w/ 1½ oz Tequila)	150	16	8
Cosmopolitan	215	24	12
Daiquiri (w/ 2 oz Rum), av. all types	140	19	4
Frozen Daiquiri (w. 2 oz Rum):			
Without fruit	155	19	6
With fruit (w/ 1½ oz Rum)	145	14	11
Gin Martini (w/ 2 oz alcohol)	140	19	0
Grasshopper	260	17	28
Greyhound (w/ 1½ oz Vodka)	170	14	17
Harvey Wallbanger (2 oz)	200	19	17
Highball (1½ oz Whiskey)	100	14	0
Irish Coffee (contains 10g fat)	205	14	2
Kahlua Mudslide: With milk (3g fat)	145	11	10
With cream (12g fat)	230	11	10
Lemon Drop, 4 fl.oz	130	14	10
Long Island Iced Tea (w/ 3 oz Cola)	270	19	32
With 3 oz Diet Cola	235	19	22
Mai Tai (w/ 2 oz Rum)	290	24	33
Manhattan	130	17	5
Margarita	160	18	7
Mint Julep (w/ 2½ oz Bourbon)	180	24	4
Mojito (w/ 2 oz rum)	170	19	9
Moscow Mule	185	14	24
Pina Colada (10g fat)	325	19	26
Red Bull & Vodka (w/ 1½ oz vodka)	210	14	28
With Sugar Free Red Bull	105	14	3
Rum & Coke (w/ 1½ oz Rum)	160	14	17
Screwdriver	160	14	15
Sex On The Beach	235	19	25
Spritzer (with 3 oz Wine)	65	8	2
Tequila Sunrise	200	14	25
Tom Collins (w/ 2 oz Gin)	210	19	18
Vodka Soda (w/ 1½ oz Vodka)	100	14	0
Vodka Tonic (w/ 1½ oz Vodka)	165	14	18
Whiskey Sour (w/ 2 oz Whiskey)	155	19	7
White Russian (10g fat)	240	19	7
Non-Alcoholic:			
Cinderella	45	0	11
Shirley Temple (w/ 6 oz Ginger Ale)	140	0	34

Liqueurs/Cordials   C   Alc   Cb

Per 1 fl.oz

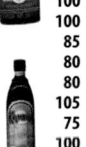

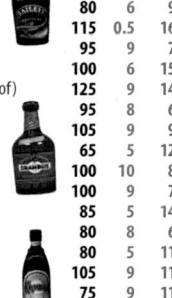

	C	Alc	Cb
Advocaat (36 Proof; 2g fat)	85	4	9
Alizé: Cognac (80 Proof)	70	9	2
Gold/Red Passion (32 Proof)	105	4	11
Amaretto (56 Proof)	100	7	14
Baileys Irish Cream (34 Proof; 5g fat)	95	4	3
Benedictine (80 Proof)	90	9	5
Chambord (33 Proof)	105	4	11
Chartreuse (80 Proof)	100	9	9
Cherry Brandy (48 Proof)	80	6	9
Coffee Liqueur (53 Proof)	115	0.5	16
Cointreau (80 Proof)	95	9	7
Creme de Cacao (54 Proof)	100	6	15
Creme de Menthe (72 Proof)	125	9	14
Curacao (70 Proof)	95	8	6
Drambuie (80 Proof)	105	9	9
Frangelico (40 Proof)	65	5	12
Galliano (86 Proof)	100	10	8
Grand Marnier (80 Proof)	100	9	7
Kahlua (40 Proof)	85	5	14
Kirsch (68 Proof)	80	8	6
Midori (42 Proof)	80	5	11
Ouzo (80 Proof)	105	9	11
Pernod (80 Proof)	75	9	11
Sambuca (84 Proof)	100	10	11
Schnapps (100 Proof)	115	12	9
Southern Comfort (70 Proof)	65	8	3

Liqueur Coffee & Hot Drinks

Per Standard Drink

	C	Alc	Cb
Liqueur Coffee: Avg. all types	200	10	10
Irish, 1½ oz Whiskey & 1 oz whip	205	9	4
Hot Toddy, with 1½ oz liquor, av. all	170	9	19
Mulled Wine (Glühwein), 4 fl.oz, av	195	14	25

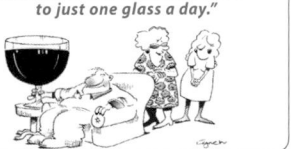

"The doctor told him to cut down to just one glass a day."

TEN TIPS TO AVOID HARMFUL DRINKING

1. **Add up the alcohol** you typically drink each day and on social occasions. How does this compare with 'low risk' amounts? (*See page 23*)

2. **Compare the alcohol content** of different drinks and select the lowest. Request half shots of alcohol in cocktails and mixed drinks. Dilute them and keep topping off with non-alcoholic drinks.

3. **Go easy on 'Light' beers.** At 4% alcohol, on average, they are still high in alcohol compared to regular beer (5% alcohol).

4. **Try low alcohol or non-alcohol** alternatives such as fruit juices and mineral water. Take your own to parties.

5. **Before drinking alcohol,** quench your thirst with water and non-alcoholic drinks – particularly after vigorous exercise or sports.

6. **Slow the rate of drinking.** Chugging or drinking fast is the major cause of illness and death from alcohol poisoning.

7. **Avoid drinking in 'rounds'.**

8. **Have a non-alcoholic 'spacer'** between drinks (e.g. mineral water, orange juice).

9. **Don't drink on an empty stomach.** Food slows the rate of alcohol absorption.

10. **Keep track of the number of drinks** and know when to stop. Stick to a set limit.

Note: Alcohol can be very dangerous when taken with prescription or street drugs, or when you are very tired.

Extra Info: www.CalorieKing.com

Cocktail Mixers & Extracts

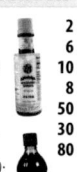

	C	Alc	Cb
Angostura Bitters, ¼ tsp	2	0	0.5
Grenadine, ½ tsp	6	0	2
Lime/Lemon Juice, 2 Tbsp, 1 oz	10	0	2
Maraschino Cherry, 1 small	8	0	2
Simple Syrup, 1 Tbsp, av.	50	0	14
Sweet & Sour Mix, 2 Tbsp, 1 oz	30	0	7
Tonic Water, 8 fl.oz	80	0	22
Flavor Extracts (*McCormick*):			
Pure Lemon (83%), 1 tsp	0	3.5	0
Pure Vanilla (35%), 1tsp	0	1.5	0

29

B Baking Ingredients

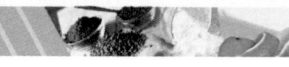

Baking Ingredients

	C	F	Cb
Almond Paste, (Marzipan), 2 Tbsp	170	7	24
Apple Pie Filling,	1	1	1
Sweetened, 9.4 oz	240	0	60
Also ~ See Page 134			
Baking Powder: Regular, 1 tsp	5	0	2
Cream of Tartar, 1 tsp	10	0	2
Baking Mix (Bisquick):			
Original, ⅓ cup, 1½ oz	160	5	26
Heart Smart, ⅓ cup, 1½ oz	140	2.5	27
Batter Mix (Golden Dipt), ¼ cup	100	0	23
Blueberries, 1 cup, 5 oz	85	0.5	21
Butter/Margarine, ½ cup, 4 oz	815	92	1
Stick (Land O' Lakes), ½ oz	100	11	0
Carob Flour, ½ cup	115	0.5	46
Chocolate Baking Bars: *Average all Brands*			
Sweet (Baker's):			
1 oz portion	120	7	16
4 oz bar	470	28	64
Semi-sweet, 1 oz	140	9	16
Bittersweet, 1 oz	140	14	14
White Baking, 1 oz	160	9	16
Unsweetened, 1 oz	140	14	8
Grated, 1 cup, 4½ oz	660	69	39
Chocolate Baking Chips: *Average all Brands*			
Milk Choc./Semi Sweet, 1 oz	140	8	18
½ cup, 3 oz	420	24	54
1 cup, 6 oz	840	48	108
Dark, 1 Tbsp, ½ oz	70	5	3
Mini Kisses (Hershey), 1 piece	5	0.5	1
Cocoa Powder:			
(Nestle): 1 Tbsp	15	1	3
⅓ cup, 1 oz	85	5	17
(Hershey's): 1 Tbsp	20	0.5	3
⅓ cup, 1 oz	115	3	17
Coconut, dried:			
Unsweetened, 1 oz	190	18	6
Sweetened/Flaked:1 oz	130	8	15
1/2 cup, 1.3 oz	195	12	22
Toasted (Baker's), 1 oz	170	13	13
Coconut Cream/Milk ~ See Page 89			
Coconut Manna (Nutiva), 1 Tbsp	100	9	3
Cornstarch, 1 Tbsp	30	0	7
Eggs: Large (1)	75	5	0
Jumbo (1)	90	6	0.5
Egg White: 1 Egg White	15	0	0
½ cup (4 egg whites), 4 oz	60	0	1
Flour: White: 1 Tbsp, 0.3 oz	25	0	5.5
1 cup, 4.2 oz	400	1	88
Whole Wheat, 1 cup, 4.2 oz	400	2	84

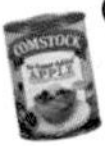

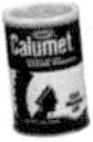

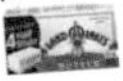

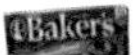

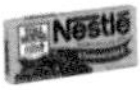

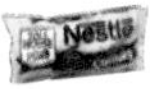

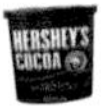

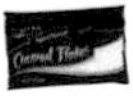

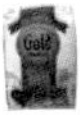

	C	F	Cb
Flavor Extracts: *Average all Brands*			
Imitation, 1 tsp	10	0	2
Pure Extract, 1 tsp	10	0	0.5
Almond, Vanilla, 1 tsp	10	0	0.5
Fruit Pectin: Swtnd, ¼ tsp	5	0	1
Unsweetened, ¼ tsp	0	0	0
Gelatin, dry, ¼ oz pkg	20	0	0
Glaze (Duncan Hines): Choc. 2 Tbsp	150	7	21
Vanilla, 2 Tbsp	140	6	22
Golden Dipt, Batter Mix			
¼ cup, 1 oz	100	0	23
Honey, ½ cup, 6 oz	515	0	140
Lemon/Orange Peel, ¼ cup	25	0	6
Lighter Bake (Sunsweet)			
(Butter & Oil replacement)			
1 Tbsp, ½ oz	35	0	9
¼ cup, 2.7 oz	140	0	36
Milk: Whole, 1 cup, 8 fl.oz	150	8	12
2%, 1 cup, 8 fl.oz	120	5	12
1%, 1 cup, 8 fl.oz	100	2.5	12
Fat-Free, 1 cup, 8 fl.oz	90	0.5	13
Pastry ~ See Page 134			
Pie Crusts ~ See Page 134			
Pie Fillings, Fruits ~ See Page 134			
Lemon Creme, ⅓ cup	130	1.5	28
Mincemeat, 3½ oz	190	5	45
Pumpkin, 1 cup, 9.3 oz	270	1.5	60
Prune Puree, ¼ cup, 3 oz	220	0	55
Raisins, ½ cup, 2.8 oz	240	0	63
Rennin, 1 pkg (11g)	10	0	2
Soy Milk ~ See Pages 49-50			
Sprinkles, all types, 1 tsp	20	1	3
Sugar: 1 Tbsp, ½ oz	55	0	14
1 oz	110	0	28
1 cup, 7 oz	775	0	195
1 lb, 16 oz	1760	0	454
Sweeteners & Sugar Substitutes ~ See Page 156			
Vinegar, average all types, 1 oz	5	0	1
Whey, sweet, dry, 1 oz	100	0.5	21
Yeast: Active, dry, ¼ oz pkg	21	0	3
Bakers, compressed, 1 oz	30	0.5	5
Fleischmann's, 0.6 oz pkg	0	0	0

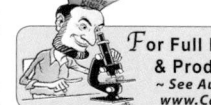

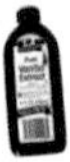

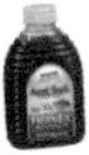

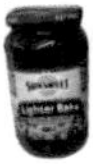

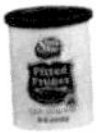

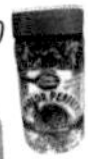

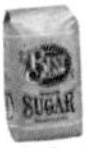

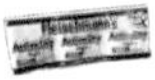

For Full Nutritional Data & Product Updates
~ See Author's Website
www.CalorieKing.com

Note: Actual weight of bars is usually 5-10% more than label Net Weight. Weigh bar and allow extra calories.

Brands

	C	F	Cb
Per Bar			
ABB, Steel Bar, all var., av., 2.5 oz	255	5	35
AdvantEdge ~ *See EAS*			
Annie's Homegrown:			
Organic Granola Bars: *Per 1 oz Bar*			
Berry Berry	120	3	20
Chocolate Chipper	120	4	19
Peanutty	120	4	17
Atkins:			
Advantage Meal: *Per 2 oz Bar*			
Chocolate Chip Cookie Dough	240	11	29
Chocolate Chip Granola	200	9	19
Chocolate Peanut Butter	250	14	23
Cookies 'n Crème	180	9	20
Advantage: *Per 1.55 oz Bar*			
Caramel varieties, av. all	170	10	21
Coconut Almond Delight	200	15	18
Dark Choc. Decadence	150	6	23
Day Break: *Per 1.25 oz Bar*			
Apple Crisp	130	5	17
Choc. Chip Crisp; Cranb. Almond, av.	145	6	16
Peanut Butter Fudge Crisp	150	7	14
Endulge:			
Caramel Nut Chew, 1.2 oz	130	8	17
Chocolate Caramel Mousse, 1.2 oz	120	4.5	23
Nutty Fudge Brownie, 1.4 oz	170	12	18
Peanut Caramel Cluster	140	9	12
Attune Bars:			
Probiotic Wellness Bars: *Per 0.7 oz Bar*			
Dark Chocolate	80	6	11
Milk Chocolate Crisp	90	6	12
Mint Chocolate	90	6	12
Balance: *Per 1.76 oz Bars*			
Original; Bare, av.	200	7	21
Carb Well, average	195	8	23
Gold, average	200	7	23
Barbara's Bakery:			
Fruit & Yogurt, av., 1.5 oz	150	3	29
Nature's Choice, av., 1.25 oz	145	2	29
Bariatrix, Proti-Bar (15g Protein),			
Crisp; Layered, average all, 1.4 oz	160	5.5	15
Cascadian Farms *(General Mills),*			
Chewy Granola, all varieties, average	140	4	25

	C	F	Cb
Per Bar			
Clif:			
Original, average, 2.4 oz	240	3.5	45
Builder's, av., 2.4 oz	270	8	30
Kid, ZBar, av., 1.25 oz	130	3.5	23
Mojo, average, 1.6 oz	195	10	23
Corazonas, Oatmeal Squares,			
all varieties, average,1.75 oz	185	6	28
Detour:			
Original, Caramel Peanut, 3 oz	350	11	32
Lean Muscle: All var. av. 1.6 oz	190	7	14
All varieties, average, 3.2 oz	395	15	33
Lower Sugar: All var., av. 1.5 oz	170	5.5	16
All varieties, average, 3 oz	345	10	32
Oatmeal, all varieties, av., 4¼ oz	460	10	60
Runner, all varieties, av., 1.75 oz	205	5.5	28
Doctor's, CarbRite Diet, av., 2 oz	195	3.5	21
dotFIT: *Per 2 oz Bar*			
Iced Oatmeal: Blueberry	220	5	29
Peanut Butter Delight	190	6	26
12 g Protein,			
Iced, all varieties, 1.75 oz	190	6	26
Note: Carb figures include 11 grams of			
Sorbitol & Malitol sweeteners			
EAS:			
AdvantEDGE:			
Carb Control: Crisp Bars, av., 2 oz	240	8	27
Other varieties, average, 2 oz	230	8	27
Myoplex:			
Carb Control, all var., av., 2.5 oz	260	8	27
Mass, Chocolate Chunk, 3.2 oz	390	20	29
Nutrition: Strength Formula,			
av., 2.65 oz	280	8	35
Lite, av. all, 2 oz	190	4.5	28
Elevate Me!: Strawb. Apple Pie	250	4.5	38
Other varieties, average, 2.35 oz	235	4.5	33
Extend Bar: Crunch, av., 1.4 oz	155	3	30
Sugar Free varieties, 1.4 oz	150	3	21
(Carbs include 4-5g sugar alcohol)			
Fiber One: Chewy, av. all, 1 oz	105	3.5	21
90-Calorie Bars, all var., av., 0.8 oz	90	3	18
FiberPlus *(Kellogg's),* Antioxidants:			
Chocolate Chip, 1.25 oz	120	4	26
Nutty Delights, all var., 1.25 oz	150	8	22
Other varieties, 1.25 oz	130	5	25
Fresh & Easy:			
Eatwell,			
90 Cal. Fiber Bars, av., 0.8 oz	90	2.5	17
Granola: *1.23 oz Bars*			
Oatmeal Raisin	130	2	27
Other varieties, average	155	5	25

Note: Actual weight of bars is usually 5-10% more than label Net Weight. Weigh bar and allow extra calories

Brands (Cont)

Per Bar	C	F	Cb
Full Bar: Regular, av. all, 1.6 oz	170	4	28
GeniSoy: *Per 1.98 oz Bar*			
Protein: Chunky PB Fudge	220	6	32
Crispy Chocolate Mint	210	4.5	33
Other varieties, av.	220	6	31
General Mills: *Per 1.6 oz Bar*			
Milk 'n Cereal Bars: Cinn Toast Crunch	180	4	33
Honey Nut Cheerios	160	4	28
Glenny's: *Per 1.1 oz Bar*			
Cashew & Almond	140	7	16
Cherry/Cranberry & Almond	150	7	17
Classic Fruit & Nut	140	6	18
Peanuts & Peanut Butter	170	13	10
Glucerna: Meal Bars, av., 2 oz	220	7	34
Snack Bars, av., 1.4 oz	145	4	23
Mini Snack Bar, av., 0.7 oz	75	2.5	12
GNC:			
Pro Performance:			
Pro Crunch, av. all, 2.3 oz	255	6	35
Lite, 1.2 oz	140	6	14
Lean Bar, av., 1.6 oz	150	5	18
(Carbs include 5g sugar alc.)			
Gnu Foods: *Per 1.6 oz Bar*			
Banana Walnut; Choc. Brownie; P'B	140	4	30
Cinnamon Raisin; Orange Cranb.	130	3	32
Good 'n Natural,			
Fruit Nuts & Seeds,			
all varieties, av., 2 oz	230	9	28
Great Value *(Walmart):*			
90 Calories, av. all, 0.8 oz	90	1.5	19
Chewy Hi Fiber, average, 1.4 oz	145	4	29
Fruit & Grain, low fat,			
all varieties, average, 1.3 oz	140	2.5	27
Granola: Choc Chunk, 0.85 oz	90	2	18
Choc Chip; PB; Smores, av., 0.8 oz	100	3	19
Peanut, 1.23 oz	180	9	19
Sweet & Salty, Almond, 1.25 oz	160	8	20
Health Valley:			
Cobbler Cereal Bars, all flav., 1.25 oz	130	2.5	27
Chewy Granola, all var., average	110	1.5	22
Herbalife, Prot. Deluxe!, av., 1.25 oz	140	4	16
HMR, Benefit Bars, av. all, 1.41 oz	155	4	27
Jenny Craig: S'mores, 1.25 oz	130	4	23
Chocolatey Caramel P'nut, 1.25 oz	140	5	19
Choc Chip Snack Bar, 1.2 oz	140	3	23
Joy Ride, Protein Bars, av., 2.8 oz	340	12	27

Per Bar	C	F	Cb
Kashi:			
Cereal Bars, av. all varieties, 1.23 oz	125	3	24
Granola: Chewy, av. all var., 1.23 oz	135	4	21
Layered, all varieties, 1.1 oz	125	4	21
Go Lean:			
Crisp!:			
Choc. Caramel, 1.58 oz	150	3	28
Choc. Peanut, 1.75 oz	180	5	30
Other varieties, av., 1.58 oz	165	4	27
Dipped: P'nut Butter Choc., 1.94 oz	200	5	32
Other varieties, average, 1.94 oz	190	5	32
Rolls, all varieties, 1.94 oz	190	5	27
Keebler,			
Granola Fudge av., 1.2 oz	150	6	25
Kellogg's:			
Cinnabon Bars, all flavors, 1.3 oz	150	4.5	26
Fiber Plus, Antiox., av. all, 1.25 oz	125	5	25
Nutrigrain ~ *See page 33*			
Special K ~ *See page 34*			
Kind: *Per 1.4 oz Bar Unless Indicated*			
Fruit & Nut: Almond & Apricot	190	11	22
Apple Cinnamon & Pecan	180	10	23
In Yogurt, average, 1.6 oz	215	12	26
Macadamia & Apricot	190	12	22
Nut Delight	210	16	14
Peanut Butter & Strawberry	190	11	18
Sesame & Peanuts with Chocolate	240	17	16
Walnut & Date	170	9	22
Plus:			
Cranberry Almond + Antioxidants	190	13	20
Almond Cashew w/ Flax & Omega 3	180	10	20
Alm. Walnut Macadamia + Protein	190	12	15
Kraft, Milk Bite Granola, av., 1.25 oz	140	6	19
Kudos, average all varieties, 0.85 oz	100	3	17
Labrada:			
Lean Body Bars:			
Cookie Roll: Choc. Chip, 2.82 oz	330	11	34
Cinn. Bun; Iced Brownie, av., 2.82 oz	300	9	34
Rockin'Roll, Hi Protein Nut, 2.47 oz	290	16	25
Whole Food:			
Banana Nut, 1.8 oz	180	4.5	21
Peanut Butter Choc Chip, 1.8 oz	190	7	20
Larabar:			
Apple Pie, 1.6 oz	190	10	24
Cherry Pie, 1.7 oz	200	8	30
Choc. Chip Brownie, 1.6 oz	200	9	31
Peanut Butter & Jelly, 1.7 oz	210	10	27
Lindora, all varieties, average, 1.6 oz	155	5	17
Luna:			
Bars For Women,			
all varieties, average, 1.7 oz	180	4.5	27
Protein, all varieties, av., 1.6 oz	185	7	20

Brands (Cont)

Per Bar	C	F	Cb
Marathon (Snickers):			
Energy: Chewy, 2 oz	215	7	26
Crunchy, av., 1.5 oz	150	4.5	22
Protein, av. all, 2.8 oz	285	10	38
Smart Stuff, av. all, 1.25 oz	140	4	22
Market Pantry (Target):			
Crunchy Granola, Oat & Honey, 1.5 oz	190	6	30
Sweet & Salty, Peanut, 1.2 oz	170	8	21
Mariani:			
Honey Bars: Cranberry, 1.4 oz	180	10	20
Granola	160	6	25
Sesame	200	14	16
Medifast: Crunch, av., 1.2 oz	110	3	12
Maintenance, av. all, 1.5 oz	160	4.5	21
Met-Rx: Per 3.53 oz Bar Unless Indicated			
Big 100, all varieties, average	375	6	49
Big 100 Colossal:			
Brownie, average	395	13	41
Chocolate Toasted Almond	410	13	46
Crispy Apple Pie	400	10	47
Protein Plus, Mud Pie, 3 oz	300	9	32
Milk Bite (Kraft), Granola, av., 1.25 oz	140	6	18
Mojo Bars – See Clif			
Muscle Milk: Regular, av., 2.5 oz	295	11	29
Light, all flavors, 1.6 oz	170	6	18
MuscleTech:			
Nitro-Tech Hardcore, 2.8 oz	310	8	29
Smart Protein: Triple Choc., 2.2 oz	270	9	26
Peanut Caramel Crunch, 2.2 oz	290	12	26
Nabisco, 100 Calorie Fruit Crisps, all varieties, 2 crisps, 0.9 oz	100	2	20
Nature's Path, Granola Bars, av. all, 1.25 oz	145	5	23
Nature Valley:			
Crunchy Granola Bars:			
Apple Crisp (2), 1.5 oz	160	6	26
Cinnamon (2), 1.5 oz	180	6	29
Other flavors (2), av., 1.5 oz	190	7	28
Chewy, Yog. coating, av., 1.2 oz	140	3.5	26
Granola Thins, Peanut Butter, 1 pouch, 0.6 oz	90	4.5	0
Protein, av., 1.4 oz bar	190	12	14
Trail Mix, Chewy, av. all, 1.25 oz	135	4	25
Nutiva: Hempseed, 1.4 oz	210	15	14
Hemp Choc.; Flax & Raisin, 1.4 oz	200	13	16
Nutrigrain (Kellogg's):			
Cereal Bars, av. all varieties, 1.3 oz	120	3	24
Fruit Fusion, w/ Antiox., 1.3 oz	130	3	26
Yogurt Bars, Strawberry, 1.3 oz	130	3.5	25

Per Bar	C	F	Cb
Nutrilite (Amway Global):			
Meal Bars. Blueb. Crunch, 1.8 oz	200	6	27
Cherry Almond, 1.8 oz	200	6	26
Chocolate Crisp, 1.8 oz	200	6	26
Lemon Twist, 1.8 oz	200	5	29
Snack Bar: Caramel Creme, 0.9 oz	100	2.5	16
Cranberry Crunch, 0.9 oz	100	3.5	14
Fudgy Brownie w/ Almonds, 0.9 oz	100	3.5	9
NutriSystem:			
Dessert Bars: Chewy Peanut	180	8	21
Chocolate Caramel	160	5	24
Odwalla: Per 2 oz Bar			
Energy: Berries GoMega	210	6	36
Blueberry Swirl	200	3	41
Choc. Chip Peanut	230	8	33
Choc. Chip Trail Mix	200	7	28
Choco-walla	210	5	39
Dark Chocolate Chip Walnut	220	7	36
Strawb. Pomegranate	200	2	42
Superfood, Original	200	3.5	39
Oh Yeah! (ISS), P'nut var., av., 3 oz	375	17	31
One Way, Protein, 3 oz	340	12	29
Optifast, 800 Bars, av., 1.6 oz	165	4	20
PowerBar:			
Energy Bars: Fruit Smoothie, all var.	220	3.5	43
Harvest, all varieties, average	245	4.5	42
Nut Naturals, all varieties, av., 1.6 oz	210	10	21
Performance, all var., av., 2 oz	240	3.5	44
Pria Bars, 110 Plus, av., 1.75 oz	110	3	16
Protein Plus, av.	300	7	37
Pure & Simple, av.	135	3	23
Triple Threat, av. all, 2 oz	225	8	31
Power Crunch (BNRG), Protein Bar, all varieties, av., 1.4 oz	205	12	10
PR Bar: Double Chocolate, 1.8 oz	200	6	22
Yogurt Berry, 1.8 oz	210	7	22
Granola, Peanut Butter, 1.75 oz	200	7	22
Premier Nutrition:			
Protein, av., 2.5 oz	280	7	24
Titan, av., 2.8 oz	325	13	32
Promax:			
Cookies 'N Cream, 2.6 oz	270	4.5	40
Chocolate Peanut Crunch, 2.6 oz	300	8	37
Double Fudge Brownie, 2.6 oz	280	7	37
Lower Sugar, Energy, av., 2.4 oz	220	7	33
Proti Bars (Bariatrix), Crisp; Layered, av., 1.4 oz	160	5.5	16
Pure Protein:			
1.75 oz Bars, av.	180	5	18
2.75 oz Bars, average	300	8	30

Note: Actual weight of bars is usually 5-10% more than label Net Weight. Weigh bar and allow extra calories.

Brands (Cont)

Per Bar	C	F	Cb
PureFit, av. all, 2 oz	220	7	25
Quaker:			
Breakfast Cookies, av., 1.7 oz	175	4.5	33
Chewy Granola Bars:			
Regular, av. 0.85 oz	100	3	18
Chewy School Days,			
Apple; Berry, 1 oz	100	2	20
Dipps, Caramel Nut	140	6	21
Fiber/Omega-3, PB. Choc, 1.25 oz	150	5	25
25% Less Sugar, Choc. Chip, 0.85 oz	100	3.5	17
90 Calories, all varieties, 1 oz	90	2	19
Stila:			
Bits, Cramberry/Apple, 0.7oz pack	80	1.5	15
Crispy Oat Cookie Bars,			
Blueberry/Strawberry, 0.9 oz bar	100	1.5	19
Revival Soy (Direct):			
Apple Cinnamon	225	3	30
Chocolate Temptation	270	7	32
Peanut Pal	240	6	28
Low Carb, all varieties, average	235	8	31
(Contains 22g sugar alc. & 3g fiber)			
Slim-Fast:			
Meal Bars:			
Chewy Chocolate Crisp	200	6	26
Chocolate Peanut Caramel	200	7	23
Sweet & Salty Chocolate Almond	200	8	23
Snack Bars:			
Chocolate Nougat Gone Nuts	100	5	14
Chocolatey Van. Blitz	100	2.5	17
Double-Dutch Choc.	100	3.5	16
SoyJoy Bars, av., 1 oz	135	6	16
Solo, GI, av. all, 1.75 oz	200	7	26
Special K:			
90 Calorie Bars, av. all, 0.8 oz	90	2	18
Cereal Bars, all varieties, av., 0.8 oz	90	1.5	18
Protein Meal, all varieties, av., 1.6 oz	180	5	25
Protein Snack Bars, av. all, 0.9 oz	110	3	16
Steel Bar (ABB), av. all, av., 2.5 oz	260	5	34

Per Bar	C	F	Cb
Supreme Protein:			
Carb Conscious: PB Crunch, 3 oz	390	18	26
Caramel Nut Chocolate, 3.4 oz	400	15	36
(Contains 14-27g Sugar alc. & 1-2g fiber)			
thinkThin:			
Protein:			
1.75 oz Bars, average	200	7	23
2.1 oz Bars, average	235	8	24
Bites, av. all, 0.9 oz	100	4	12
(Contains between 5-14g Sugar Alc)			
Tiger's Milk:			
Protein Rich, 1.2 oz	140	5	18
Peanut Butter, 1.2 oz	150	6	18
King Size, all varieties, av., 2 oz	225	9	28
Toaster Strudel ~ *see page 64*			
Trader Joe's:			
Chewy Granola Bars, 6-Packs:			
Chocolate Chip, 1.25 oz	150	4	26
Peanut Butter, 1.25oz	170	8	19
Vanilla Almond, 1.25 oz	150	6	22
Fruit Bars: Fig 1.5 oz	120	2	24
Other varieties, average, 1.5 oz	140	2.5	27
Granola Bars, 6-packs:			
Fruit & Nut Trek Mix, 1.25 oz	130	2.5	25
Trail Mix, 1.25 oz	150	5	23
Tri-O-Plex (Chef Jay's):			
High Protein, Ban. Walnut, 4.2 oz	405	14	40
Duo: Caramel Peanut Butter, 3.5 oz	340	8	45
Peanut Butter & Jelly, 3.5 oz	360	11	41
Usana:			
Nutrition Bars: Oatmeal Raisin, 2 oz	170	3	30
Peanut Butter Crunch, 1.5 oz	160	5	19
Wheaties, Fuel Energy Bars:			
Chocolate Peanut Butter, 2.25 oz	290	12	30
Double Chocolate, 2.25 oz	280	10	34
Zoe's, Omega-3's, Choc. Delight	190	7	27
Zone Perfect:			
Classic, av., 1.76 oz	210	7	24
Cookie Dough, all var., av., 1.5 oz	185	6	23
Dark Chocolate, all var., av., 1.5 oz	190	6	22
Fruitified, all varieties, av., 1.75 oz	195	5	25
Perfectly Simple, all var., av., 1.6 oz	180	6	22
Sweet & Salty, all var., av., 1.5 oz	200	7	22

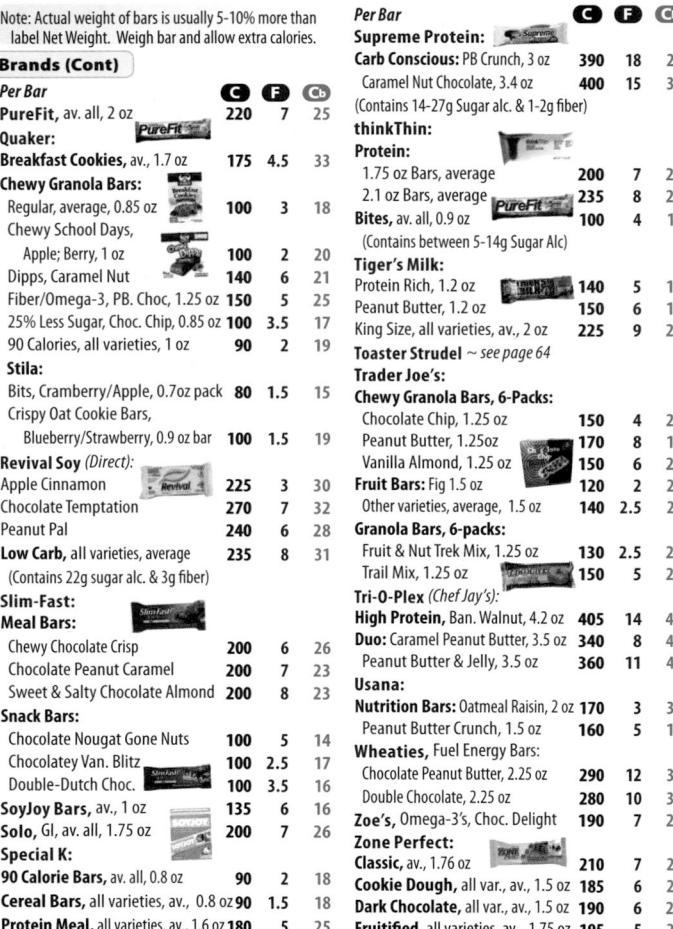

Cocoa & Hot Chocolate | C | F | Cb

Cocoa:
	C	F	Cb
Small (8 fl.oz): With Whole Milk	205	8.5	22
With Nonfat Milk	145	1	23
Tall (12 fl.oz): With Whole Milk	280	12	26
With Nonfat Milk	185	1	28

Hot Chocolate:
	C	F	Cb
Small (8 fl.oz): With Whole Milk	180	7	26
With Nonfat Milk	140	2	17
Tall (12 fl.oz): With Whole Milk	260	10	36
With Nonfat Milk	190	2	37
Cinnabon, Mochalatta Chill, 16 oz	420	17	63
Swiss Miss, Mixes, av., 1 packet	120	2.5	22

Cocoa - Chocolate Mixes

Add extra cals/fat/carbohydrate for milk
Carnation Breakfast Drinks ~ See Page 38
	C	F	Cb
Carnation: Per 3 Tbsp			
Malted Milk: Original	90	2	15
Chocolate	90	1	18
Ghirardelli:			
Choc. Mocha, 4 Tbsp, 1.2 oz	135	1.5	33
Double Chocolate, 4 Tbsp, 1.4 oz	140	1.5	34
White Mocha, 2 Tbsp, 0.8 oz	100	0	24
Hershey's, Cocoa, Natural, 1 Tbsp, 0.2 oz	10	0.5	3
Land O Lakes, Mint/Raspberry/Supreme, 1.25 oz	140	3.5	26
Nestle: Per Per Single Serve Envelope			
/ Vitamins & Minerals	80	3	14
Dark Chocolate	100	3	19
Rich Milk Chocolate:			
Regular	80	3	14
Fat Free	25	0	5
No Sugar Added	50	0	9
Nesquik Powder: Per 2 Tbsp			
Choc.; Strawberry, 25% less sugar	60	0	15
Chocolate; Strawb., No Added Sugar	35	1	7
Ovaltine, All Natural Cocoa Mixes, all varieties, average, 2 Tbsp	40	0	10
Swiss Miss: Per Single Serve Envelope			
Breakfast Blends: Great Start	60	1	11
Pick Me Up	110	2	23
Classics: French Vanilla	115	2	23
Marshmallow	110	2	23
Marshmallow Lovers	120	2.5	23
Milk Chocolate	120	2	23
Rich Chocolate	120	2	23
Fat-Free: Original	50	0	10
Marshmallow Lovers	70	0	13

Instant Coffee | C | F | Cb

	C	F	Cb
Powder/Granules: Regular or Decaffeinated,			
1 level tsp	2	0	0.5
1 rounded tsp	4	0	1
Ground, 3 tsp	7	0	1
Brewed/Percolated, 1 cup, 8 fl.oz	4	0	1
Coffee With Milk/Cream/Creamers: Per 8 oz Cup			
Black:	4	0	1
With Whole Milk: Dash, 1 Tbsp	15	0.5	2
2 Tbsp, 1 fl.oz	25	1	2.5
With 2% Milk, 2 Tbsp	20	0.5	2.5
With 1% Milk, 2 Tbsp	20	0.5	2.5
With Fat Free Milk, 2 Tbsp	15	0	2.5
With Soy Milk: 1 Tbsp	10	0	1.5
2Tbsp, 1 oz	15	0.5	2
With Half & Half: 2 Tbsp	50	3	3
¼ cup, 2 fl.oz	90	6	4
With Cream (light coffee), 2 Tbsp	65	6	2
With Coffee Mate: Liquid, reg., 1 T.	20	1	3
Liquid Fat Free, 1 Tbsp	25	0	2
Powder, 1 heaping tsp	15	1	2
Sugar ~ Add Extra: 1 heaping tsp	25	0	6
Single portion, 1 package	25	0	6
Sweeteners, (Equal/Splenda/Sweet N Low), Powder, 1 package	0	0	0

Flavored Coffee Mixes

	C	F	Cb
Chicory:			
Instant Coffee, 1 tsp	5	0	1
Coffee Essence, 1 tsp	15	0	4
Caffé D'Vita: Mixes, 3 tsp	60	1.5	11
Sugar Free Mixes, 2 tsp	35	2	3
General Foods International:			
All varieties, average· 1/2 oz	60	3	10
Sugar-free, all var., av., 1 tsp	30	2.5	2
Cappuccino Coolers, all, ½ oz	60	0	15
Hills Bros, Cappuccino, Fr. Vanilla, 3 Tbsp, 1 oz	120	4.5	19
Nescafé, Latte; Mocha, av., 1oz	115	3.5	21
Starbucks, VIA® Iced Coffee, 1 stick	100	0	24

Coffee Shops/Restaurants

Per 8 fl.oz Cup (Unless Indicated)

	C	F	Cb
Coffee, Regular/Percolated/Filtered	5	0	0
Americano Drip Coffee, 1 cup	7.5	0	1
Cafe Au Lait: 1 cup, 8 fl.oz	60	3.5	5
Nonfat Milk, 1 cup, 8 fl.oz	35	0	5
Caffe Latté:			
8 fl.oz cup: With Whole Milk	110	6	9
With 2% Milk	100	3.5	9
With Nonfat Milk	70	0	9
12 fl.oz: With Whole Milk	180	9	14
With Nonfat Milk	100	0	15
16 fl.oz: With Whole Milk	220	11	18
With Nonfat Milk	130	0	19
Cafe Mocha (Mochaccino): 8 fl.oz	150	6	20
12 fl.oz	230	9	31
16 fl.oz	290	12	41
Cappuccino:			
8 fl.oz cup: With Whole Milk	90	3.5	7
With 2% Milk	80	3	8
With Nonfat Milk	50	0	8
12 fl.oz: With Whole Milk	110	6	9
With 2% Milk	90	3.5	9
With Nonfat Milk	60	0	9
16 fl.oz: With Whole Milk	140	7	11
With 2% Milk	120	3.5	11
With Nonfat Milk	80	0	12
Mocha: *With Cream*			
8 fl.oz: With Whole Milk	200	11	22
With Nonfat Milk	160	6	22
12 fl.oz: With Whole Milk	290	15	33
With Nonfat Milk	230	8	34
Iced Mocha: *Without Cream*			
12 fl.oz: With Whole Milk	170	6	26
With Nonfat Milk	130	2	27
Espresso: Single (Solo), 1 fl.oz	5	0	1
Doppio (Double), 2 fl.oz	10	0	2
Espresso con Panna,			
(w/ dollop wh. cream), solo, 1 fl.oz	30	2.5	1
Espresso Macchiato, solo, 1 fl.oz	10	0	1
Frappuccino: Tall, 12 fl.oz	180	2.5	37
Grande, 16 fl.oz	240	3	48
Frappuccino Mocha:			
(With Cream): Tall, 12 fl.oz	280	11	43
Grande, 16 fl.oz	380	15	57

Iced Latte: Similar to Caffe Latte
McCafe (McDonald's) ~ *See Fast Food, Page 216*
Starbucks ~ *See Fast-Foods Section , Page 243*

Coffee Substitute Mixes

	C	F	Cb
Roasted Cereal Beverages ~ *(No Caffeine)*			
Cafix, Instant Beverage, 1 tsp	5	0	1
Kaffree Roma, Instant Beverage, 1 tsp	10	0	2
Teeccino, Herbal Coffees, 1 tsp	10	0	2

Irish & Liqueur Coffees

	C	F	Cb
Irish Coffee, without sugar	175	10	0
Liqueur Coffee,			
with cream, all varieties, av., 1 fl.oz	100	5	7

Coffee Extras

	C	F	Cb
Chocolate (Cocoa) Topping, ½ tsp	5	0	1
Flavored Syrups: Regular, 2 Tbsp	80	0	20
Sugar-free, 2 Tbsp	0	0	0
Half & Half Cream: 2 Tbsp	40	3.5	1
Single serve pkg, ⅜ fl.oz	15	1.5	0.5
Light whipped cream, 2 Tbsp	15	1.5	1
Marshmallows, miniature (2)	5	0	1
Sugar:			
1 single portion package	20	0	5
1 level tsp	15	0	4
1 heaping tsp	25	0	6
Equal/Splenda/Sweet 'N Low	0	0	0

Coffee Shop ~ Cakes, Cookies

	C	F	Cb
Cookies:			
Biscotti, 1 oz	140	6.5	18
Chocolate Chip, 3 oz	350	15	54
Oatmeal Raisin, 3 oz	350	12	56
Peanut Butter, 3 oz	410	25	39
White Chocolate Macadamia, 3.33 oz	420	20	55
Cakes/Pastries:			
Almond Croissant, 5 oz	620	35	67
Apple Danish, 5 oz	450	18	67
Banana Walnut, 4.5 oz	410	17	60
Brownie, 3 oz	390	24	42
Bundt, Chocolate, 4 oz	440	21	61
Carrot Cake, 4 oz	400	22	45
Chocolate Cake, 5 oz	530	28	66
Crumble Coffee Cake, 4.5 oz	500	25	65
Cupcake, 3 oz	330	16	43
Pound Cake, av., 3 oz	330	17	40
Cinnamon Roll, 6 oz	500	15	83
Donuts:			
Sugared, 1.75 oz	220	11	27
Glazed, 2 oz	250	12	34
Pretzel, large, 4 oz	290	5	52

Starbucks Bakery Items ~ *See Page 244*

Beverages ~ Coffee ◇ Caffeine Counter (B)

Ready To Drink Coffee

	C	**F**	**Cb**
Chilled:			
Adina. Per 8 fl.oz can			
Double XXpresso	100	2	18
Mayan Mocha	130	2.5	24
Mocha Madness	110	2.5	20
Coffee Bean & Tea Leaf,			
Cafe Latte/Mocha/Vanilla, 9.5 fl.oz	200	3	33
Full Throttle Coffee & Energy ~ *See Page 38*			
International Delight,			
Iced, all varieties, 8 fl.oz	150	25	29
Java Monster Energy ~ *See Page 39*			
Kahlua, Cappuccino Shake, 10.5 fl.oz	130	2	24
RealBeanz: Per 9.5 fl.oz			
Iced Coffee: All varieties	140	2	27
Diet, Trim & Fit, Cappuccino	60	2	16
Shock Coffee:			
Triple Latte, 8 fl.oz	150	3.5	28
Triple Mocha, 8 fl.oz can	150	3.5	28
Starbucks: *Per Bottle*			
Frappuccino:			
Coffee, 9.5 fl.oz	200	3	37
Mocha, 9.5 fl.oz	180	3	33
Vanilla: 9.5 fl.oz	200	3	37
Light: 9.5 fl.oz	100	3	12
DoubleShots:			
Espresso & Cream: Regular, 6.5 fl.oz	140	6	18
Light, 6.5 fl.oz	70	4	6
Starbucks Coffee & Energy ~ *See Page 40*			
Trader Joe's,			
Caffe Latte; Caffe Mocha, 6.5 fl.oz	120	1.5	25

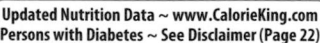

CALORIE KING TIP!

Reduce the Calories in Your Coffee Drinks:

- Request non-fat milk in place of whole or 2% milk
- Downsize to 8 fl.oz or 12 fl.oz
- Avoid cream on frappuccinos
- Replace sugar with Equal, Splenda Stevia or Sweet 'N Low
- Avoid syrup add-ons

CAFFEINE COUNTER

Moderate caffeine intake is not harmful to healthy adults. However, frequent large amounts (over 350mg/day) may cause dependency ('caffeinism') and adversely affect health. To be safe, limit caffeine to 200mg/day. Avoid if pregnant, breast feeding, a child under 8, have sleep problems, an overactive bladder or heart arrhythmia.

	Caffeine (mg)
Coffee: Instant, weak, 1 level teaspoon	30
Medium, 1 rounded teaspoon	60
Strong, 1 heaping teaspoon	100
Decaffeinated, 1 round teaspoon	2
Bags (Folgers), 1 bag (6-8 fl.oz)	115
Ground, 1 Tbsp, 0.2 oz	60
Bottled (Ready-To-Drink), 9.5 fl.oz	70
Coffee Shop: Brewed, 8 fl.oz	110 -150
Cappuccino: 1 cup, 8 fl.oz	75
Tall, 12 fl.oz	110
Large, 16 fl.oz	150
Decappuccino, decaffeinated	5
Espresso: Regular/Solo	75
Double (Doppio)	150
Iced Coffee, 12 fl.oz	140
Latte, 1 cup, 8 fl.oz	75
Mocha, 1 cup, 8 fl.oz	90
Hot Chocolate, 8 fl.oz	15
Tea (Black/Green): Weak, 1 cup	20
Medium Strength, 1 cup	40
Strong, 1 cup	70
Decaffeinated Tea	0-5
Herbal Tea	0
Iced Tea, tall glass/can, 12 fl.oz	25-30
Soft Drinks: Per 12 fl.oz Can	
Coca-Cola, Pepsi (Regular/Diet)	35
Diet Coke; TAB; RC Cola (Regular)	45
Dr. Pepper, Sunkist Orange	40
Pepsi One; Mountain Dew; Mellow Yellow; Surge	55
Pepsi Max (Regular/Diet) Sun Drop (Reg/Diet)	70
7-Up, Fanta, Sprite, Fresca, Diet Rite Cola	0
Energy Drinks (with added caffeine):	
(AMP, Adrenaline Rush, Full Throttle Monster, No Fear, Red Bull, Rockstar)	
Average all brands: 8 fl.oz	80
16 fl.oz	160
NOS Energy, 16 fl.oz	260
Chocolate Bars: Milk Chocolate, 2 oz	20
Dark Chocolate, 2 oz	30
Choc Chip Cookies, 2 medium, 2 oz	6
Chocolate Syrup, 2 Tbsp, 1.4 oz	5
Medicinals: Excedrin, Extra Strength (2)	130
NoDoz Maximum, 1 tablet	200

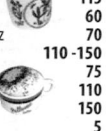
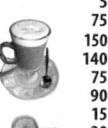
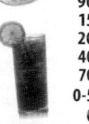
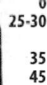
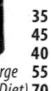

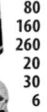

Energy/Protein Drinks

	C	F	Cb
5-hour Energy, 2 fl.oz	4	0	1
ABB:			
Anytime, Turbo Tea, 18 fl.oz	150	0	38
Energy: Speed Shot, 8.5 fl.oz	0	0	0
Ripped Force, 18 fl.oz	90	0	23
Hi-Pro:			
Pure Pro Shake, Chocolate, 12 fl.oz	160	0.5	5
Pure Pro 50, 14.5 fl.oz	240	1.5	7
Recovery,			
Maxx Recovery, Grape, 18 fl.oz	480	0.5	6
AdvantEDGE (EAS),			
Carb Control, av. all, 11 fl.oz	110	3	4
AllSport,			
Body Quencher, all flav., 20 fl.oz	150	0	40
AMP: Per 16 fl.oz Can			
Elevate; Energy Drink, average	225	0	58
Other varieties, average	225	0	58
Arizona: AM Awake Fast Shot, 2 fl.oz	10	0	3
Caution Energy, 11 fl.oz	160	0	40
Atkins, Advantage Shakes, av., 11 oz	160	10	4
Bariatrix: Pudding Shakes (1), av.	100	2	7
Ready To Serve Drinks (1), average	110	4	4
Bawls: Guarana, 10 fl.oz	120	0	32
Blue Sky,			
Blue Energy, 8.3 fl.oz	120	0	29
Body Fuel, (w. NutraSweet),			
1 scoop	80	0	20
Bolthouse: Per 8 fl.oz			
Protein Plus:			
Blended Coffee	190	2.5	26
Chocolate; Mango, average	200	2	30
Boost: Per 8 fl.oz			
Original, all varieties	240	4	41
High Protein, all varieties	240	6	33
Glucose Control, all varieties	190	7	16
Plus, all flavors	360	14	45
Carnation, Breakfast, Essentials:			
Powder:			
All varieties, 1 envelope, 1.3 oz	130	1	27
No Sugar Added, av. all, 0.7 oz	60	1	12
Ready-To-Drink, av. all, 11.5 fl.oz	260	5	41
Celebrity, Juice Diet, 4 fl.oz	60	0	14
Celestial Seasoning, Shots,			
Green Tea/ Kombucha, all var., 2 oz	30	0	8
CeraSport, EX1 pdr, ½ pkt, 8.5 fl.oz	20	0	5
Champion Lyte, Sports Drink	0	0	0

	C	F	Cb
Champion Nutrition:			
Heavywt Gainer 900, av., 4 scps, 5.4 oz	600	6	102
Ultramet: Original, 1 packet, 2.7 oz	280	2	24
Low Carb, 1 packet, 2 oz	230	6.5	6
Clif Shot, Energy Gel, 1.1 oz pkt	100	0	24
Cocaine, Energy, 8.4 fl.oz can	70	0	18
Curves, Protein Drink:			
Choc.,; Vanilla, 2 scps, 1 oz	120	1	12
With skim milk, 8 fl.oz	200	2	24
CytoSport, Muscle Milk, 2 scps	300	12	16
Drank, Anti Energy, 8 fl.oz	110	0	27
EAS ~ See AdvantEdge/Myoplex			
Ensure:			
Clear, 10 fl.oz	180	0	35
Clinical/Plus, 8 fl.oz bottle	350	11	50
High Protein Shake, 14 fl.oz	210	2.5	23
Muscle Health, 8 fl.oz	250	8	32
Nutrition Shake, all flavors, 8 fl.oz	250	8	40
Enterex, Diabetic, 8 fl.oz	235	9	27
FRS, Energy, Orange Cream, 12 fl.oz	190	2.5	11
Fruit₂0 (Verifine)	0	0	0
Full Throttle: Per 16 fl.oz			
Energy, Citrus	220	0	58
Coffee & Energy:			
Caramel	230	0	58
Mocha	270	7	50
Fuze: Refresh, 8 fl.oz	95	0	25
Slenderize, 8 fl.oz	10	0	2
Vitalize, 8 fl.oz	100	0	25
Gatorade:			
G Series: Ready To Drink			
Perform: Original G, all var., 8 fl.oz	50	0	14
G2, low calories, all varieties, 8 fl.oz	20	0	5
Prime, all varieties, 4 fl.oz pouch	100	0	25
Recover: 03 Drink, all var., 8 fl.oz	110	0	20
03 Shake, all var., 330 ml carton	270	1.5	45
Fit: 02, Perform, all var., 8 fl.oz	10	0	2
03, Recover, all varieties, 11 fl.oz	100	0	12
Pro: 01, Prime, all var., 4 fl.oz pouch	120	0	30
02, Perform, all var., 8 fl.oz	50	0	14
03, Recover, all var., 8 fl.oz	110	0	20
Natural:			
G Series, 02, Thirst Quencher,			
Orange Flavor, 8 fl.oz	50	0	14
G2, Thirst Quencher,			
Berry, 8 fl.oz	20	0	4
Genisoy:			
Ultra XT, 3 Tbsp	150	1	20
Protein Powder, Chocolate; Vanilla,			
average, 1.25 oz scoop	125	0	18
Glaceau:			
Smartwater, 8 fl.oz	0	0	0
Vitaminwater, 20 fl.oz	125	0	33
Glucerna, Shakes, all var., 8 fl.oz	200	7	27

	C	F	Cb
GNC:			
Lean Shake:			
Powder, all varieties, 2 scoops	200	3	17
Drinks, av. all, 14 fl.oz bottle	170	6	6
Pro Performance			
100% Whey Protein, all, 1 oz	130	2	8
50 Gram Slam, Choc., 15 fl.oz	250	2	9
Amplified: Mass XXX, Strawberry, 4 level scoops	750	6	124
Wheybolic Extreme 60, all varieties, 3 scoops	280	1	7
Golanzo:			
Sports Energy: All flav., 12 fl.oz	90	0	22
Sug. Free, Mango Lime, 12 fl.oz	10	0	5
Sports Hydration, 20 fl.oz bottle			
Mandarin	90	0	23
Other flavors, average	115	0	30
GU, Energy Gel, av. all, 1 packet	100	2	25
Guru, Energy: Regular, 8.3 oz can	100	0	25
Lite, 8.3 oz can	10	0	2
Hammer, Gel, all flav., av., 2 T., 1¼ oz	90	0	21
Hansen's: Energy Pro, 8 fl.oz	120	0	32
Energy Diet Red, 8 fl.oz	10	0	3
Rumba, 8 fl.oz	130	0	32
Herbalife: Nutritional Shake, 1 pkt	90	1	13
With 8 fl.oz non-fat milk	180	1	26
Holistics (Adina), Herbal Blends, Av. all, 14 fl.oz bottle	90	0	22
Hollywood Miracle Diet, ½ cup	100	0	25
Hype:			
Energy: Regular; Organic, av., 8.4 fl.oz	110	0	28
Enlite, 8.4 fl.oz	25	0	4
Shot, 2.5 fl.oz	35	0	8
Jarrow: Whey Protein, av., 1 scoop	95	2	2
Berry High, 1 scoop, 0.2 oz	25	0	5
Muscle Optimeal, 2 scoops, 1.65 oz	180	2	17
Java Monster: Per 15 fl.oz Can			
Average all flavors	190	3	33
Vanilla Light	95	3	13
Jolt, av. all flav., 16 fl.oz can	200	0	52
Orange Burst, 16 fl.oz	210	0	54
Knudsen: Recharge, av., 8 fl.oz	70	0	23
Simply Nutritious, av. all, 8 fl.oz	120	0	30
Kombucha, Wonder Drink, 8.5 fl.oz	60	0	16
La Brada:			
Powders: Lean Body, 2.8 oz	330	8	24
Lean Body, Mass 60, 6 oz	615	7	76
Carb Watchers, 2.3 oz	250	4.5	12
RTD, Lean Body, 17 fl.oz	260	9	9
Lipovitan, B3, 8.6 fl.oz	130	0	30
Liquid Ice: Regular, 8.3 fl.oz	130	0	32
Sugar Free, 8.3 fl.oz	15	0	0
Liquid Lightning, Reg., 8.4 fl.oz	90	0	22
Max Velocity: Reg., 8.45 fl.oz can	130	0	33
16 fl.oz can	240	0	62
Sugar Free, 16 fl.oz can	15	0	1

	C	F	Cb
Met-Rx:			
Colossal RTD 15Z, 15 fl.oz can	380	14	28
Meal Replacement, av. all, 1 pkt	250	2	21
Protein Plus, Choc., 2 scoops	220	1.5	7
Metabol: Endurance, 2 sc., 1.83 oz	200	5	24
GlyProXTS, 1 scoop, 0.2 oz	20	0	4
Met, 2 scoops, 2 oz	260	3	40
Met Max, mix, 2 scoops, 2.2 oz	230	2.5	11
MiO Energy, 1 serving	0	0	0
MLO, Mus-L Blast, Choc., 4 scoops	570	3.5	112
Monster, Energy: 16 fl.oz can	180	0	44
18.6 fl.oz (550ml) can	205	0	50
Lo-Carb, 16 fl.oz	20	0	5
M-80, 16 fl.oz	180	0	46
Mixxd (with Juice), 16 fl.oz	220	0	54
MRM: Low Carb Protein, 1 scoop	120	2.5	2
Iso-bolic, 1 scoop, 1 oz	115	1.5	2
Metabolic Whey, 1 scoop, 1 oz	115	2	2
Muscle Milk (Cytosport):			
Powders: Regular, 2 scoops, 2.5 oz	300	12	16
Light, 2 scoops, 1.75 oz	195	6	11
Naturals, 2 scoops, 2.65 oz	350	18	12
Ready To Drink ~ See Page 48			
Muscle Tech: Meso-Tech Comp. 1 pkt	275	3	31
Mass Tech Weight Gain, 5 scoops	870	4	168
Nitro Tech Hard Core, RTD, 15 fl.oz	195	1	6
Myoplex (EAS):			
Original Shakes, av., 17 fl.oz	300	7	19
Carb Control, 11 fl.oz	150	3.5	5
Lite, 11 fl.oz	170	2	20
Powder: Original Choc. 1 pkt	300	6	22
Deluxe Powder, 1 pkt, 3.4 oz	330	3	29
Lite, 1 packet, 1.9 oz	180	2	24
Naturade:			
Powders: 100% Whey, Choc., 1 oz	110	1	11
100% Soy Natural, ⅓ cup	110	1	0
Nature's Best:			
Isopure: Original, 20 fl.oz	260	0	25
Endurance, 20 fl.oz	320	0	60
Zero Carb, 20 fl.oz	160	0	0
Carbo Power, 16 fl.oz	400	0	100
No-Fear: 16 fl.oz	200	0	72
Sugar Free, 16 fl.oz	20	0	2
Noni: Tahitian/Pacific, 2 Tbsp	10	0	3
Liquid Hawaiian/Tahiti, 1 Tbsp	30	0	8
NOS: 16 fl.oz can, all varieties	210	0	54
Sugar Free, 16 fl.oz can	10	0	0
Nutrament (Nestle) 12 fl.oz	360	10	52
Nutrilite (Amway):			
Protein Shakes, 11.5 fl.oz	170	6	6
Sports Drinks, Regular, 16 fl.oz	120	0	28
Whey Protein Powder, Chocolate, 1.27 oz sachet	130	2	5

Energy/Protein Drinks (Cont)

	C	F	Cb
Optifast 800:			
High Protein Powder, 1 pkg	200	6	10
Powder 800 Formula, 1 pkg	160	3	20
Ready To Drink Shakes, 8 fl.oz	160	3	20
Optimum Nutr.: 100% Whey, 1 oz	120	1	3
100% Oats & Whey, 1 sc., 1.85 oz	200	1.5	22
100% Soy Protein, 1.1 oz Scoop	120	1.5	1
Piranha (EAS), Energy, 8.4 oz	140	0	35
Powerade:			
ION4: 12 fl.oz, all flav., av.	75	0	23
20 fl.oz bottle, all flav., av.	125	0	35
Zero,	0	0	0
PowerBar:			
Endurance, 1 scoop, 0.7 oz	70	0	17
Power Gel, av. all, 1.5 oz package	110	0	27
Pro-Cal 100 (R-Kane), 1 packet	100	1.5	7
Propel, Enhanced Water,			
all flavors, 20 fl.oz	25	0	5
Radioactive: Regular, 10.5 oz	150	0	37
16 oz	220	0	56
Sugar Free, all sizes	0	0	0
Red Bull:			
Energy Drink: 8.4 fl.oz	110	0	28
12 fl.oz can	160	0	40
Sugar-Free, 8.4 fl.oz	10	0	3
Shots: 2 fl.oz	25	0	6
Sugar Free, 2 fl.oz	2	0	0
Resource (Nestle):			
Breeze, 8 fl.oz	250	0	54
Diabetishield, 8 fl.oz	150	0	30
Health Shake: 4 fl.oz	200	4	35
No Added Sugar, 4 fl.oz	200	9	22
Shake Plus, 8 fl.oz	480	16	69
Revenge (Champion Nutrition):			
Pro-Score 100, Choc., 2 scoops, 1.4 oz	150	2	3
Sport, 1 scoop, 0.9 oz	90	0	23
Revival: Soy Mix, unsweetened:			
Plain, 2 scoops, 0.8 oz	90	1	0.5
Chocolate Day Dream, 1 package	120	2.5	4
Other varieties, average, 1 pkg	115	2	4
Rhino's, Energy Drink, 100ml	50	0	11
Rip It, Energy Fuel, Citrus X, 16 fl.oz	260	0	66
Rockstar: Per 16 fl.oz Can			
Energy Drink: Reg.; Punched, av.	270	0	62
Sugar Free	20	0	0
Rush: Per 8 fl.oz			
Energy Drink: Regular	140	0	31
Lite	0	0	0
SK Energy, all flavors, 2 oz	0	0	0
Slim-Fast: Per 10 fl.oz			
Shake (Ready To Drink):			
Cappuccino; High Protein, av.	190	6	25
Lower Carb Diet, average	180	9	3.5
Powder Shake Mix, av. all, 0.9 oz	110	3	18

	C	F	Cb
Snapple, LYte Water,			
all flavors, average, 8 fl.oz	0	0	0
SoBe: Per 20 fl.oz Can/Bottle			
Energize, Citrus Energy	270	0	67
Lifewater: All flavors	100	0	42
0-Cal, all flavors	0	0	6
Vita Boom: Per 20 fl.oz			
Cranberry Grapefruit	260	0	66
Orange-Carrot	220	0	57
Solixir, Energy Drink, av. all, 12 fl.oz	55	0	13
Spiru-Tein, Powder: Per 1.2 oz			
Banana; Cappuccino	100	0	10
Black Cherry Chocolate	110	1	13
Starbucks,			
Refreshers, all flavors, 12 fl.oz	60	0	20
Steaz: Energy, 12 fl.oz	135	0	35
Zero Calorie, Berry, 12 fl.oz	0	0	0
The Sports Club/LA:			
Beachbody Whey Protein Pdr,			
Chocolate; Vanilla, 2 scoops, 1.4 oz	130	4	7
Trader Joe's,			
Enhanced Water, 33.8 fl.oz	0	0	0
Twin Lab:			
Endurance Fuel, 1 sc., 1.1 oz	110	0	20
Energy Fuel, 250ml can	0	0	0
Ukon, Power, 3.4 fl.oz can	5	0	5
Venom: Energy, av., 16.9 fl.oz	250	0	60
Low Carb, 16.9 fl.oz	60	0	8
Verve, Energy, 8.3 fl.oz can	70	0	18
Sugar Free	5	0	1
Vitamin Water ~ See Glaceau			
Weider:			
Creatine ATP, powder, ½ cup, 1.7 oz	210	0	37
Mega Mass 4000, powder, av., 1½ c.	570	3.5	105
Muscle Builder, powder, 1½ oz	170	1	22
Pure Pro Shake: Chocolate, 11.5 fl.oz	170	0.5	7
Vanilla, 11.5 fl.oz	160	0	6
Ultra Whey Pro, ⅓ cup, 1 oz	110	1.5	6
Weight Gainer, 4 scoops, 3.4 oz	380	2	71
Worldwide:			
Carbo Rush, 20 fl.oz	270	0	68
Pure Protein Shakes,			
35g Protein, 11 fl.oz	165	1	3
Worx, Energy,			
Original; Extra Strength, 2 fl.oz	0	0	0
XS (Quixtar), Energy Drink, 8.4 oz	10	0	1
Zico, Coconut Water, all flav., 11 fl.oz	60	0	13
Zola, Acai, Original Juice, 12 fl.oz	185	3	39

Quick Guide   C F Cb

Orange Juice
Average ~ Fresh

	C	F	Cb
½ Cup, 4 fl.oz	55	0	13
Small Glass, 6 fl.oz	85	0	19
Regular Glass, 8 fl.oz	110	0.5	26
8¾ fl.oz Box	120	0.5	28
10 fl.oz Bottle	140	0.5	32
11½ fl.oz Can	160	0.5	37
16 fl.oz Bottle	225	1	52
20 fl.oz Bottle	280	1	64
64 fl.oz, ½ Gallon	895	4	206

Juices ~ Generic

Average All Brands

	C	F	Cb
Aloe Vera Juice, unsweetened, 2 oz	10	0	0
Apple Juice: 8 fl.oz	120	0	29
10 fl.oz Bottle	145	0.5	36
16 fl.oz	235	0.5	58
Carrot Juice: Fresh, 6 fl.oz	35	0	8
Sweetened, 6 fl.oz	75	0	17
Coconut Water, 8 fl.oz	50	0.5	9
Cranberry Juice, Cocktail/Blend	140	0	34
Fruit Blends, av. all, 8 fl.oz	110	0	29
Fruit Nectars, av. all, 8 fl.oz	140	0	36
Grape Juice, 8 fl.oz	155	0	38
Grapefruit Juice, 8 fl.oz	95	0	22
Lemon/Lime Juice: 1 Tbsp	3	0	1
1 cup, 8 fl.oz	50	0.5	16
Concentrate, 1 tsp	0	0	0
Noni Juice:			
Tahitian, 2 Tbsp, 1 fl.oz	5	0	1
Tahiti Traders, 1 fl.oz	20	0	5
Passion Fruit Juice (Fresh):			
Purple, 1 cup, 8 fl.oz	125	0	34
Yellow, 1 cup, 8 fl.oz	80	1.5	14
Papaya/Peach Nectar, av., 8 fl.oz	140	0	36
Pear Nectar, 8 fl.oz	150	0	40
Pineapple Juice, 8 fl.oz	130	0	32
Pomegranate Juice, 8 fl.oz	160	0	40
Prune Juice, 8 fl.oz	180	0	45
Strawb./Raspberry Juice, 8 fl.oz	100	0	24
Tangerine Juice, 8 fl.oz	105	0.5	25
Tomato Juice, 8 fl.oz	40	0	10
Vegetable Juice, 8 fl.oz	45	0	11
Wheat Grass Juice: 1 fl.oz 'Shot'	10	0	1.5
2 fl.oz 'Shot'	20	0	3

Quick Guide   C F Cb

Fruit Smoothies (Jamba Juice; Smoothie King)
Average All Brands

Fruit Only: 8 fl.oz	C	F	Cb
	115	0.5	29
12 fl.oz	175	1	43
16 fl.oz	230	1	58
24 fl.oz	350	1	78
Fruit + Non-Fat Milk/Soy:			
12 fl.oz	135	0	29
16 fl.oz	155	0	37
24 fl.oz	265	1	59
Fruit + Non-Fat Frozen Yogurt/Sherbet:			
12 fl.oz	200	0.5	47
16 fl.oz	265	1	63
24 fl.oz	395	1.5	95

Juice Brands   C F Cb

Per 8 fl.oz Unless Indicated

	C	F	Cb
Apple & Eve:			
Naturally Cranberry	130	0	32
Cranberry Grape	140	0	34
Fruitables, all varieties, av., 6.75 fl.oz	70	0	16
Bolthouse: *Per 8 fl.oz*			
100% Juices: Carrot	70	0	14
Orange & Carrot	120	0	27
Fruit Smoothies:			
Berry Boost	130	0	31
Blue Goodness	160	0	34
C-Boost	160	0.5	40
Green Goodness	140	0	33
Strawberry Banana	130	0	32
Bom Dia: *Per 8 fl.oz*			
Acai: Original	110	0	27
+ 10 Superblend	120	0	31
Mango Coconut Splash	60	0	15
Pomegranate	170	0	42
Bossa Nova: *Per 10 fl.oz Bottle*			
Acai Juice: Original	90	0	24
Other varieties, average	90	0	23
Acerola Red Peach	90	0	24
Bright & Early *(Minute Maid),*			
Orange Juice (Chilled/Frozen)	110	0	29
Campbell's:			
Tomato Juice: 5.5 fl.oz can	30	0	7
8 fl.oz	50	0	10
Capri Sun: *Per 6.75 fl.oz*			
Juice Drinks (25% Less Sugar),			
all varieties, average	70	0	19
100% Juice, all varieties, av.	100	0	24

Juice Brands (Cont) C F Cb

Per 8 fl.oz Unless Indicated

	C	F	Cb
Clamato,			
Tomato Cocktail, average	50	0	11
Crystal Geyser:			
Juice Squeeze: *Per Bottle (12 fl.oz)*			
Blackberry Pomegranate	170	0	43
Ruby Grapefruit	150	0	36
Other flavors, average	140	0	32
Dannon:			
Frusion Smoothie, av., 7 fl.oz	180	2.5	35
Light & Fit, 7 fl.oz bottle	70	0	14
Dole:			
Aguas Frescas, all varieties, average	110	0	26
Blended Juices:			
Orange Peach Mango	120	0	29
Pina Colada	120	0	29
Pineapple Juice	130	0	30
Pineapple-Orange Banana	120	0	30
Strawberry Kiwi	120	0	31
Other flavors, average	120	0	29
Frozen Concentrates 100%,			
average all flavors, ¼ cup	125	0	31
Five Alive (Minute Maid),			
Frozen Concentrate,			
prepared, 8 fl.oz	110	0	29
Florida's Natural:			
Apple Juice	120	0	29
Cranberry Ruby Red	130	0	32
Orange: Original	110	0	26
Mango	110	0	27
Pineapple	130	0	31
Strawberry	110	0	26
Raspberry Lemonade	110	0	28
Ruby Red Grapefruit, Orig.,	90	0	22
Fuze: *Per 16.9 fl.oz*			
Original, all flavors	160	0	38
Slenderize, all flavors, av.	15	0	3
Goya:			
5% Juice:			
Guanabana, 12 fl.oz	230	0	57
Passion & Pineapple, 12 fl.oz	220	0	55
Nectar, Mango, 12 fl.oz	230	0	56

Per 8 fl.oz Unless Indicated

	C	F	Cb
Hansen's:			
Juice Slam: *Per 6.75 fl.oz Box*			
Awesome Apple	90	0	23
Strawberry Banana	110	0	27
Other flavors	100	0	24
Junior Juice,			
100% Juice, all flav., 4.23 oz box	60	0	15
Natural, (64 fl.oz Bottles): *Per 8 fl.oz*			
Apple	120	0	28
Apple Strawberry	110	0	27
Grape	120	0	33
Ruby Red Grapefruit Cocktail	100	0	25
White Grape	140	0	36
Smoothie Nectar, av., 12 fl.oz	180	0	44
Hawaii's Own: *Per 8 fl.oz Prepared*			
Frozen Concentrate,			
10% Juice, all varieties, average	110	0	28
Hi-C Juice Drinks: *Per 6.75 fl.oz Box*			
Flashin' Fruit Punch	90	0	26
Orange Lavaburst	90	0	26
Poppin' Lemonade	100	0	26
Hood: Apple, 8 fl.oz	120	0	31
Fruit Punch; Orange, 8 fl.oz	120	0	30
Jamba Juice ~ *See Fast-Foods Section*			
Juicy Juice (Nestle):			
All flav., av., 6.75 fl.oz box	100	0	24
4.23 fl.oz box, average	60	0	15
Kerns:			
Nectars: *Per 11.5 fl.oz Can*			
Pear	220	0	54
Pineapple Coconut	280	8	53
Other flavors, average	215	0	52
Kool Aid:			
Jammers: Grape; Cherry	70	0	19
Other varieties	70	0	19
Kroger/Ralph's Smoothies:			
Active Lifestyle, all flavors, average	130	0	25
Regular, all flavors, average	200	2.5	38
L & A: *Per 8 fl.oz*			
All Cherry	180	0	45
All Prune Juice	180	0	41
Mixed Berry	120	0	30

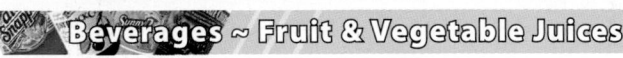
Juice Brands (Cont)   C   F   Cb

Per 8 fl.oz Unless Indicated

Lakewood Organic: *Per 8 fl.oz*

	C	F	Cb
Acai Amazon Berry	125	3.5	28
Banana Strawberry	115	0	30
Blueberry Blend	110	0	27
Cranberry Lemonade	75	0	20
Fruit Garden: Summer Gold, av.	100	0	20
Blue/Purple/Red Pomegr., average	110	0	24
Goji	90	0	20
Lemonade	80	0	20
Pomegranate Blend	125	0	31
Pure: Apple	110	0	27
Blueberry	90	0	22
Carrot	80	0	19
Pink Grapefruit	90	0	22
Prune	170	0	42
Super Veggie	55	0	13
Light: Lemonade	40	0	10
Other flavors, average	60	0	21

(Note: Carbs include Erythritol natural sweetener)

Langers: *Per 8 fl.oz*

100% Juice (No Sugar Added):

	C	F	Cb
All Pomegranate	140	0	34
Apple Cider	120	0	28
Apple Juice	120	0	28
Mixed Berry	120	0	30
Pineapple Coconut	140	3	28
Red/White Grape Juice	160	0	40

Diet Low-Carb (25-50% Juice):

	C	F	Cb
Apple Juice Cocktail	60	0	14
Cranberry	30	0	8
Pomegranate	40	0	9

Juice Cocktails (27% Juice):

	C	F	Cb
Blueberry Cranberry	135	0	34
Cranberry	140	0	35
Cranberry Grape	165	0	41
Cranberry Raspberry	150	0	36
Pomegranate	140	0	34
Pomegranate Blueb./Cranberry	140	0	34
Strawberry Peach (20% Juice)	120	0	30
White Cranberry	120	0	28
White Cran-Raspberry	120	0	28

Martinelli's, Sparkling Apple Juice,

	C	F	Cb
Single Serve Size, 10 fl.oz bottle	180	0	43

Per 8 fl.oz Unless Indicated

Minute Maid: C   F   Cb

	C	F	Cb
Apple Juice, 15.2 fl.oz bottle	210	0	52
Cranb. Apple, Rasp.,15.2 fl oz bottle	230	0	63
Orange Juice:			
100% Original: 8 fl.oz	110	0	27
15.2 fl.oz bottle	210	0	51
Light, 42%, 8 fl.oz	50	0	12
Fruit Punch, 6.75 fl.oz	100	0	24
Pineapple Orange, Apple	120	0	29
Kids+Orange Juice, 6.75 fl.oz	100	0	23
Enhanced: *Per 8 fl.oz*			
Pomegranate Blueberry	120	0.5	31
Pomegranate Lemonade	110	0	31
Boxed Juices, av., 6.75 fl.oz	100	0	22
Soft Frozen, Limeade, 3 fl.oz	70	0	19

MonaVie:

Acai Blends,

	C	F	Cb
Original; Active, 4 fl.oz	120	2	20

Mott's:

	C	F	Cb
100% Original Juice: Apple	120	0	29
All other varieties, 6.75 fl.oz	100	0	25
Garden Blend	45	0	9
Natural Juice, Apple	110	0	27
Medley Juice: Apple & Carrot	110	0	25
Other varieties, average	140	0	33

Mott's For Tots (47-54% Juice):

	C	F	Cb
All varieties, 6.75 fl.oz	50	0	13
8 fl.oz	60	0	15

Mott's Plus For Kids:

	C	F	Cb
100%: Apple	130	0	32
Apple Punch	120	0	30
Plus Light, Apple	60	0	15

Naked Juice:

Antioxidants:

	C	F	Cb
Pomegranate Acai	160	1	36
Pomegranate Blueberry	150	0	36
Protein Zone: Mango	220	1	35
Pineapple, Coconut & Banana	220	2	34
Pure Juice (100%): O-J	110	0	27
Coconut Water, 11 fl.oz	60	0	14
Well Being: Berry Blast	130	0	29
Mighty Mango	150	0	36
Orange Carrot	120	0	29
Orange Mango	130	0	31
Strawberry Banana	130	0	31

Juice Brands (Cont)

C **F** **Cb**

Per 8 fl.oz Unless Indicated

Naked Juice (Cont):

Superfood Smoothies: *Per 15.2 fl.oz*

	C	F	Cb
Acai Machine	305	5	58
Berry Veggie	245	1	70
Blue Machine	320	0	76
Gold/Green Machine, av.	265	0	63
Power C Machine	230	0	55
Red Machine	320	8	58

Nantucket Nectars:

100% Juice: *Per 17.5 fl.oz Bottle*

Peach Orange	285	0	70
Pineapple Orange Banana	305	0	74
Pomegranate Cherry	265	0	63
Premium Orange Juice	240	0	57
Pressed Apple	260	0	65

Juice Cocktails: *Per 17.5 fl.oz Bottle*

Big Cranberry	285	0	70
Grapeade	305	0	72
Other varieties, average	260	0	65
Nectar, Squeezed Lemonade	240	0	61

Newman's Own: *Per 8 fl.oz*

Lemonade: Regular; Pink	110	0	27
Limeade	140	0	34

Fruit Juice Cocktail:

Gorilla Grape	140	0	34
Orange Mango Tango	130	0	33

Northland:

100% Juice:

Cranberry Blackberry/Raspberry	140	0	34
Cranberry Grape	140	0	36

Ocean Spray: *Per 8 fl.oz*

Juice Cocktails:

Cranberry Juice Cocktail	120	0	30
With Calcium	130	0	31
Ruby Tangerine	120	0	31
Ruby Red Grapefruit	110	0	28

100% Juice Blends:

Cranberry & Concord Grape	150	0	37
Cranberry Blueberry	140	0	36
Cranberry Blends	140	0	35

Juice Drinks:

CranApple	130	0	32
CranGrape	120	0	31
CranRaspberry/Strawberry	110	0	27

Per 8 fl.oz Unless Indicated

Ocean Spray (Cont): *Per 8 fl.oz*

	C	F	Cb
Light Juice Drinkjs, all flavors	40	0	10
Diet Juice Drinks, Sprays, all varieties	5	0	2

Odwalla: *Per 12 fl.oz Bottle*

Blueberry B	210	0.5	50
Carrot Juice	100	0.5	20
Mo'Beta	170	0	40
Pink Poetry	210	0	48
PomaGrand, Pomeg. Limeade	180	0	44
Protein Monster, Chocolate	320	6	40
Strawberry C Monster	240	0	56
Super Food, Original	190	0.5	40
Super Protein, Original	290	1	52
Tropical Energy	240	0	59

Orange Julius:

Originals, Orange:

Small, 16 fl.oz	230	0	62
Medium, 20 fl.oz	290	0	77
Large, 32 fl.oz	470	0	123

Smoothies ~ *See Fast-Foods Section*

Pom Wonderful: *Per 8 fl.oz*

100% Pomegranate Blend:

Blueberry; Cherry, average	155	0	39
Kiwi	150	0	36
Mango	140	0	36
Nectarine	130	0	31
Light, all varieties, average	80	0	20

R.W. Knudsen:

Natural Juices: 100% Apple

	120	0	30
Cranberry Raspberry	130	0	32
Grape	150	0	37
Hibiscus Cooler	100	0	25
Kiwi Strawberry	120	0	29
Mango Peach	120	0	31
Razzleberry	120	0	30
Rio Red Grapefruit	140	0	35
Other varieties, average	120	0	30

Just Juice:

Just Black Currant	100	0	15
Just Black Cherry	160	0	37
Just Blueberry	100	0	24
Simply Nutritious: Mega C	140	0	34
Other varieties, average	125	0	30

Juice Brands (Cont) C F Cb

Per 8 fl.oz Unless Indicated

R.W. Knudsen (Cont):

	C	F	Cb
Sparkling Essence:			
all varieties, average, 10.5 fl.oz	0	0	0
Spritzers: *Per 12 fl.oz Bottles*			
100% Juice: Black Cherry	180	0	46
Mango	170	0	42
Red Raspberry; Tangerine	200	0	47
Very Veggie, Orig, 8 fl.oz	50	0	11
RealLemon – RealLime:			
Lemon/Lime Juice (from concentrate)			
1 teaspoon	0	0	0
2 Tbsp, 1 fl.oz	8	0	2.5
Santa Cruz: *Per 8 fl.oz*			
100% Juice:			
Apple Juice	120	0	30
Concord Grape; White Grape	160	0	40
Orange Mango	130	0	32
Strawberry Kiwi	120	0	30
25% Juice Drink Boxes:			
Lemon	120	0	29
Orange; Grape, average	100	0	24
Tropical	110	0	27
Champagne Style:			
Sparkling Lemonade	110	0	27
Sparkling Limeade	100	0	26
Nectars: Cranberry	110	0	27
Passionfruit	150	0	40
Other varieties, average	120	0	30
Sparkling Beverages: *Per 10.5 fl.oz Can*			
Lemon Lime	130	0	32
Root Beer	130	0	32
Seismic:			
Super Juices: *Per 10 fl.oz Bottle*			
Citrus; Berry	180	0	44
Low Sugar Cherry	100	0	26
Simply Orange:			
Lemonade; Limeade	120	0	30
Orange Juice, all varieties, average	110	0	26
Snap•E• Tom,			
Tomato & Chili Cocktail, 8 fl.oz	50	0	11
Snapple:			
Juice Drink Blends:			
Grapeade; Orangeade	100	0	26
Other flavors, average	110	0	27
Diet: Cranberry Raspberry	10	0	2
100% Juiced,			
(added vitamins), 11.5 fl.oz	170	0	40

Per 8 fl.oz Unless Indicated

	C	F	Cb
Sips, Juice Drinks,			
all varieties, average, 6 fl.oz box	70	0	18
Stonyfield Farm: *Per 10 fl.oz Bottle*			
Smoothies: Berry; Strawberry	230	3	39
Peach	230	3	41
Sunsweet:			
Plum Smart: Orig., 8 fl.oz	160	0	36
Light, 8 fl.oz	60	0	15
Prune Juice: Original, 8 fl.	180	0	43
Light, 8 fl.oz	100	0	26
With Pulp, 8 fl.oz	150	0	44
Trader Joe's:			
Refrigerated, 64 fl.oz bottle: *Per 8 fl.oz:*			
Grapefruit	100	0	23
Lemonade, with Pulp	110	0	27
Orange	110	0	26
Orange Peach Mango	120	0	29
Pineapple	130	0	30
Tangerine	110	0	25
Organic, 32/64 fl.oz Bottle: *Per 8 fl.oz*			
100% Pomegranate	140	0	35
Apple Juice	120	0	30
Concord Grape Juice	160	0	39
Cranberry	70	0	18
Grapefruit Sunset; Lemonade	120	0	30
Mango Nectar	130	0	32
Pink Lemonade	130	0	32
Strawberry Lemonade	120	0	29
White Grape Juice	160	0	40
All Natural Pasteurized, 32/64 fl.oz Bottle: *Per 8 fl.oz*			
100% Cranberry	70	0	18
Blueberry Pomegranate	140	0	34
Just Blueberry	100	0	24
Just Pomegranate	150	0	37
Mango PassionFruit	130	0	32
Omega Orange Carrot	110	0	26
Joe's Kids: *Per 6.75 oz Box*			
100% Juice: Apple	90	0	23
Apple Grape	100	0	24
White Grape	120	0	30
10% Juice, Lemonade	90	0	22
Sparkling Juices, 25.4 fl.oz Bottle: *Per 8 fl.oz*			
Blueberry	120	0	30
Cranberry	140	0	35
Pomegranate	130	0	31

Juice Brands (Cont) **C** **F** **Cb**

Per 8 fl.oz Unless Indicated

Tree Top:

	C	F	Cb
100% Juice From Concentrates:			
Apple Berry/Grape., av	125	0	32
Apple Pear, 6.75 fl.oz box	100	0	25
Apple Cider	120	0	29
Kiwi Strawberry, 10 fl.oz	130	0	32
Mango Peach, 10 fl.oz	160	0	39
Ochango, 10 fl.oz	170	0	42
Orange, 6.75 fl.oz	110	0	27
Orange Passionfruit	110	0	26
Pineapple Orange	120	0	29
100% Juice Fresh Pressed,			
3 Apple Blend	120	0	30
Fiber Rich: Apple	140	0	35
Apple Apricot	160	0	37
Trim, all varieties, average	60	0	16

Tropicana:

	C	F	Cb
Chilled: Pure Prem. Orange Juice	110	0	26
Light Drinks, all varieties	10	0	2
Punches, all flavors, average	125	0	31
Non-Refrigerated: 100% Juice,			
all varieties, average	115	0	22
Trop50 (50% less sugar,) all flav., av.	50	0	12
Tropics, all varieties, average	120	0	30
Twisters, all varieties, average, 8 fl.oz	120	0	29

V8 Juices & Drinks:

	C	F	Cb
100% Vegetable Juice:			
5.5 fl.oz can	35	0	7
8 fl.oz cup	50	0	10
11.5 fl.oz can	70	0	14
12 fl.oz bottle	75	0	15
V8 Spicy Hot, 12 fl.oz	70	0	14
V8 Splash, av. all, 8 fl.oz	70	0	19
V8 Splash Smoothies: Strawberry	90	0	20
Tropical Colada, 8 fl.oz	100	0	21
Diet V8 Splash, all varieties, 8 fl.oz	10	0	3
V-Fusion: Grape Raspberry	140	0	35
Other flavors, av.	110	0	27
12 fl.oz bottle	165	0	40
Light varieties; Green Tea	50	0	13
Smoothies, all flavors, av.	125	0	31
Sparkling, all flav., av., 8.4 fl.oz	55	0	13

Per 8 fl.oz Unless Indicated **C** **F** **Cb**

Veryfine:

	C	F	Cb
Apple Juice (100%)	120	0	29
Orange Juice (100%)	120	0	30

Walnut Acres:

	C	F	Cb
Organic: Apple	110	0	29
Apricot; Raspberry	130	0	32
Cherry	140	0	34
Cranberry	110	0	26
Incredible Vegetable	50	0	12
Mango Nectar	120	0	29

Welch's:

	C	F	Cb
100% Juice: Red Grape	170	0	43
White Grape Cherry	140	0	35
White Grape Peach	160	0	39
Cocktails, (Refrigerated, 64 fl.oz Ctn):			
Guava Pineapple	140	0	35
Mango Twist	150	0	38
Strawberry Breeze	130	0	33
Light Juice, (52 fl.oz Bottle),			
Concord/WhiteGrape	45	0	12
Sparkling Juice Cocktail,	160	0	40
Concentrates, (100% Juice),			
all flavors, ¼ cup, 2 fl.oz	160	0	41

Zola: *Per 12 fl.oz Bottle*

	C	F	Cb
Acai: Original	185	2	44
With Blueberry Juice	180	3	38

CALORIEKING PORTION WATCH

ORANGE JUICE	C	Cb
8 fl.oz	110	26
16 fl.oz	220	52
24 fl.oz	330	78
32 fl.oz	440	104

Quick Guide **C** **F** **Cb**

Cow's Milk ~ *Average All Brands*

Whole (3.25% fat):

	C	F	Cb
2 Tbsp, 1 fl.oz	20	1	1.5
1 Cup, 8 fl.oz	150	8	12
1 Large Glass, 12 fl.oz	220	12	17
1 Pint, 16 fl.oz	295	16	22
1 Quart, 946 ml	590	32	44

Reduced-Fat (2% fat):

2 Tbsp, 1 fl.oz	15	0.5	1.5
1 Cup, 8 fl.oz	120	5	12
1 Large Glass, 12 fl.oz	180	7.5	18
1 Pint, 16 fl.oz	245	10	23
1 Quart, 946 ml	490	20	46

Light/Low-Fat (1% fat):

2 Tbsp, 1 fl.oz	13	0.3	1.5
1 Cup, 8 fl.oz	100	2.5	12
1 Large Glass, 12 fl.oz	150	4	18
1 Pint, 16 fl.oz	205	5	25
1 Quart, 946 ml	410	10	49

Fat Free/Skim:

2 Tbsp, 1 fl.oz	10	0	1.5
1 Cup, 8 fl.oz	90	0.5	13
1 Pint, 16 fl.oz	180	1	26
Protein Fortified			
1 cup	100	0.5	14

Buttermilk: *Average All Brands*

Reduced-Fat (2%), 1 cup, 8 fl.oz	120	5	10
Low-Fat (1%), 1 cup, 8 fl.oz	100	2.5	12

Lactose-Free: *Per 8 fl.oz*

Dairy Ease: Whole	160	9	11
2% Reduced-Fat	130	5	12
Fat-Free	90	0	12
Lactaid 100: Whole	150	8	12
2% Reduced-Fat	130	5	12
1% Low-Fat	110	2.5	13
Fat-Free; Calcium Fort.	80	0	13
Real Goodness, 2% Fat	120	5	7
Smart Balance,			
FF + Omega-3s & Vit. E	110	1	14

Lower Calorie Dairy Drinks: *Per 8 fl.oz Cup*

Calorie Countdown *(Hood):*			
2% Reduced-Fat	90	5	3
2% Reduced-Fat, Chocolate	90	5	5
Fat-Free	45	0	3

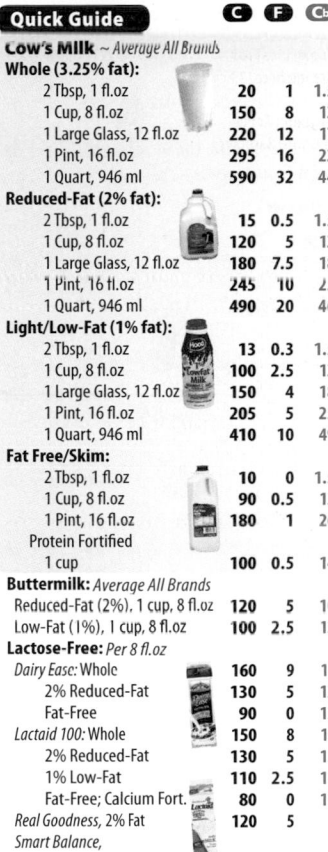

Goat/Sheep Milk, Kefir

Goat's Milk (Meyenberg):	C	F	Cb
Whole, 1 cup, 8 fl.oz	140	7	11
Light/Low-Fat (1%), 8 fl.oz	100	2.5	11
Evaporated, reconst., 8 fl.oz	150	8	11

Kefir (Cultured Milk): Per 8 fl.oz

Lifeway: Original	150	8	12
Greek Style	210	14	12
Green	170	2	25
Lowfat, all flavors, average	140	1.5	20
Nancy's: Plain	110	3	14
Fruit flavors, average	180	2.5	34
Trader Joe's: Plain	110	2.5	8
Strawberry	160	2	21
Sheep's Milk, Whole, 1 cup	265	17	13

Canned & Dried Milk

Condensed: Reg. 2 Tbsp, 1 fl.oz	130	3	23
Low Fat, 2 Tbsp	120	1.5	23
Fat-Free, 2 Tbsp	110	0	24
Evaporated: Whole, 2 Tbsp	40	3	3
Whole, ½ cup, 4 fl.oz	170	10	13
Low-Fat *(Carnation):* 2 Tbsp, 1 oz	25	0.5	3
½ cup, 4 fl.oz	115	2.5	14
Fat-Free, 2 Tbsp, 1 oz	25	0	4
Dried: Whole, ¼ cup, 1 oz	160	9	12
Skim/Non-Fat, ⅓ cup	80	0	12
Made-up, 1 cup, 8 fl.oz	80	0	12
Buttermilk (sweet cream): 1 oz	110	2	14
Non-Fat, 1 Tbsp	25	0	3
Carnation, Malted, dry, 1 tbsp	30	0.5	6
Horlick's, Malt Powder, dry, 1 oz	180	4	27

Soy/Non-Dairy Drinks ~ *See Page 49*

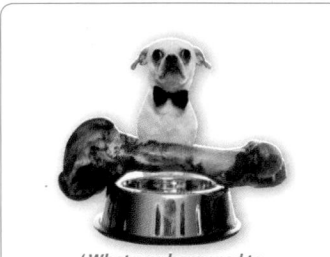

'Whatever happened to sensible portion size?!'

Quick Guide	**C**	**F**	**Cb**

Chocolate Milk:

Average All Brands: Per 8 fl.oz Cup

	C	**F**	**Cb**
Whole Milk, (3.3%): 1 cup	210	8	26
1 Pint, 16 fl.oz	415	17	52
Reduced-Fat, (2%): 1 cup	190	5	30
1 Pint, 16 fl.oz	380	10	60
Low-Fat, (1%): 1 cup	160	2.5	26
1 Pint, 16 fl.oz	315	5	52

Brands ~ Flavored Milk

Ready-To-Drink: Per 8 fl.oz Cup Unless Indicated

	C	**F**	**Cb**
Albertson's, Choc Milk	200	2.5	34
Alta Dena: Chocolate: 8 fl.oz	260	9	37
16 fl.oz	520	18	74
Low-Fat Chocolate: 8 fl.oz	200	3	32
16 fl.oz	400	6	64
Hood: Chocolate	230	9	31
Low-Fat (1%), Chocolate	170	3	28
Horizon Organic,			
Low-Fat, all flavors, average	150	2.5	22
Kroger, Choc Milk, Low-Fat, 1%	180	2.5	33
Land O Lakes:			
Grip 'n Go: Choc. (2% red-fat), 12 fl.oz	285	8	39
Strawberry (whole milk),12 fl.oz	285	12	33
Magic Straws, av. all flavors (1)	15	0	4
Muscle Milk (Cytosport), Hi Protein:			
17 fl.oz Box: Chocolate	340	16	17
Other flavors, average	310	12	16
11 fl.oz Box: Choc./Choc Malt, av.	230	11	11
Other flavors, average	210	10	9
14 fl.oz Bottle: Chocolate	240	9	14
Other flavors, average	220	9	11
Lite: Chocolate	170	4.5	12
Cafe Late; Vanilla, average	160	4.5	11
Nesquik:			
Chocolate: Low Fat, 16 fl.oz	340	5	58
No Sugar Added, 8 oz	100	2	13
Fat-Free, 16 fl.oz	300	0	58
Strawberry, Low Fat, 16 fl.oz	360	5	62
Prairie Farms, Choc., 16 fl.oz	440	16	58
Quaker, Milk Chillers, 14 fl.oz	245	9	32
Ralphs, Chocolate, Low-Fat, 8 fl.oz	210	2.5	36
Skinny Cow, Chocolate, Fat-Free	150	0	26
TruMoo, Choc.; Strawb., av, 8 fl.oz	150	2.5	24

Flavored Milk (Cont)	**C**	**F**	**Cb**

Ready-To-Drink: Per 8 fl.oz Cup Unless Indicated

Starbucks,

	C	**F**	**Cb**
Vanilla Frappuccino, 9.5 fl.oz	200	3	37

Yoo-Hoo,

	C	**F**	**Cb**
Chocolate,15.5 fl.oz bottle	260	2	57

Bottle Coffee Drinks ~ See Page 37

Shakes

Arby's:

	C	**F**	**Cb**
Chocolate; Jamocha, 16.5 oz	565	15	99
Vanilla, 15 oz	470	15	75
Burger King:			
Chocolate:			
Small, 12 fl.oz	580	17	97
Medium, 16 fl.oz	760	21	131
Large, 20 fl.oz	980	24	174
Other flavors ~ See Page 186			
Denny's: Per 14 oz			
Chocolate; Strawberry	580	25	68
Vanilla	580	25	68
Dreyers:			
Slow Churned: Prep'd with ⅓ cup FF Milk			
Choc./Strawb./Vanilla, av, 8.1 oz	220	5	38
Cookies n' Cream	270	6	45
Hardees, all flavors, av., 16 fl.oz	700	33	86
McDonalds, McCafe Shakes:			
Average all flavors:			
12 fl.oz cup	555	17	88
16 fl.oz cup	695	21	113
22 fl.oz cup	845	25	137

Other Restaurants ~ See Fast-Foods Section

Smoothies

Made Up Ready-To-Drink:
8 fl. oz Milk/Soy + Fruit: Per 12 fl.oz

Average all types:

	C	**F**	**Cb**
With Whole Milk	300	8	50
+ Ice Cream, 1 scoop	400	13	62
With Non-Fat Milk	240	0	50

Fruit Smoothies ~ See Page 41

Freshens; Jamba Juice; TCBY ~ See Fast-Foods

Rice & Cereal Drinks

Per 8 fl.oz Cup **C** **P** **Ca**

	C	P	Ca
Almond Breeze (Blue Diamond):			
Refrigerated/Shelf Stable:			
Original	60	2.5	8
Chocolate	120	3	22
Vanilla	90	2.5	16
Unsweetened: Orig.; Vanilla, av.	40	3.5	3
Chocolate	45	3.5	3
Almond Dream:			
Shelf Stable			
Enriched: Original	50	2.5	6
Unsweetened	50	3.5	3
Amazake, Oh So Original	150	0	34
Better Than Milk:			
Rice Vegan Powder Mix:			
Original; Vanilla, 2 Tbsp, 0.67 oz	70	0	17
Cacique,			
Horchata Rice Drink	160	3.5	31
Don Jose:			
Cereal Match	100	3	17
Horchata Rice Drink	140	4	25
EdenBlend, Rice & Soy	120	3	18
Pacific:			
Rice Drinks,			
Low-Fat Plain/Vanilla	130	2	27
Organic Oat, Original/Vanilla, av.	130	2.5	25
Nut Drinks: Hazelnut, Original	110	3.5	19
Chocolate	120	5	19
Organic Almond:			
Original, Low-Fat	60	2.5	8
Vanilla, Low-Fat	70	2.5	11
Chocolate, single serve container	100	3	19
Rice Dream:			
Refrigerated, Enriched, Original	120	2.5	23
Shelf Stable: Classic Carob	150	2.5	30
Classic/ Enriched Vanilla, average	130	2.5	27
Heartwise, Original/Vanilla, av.	135	2	29
Supreme: Chocolate Chai	160	3	35
Vanilla Hazelnut	140	2.5	29
Trader Joe's:			
Rice Drinks:			
Original, Organic	120	2.5	23
Vanilla	130	2.5	26
WestSoy, Rice, Plain; Vanilla	110	2.5	20

Note: Rice/Oat/Nut drinks are very low in protein. Unless enriched with protein (and calcium), they are not suitable for infants as a substitute for milk or calcium-enriched soy drinks.

Soy Milk ~ Ready-To-Drink

Per 8 fl.oz Cup **C** **F** **Ca**

	C	F	Ca
365 Organic (Whole Foods):			
Original, unsweetened	70	4	4
Chocolate	140	3.5	22
Vanilla	90	3.5	10
Light: Original	70	1.5	10
Vanilla	70	1.5	10
8th Continent:			
Original	80	2.5	7
Complete Vanilla	80	2.5	8
Vanilla	100	2.5	11
Fat-Free: Original	60	0	8
Vanilla	70	0	11
Light: Original	50	2	2
Chocolate	90	1.5	12
Vanilla	60	2	5
Bolthouse Farms:			
Cafes Perfectly Protein:			
Mocha Cappuccino	160	2.5	29
Vanilla Chai Tea	160	3	27
EdenBlend, Organic	120	3	18
Edensoy: *Per 32 fl.oz Container*			
Organic: Original	140	5	14
Unswseetened	120	6	5
Carob; Chocolate, average	175	4	28
Vanilla	150	3	24
Extra: Original	130	4	13
Vanilla	150	5	23
Kidz Dream:			
Smoothies: Berry Blast	100	2	17
Orange Cream	120	2	21
O Organics (Safeway):			
Plain	90	3.5	8
Chocolate	150	4	23
Vanilla Soy	90	3	9
Odwalla:			
Super Protein: *Per 12 fl.oz Bottle*			
Original	290	1	52
Vanilla Al'Mondo	290	8	37
Protein Monster: *Per 12 fl. oz Bottle*			
Strawberry	240	5	28
Vanilla	290	5	36
Pacific:			
Select Soy: Original	70	2.5	9
Vanilla	80	2.5	11
Organic, Original, Unsweetened	90	4.5	4
Ultra (Extra Protein/Calcium): Plain	140	5	12
Vanilla	140	5	14

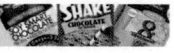

Soy Milk ~ Ready-To-Drink (Cont)

Per 8 fl.oz Unless Indicated

	C	F	Cb
Silk:			
Refrigerated:			
All Natural: Original	90	3.5	8
Chocolate	140	3.5	23
Vanilla	100	3.5	11
Very Vanilla	130	3.5	19
Light: Original	60	1.5	6
Chocolate	90	1.5	15
Vanilla	70	1.5	7
Shelf Stable: Original	100	4	8
Plus DHA Omega-3, Plain	110	5	8
Unsweetened	80	4	4
Fruit & Protein, all flavors, 8.45 fl oz	150	1.5	29
Slim-Fast (Soy-Based) ~ *See Page 40*			
Soy Dream			
Refrigerated: Original	130	4	16
Enriched: Original	100	3.5	9
Vanilla	120	3.5	14
Shelf Stable:			
Classic Vanilla	140	4	18
Enriched: Original	100	4	8
Chocolate	150	4	21
Vanilla	120	4	14
Soy Slender,			
all flavors, av.	70	3	4
Trader Joe's:			
Soy Milk: Original	110	2	13
Chocolate	130	2.5	23
Vanilla	100	2	16
Organic: Original	130	3	17
Chocolate	120	3	17
Vanilla	130	3	19
Unsweetened	70	3.5	3
WestSoy:			
Low-Fat: Plain	90	2	15
Vanilla	120	1.5	21
Non-Fat: Plain	70	0	10
Vanilla	80	0	12
Longevity, Plain	90	3.5	10
Organic Plus, (25% Less Sugar):			
Plain	110	4.5	11
Vanilla	110	4.5	11
Unsweetened: Plain	90	4.5	5
Chocolate; Vanilla, average	100	4.5	6

Soy Powder Mix

	C	F	Cb
1 oz (¼ cup) mix makes 8 fl.oz Cup			
Soy Protein Isolate, dry, 1 oz	95	1	2
Better Than Milk:			
Original, 2 Tbsp	90	1.5	18
Vanilla, 2 Tbsp	90	1.5	18
Genisoy: *Per Scoop*			
Natural, unflavored, 1 oz	100	0	0
Chocolate, 1.2 oz	120	0	17
Vanilla, 1.2 oz	130	0	18
Now:			
Soy Protein Isolate:			
Plain, ⅓ cup, 0.8 oz	90	0.5	0.5
Chocolate, 1 level scoop, 1.58 oz	160	1.5	9
Revival: *Per Packet*			
Unsweetened Shakes: Plain	90	1	0.5
Vanilla Pleasure	120	2	6
Other flavors, average	115	2	4
Whole Foods:			
Choc. with Spirulina, 1 oz	100	1	10
Vanilla, with Spirulina, 1 oz	100	0	11

Coconut Milk Drink

	C	F	Cb
So Delicious: *Per 8 fl.oz cup*			
Shelf Stable: Original	80	5	7
Original, Unsweetened	50	5	1
Vanilla	90	5	9
Trader Joes: *Per 8 fl.oz cup*			
Unsweetened	60	5	1
Vanilla	90	5	9
(Enriched with calcium + vitamins D & B12)			

Confucious say:
"Man who eat with one chopstick never have problem with obesity"

Quick Guide

Cola Drinks:
Average All Brands
Includes Coca-Cola and Pepsi

	C	F	Cb
8 fl.oz Cup/Can	100	0	26
12 fl.oz Can	150	0	39
16 fl.oz Bottle	200	0	52
20 fl.oz Bottle	250	0	65
24 fl.oz (Pepsi)	300	0	84
1-Liter Bottle (34 fl.oz)	400	0	100
2-Liter Bottle (68 fl.oz)	800	0	200

Other Soda Drinks: *Av. All Brands, Per 12 fl.oz*

	C	F	Cb
Club Soda	0	0	0
Cream Soda	190	0	48
Diet/Low Cal Drinks	5	0	1
Dr Pepper Type	150	0	38
Ginger Ale	125	0	31
Grape	160	0	42
Lemonade, Regular/Pink	180	0	45
Orange	180	0	45
Root Beer	150	0	39
Tonic Water	125	0	32
Mineral Water: Plain	0	0	0
Sweetened/flavored	150	0	37
With Fruit Juice	120	0	30
Soda Water/Seltzer: Plain/Diet	0	0	0
Sweetened/flavored	155	0	39
With Fruit Juice	160	0	40

Fountain, Movie Theater & Take-Out

Average All Flavors

	C	F	Cb
Small Cup, 12 fl.oz: No Ice	160	0	40
With ⅓ Ice	120	0	30
Regular, 16 fl.oz: No Ice	215	0	53
With ⅓ Ice	160	0	40
Medium, 22 fl.oz: No Ice	295	0	73
With ⅓ Ice	220	0	55
Large, 32 fl.oz: No Ice	430	0	105
With ⅓ Ice	320	0	80

(Note: ⅓ Cup of Ice = ¼ Cup Liquid)

Soft Drink Brands

Per 12 fl.oz Unless Indicated

	C	F	Cb
A&W, Root Beer	170	0	47
Albertson's:			
Super Chill: Cola	160	0	43
Root Beer	180	0	48
Barq's, Root Beer	160	0	45
Big Red, Soda, 20 fl.oz	250	0	63
Blue Sky:			
Natural Soda: Black Cherry	140	0	37
Cola; Orange Creme, av.	160	0	43

Soft Drink Brands (Cont)

Per 12 fl.oz Unless Indicated

	C	F	Cb
Bubble Up, Soda, 8 fl.oz	110	0	28
Cactus Cooler, 12 fl.oz	150	0	40
Canada Dry: *Per 8 fl.oz*			
Club Sod; Diet Ginger Ale	0	0	0
Ginger Ale; Tonic Water, av.	90	0	25
Capri Sun,			
Juice Drinks, all flavors, 6 fl.oz	60	0	16
Cheerwine, 12 fl.oz	150	0	42
Coca-Cola:			
Classic/Caffeine Free	140	0	39
Diet Coke, all flavors	0	0	0
Cherry Coke/Vanilla Coke	150	0	42
Zero	0	0	0
Country Time *(Dr Pepper/Snapple),*			
Lemonade, all varieties, 20 fl.oz	230	0	58
Crush:			
Orange/Grape: 12 fl.oz	160	0	43
20 fl.oz bottle	270	0	72
Diet Orange, 20 fl.oz	0	0	0
Strawberry, 20 fl.oz	290	0	77
Dad's: Orange Cream Soda	180	0	46
Root Beer	165	0	41
Diet Rite, Pure Zero	0	0	0
Dr Pepper: Regular	150	0	40
Cherry	165	0	44
Diet, all flavors	0	0	0
Ten, 8 fl.oz	10	0	2
Fanta, all flavors, average	175	0	48
Fresca, all flavors	0	0	0
GuS, all flavors, average	95	0	23
Hansen's:			
Diet Soda	0	0	0
Natural Cane Sugar:			
Creamy Root Beer	160	0	43
Pomegranate	130	0	35
Hawaiian Punch, Fruit Juicy Red	105	0	26
Henry Weinhard's: Root Beer	170	0	43
Cream flavors, average	175	0	42
Hires, Root Beer	170	0	46
IBC: Root Beer	160	0	43
Cream Soda; Black Cherry	180	0	48
Icee: Coca-Cola	100	0	27
Fanta, Lemon Lime	90	0	24
Minute Maid, Raspb. Lemonade	100	0	27
Jarritos, all flav., 12.5 fl.oz	110	0	28
Jelly Belly, all flavors	180	0	28
Jolt, Power Cola, 16 fl.oz	200	0	54

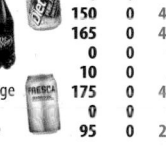

Soft Drink Brands (Cont)

Per 12 fl.oz Unless Indicated

	C	F	Cb
Jones Soda: Cola	170	0	40
Whoopass, 16 fl.oz	220	0	52
Other flavors, average	185	0	46
Kool Aid, Bursts, all flavors, av.	35	0	9
Mello Yello, Regular	170	0	47
Minute Maid: Fruit Punch	160	0	44
Lemonade, Regular:			
12 fl.oz can	150	0	42
20 fl.oz bottle	250	0	70
Orangeade, 20 fl.oz bottle	275	0	73
Mountain Dew: Original	165	0	47
Live Wire; Code Red	170	0	46
Voltage; White Out	170	0	46
Diet flavors	0	0	0
Mug, Root Beer	160	0	43
Natural Brew:			
Draft Root Beer	180	0	44
Outrageous Ginger Ale	170	0	42
Vanilla Cream	170	0	42
Nehi, Royal Crown Peach	190	0	51
Orangina, Regular	160	0	39
Pepsi: Regular; Caffeine Free	150	0	41
Diet Pepsi; Jazz; Pepsi One	0	0	0
Pepsi Next	60	0	16
Wild Cherry; Vanilla	160	0	42
Perrier, Carbonated Water	0	0	0
Pibb, Xtra	150	0	39
RC Cola, Regular	160	0	43
Reed's, Ginger Brew, average all varieties	145	0	38
7-UP: Regular; Cherry	150	0	39
Diet varieties	0	0	0
Safeway: *Per 8 fl.oz*			
Refreshe: Cola	110	0	29
Grape	140	0	36
Lemon Lime	110	0	27
Mountain Breeze	120	0	32
Strawberry	120	0	29
Santa Cruz, Sparkling, av., 10.5 fl.oz	135	0	33
Schweppes: Seltzer	0	0	0
Tonic Water; Ginger Ale, average	130	0	35
Shasta: Cream Soda	190	0	47
Cherry Cola	180	0	45
Dr. Shasta	150	0	38
Club Soda; Diet, all flavors	0	0	0
Tiki Punch; Pineapple; Or.	200	0	50
Ginger Ale	130	0	33
Other flavors, average	170	0	41
Sierra Mist, Lemon Lime	140	0	37
Slurpee ~ *See Page 236*			
Sprite: Regular	140	0	38
Zero	0	0	0
Squirt, Ruby Red	170	0	45

Per 12 fl.oz Unless Indicated

	C	F	Cb
Stewarts: Root Beer	160	0	41
Grape; Orange 'n Cream	190	0	48
Sun Drop: Citrus Soda, 20 fl.oz	290	0	76
Cherry Lemon, 12 fl.oz	180	0	46
Diet Citrus Soda, 12 fl.oz	10	0	1
Sunkist, Orange, 12 fl.oz	165	0	45
20 fl.oz	270	0	74
SunnyD:			
Original: *Per 64 fl.oz Ctn*			
All varieties, 8 fl.oz	90	0	22
Blends: *Per 64 fl.oz Containers*			
Fused, all flavors, 8 fl.oz	80	0	20
Fruit Punch, 8 fl.oz	80	0	21
Baja Juice: *Per 12 fl.oz Bottles*			
Red Punch	170	0	43
Other flavors	190	0	46
TAB	0	0	0
Tampico, Punch, av., 8 fl.oz	110	0	25
Thomas Kemper, Average all varieties	160	0	40
Trader Joe's:			
Sparkling:			
French Berry Lemonade, 1 cup, 8 fl.oz	130	0	31
1 bottle, 33.8 fl.oz	520	0	124
Lime Ade, 1 cup, 8 fl.oz	110	0	28
1 bottle, 33.8 fl.oz	440	0	108
Pink Lemonade, 1 cup, 8 fl.oz	130	0	31
1 Bottle, 33.8 fl.oz	520	0	124
Vernor's, Ginger Soda	140	0	39
Virgil's, Root Beer	160	0	42
Walgreens: *Per 20 fl.oz*			
Orchard Grape Soda	300	0	84
Cola; Zesty Lem. Lime, av.	225	0	65
Root Beer	225	0	75
Welch's, Sparkling Grape Juice C'tail	240	0	60
365 Organic *(Whole Foods)*, Spritzers, all flavors	110	0	28

Powdered Soft Drink Mix

Per 8 fl.oz Prepared, Unless Indicated

	C	F	Cb
Country Time *(Kraft)*:			
Lemonade; Pink Lemonade	60	0	16
Average other flavors	80	0	19
Lite	35	0	8
Crystal Light: Orig., 8 fl.oz	5	0	0
Pure, all flav., av., 0.3 oz pkt	15	0	4
Flavor Aid, ⅛ package	0	0	0
Kool-Aid, all flavors	60	0	16
Propel, Fit, 3 grams	10	0	3
Tang, Regular, 2 Tbsp, 1 oz	105	0	28

Quick Guide

Teas

	C	F	Cb
Regular: Bag, Loose or Instant Brewed, 1 cup, 8 fl.oz (Add extra for sugar/milk)	2	0	0.5
Herbal: All flavors, average, 1 cup	2	0	0.5
Bigelow, all flavors	0	0	0
Celestial Seasonings, all flavors	0	0	0
Bubble Milk Tea, w/ Pearls, 8 fl.oz	175	0	41
Chai Tea *(Cafe D' Vita),* 2 Tbsp	120	3.5	21
Starbucks ~ *See Fast-Foods Section*			

Iced Tea
Average All Brands

	C	F	Cb
Sweetened: 8 fl.oz	90	0	22
12 fl.oz	140	0	34
16 fl.oz	180	0	46
Unsweetened, 8 fl.oz	2	0	0.5

Iced Tea Mixes

Per 8 fl.oz Made-Up

	C	F	Cb
4C Iced Teas:			
Sweetened, average	70	0	18
Totally Light, all flavors	0	0	0
Crystal Light, sugar free	5	0	0
Lipton: Iced Tea To Go	0	0	0
Instant, unsweetened	0	0	0
Instant Raspberry	80	0	19
Lemon, sweetened	70	0	18
Peach; Raspberry, Sugar Free	5	0	1
Nestea:			
Lemonade Tea, 1⅓ Tbsp	60	0	15
Lemon flavored Iced Tea, 1⅓ Tbsp	60	0	15
Sugar Free Lemon Iced Tea, 2 tsp	5	0	2
Unsweetened Tea, 2 tsp	0	0	0

Bottled & Canned Teas

	C	F	Cb
Arizona: *Per 8 fl.oz*			
Black: Cranberry	80	0	22
Sweet	90	0	23
With Ginseng	60	0	15
Green Tea: Flavored, av.	70	0	18
Diet Blueberry	5	0	2
Lite, Half & Half Lemonade	50	0	14
Fuze, average all flavors, 16 fl.oz	120	0	30
Gold Peak, Lemon, 18.5 fl.oz	185	0	48

Bottled & Canned Teas (Cont)

	L	H	Cb
Honest Tea, Black Forest Berry/Peach, 16 fl.oz	65	0	17
Lipton:			
Brisk, average all flavors:			
12 fl.oz can	120	0	34
20 fl.oz bottle	210	0	55
Iced Tea:			
Lemon; White, w/ Raspb., 16.9 fl.oz	110	0	29
Diet, 16.9 fl.oz	5	0	0
Natural Green Tea, w/ Citrus:			
16.9 fl.oz Bottle	110	0	28
Diet, 16.9 fl oz bottle	5	0	0
20 fl.oz bottle	130	0	34
Diet, 20 fl.oz bottle	5	0	0.5
Sweet Iced Tea, 16.9 fl.oz	180	0	49
Sparkling, Strawberry Kiwi, Diet, 16.9 fl.oz	5	0	0
Minute Maid, Pomeg. Tea, 8 fl.oz	40	0	9
Nantucket, Lemon Tea 17.5 fl.oz	190	0	47
Nestea:			
Iced Tea, with Lemon:			
8 fl.oz	80	0	22
17 fl.oz bottle	180	0	45
20 fl.oz bottle	210	0	56
Diet, Green/Lemon	0	0	0
POMx:			
Antioxidant Super Tea: *Per 16 fl.oz*			
Pomegranate: Blackberry	160	0	40
Lychee	140	0	36
Peach Passion	160	0	38
Snapple:			
Green Tea	120	0	31
Diet Green Tea	0	0	0
Lemon/ Raspberry Tea	150	0	37
Diet Lemon/Raspberry Tea	10	0	0
Peach	160	0	40
Diet Peach	10	0	0
SoBe, Energize, Green Tea, 20 fl.oz	200	0	52
Ssips, Lemon Iced, 6.75 fl.oz	80	0	20
Steaz, Green Tea, Peach/Mint, 16 fl.oz	80	0	20
Tazo, Sweet Organic Black, 14 fl oz	60	0	15
TeaZazz: Original; Peach, 20 fl.oz	50	0	12
Green Tea Lemon, 20 fl.oz	60	0	15
Trader Joe's: *Per 8 fl.oz*			
Organic Tea & Lemonade	100	0	25
Pomegranate Green Tea	60	0	15
Unsweetened *(Kettle/Green)*	0	0	0
Turkey Hill: Iced Tea, 16 fl.oz	180	0	42
Fruit flavors, av., 16 fl.oz	205	0	50
365 Organic *(Whole Foods):*			
Unsweetened: Black Tea	0	0	0
Green Tea	0	0	0

Note: Most breads have similar calories on a weight basis. However, volume may vary.

For example, 1 oz of bread may equal 1 slice regular bread or 2 slices of a lighter bread.

It is best to weigh bread used and calculate using: 1 oz bread = 70 calories, 14g carb.

Quick Guide

Bread	C	F	Cb
White or Wheat: *Average Per Slice*			
Thin or Light, ¾ oz	50	0.5	9
Sandwich slice, 1 oz	70	1	12
Thick or Large, 1½ oz	105	1.5	18
Thick, 2 oz	140	2	23
Extra Thick, 3 oz	210	3	35
Whole Loaf, 16 oz	1120	15	185
24 oz Loaf	1680	24	280
Multi Grain/Whole Grain: *Per Slice*			
Sandwich Slice, 1 oz	75	1.5	12
Thick Slice, 2 oz	150	2.5	25

Toast: *Based on same counts as White/Wheat as shown above*

1 Slice (1 oz fresh):			
With 1 tsp butter/margarine	105	5	12
With 1 tsp "light" butter/marg.	90	3.5	12
With 2 tsp butter/margarine	140	9	12
With 2 tsp "light" butter/marg.	110	6	12

Breads

Per Slice Unless Indicated

12-Grain, 1.5 oz	110	1.5	22
Bran style/Dark, 1 oz	70	1	14
Buttermilk, average, 1.5 oz	110	1	22
Challah, ¾ oz	85	1.5	17
Chapati, 1 oz	110	3	18
Ciabatta, 2 oz	130	1	26
Cornbread, average, 3 oz	220	6	37
Cracked Wheat Sourdough, 1.5 oz	130	0.5	27
Croissants ~ *See Page 134*			
Crustless Bread, regular, slice, ¾ oz	40	0.5	8.5
Crusts Only, regular slice, ¼ oz	30	0	7
English Toasting, 2 oz	140	1.5	27
Flax & Grain, 1.5 oz	120	3	19
Foccacia: Plain, 2 oz serve	150	2.5	28
Cheese & Garlic; Pesto, 2 oz serve	160	6	21
Tomato & Olive, 2 oz serve	150	5	21

Per Slice Unless Indicated

French Stick/Baguette, 1 oz	70	1	15
French Toast: Slices, 1.5oz	140	2	26
Sticks *(Aunt Jemima)*, av., 2 oz	110	2	18
Garlic Bread/Toast:			
Small slice + 1 tsp spread, ¾ oz	80	5	7
Medium slice + 2 tsp spread, 1½ oz	160	10	14
Thick slice + 3 tsp spread, 1.8 oz	220	14	20
Pepperidge Farm, 1 slice, 1.4 oz	160	10	15
Hemp Bread, 1.2 oz	95	2	12
Italian Bread, 2 oz	140	1	28
Lower Carb, (higher protein/fiber), average all brands, 1 oz	60	1.5	9
MultiGrain, 1.5 oz	100	2	21
Naan Flatbread, 2 oz	160	3.5	29
Nut/Health Nut, 1.35 oz	90	1.5	18
Oatmeal/Oatbran Bread, 1.5 oz	90	0.5	19
Pita: Average all types:			
Small (4" diam), 1 oz	90	0	18
Large (6½" diam), 2 oz	140	1.5	27
Extra Large (9" diam), 4 oz	300	1.5	60
Popovers, (1), without butter	130	2	18
Pumpernickel:			
Cocktail/Party size	30	0.5	6
Large slice, 1.35 oz	80	0	15
Raisin Bread, 1 oz	80	1	15
Rye: 1 thin slice, av., 1 oz	80	1	14
1 thick slice, 2 oz	150	2	25
Cocktail size, 0.4 oz	25	0.5	4
Sandwich Pockets, 2 oz	140	1.5	27
Sourdough: Regular, 1½ oz	120	1	25
French Style, 1 oz	75	0	14
Spelt, 1.6 oz	130	1	26
Sprouted 7-Grain, 1.5 oz	110	0.5	18
Squaw, 1.1 oz	85	0.5	13
Sweet Hawaiian Bread, 1.5 oz	110	2	19
Tacos/Tortillas ~ *See Page 172*			
Turkish/Middle Eastern, 1 oz	80	1.5	16
Wheat-Free Breads: Spelt, 1.6 oz	130	1	26
Rice w/ Fruit Juice, 1.5 oz	110	2	21
Healthseed Rye, 1.6 oz	90	1	20
Millet, 1.5 oz	100	1	20

Bread Brands

C F Cb

Per Slice Unless Indicated

	C	F	Cb
Ener-G: Gluten-Free Breads:			
Brown Rice Loaf: Regular, 1.3 oz	100	3	16
Light, 0.7 oz	50	2	7
Corn Loaf, 0.7 oz	40	2	7
Tapioca: Regular, 1.34 oz	100	4.5	15
Light, 0.7 oz	45	1.5	7
Ezekiel:			
Sprouted Grain: Flax, 1.2 oz	80	1	14
Sesame, 1.2 oz	80	0.5	14
Whole Grain, 1.34 oz	80	0.5	15
French Meadow: *Per 1.2 oz Slice*			
Flax & Sunflower	90	1.5	15
Hemp	100	2.5	12
Men's Bread	100	4	10
Spelt	85	0.5	17
Francisco International,			
Sourdough, Sliced Loaf, 1.45 oz	120	0.5	22
Nature's Path: *Per 2 oz Slice*			
Manna: Carrot Raisin; Millet Rice	130	0	27
Cinnamon Date	150	0	29
Sunseed	160	2	29
Oroweat:			
3 Seed Oatnut, 1.34 oz	110	2.5	18
100% Whole Wheat, 1.35 oz	90	1	17
Country Buttermilk, 1.35 oz	100	1	19
Honey Wheat Berry, 1.2 oz	80	1	17
Pepperidge Farm:			
Farmhouse, Hearty White	120	1.5	22
Goldfish:			
White/Wheat (2), av.	100	1.5	21
Brown Sugar/Cinnamon (2)	130	1.5	24
Frozen Breads:			
Garlic Bread:			
Five Cheese, 2.25 oz	200	10	20
Parmesan, 21/2″	180	8	21
Premium: Roasted Garlic Toast	150	7	18
Tuscan Inspired Sourdough	170	7	22
Light Style, average	130	1	26
Small slices, 15 Grain	70	1.5	13
Very Thin, 100% Whole Wheat, 3 sl.	75	12	13
Roman Meal: Orig. Multigrain (2)	130	1.5	25
Honey Wheatberry, 1.5 oz	100	1.5	19
Sara Lee: Honey Wheat, 1 oz	75	1	15
100% Whole Wheat, 1 slice, 1 oz	70	1	13
45 Cals & Delightful Wheat	45	0.5	9
Schwan's, Frozen:			
Cheese Stuffed Breadsticks, 2 oz	160	7	18
French Baguette, ¼ loaf, 1.7 oz	130	0	25
Trader Joe's: Gourm. White, 1.5 oz	120	3.5	19
Soft 10 Grain, 1.5 oz	90	1.5	16
Sprouted Rye, 1.2 oz	90	1	15

Biscuits, Bread Rolls & Buns

C F Cb

	C	F	Cb
Biscuits: *Average, 2½″ diameter*			
Plain/B'Milk:			
Prepared from Recipe	210	10	27
Refrig. Dough, Baked	95	4	13
Brown 'n Serve, av., 1 oz	70	1	13
Refrigerated Dough:			
Buttermilk Biscuit *(Pillsbury)*,			
(3), 2¼ oz	150	2	30
Buns:			
Frankfurter/Hot Dog: 1.25 oz	110	1.5	21
1.5 oz size	130	2	25
Hamburger: Regular, 1.5 oz	110	1.5	22
Large, 3 oz	210	3	40
Hoagie/Submarine, Plain, 2⅓ oz	200	1	38
Rolls:			
Ciabatta Roll, 3.5 oz	230	4	41
Crescent Roll, Original, 1 oz	100	6	11
Dinner:			
1 small, 1 oz	90	1.5	17
1 medium (3″ diam), 1.5 oz	110	1	23
French: 1 med, 1.3 oz	110	1.5	22
1 large, 3 oz	230	2.5	42
Kaiser:			
Small, 2 oz	200	2.5	35
Large, 3.5 oz	350	4	61
Plain, 6″, average all, 2.5 oz	200	1	38
Sourdough, 1.25 oz	110	1	21
Wheat Rolls: Small, 1.2 oz	100	1	17
Medium, 1.75 oz	130	1.5	23
Large, 3.5 oz	260	3	46

Breadsticks, Croutons

	C	F	Cb
Breadsticks:			
Salt Sticks, plain, 1 oz	110	1	20
Fresh baked (1), 2 oz	180	2.5	34
Stella D'oro: Original (1)	45	1	7
Sesame (1)	50	2	7
Croutons: Seasoned, 2 Tbsp, ¼ oz	35	1.5	4
Zesty Italian *(Pepp. Farm)*, 6 croutons	30	1	5

Bread Products

	C	F	Cb
Bread Crumbs, dry:			
Plain or seasoned: 1 oz	110	1.5	20
1 cup, 3½ oz	385	5	70
Corn Flake Crumbs, 1 oz	120	0	29
Graham Cracker Crumbs *(Keebler)*,			
1 oz	110	2.5	20
Bread Dough: Frozen, 1 sl., 2 oz	140	2	26
Refrigerated: French, 1″ slice	60	1	13
Wheat; White, 1″ slice	80	2	14
Coating Mixes, av., 2 Tbsp., 1 oz	100	0.5	20
Stuffing: Dry mix, average, all, 1 oz	110	1	10
Prepared, ½ cup, 4 oz	180	9	11

Quick Guide

Bagels

	C	F	Cb
Average All Brands			
Plain/Onion:			
1 mini/bagelette, 1 oz	65	0.5	13
1 small bagel, 2 oz	145	1	29
1 medium bagel, 3 oz	220	1.5	43
1 large bagel, 4 oz	290	2	57
Bagel Chips, 1 oz	130	4.5	19
Pizza Bagel Bites *(Bagel Bites)*, average all ,4 pieces, 1 oz	190	5.5	27
Bagel Crisps *(New York Style)*, average all, 6 crisps, 1 oz	130	5	17
Bagel Thins *(Thomas')* 1, 1.5 oz	110	1	25

Bagel Brands

Per Bagel

	C	F	Cb
Bubba's: Plain; Onion, average	220	1.5	46
Blueberry	230	2	49
Cinnamon Raisin	230	1.5	48
Costco Bakery: Plain	330	1.5	70
Cinnamon Raisin	340	1.5	73
Whole Grain	300	5	56
Lender's: Fresh, NY Style: Plain, 3.3 oz	240	2	46
Blueberry, 2 oz	150	0.5	32
Other flav., 3.3 oz	250	1.5	51
Whole Grain, 3.3 oz	250	1.5	49
Whole Wheat, 3.3 oz	210	1.5	41
Panera Bread: Plain	290	1.5	59
Cinnamon & Raisin Swirl, 3.75 oz	320	2	65
Everything, 4 oz	300	2.5	59
Whole Grain, 4.25 oz	340	2.5	67
Sara Lee: Mini, average, 1.3 oz	100	0.5	20
Plain, 3.35 oz	260	1	50
Blueberry, 3.7 oz	280	1	54
Cinnamon Raisin, 3.7 oz	270	1	54
Everything, 3.7 oz	280	3.5	50
Onion, 3 oz	270	1	52
Western, The Alternatives, av., 2 oz	110	0	25

Bagel Spreads

	C	F	Cb
Cream Cheese:			
Plain: 2 Tbsp, 1 oz	100	9	1
2 oz mini-tub	200	18	2
Reduced Fat: 2 Tbsp, 1 oz	60	5	2
2 oz mini-tub	120	10	4
Flavors: Lox, 1 oz	90	8	2
Honey Nut, 1 oz	80	7	4
Strawberry, 1 oz	90	7	5
Sundried Tomato, 1 oz	80	7	2
Vegetable, 1 oz	90	8	2

English Muffins

	C	F	Cb
Average All Brands			
Plain/Whole Wheat:			
Regular, 2 oz	135	1.5	26
Heavier, 2½ oz	155	2	31
Super Size, 3.2 oz	190	2	38
Raisin-Cinnamon, 2.2 oz	150	1	30

Note: *Actual weight of packaged muffins can be 10-15% heavier than stated net weight.*

Rice Cakes

	C	F	Cb
Reg. size, av.1 cake, 0.32 oz	35	0.5	7.5
Hain, Mini, plain, 10 pcs	70	2	15
Lundberg, all types, 0.65 oz	70	0.5	14
Quaker, Apple Cinnamon, 0.45 oz	50	0	11

Tortillas & Shells

	C	F	Cb
Corn Tortilla: *Per Single Tortilla*			
White/Yellow: 6", 1 oz	55	1	11
7", 1.2 oz, average	75	1	11
Flour Tortilla: *Per Single Tortilla*			
6", 1.2 oz	100	3	16
8", 1.4 oz	130	4	20
10", 2.3 oz	200	6	31
12", 3.3 oz	300	9	46
Shells: *Per Single Shell, Without Fillings*			
Taco Shells:			
Mini, 3", 0.2 oz	25	1	3
Medium, 5", 0.5 oz	60	2.5	8
Large, 6½", 0.7 oz	100	4.5	13
Extra Large, Salad Shell/Bowl *(Taco Bell)*, Fried, 10", 2.4 oz	360	21	40
Tostada Shells:			
White Corn, 5½" diam. 0.4 oz	55	2.5	8
Yellow Corn, 5½" diam. 0.5 oz	80	3.5	11
Sopes, 1 shell, 4", 2 oz, av.	110	1.5	23
La Tortilla Factory:			
Hand Made Style, Corn, av., 1.45 oz	90	1	14
100 Calorie, Traditional, 2 oz	100	1.5	24
Mission Foods:			
Homestyle, 1 Tortilla, 2.2 oz	190	4.5	32
Yellow/White Corn:			
2 Tortillas, 1.48 oz	90	1	18
Super Size, 1 Tortilla, 1.15 oz	70	1	14
Flour: Large, 1 Tortilla, 2.47 oz	210	4.5	36
Medium, Soft , 1 Tortilla, 1.73 oz	140	3	25
Small, 1 Tortilla, 1.27 oz	110	2.5	19
Smart & Delicious:			
Low Carb: Orig, 1.27 oz	50	2	10
Large, 2.19 oz	80	3	18
Sonoma, Yellow Corn (2), 2.4 oz	120	1.5	25

Quick Guide

Cooked Cereals

	C	F	Cb
Barley, pearled, cooked, 1 cup	195	0.5	44
Buckwheat Groats, roasted:			
Dry, ½ cup, 3 oz	285	2	61
Cooked, 1 cup, 6 oz	155	1	34
Bulgur: Dry, ½ cup, 2½ oz	240	1	53
Cooked, 1 cup, 6½ oz	150	0.5	34
Corn/Hominy Grits:			
Dry: Regular, ¼ cup, 1.4 oz	140	0.5	32
Instant: 0.8 oz packet	75	0	18
W/ Imitation Bacon Bits, 1 oz	100	0.5	22
Cooked, ¾ cup, 6½ oz	110	0.5	23
Cream of Rice, cooked, ¾ cup, 6½ oz	95	0	21
Cream of Wheat:			
Cooked: Regular, ¾ cup, 6½ oz	95	0.5	20
Instant, ¾ cup, 6½ oz	105	0.5	21
Quick, ¾ cup, 6½ oz	100	0.5	22
Farina, cooked, ¾ cup, 6 oz	95	0.5	19
Millet, dry, ¼ cup, 1¾ oz	190	2	36
Oat Bran: Raw, ⅓ cup, 1 oz	70	2	19
Cooked, ½ cup, 3¾ oz	45	1	13
Oatmeal:			
Dry: Regular, ⅓ cup, 1 oz	100	1.5	18
Instant: Regular, average, 1 oz	105	1.5	18
Flavored, average, 1½ oz	165	2	34
Cooked: Regular, ¾ cup, 6 oz	125	2.5	21
1 cup, 8 oz	165	3.5	28
Whole Wheat, cooked, ¾ cup, 6.4 oz	115	0.5	25

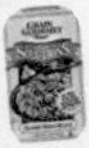

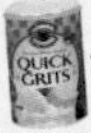

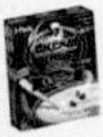

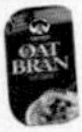

Brans, Wheat Germ, Add-Ons

	C	F	Cb
Bran:			
Oat Bran: Raw, 1 Tbsp, 0.18 oz	10	0.5	4
⅓ cup, 1 oz	70	2	19
Rice Bran: Raw, 1 Tbsp, 0.18 oz	15	1	2.5
¼ cup, 1 oz	95	6	15
Wheat, unprocessed,			
1 Tbsp, 0.10 oz	5	0	2
Wheat Germ: Raw, 1 Tbsp, ¼ oz	25	0.5	4
¼ cup, 1 oz	105	3	15
Bee Pollen Granules, 1 Tbsp, 0.28 oz	25	1	2
Fruit: Dried, average, 1 oz	70	0	18
Banana, ½ medium	55	0	14
Prunes in Syrup (5), 3 oz	90	0	23
Honey, 1 Tbsp, ¾ oz	65	0	17
Lecithin Granules, 1 Tbsp, 0.35 oz	55	4	0.5
Nuts, Almonds (6), ¼ oz	40	4	1.5
Psyllium Husks, 1 Tbsp, 0.18 oz	15	0	4

Hot/Cooked Cereals ~ Brands
Per Serving, Dry Mix only

	C	F	Cb
Albers Grits,			
¼ cup, 1.4 oz	140	0.5	31
B&G,			
Cream of Wheat: Instant Orig., 1 oz	100	0	19
Instant Maple Brown Sugar, 1.23 oz	130	0	28
Bobs Red Mill,			
10 Grain, ¼ cup, 1.6 oz	140	1	28
Country Choice,			
Quick Oats, ½ cup, 1.4 oz	150	3	27
Dr McDougall's:			
Big Cup Organic Oatmeal: *Per Cup*			
Grains: With Cranb. Muesli, 3.1 oz	320	4	62
With Peach Raspberry, 3 oz	300	4	62
4 Grain with Real Maple, 2.55 oz	260	3	52
Organic Instant Oatmeal: *Per Cup*			
Original, 1 oz	120	2	21
Light Apple Cinnamon, 1.95 oz	120	1.5	24
Light Maple Brown Sugar, 1.34 oz	150	2	29
Great Value *(Walmart):*			
Instant Oatmeal: Original, 1 oz	100	2	19
Maple & Brown Sugar, 1 oz	160	2	33
Apple & Cinn.; Peaches & Crm, 1.23 oz	130	1.5	27
McCann's:			
Instant Irish Oatmeal:			
Regular, 1 oz package	100	2	19
Apple & Cinnamon, 1.23 oz	130	1.5	27
Maple & Brown Sugar, 1.5 oz	160	2	32
Malt-O-Meal: Orig., 3Tbsp, 1.2 oz	130	0.5	27
Maple Brown Sugar, ¼ cup	170	0	37
Natures Path:			
Oatmeal:			
Apple Cinnamon, 1.7 oz	210	2.5	40
HempPlus, 1 pkt, 1.4 oz	160	2.5	30
Maple Nut, 1.7 oz	210	4	38
NutriSystem:			
Oatmeal, Apple Cinnamon, 1 pkt	130	1.5	26
Quaker:			
Instant Oatmeal: *Per Packet Unless Indicated*			
Regular, Organic 1 oz	100	2	19
Cinn. & Spice, 1.5 oz	160	2.5	32
Maple Brown Sugar, 1.5 oz	160	2.5	32
Peaches & Cream, 1.23 oz	130	2	27
Old Fash'nd/Quick Oats, ½ c., 1.4 oz	150	3	27
Real Medleys: Summer Berry, 2.5 oz	250	3	51
Other varieties, av., 2.6 oz	290	8	51
Grits:			
Instant, all flavors, average, 1 oz	100	2	22
Quick, Original, ¼ cup, 1.3 oz	130	0.5	29
Wegmans:			
Instant Oatmeal: Regular, 1oz pkt	100	2	19
Lower Sugar Maple & Brn Sgr, 1 pkt	120	2	24

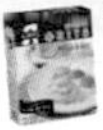

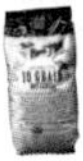

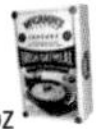

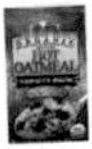

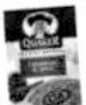

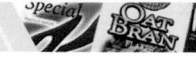

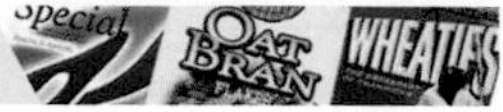

Quick Guide

Cold Cereals
Average All Brands

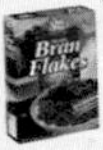

	C	F	Cb
Bran Flakes, ¾ cup, 1 oz	95	0.5	24
Corn Flakes, 1 cup, 1 oz	100	0	22
Frosted Flakes, ¾ cup, 1 oz	110	0	27
Granola, 100% Nat., ½ cup, 1.7 oz	205	6	35
Oat Bran Cereal, ½ cup, 1½ oz	145	3	25
Puffed Rice, 1 cup, ½ oz	55	0	13
Puffed Wheat, 1 cup, ½ oz	45	0	10
Raisin Bran, ½ cup, 1 oz	90	0.5	22
Rice Crisps, 1 cup, 1 oz	105	0.5	24
Shredded Wheat, 1 biscuit, 1 oz	85	0.5	20
Wheat Flakes, ¾ cup, 1 oz	105	1	24

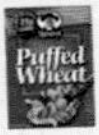

Breakfast/Cereal Bars ~ *See Page 31*

Ready-To-Eat Cereal

	C	F	Cb
Arrowhead Mills: *Per Cup*			
Flakes: Amaranth, 1.2 oz	140	2	26
Kamut, 1.1 oz	120	1	25
Maple Buckwheat, 1.5 oz	170	1	35
Oat Bran, 1.2 oz	140	2.5	24
Rice, sweetened, 1.7 oz	180	1	40
Spelt, 1.1 oz	120	1	24
Breadshop Granola:			
Crunchy Oat Bran, w/ Almonds, 1.7 oz	210	8	33
Triple Berry Crunch, ½ cup, 1.75 oz	210	8	34
Puffed: Corn, ½ oz	60	1	12
Kamut, ½ oz	50	0	11
Millet, ½ oz	60	0.5	11
Rice, ½ oz	60	0	14
Wheat, ½ oz	60	0	12
Shredded Wheat:			
Bite Size, 1.7 oz	190	1	38
Sweetened, 1.8 oz	200	1	42
Back to Nature: *Per ½ Cup, Unless Indicated*			
Granola: Apple Blueberry, 1.75 oz	200	2.5	39
Blueberry Walnut, 1.5 oz	190	6	30
Chocolate Delight, 1.75 oz	220	6	37
Classic, 1.8 oz	200	3	39
Cranberry Pecan, 1.65 oz	180	4.5	36
Honey Almond, 1.48 oz	190	7	29
Organic Cherry Vanilla, 1.75 oz	200	4	38
Sunflower & Pumpkin Seed, 1.75 oz	210	7	30

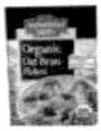

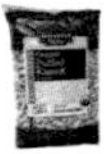

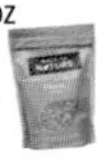

	C	F	Cb
Barbara's Bakery:			
Classics, Organic & Sweetened:			
Brown Rice Crisps, 1 oz	120	1	25
Corn Flakes, 1 cup, 1 oz	110	1	25
Hole n' Oats, Honey Nut, 1 oz	120	2	24
High Fiber:			
Original, 1.94 oz	180	1.5	42
Cranberry, 2 oz	190	1.5	42
Flax & Granola, 1 cup, 2 oz	200	3	42
Puffins:			
Original, ¾ cup, 0.95 oz	90	1	23
Cinnamon, ⅔ cup, 1 oz	90	1	26
Multigrain, ¾ cup, 1 oz	110	0	25
PB/PB & Choc., av., ¾ cup, 1 oz	110	2	24
Puffs: Crunchy Cocoa, ¾ cup, 1 oz	120	1	24
Fruit Medley, ¾ cup , 1.1 oz	120	1	26
Shredded:			
Oats: Original, 1.25 cups, 2 oz	220	2.5	46
Cinnamon Crunch, 1 cup, 2 oz	230	3	43
Vanilla Almond, 1 cup, 2 oz	220	3	42
Spoonfuls, Multigrain, ¾ cup, 1.1 oz	120	1.5	25
Cascadian Farm:			
Cinnamon Crunch, 1 cup, 0.95 oz	110	3	22
Granola: Ancient Grains, 1c., 1.94 oz	210	5	38
French Van. Almond, 1.76 oz	210	5	38
Oats & Honey, ⅔ cup, 2 oz	230	6	42
Hearty Morning, ¾ cup, 1.94 oz	200	3	43
Honey Nut O's, 1 cup, 1 oz	110	1	25
Multi Grain Squares, ¾ cup, 1 oz	110	1	25
Raisin Bran, 1 cup, 1.94 oz	180	1	43
Emerald:			
Breakfast on the Go:			
B'fast/Berry Nut Blend, av., 1.5 oz	180	8	26
S'mores Nut Blend, 1.5 oz	200	10	24
Ener-G, Rice Bran, ½ cup, 2.36 oz	220	14	34
EnviroKidz: *Per 1 oz*			
Amazon Frosted Flakes, ⅔ cup	120	0	26
Gorilla Munch, ¾ cup	120	0	27
Koala Crisp, ¾ cup	110	1	25
Leapin Lemur, ¾ cup	120	1.5	25
Panda Puffs, ¾ cup	130	2.5	24
Erewhon:			
Corn Flakes, 1 cup, 1.2 oz	130	0	30
Crispy Brown Rice: Original, 1 oz	110	0.5	25
W/ Mixed Berries, 1 c., 1 oz	120	0.5	27
Gluten Free, 1 oz	110	0.5	25
Raisin Bran, 1 cup, 1.83 oz	180	1	40
Rice Twice, ¾ cup, 1 oz	120	0	26

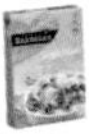

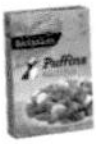

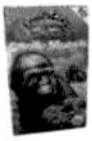

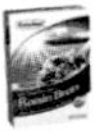

Ready-To-Eat (Cont)

	C	F	Cb
Ezekiel 4.9:			
Sprouted Whole Grain Cereals:			
Original, ½ cup, 2 oz	**190**	**1**	40
Almond, ½ cup, 2 oz	**200**	**3**	38
Cinnamon Raisin, 2 oz	**190**	**1**	41
Golden Flax, ½ cup, 2 oz	**180**	**2.5**	37
F-Factor, Skinnys 'n Fruit, ½ cup	**70**	**1**	27
General Mills:			
Cheerios: *Per ¾ Cup Unless Indicated*			
Original, 1 cup, 1 oz	**100**	**2**	20
Apple Cinnamon, 1 oz	**120**	**1.5**	24
Banana Nut, 1 oz	**100**	**1**	24
Cinnamon Burst, 1 cup, 1.2 oz	**110**	**2**	27
Chocolate; Dulce de Leche, 1 oz	**100**	**1.5**	22
Frosted, 1 oz	**100**	**1**	22
Fruity, 1 oz	**100**	**1.5**	23
Honey Nut, 1 oz	**110**	**1.5**	22
Multi Grain, 1 cup, 1 oz	**110**	**1**	23
Oat Cluster Crunch, 1.1 oz	**100**	**1**	22
Yogurt Burst, Strawberry, 1 oz	**120**	**1.5**	24
Chex: Corn, 1 cup, 1.1 oz	**120**	**0.5**	26
Apple Cinn; Choc., average, 1.1 oz	**130**	**2.5**	26
Honey Nut, ¾ cup, 1.1 oz	**120**	**0.5**	28
Multi-Bran, ¾ cup, 1.65 oz	**160**	**1.5**	39
Rice, 1 cup, 1 oz	**100**	**0**	23
Wheat, ¾ cup, 1.65 oz	**160**	**1**	39
Cinn. Toast Crunch, ¾ cup, 1.1 oz	**130**	**3**	25
Count Chocula, ¾ cup, 1 oz	**100**	**1.5**	23
Fiber One: Original, ½ cup, 1 oz	**60**	**1**	25
Honey Clusters, 1 cup, 1.83 oz	**160**	**1.5**	44
80 Calorie Honey Squares, ¾ c., 1 oz	**80**	**1**	25
Kix: Original, 1¼ cups, 1 oz	**110**	**1**	25
Berry; Honey, 1¼ cups, 1.16 oz	**120**	**1.5**	28
Lucky Charms, average, ¾ cup, 1 oz	**110**	**1.5**	23
Total: Original, ¾ cup, 1 oz	**100**	**0.5**	22
Plus Omega-3s, 1.8 oz	**200**	**3.5**	39
Raisin Bran, 1 cup, 2.1 oz	**190**	**1**	46
Trix, 1 cup, 1.1 oz	**120**	**1.5**	27
Wheaties: Original, ¾ cup, 1 oz	**100**	**0.5**	22
Fuel, ¾ cup, 1.94 oz	**190**	**3**	46

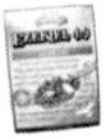
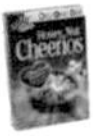
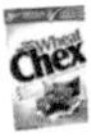
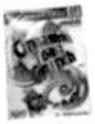
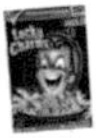

Updated Nutrition Data ~ www.CalorieKing.com
Persons with Diabetes ~ See Disclaimer (Page 22)

	C	F	Cb
Great Value *(Walmart):*			
Apple Blasts, 1 cup, 1.16 oz	**120**	**0**	29
Crunch Honey Oats, w/ Almonds ¾ cup, 1.1 oz	**130**	**1.5**	26
Frosted Shredded Wheat, 1.83 oz	**180**	**1**	42
Fruit Spins, 1 cup, 1 oz	**110**	**1**	25
Honey Crunch, ¾ cup, 1 oz	**100**	**0**	24
Raisin Bran, extra raisin, 1 cup, 2 oz	**200**	**1**	43
Health Valley:			
Cranberry Crunch, ¾ cup, 1.8 oz	**190**	**4**	38
Crunch-Ems!, Rice, 1¼ cups, 1 oz	**110**	**0**	26
Golden Flax, 1 cup, 1.75 oz	**190**	**3.5**	37
Heart Wise, 1 cup, 1.94 oz	**200**	**3**	37
Organic Flakes:			
Amaranth, 1¼ cups,1.94 oz	**210**	**2**	43
Fiber 7, Multigrain , 1 cup, 1.75 oz	**160**	**1**	37
Oat Bran: 1 cup, 1.75 oz	**190**	**1.5**	39
With Raisins, 1 cup, 1.87 oz	**200**	**1.5**	43
Heartland:			
Granola: Original, ½ cup, 2.25 oz	**240**	**6**	40
Balanced Blend, ⅔ cup, 1.8 oz	**210**	**3**	41
Low-Fat Raisin, ½ cup, 2 oz	**210**	**3**	40
Kashi:			
7 Whole Grain: Flakes, 1 c., 1.8 oz	**180**	**1**	41
Honey Puffs, 1 cup, 1.1 oz	**120**	**1**	25
Nuggets, ½ cup, 2 oz	**210**	**1.5**	47
Puffs, 1 cup, 0.67 oz	**70**	**0.5**	15
Blackcurrant & Walnuts, 1 cup,1.9.oz	**210**	**3.5**	43
GoLEAN: Original, 1 cup, 1.8 oz	**140**	**1**	30
Crunch!: Original, 1 cup, 1.9 oz	**190**	**3**	39
Honey Almond Flax, 1 cup, 1.9 oz	**200**	**4.5**	36
Good Friends, Orig., 1 cup, 1.9 oz	**160**	**1.5**	42
Granola: Cocoa Beach, ½ cup, 1.9 oz	**220**	**8**	35
Mountain Medley, ½ cup, 1.9 oz	**230**	**6**	41
Heart to Heart:			
Honey Toasted Oat, ¾ cup, 1.2 oz	**120**	**1.5**	26
Oat Flakes & Blueb. Clusters, 1 cup, 1.9 oz	**200**	**2**	44
Warm Cinnamon Oat, ¾ cup, 1.2 oz	**120**	**1.5**	25
Whole Wheat Biscuit:			
Autumn Wheat, 29 Biscuits, 1.9 oz	**180**	**1**	43
Cinnamon Harvest, 28 Bisc., 1.9 oz	**180**	**1**	43
Island Vanilla, 27 Biscuits, 1.9 oz	**190**	**1**	44

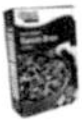
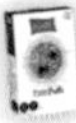

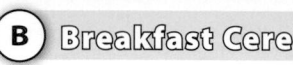
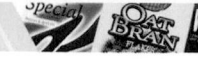

Ready-To-Eat (Cont) — C F Cb

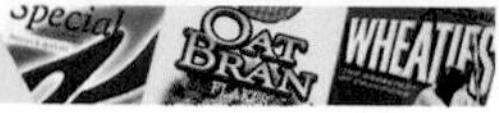

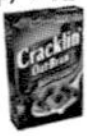

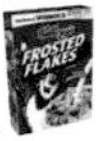

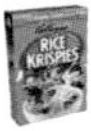

Kellogg's:

	C	F	Cb
All-Bran: Original, ½ cup, 1.1 oz	80	1	23
Bran Buds, ⅓ cup, 1.1 oz	80	1	24
Complete Wheat Flakes, ¾ cup, 1.1 oz	90	0.5	24
Apple Jacks, 1 cup, 1 oz	110	1	25
Cinnabon, 1 cup, 1 oz	120	2	25
Cocoa Krispies, ¾ cup, 1.1 oz	120	1	25
Corn Flakes, Original, 1 cup, 1 oz	100	0	24
Corn Pops, 1 cup, 1.1 oz	120	0	28
Cracklin' Oat Bran, ¾ cup, 1.8 oz	200	7	35
Crispix, Original, 1 cup, 1 oz	110	0	25
Crunchy Nut:			
Caramel Nut, ¾ cup, 1.1 oz	120	1	26
Roasted Nut & Honey, ¾ cup, 1oz	100	1	23
Fiber Plus, Caramel Pecan, ¾ cup, 1.7 oz	170	1.5	43
Fiber Plus Antioxidants, Berry Yogurt Crunch, 1 cup	180	1	46
Fruit Loops: Original, 1 cup, 1 oz	110	1	26
Marshmallow, 1 cup, 1.1 oz	110	1	26
Frosted Flakes: Orig., ¾ cup, 1.1 oz	110	0	27
With Fiber, Less Sugar, 1 cup, 1.1 oz	110	0	26
Granola, Low-Fat:			
With Raisins, ⅔ cup, 2.1 oz	230	3	48
Without Raisins, ½ cup, 1.7 oz	190	3	40
Honey Smacks, ¾ cup, 1 oz	100	0.5	24
Mini-Wheats: Frosted Big Bite (7)	200	1	47
Frosted: Bite Size (21), 1.9 oz	190	1	46
Blueberry Muffin (25), 1.94 oz	190	1	47
Touch of Fruit In Middle, Raspberry (24), 1.94 oz	190	1	45
Unfrosted (30), 1.94 oz	190	1	45
Little Bites: Original (42), 2 oz	200	1	47
Chocolate (42)	190	2	45
Mueslix, ⅔ cup, 2 oz	200	3	41
Nutri-Grain Bars ~ *See Page 31*			
Product 19, 1 cup, 1.1 oz	110	0	25
Raisin Bran: Regular, 1 cup, 2.1 oz	190	1	46
Crunch, 1 cup, 1.87 oz	190	1	45
Rice Krispies:			
Original, 1¼ cups, 1.15 oz	130	0	29
Cocoa, ¾ cup, 1.1 oz	120	1	27
Frosted, ¾ cup, 1.1 oz	110	0	27
Gluten Free, 1 cup, 1.1 oz	110	0.5	25
Treats, ¾ cup, 1.1 oz	120	1	26

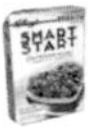

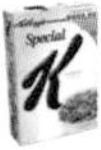

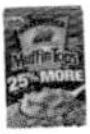

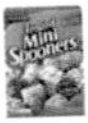

Kellogg's (Cont):

	C	F	Cb
Smart Start, Antioxidants, 1 cup, 1.8 oz	180	1	43
Special K: Original 1 cup, 1.1 oz	120	0.5	23
Blueberry, ¾ cup, 1.1 oz	110	0	26
Fruit & Yogurt, ¾ cup, 1.1 oz	120	1	27
Low Fat Granola, ½ cup, 1.8 oz	190	3	39
Red Berries, 1 cup, 1.1 oz	110	0	27
Vanilla Almond, ¾ cup	110	1.5	25
Malt-O-Meal:			
Apple Zings, 1 cup, 1.15 oz	130	1	30
Blueb. Muffin Tops, ¾ cup	130	3.5	24
Cocoa Dyno-Bites, ¾ cup	120	1	26
Coco Roos, ¾ cup, 1 oz	120	1.5	26
Colossal/Berry Crunch, ¾ cup, 1.1 oz	120	1.5	26
Frosted Flakes, ¾ cup, 1 oz	120	0	28
Frosted Mini Spooners, 1 c.	190	1	45
Golden Puffs, ¾ cup, 0.95 oz	110	0	26
Honey Nut Scooters, 1 cup, 1.1 oz	110	1.5	24
Raisin Bran, 1 cup, 2.08 oz	220	1.5	45
Nature's Path:			
Flax Plus: Maple Pecan Cr., ¾ cup	220	7	38
Pumpkin Raisin Crunch, ¾ cup	210	4.5	40
Raisin Bran Flakes, ¾ cup, 2 oz	190	2.5	41
Heritage Flakes, ¾ cup, 1 oz	120	1	24
Honey'd Cornflakes, ¾ cup, 1 oz	120	0	27
Kamut Puffs, 1 cup, ½ oz	50	0	11
Multigr. Oatbran Flakes, ¾ cup, 1 oz	110	1	24
Qi'a, all varieties, av., 2Tbsp, 1 oz	135	6.5	14
Optimum: Banana Almond, 1.9 oz	190	6	35
Blueb. Cinnamon Flax, 1 cup 2 oz	200	3	38
New England Natural Bakers:			
Granola Pouches:			
Organic Crispy Fruity, ⅔ cup, 1.9 oz	250	9	39
All Natural:			
Banana Walnut, ½ cup, 1.95 oz	260	12	34
Honey Nut Cinn., ½ cup, 2.1 oz	270	12	35
Organic Muesli, ½ cup, 2.1 oz	220	5	40
New Morning:			
Fruit-e-O's, Organic, 1 cup, 1 oz	120	1.5	25
Grahams, Cinn./Honey (2), av., 1.1 oz	130	2.5	24
Oatios, Original, 1 cup, 1 oz	110	2	22

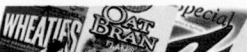

Ready-To-Eat (Cont) | C | F | Cb

NutriSystem: *Per Packet*

	C	F	Cb
Granola, Low-Fat	160	2.5	31
NutriFlakes (40% Bran Flakes)	110	1	23
Whole Grain O's	110	2	19

Peace:

	C	F	Cb
Clusters & Flakes:			
All varieties, average, 1.95 oz	225	2.5	46
Low Fat:			
Hearty Raisin Bran, 1.95 oz	190	2	44
Mango Peach Passion; Wild Berry,			
1 cup, 1.94 oz	225	3	45
Crispy Rice & Flakes,			
Blueberry Pomegranate, 1.95 oz	240	6	41
Granola, all varieties, av., ⅔ cup	240	6	41

Post:

	C	F	Cb
Alpha Bits, 1 cup, 1 oz	110	1	23
Bran Flakes, ¾ cup, 1.1 oz	100	0.5	24
Grape-Nuts: Original, ½ cup	200	1	48
Flakes, ¾ cup, 1 oz	110	1	24
Great Grains:			
Banana Nut Crunch, 1 cup, 2.1 oz	240	6	43
Cranb. Alm. Crunch, ¾ cup, 1.7 oz	180	3	37

Honey Bunches of Oats:

	C	F	Cb
With Almonds, ¾ cup	130	2.5	26
With Vanilla Bunches, 1 cup	220	3	46
Raisin Medley, 1 cup	200	2	42
Honeycomb, Original, 1½ cups	130	1.5	29
Pebbles, all varieties, ¾ cup	120	1	26
Raisin Bran, 1 cup	190	1	46
Selects: Blueberry Morning, 1¼ c.	220	3	45
Maple Pecan Crunch, ¾ cup, 1.83 oz	210	4.5	40
Waffle Crisp, 1 cup, 1 oz	120	2.5	26

Quaker:

	C	F	Cb
Natural Granola:			
Apple Cranberry Almond, 1.7 oz	200	5	37
Oats, Honey, & Alm., ½ cup, 1.7 oz	200	6	35
Honey Graham Oh's, ¾ cup, 0.95 oz	110	2	23
King Vitamin, 1½ c., 1.1 oz	120	1	26
Life, all types, ¾ cup, 1.1 oz	120	1.5	25
Oatmeal Squares:			
Brown Sugar, 1 cup, 2 oz	210	2.5	44
Shredded Wheat, 3 Biscuits, 2.22 oz	220	1.5	50
Whole Hearts, ¾ cup, 1 oz	110	1.5	23

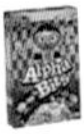

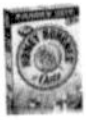

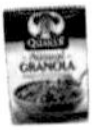

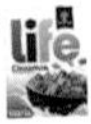

Sweet Home Farm:

	C	F	Cb
Honey Nut Granola,			
½ cup, 1.9 oz	250	10	37
Low-Fat Granola,			
½ cup, 1.9 oz	210	3	44

Stop & Shop:

	C	F	Cb
Oats & O's, ½ cup, 1.8 oz	110	1.5	22
Raisin Bran, 1 cup, 2 oz	190	1	46

Trader Joe's:

	C	F	Cb
Clusters: Raisin Bran, 1 cup, 2 oz	190	3	41
Super Nutty Toffee, ¾ cup, 2 oz	250	9	38
Other flavors, av., ⅔ cup, 1.3 oz	145	3.5	26
Cornflakes, 1.1 oz	110	0	26
Golden Flax Cereal, ¾ cup 1.7 oz	200	3.5	37
Granola: Mango Passion, 2 oz	240	8	37
Pecan Praline, ½ cup, 1.65 oz	210	7	31
Trek Mix, ⅔ cup, 2 oz	240	8	37
High Fiber, ⅔ cup, 1 oz	80	0.5	23
Honey Nut O's, ¾ cup, 1 oz	120	1.5	24
Joe's O's, 1 cup, 1 oz	110	1.5	22
Morning Lite, 1 cup, 1.85 oz	170	2.5	40
Shredded Wheats, Bite Size, 1 c., 1.7 oz	180	1	38
Triple Berry O's, ¾ cup, 1 oz	110	1	25
Toasted Oatmeal Flakes, ¾ cup, 1.1 oz	110	1	23
Wheats, average, 1 cup, 2 oz	200	1	42
Twigs, Flakes & Clusters, 1 c., 1.9 oz	170	1.5	41

Uncle Sam:

	C	F	Cb
Original, ¾ cup, 1.95 oz	190	5	38
Strawberry, ¾ cup, 2.1 oz	240	5	40

Weetabix:

	C	F	Cb
2 biscuits, 1.3 oz	130	1	29

Wegmans: *Per ¾ Cup Unless Indicated*

	C	F	Cb
Chocolaty Rice Crisps, 1 oz	120	1	26
Frosted Flakes, 1 oz	120	0	28
Granola, ½ cup, 1.7 oz	230	9	31
Oats & Honey, with Almonds, 1 oz	130	2	26
Raisin Bran, 1 cup, 2 oz	190	1	46
Squares, Blueberry/Cinnamon, 1 oz	130	3.5	24

Whole Foods (365):

	C	F	Cb
Corn Flakes, 1 cup, 1 oz	110	0	26
Frosted Flakes, ¾ cup, 1 oz	110	0	27
Honey Flakes & Oat Clusters,			
¾ cup, 1 oz	120	1	25
Protein & Fiber, 1 cup, 1.8 oz	190	1	33
Raisin Bran, 1 cup, 2 oz	180	1	44
Wheat Squares:			
Bite Sized, 1.7 oz	180	1	38
Frosted, 1 cup, 1.9 oz	210	1	45

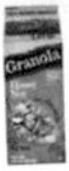

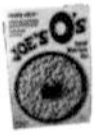

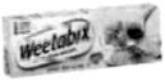

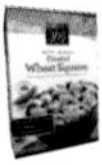

Ready-to-Eat	C	F	Cb
Per Piece/Slice			
Angel Food: Plain: W/out oil, 2 oz	145	0	33
With oil, 2 oz	145	1	27
With Cream Frosting	255	7	45
Almond Croissant, 5 oz	620	35	67
Apple Danish, 5 oz	450	18	67
Apple Pie ~ *See Pies/Tarts Page 134*			
Baklava, 1½" square, 1.75 oz	200	10	27
Banana Cake, w/ Butter Crm, 2 oz	230	9	37
Banana Walnut Cake, 3 oz	270	11	40
Bear Claw, 4.5 oz	540	24	71
Black Forest, 3 oz, (½ cake)	345	11	59
Brownie: Small, 2" Square, 1 oz	130	8	14
Large, 3 oz	390	24	42
Bundt Cakes, average all types:			
3 oz, (⅒ cake)	300	13	42
Mini-Bundt, 5 oz	500	22	70
Cannoli	375	17	44
Carrot Cake: Plain, 3 oz	300	16	37
With Cream Cheese Frosting	400	22	48
Cheesecake: Small serving, 3 oz	235	13	26
Large serving, 5 oz	395	21	44
With Low-Fat Cheese/Fruit, 3 oz	170	4	28
Denny's, NY Style, 5oz	510	34	43
Chocolate Cake:			
With Chocolate Frosting, 4 oz	415	18	62
Without Frosting, ½ of 9", 3.5 oz	340	14	51
Chocolate Croissant, 4.25 oz	470	26	54
Chocolate Eclair, w/ Custard, 3.5 oz	260	16	24
Chocolate Fudge Cake, 3 oz	270	12	40
Chocolate Meringue, ⅙ pie	320	13	48
Churros, 1 stick, 1.5 oz	165	8	21
Cinnamon Crumb Cake, 2.5 oz	260	9	40
Cinnamon Rolls: Small, 2 oz	220	8	34
Regular, 4 oz	440	16	68
Large, 6 oz	660	24	102
Brands ~ *See Page 67*			
Coffee Cake, 2 oz	180	6	30
Concha: Small, 2 oz	240	9	33
Large (5" diameter), 5.5 oz	615	23	85
Cream Puff, (custard fill) 4.6 oz	335	20	30
Cream Horn, 3 oz	210	5	36
Crumble Coffee Cake, 4.5 oz	500	25	65
Danish Pastries:			
Small, 2.5 oz	250	14	25
Large, 5 oz	500	28	50
Donuts ~ *See Page 66*			
Eclair, Chocolate, Custard fill, 3.5 oz	260	16	24
Fig Bars, average	160	3	31

Ready-to-Eat (Cont)	C	F	Cb
Per Piece/Slice			
Fruit Cake, Dark/Light, 2 oz	185	5	34
Fudge Nut Brownie, (1), 3.5 oz	380	18	54
Gingerbread, from mix, 3" square	210	4	41
Honey Bun, 2.7 oz	310	15	39
Jelly Roll, ½ roll, 1.8 oz	150	2	32
Key Lime Pie, 4.3 oz	400	25	41
Lady Finger, 3 oz	310	4.5	59
Lemon Cake, 4 oz	440	24	49
Lemon Poppy Seed Creme, 1.6 oz	180	9	23
Marble Cake, 4 oz	430	23	50
Mississippi Mud Pie, 4 oz	480	22	67
Mud Cake, 4.5 oz	380	20	44
Muffins ~ *See Page 67*			
Palmier Cookie, large, 4.5 oz	490	25	62
Pineapple Upside Down Cake,			
2.5 oz	230	9	36
Peach Melba, 3.5 oz	300	8	52
Pecan Sticky Roll, 6.5 oz	690	22	91
Pecan Twirls, 1.3 oz	170	7	26
Pies & Tarts ~ *See Page 134*			
Pound Cakes: Iced Lemon, 3.5 oz	360	17	50
Marble, 3.75 oz	350	13	53
Raspberry Rugulah,			
1.2 oz	110	9	7
Scone, fruit, 2 oz	200	9	30
Sponge Cake: Plain, 2.5 oz	220	10	33
With Chocolate Frosting	290	12	45
With Cream & Strawberry Jam	390	12	69
Starbucks Cakes ~ *Page 244*			
Strawberry Creme Cake, 4.7 oz	400	27	33
Strudel Bites, ¾ oz	60	2.5	9
Strudel, fruit, av., 4.4 oz	300	17	32
Swiss Rolls,	135	6	19
Tiramisu, 4.4 oz	440	22	34
Turnovers, fruit, average, 3 oz	290	15	35

Cupcakes	C	F	Cb
Average all Varieties			
Regular:			
Cake only, 1.5 oz	140	5.5	20
Cake + Icing, 2.5 oz	260	13	34
Large, (Muffin Size):			
Cake only, 2.5 oz	235	9	34
Cake + Icing, 5 oz	520	27	67
Mini, (2-Bite):			
Cake only, 0.4 oz	40	1.5	5.5
Cake + Icing, 1 oz	110	5.5	13
Icing Only: Per 1 oz	115	7	13
Thick/Tall amount, 2.5 oz	290	17	32

Cakes ~ Brands (C) (F) (Cb)

Albertson's Bakery:

Ring Cakes: *Per 1/6 Cake*

	C	F	Cb
Angel Food, 2 oz	160	0	36
Butter, 3 oz	310	16	39
Chocolate, 3 oz	300	14	38

Cake Slices:

	C	F	Cb
Banana Nut Loaf	330	17	39
Butter Creme	110	6	20
Creme Cake (2), 3.17 oz	300	12	43
Cinnamon Streusel (2), 3.17 oz	350	18	43

Bimbo Bakery:

	C	F	Cb
Concha, Vanilla, 2.1 oz	260	11	35
Pound Cakes: Mini 1.76 oz	170	4.5	29
Pecan, 2.25 oz	260	11	36
Raisin, 2.25 oz	240	9	38

Bon Appetit Bakery:

	C	F	Cb
Banana Bread	440	25	49
Cream Cheese Cake, 4 oz slice	430	24	49
Danish: Apple (1), 5 oz	420	22	50
Bear Claw (1), 5 oz	480	26	54
Cheese & Berries (1), 5 oz	500	28	52
Vienna Cream (1), 5 oz	480	28	54
Sliced: Cheesecake, 4 oz	430	24	49
Lemon Cake, 4 oz	430	24	49
Marble Cake, 4 oz	430	24	50
Walnut Brownie, 3.5 oz	380	18	54

Cheesecake Factory ~ *See Fast-Foods Section*

Entenmann's: *Per Slice*

	C	F	Cb
Crumb Cakes: All Butter French, 1.75 oz	210	10	29
Other varieties, average, 2 oz	255	13	34
Danish: Pecan Danish Ring, 2 oz	240	15	24
Cheese-Filled Crumb Coffee, 1.9 oz	200	10	25
Raspberry Danish Twist, 2 oz	220	11	29
Dessert Cakes: Ban. Crunch, 1.75 oz	200	9	29
Carrot, Iced, 2.36 oz	260	12	37
Chocolate Fudge, 2.25 oz	240	10	37
Iced Cake, Red Velvet, 1/8 cake	270	14	36
Loaf Cakes: Chocolate, 1/6 loaf	190	8	29
Cinnamon Crunch, 1/6 loaf	270	14	33

Muffins/Sweet Rolls ~ *See Page 67*

Glenny's: (C) (F) (Cb)

100 Calorie:

	C	F	Cb
Blondie, 1.45 oz	100	4	15
Brownies: Chocolate Chip, 1.45 oz	100	4	12
Peanut Butter, 1.45 oz	100	4	15

Great American Cookies:

Cookie Cakes: *Per Slice*

	C	F	Cb
By the Slice, 4.6 oz	580	27	83
Heart Shaped, 3.5 oz	440	21	64
M&M, 1 slice, 4 oz	500	24	73

Great Value *(Walmart)*:

	C	F	Cb
Devil's Food Cake (1)	160	7	23
Fudge & Crème Soft Cookies (1), 1.2 oz	150	6	22
Swiss Rolls (2), 2.2 oz	250	10	38

Little Debbie:

	C	F	Cb
100 Calories: Choc. Cake (1), 1 oz	100	3	17
Yellow Cake with Icing (1), 1 oz	100	3	18
Brownie: Choc Chip (1), 2.2 oz	270	11	41
Fudge (1), 2.15 oz	280	12	40
Choc. Cup Cake (1)	210	8	33
Cocoa Creme (1), 1.4 oz	170	8	24
Coffee Cake (1)	190	5	35
Devil Creme (1), 1.65 oz	200	9	29
Devil Squares (2), 2.2 oz	260	11	38
Fancy Cake (2)	300	13	44
Frosted Fudge Cake, 1.5 oz	190	9	27
Star Crunch (1)	150	6	22
S'mores (1)	190	7	30
Strawberry Shortcake Roll, 2.1 oz	240	9	40
Swiss Cake Roll (2), 2.15 oz	270	12	38
Zebra Cake (2), 2.6 oz	320	14	48

Nemo's:

	C	F	Cb
Brookie, (1), 1.5 oz	160	7	26
Cake Squares: Banana, 3 oz	300	12	45
Carrot, 3.6 oz	390	21	47
Chocolate, 3 oz	300	12	44
Crumble Cake: Blueb. (1), 3.9 oz	390	17	54
Cinnamon Streusel (1), 3.9 oz	420	18	59
Lemon Raspberry (1), 3.9 oz	400	19	55

Oreo:

	C	F	Cb
Brownie, Creme Filled, 1.5 oz	190	9	25

Soft Cakesters:

	C	F	Cb
Chocolate (2), 2 oz	250	12	36
Double Stuf (2), 2.65 oz pkt	350	18	48
Golden (2), 1.76 oz	220	10	32

C · Cakes, Pastries ~ Packaged

Cakes ~ Brands (Cont)

	C	F	Cb
Pepperidge Farm:			
3-Layer Cakes: *Per ⅛ Cake*			
Devil's Food	220	9	34
Key Lime	230	11	31
Orange Cream	210	9	32
Other varieties, av.	240	11	33
Turnovers (Frozen):			
Apple; Cherry (1)	260	13	31
Peach; Raspberry (1)	270	13	34
Pop Tarts *(Kellogg's):*			
Fruit/Frosted, average	200	5	36
Whole Grain & Fiber, low fat, all varieties, av., 1.75 oz	180	3	37
Mini Crisps, all flavors, 1 pouch	100	2.5	18
Safeway Select,			
Molten Choc. Lava Cake, 4.5 oz	440	26	50
Sara Lee:			
Cakes: Carrot, ⅙ cake	340	18	41
Cheesecake: *Per Slice*			
Original Cream, ¼ cake, 4.2 oz	340	18	38
Original Cream, Strawberry ⅙ cake, 4.8 oz	310	11	49
French, with Strawberry Topping, ⅙ cake, 4.3 oz	320	18	37
New York Style Classic, ⅙ cake, 5 oz	480	29	48
Pound Cakes:			
Butter, ¼ cake	300	16	35
Individually Wrapped Slices, Orig.; Double Choc.,1 slice, av.	170	6	27
Smart Ones *(Weight Watchers):*			
Smart Delights: *4 Pack*			
Brownie à la Mode, 2.15 oz	130	2.5	24
Chocolate Fudge Brownie, 2.1 oz	140	3.5	24
Double Fudge Cake, 1.94 oz	140	3	26
Key Lime Pie, 2.92oz	150	2.5	28
Raspb. Cheesecake	130	3.5	22
Strawb. Shortcake, 2.36 oz	120	4	19
Sundaes, all varieties, average	140	3	25
Special K, Pastry Crisps (2), all varieties, 0.9 oz	100	2	20

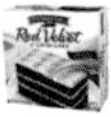

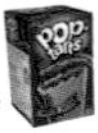

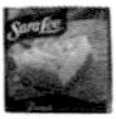

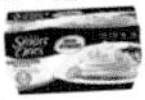

	C	F	Cb
Tastykake:			
Cream Filled Cupcakes: *Per 3 Cakes*			
Chocolate, w/ Vanilla Icing, 3.5 oz	390	15	60
Crumb Topped Koffee, 3.5 oz	370	17	52
Kandy Kake, Peanut Butter (3) 2 oz	270	16	30
Krimpets, Butterscotch (3), 3 oz	350	10	60
Toaster Strudel *(Pillsbury):* *Per 2 oz*			
Boston Cream Pie	170	7	25
Cream Cheese, av.	185	9	24
Fruit flavors, all var.	170	7	25
Trader Joe's:			
Bakery:			
Apricot Almond Tart, ⅙, 4 oz	450	24	56
Cheesecake Brownie Bites (1)	110	7	9
Chocolate Ganache Cake, ⅛ 3 oz	390	22	44
Flourless Chocolate Cake, 1 piece, 2 oz	260	17	23
Lemon Cake, ⅛, 3.25 oz	350	19	43
Mini Bundt, Triple Choc., ½ cake	340	21	41
Mini Carrot Cake, 5 oz	450	19	68
Whoopie Pie (1), 2.5 oz	350	14	54
Bread Cake:			
Banana Bonanza, ⅙, 2.65 oz	250	9	39
Pumpkin Nut, ⅟₇, 2.65 oz	270	10	43
Walnut Streusel Coffee, ⅟₁₂, 2 oz	180	8	25
Zucchini Carrot, ⅛, 2 oz	200	7	32
Loaf Cakes:			
Cranberry Pumpkin, ⅛, 2 oz	140	2	30
Pumpkin Nut, ⅟₇, 2.65 oz	270	10	43
Frozen Dessert:			
Apple Raspb. Turnovers, 3.17 oz	280	14	34
Chocolate Dilemma Cheesecake:			
Plain, 3.5 oz	320	19	30
Choc. Chip; Triple Choc, 3.5 oz, av.	345	20	35
Tuxedo, 3.5 oz	320	17	34
Choc Lava Cake (1), 3.8 oz	360	23	40
Karat Cake, ⅛, 2.9 oz	320	19	37
N.Y. Style Cheesecake, ⅟₇, 4.5 oz	400	28	32
Tiramisu Torte, ⅟₇, 3.2 oz	230	12	24
Tarts: Pear, ⅙, 3.5 oz	250	9	39
Raspberry, ¼, 4.83 oz	290	10	51
Wild Blueberry, ⅙, 3.5 oz	260	6	52

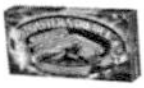

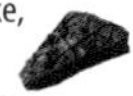

Cakes ~ Mixes

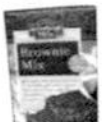

Prepared as Directed	C	F	Cb
Arrowhead Mills:			
Brownie Mix:			
Chocolate Chip, 1/20 pkg	150	7	21
Gluten Free, 1/20 pkg	160	8	21
Cake Mix: Choc., org., 1/12, 1.55 oz	260	11	39
Vanilla, 1/12, 1.73 oz	260	10	41
Betty Crocker:			
Bars: Caramelita, 1/16 pkg	190	8	28
Reese's, 1/15 pkg	180	13	20
Sunkist Lemon, 1/16 pkg	140	4	24
Brownie Mix: *Per 1/20 Pkg Unless Indicated*			
Dark Chocolate Fudge	160	7	24
Fudge	170	8	23
Low-Fat Fudge, 1/18 pkg	140	3	28
Premium: Choc. Chunk	170	7	27
Original Supreme	160	6	27
Peanut Butter; Walnut, average	160	6	25
Triple Chunk	170	6	28
Cake Mixes:			
Decadent Supreme:			
Chocolate Molten Lava, 1/8 pkg	290	14	38
Cinnamon Swirl, 1/12 pkg	240	9	39
SuperMoist: *Per 1/10 Pkg, 1.5 oz Mix*			
Butter Recipe Yellow	240	9	38
Carrot	310	18	35
Cherry Chip	280	14	36
Devil's Food	280	14	35
Milk Chocolate, 1/10 pkg	250	10	35
Other Choc. varieties, average	280	14	35

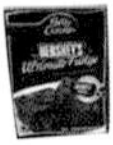

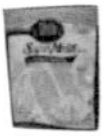

If using No-Cholesterol Recipe, deduct 40 cals and 4g fat.

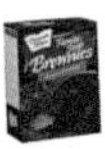

	C	F	Cb
Cupcakes:			
FUN da-Middles: *Per 0.8 oz Mix & 0.42 oz Filling*			
Choc./Yellow Cake, Van. Filling	200	9	27
Yellow Cake, Choc Filling	190	9	25
Duncan Hines:			
Brownie Mix: *Per 1/20 Pkg Unless Indicated*			
Decadent, Caramel Turtle, 1/16	150	7	23
Premium: Chewy Fudge	180	8	24
Snack Size, 1/12 pkg	140	7	20
Milk Chocolate	160	8	21
Cake Mix: *Per 1/12 Pkg*			
Classic, Dark Chocolate Fudge, 1/12 pkg, 1.4oz	220	11	28

Updated Nutrition Data ~ www.CalorieKing.com
Persons with Diabetes ~ See Disclaimer (Page 22)

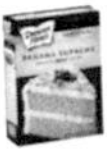

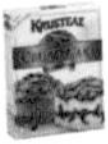

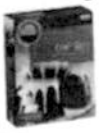

Prepared as Directed	C	F	Cb
Duncan Hines Cont:			
Decadent: Apple Caramel	280	12	39
Classic Carrot; Triple Chocolate, av.	265	11	39
Signature:			
Banana Supreme	270	12	36
Coconut Supreme	250	11	34
French Vanilla	270	12	34
Jell-O:			
No Bake Cheesecake:			
Cherry, 1/9 pkg, 2.43 oz	290	11	48
Homestyle, 1/6 pkg, 2 oz	360	15	51
Strawberry, 1/9 pkg, 2.43 oz	290	10	48
Krusteaz: Cinn. Crumb Cake, 2"	220	5	40
Lemon; Key Lime Bar, 2½x2" bar	160	4.5	29
Pillsbury:			
Brownies, Premium Mix: *Dry Mix Only*			
Caramel Swirl, 1/12 pkt, 1.2 oz	130	3	26
Cheesecake Swirl, 1/18 pkt, 0.85 oz	100	2.5	19
Chocolate Extreme, 1/16 pkt, 1 oz	120	3	22
Minis, with Caramel Filling			
2 Brownies, 1/6 package	140	4	25
Cakes, Moist Supreme: *Per 1/10 Pkg, Dry Mix Only*			
Classic White/Yellow, 1.52 oz	160	4	34
Devils Food, Regular, 1.52 oz	160	3	34
Supreme Collection: *Per 1/12 Pkg, Dry Mix Only*			
Apple Spice, 1.83 oz	160	3.5	33
Fudge Truffle, 1.83 oz	200	4.5	40
Red Velvet, 1.83 oz	200	5	41

Cake Frostings

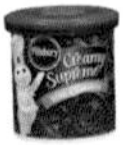

	C	F	Cb
Betty Crocker:			
Rich & Creamy, av., 2 T., 1.15 oz	140	6	23
Whipped, all var., av., 2 T., 0.85 oz	100	4.5	15
Duncan Hines:			
Creamy Homestyle, all var., av., 2T.	140	6	23
Whipped, all varieties, av., 3 Tbsp	150	8	23
Pillsbury: *Per 2 Tbsp*			
Creamy Supreme:			
Choc Fudge; Milk Choc., 1.15 oz	130	6	20
Classic White, 1.15 oz	140	5	22
Vanilla; Vanilla Funfetti, 1.2 oz	140	5	22
Sugar Free, Chocolate Fudge	100	6	18
Whipped Supreme, av. all flavors	100	5	14

Quick Guide

Donuts	C	F	Cb
Average All Brands			
Cake: Plain, 1¾ oz	205	12	23
Chocolate Iced, 2 oz	255	14	29
Sugared 1¾ oz	205	10	29
Non-Cake, Glazed, 2 oz	225	11	29

Donuts ~ Brands

	C	F	Cb
Albertson's:			
Donut Holes:			
Glazed Old Fashioned (4)	240	12	31
Powdered Sugar (4), 1.7 oz	210	12	24
Gem Donuts: Plain Cake (3), 1.6 oz	190	12	20
Cinnamon Sugar (3), 1.8 oz	240	15	23
Glazed (1), 1.6 oz	140	6	21
Bon Appetit:			
Mini Donuts: Chocolate (4)	290	17	31
Crumb (4), average	270	13	36
Powdered (4)	240	12	32
Dolly Madison:			
Regular, 1.75 oz	270	12	40
Donut Gems,			
Powdered Mini's (4), 2 oz	230	11	31
Dunkin' Donuts:			
Apple Crumb	490	18	80
Apple N' Spice	270	14	32
Barvarian Kreme	270	15	31
Blueberry Cake	340	17	44
Blueberry Crumb	500	18	84
Boston Kreme	310	16	39
Bow Tie	310	15	39
Chocolate Frosted Cake	370	23	45
Chocolate Frosted Cocoa	270	13	32
Chocolate Glazed Cake	370	24	35
Cinnamon Cake	340	22	38
Cocoa Boston Kreme	300	16	37
Cocoa Butternut	280	13	37
Cocoa Glazed	260	13	32
Glazed Cake	360	22	44
Jelly Filled	290	14	36
Old Fashioned Cake	320	22	33
Powdered Cake	340	22	38
Sugar Raised	230	14	22
Vanilla Kreme Filled	380	23	42

Donuts ~ Brands (Cont)

	C	F	Cb
Entenmann's:			
8 Pack: Per Donut			
Chocolate Lovers, 2 oz	300	20	31
Crumb, 2 oz	250	12	36
Frosted Devil's, 2.35 oz	310	18	36
Glazed Buttermilk, 2.25 oz	270	13	37
Rich Frosted, 2 oz	300	20	30
Pop'ems (bite size):			
Frosted (4), 2 oz	320	23	28
Powdered (4), 2 oz	250	13	31
Great Value (Walmart):			
Minis: Chocolate Frosted (4)	280	16	32
Powdered (4)	210	10	30
Krispy Kreme:			
Apple Fritter	210	14	18
Baseball Donut	290	17	33
Chocolate Iced Cake	280	15	34
Chocolate: Iced Custard Filled	310	17	36
Iced Glazed Cruller	260	12	38
Iced Glazed	240	11	33
Iced Kreme Filled	360	21	40
Iced Glazed w/ Sprinkles	250	11	35
Cinnamon Twist	240	15	23
Glazed Cruller	220	12	27
Glazed Doughnut Holes:			
Original (4)	200	11	26
Blueberry	190	8	26
Chocolate Cake	190	9	25
Glazed Kreme Filled	340	20	38
Maple Iced Glazed	230	11	32
New York Cheesecake	350	21	36
Original Glazed	190	11	21
Powdered Cake	220	11	27
Traditional Cake	190	12	19
Little Debbie,			
Donut Sticks (1), 1.65 oz	230	14	25
Tastykake:			
Cinnamon, 1.8 oz	210	11	26
Mini: Coated, 3 oz	380	22	42
Powdered Sugar (6), 2.5 oz	280	13	37

Quick Guide | C | F | Cb

Muffins: Ready-To-Eat
Average All Types:

	C	F	Cb
Small, 1 oz	90	3.5	14
Medium, 2 oz	185	6.5	28
Large, 3 oz	275	10	42
Extra Large, 4 oz	365	13	57
Giant, 6 oz	550	20	84
Super Size, 8 oz	730	27	112

Brands ~ Ready-To-Eat

	C	F	Cb
Albertsons:			
Minis: Banana Nut (2)	200	12	20
Blueberry (2)	180	10	21
Honey Raisin Bran (2)	170	7	24
Entenmann's: *Per Muffin*			
Individually wrapped, all varieties	190	9	26
Little Bites, all varieties, 1.65 oz	180	8	25
Fiber One *(General Mills):*			
4-Pack, av., 1 muffin, 2.3 oz	175	4.5	35
3-Pack, av., 1 muffin, 2.3 oz	195	4	36
Great Value *(Walmart),*			
Double Blueberry (1), 4 oz	430	16	65
Little Debbie: Banana Nut (1), 1.9 oz	210	9	30
Blueberry (1), 1.9 oz	190	8	27
Chocolate Chip (1), 1.9 oz	210	9	28
My Favorite Muffin: *Per 6 oz Muffin*			
Banana Nut	585	33	63
Blueberry	505	24	66
Boston Cream Pie	530	21	78
Chocolate Chip	635	33	81
Lemon Poppyseed	605	30	75
Otis Spunkmeyer: *Per 4 oz Muffin*			
Banana Nut	440	22	58
Chocolate Chip	420	24	54
Wild Blueberry	400	16	56
Starbucks ~ *See Fast-Foods Section*			
Trader Joe's: *Per Muffin*			
Apple Cranberry, 4.8 oz	220	5	38
Banana Chocolate Chip, 4 oz	400	18	57
Carrot, 4 oz	320	11	52
Triple Berry (1), 4 oz	310	11	49
Vitalicious:			
VitaMuffins: All varieties, av., 2 oz	100	1	24
Large, all varieties, av., 4 oz	200	2	50
Sugar-Free, Banana Nut, 2 oz	90	2.5	21
VitaTops: All varieties, av., 2 oz	100	1.5	24
Sugar free, all varieties, av., 2 oz	90	2.5	22
Weight Watchers,			
Blueb.; Double Choc, av., 2.5 oz	185	2.5	42

Muffin Mixes | C | F | Cb
Per Muffin, Prepared

	C	F	Cb
Betty Crocker: Banana Nut	210	9	27
Cinnamon Streusel	210	9	30
Wild Blueberry	180	7	26
Pouch Mix:			
Banana Nut	120	3	23
Blueberry	120	2.5	23
Choc Chip	130	3.5	22
Triple Berry	120	3	23
Krusteaz: Banana Nut	250	13	29
Choc Chunk	260	13	32
Lemon Poppyseed	170	4.5	30
Oat Bran	180	4.5	31
Trader Joe's, Triple Berry	150	2	28

Sweet Rolls & Buns | C | F | Cb

Note: It is best to weigh for accuracy as actual weight can be 10-50% higher than label weight

	C	F	Cb
Bimbo, Bimbolete (1), 2.2 oz	240	9	36
Bon Appetit,			
Cinnamon Roll, 2.5 oz	230	8	34
Cinnabon: Classic	880	36	127
Caramel Pecanbon	1080	50	147
Cloverhill Bakery,			
Jumbo Honey Bun, 4.75 oz	600	35	64
Entenmann's,			
Cinnamon Swirl Bun (1), 3 oz	320	14	44
Little Debbie: Honey Buns, 1.75 oz	230	13	26
Pecan Spinwheels, 1 oz	100	4	16
McDonald's,			
Cinnamon Melts, 4 oz	460	20	66
Pillsbury:			
Sweet Rolls, Refrigerated:			
Cinnamon, with Icing:			
All varieties (1)	140	5	23
Red. Fat (1)	130	3.5	24
Mini-Bites w/ Icing (3)	160	4.5	27
Orange Flavored (1), 1.7 oz	160	6	26
Twists, Flaky Cinnamon, w/ Icing (1)	160	7	23
Grands:			
Cinnabon with Cream Cheese (1)	300	8	54
Other Varieties (1), 3.5 oz	300	8	54
Flaky Supreme Cinnabon,			
all varieties (1), 3.5 oz	360	17	48
7-Eleven, Iced Honey Bun, 4.75 oz	520	24	71
Sara Lee, Cinnamon Rolls, 1 roll	260	12	33

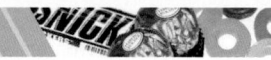

Quick Guide

Chocolate

	C	F	Cb
Average All Brands			
Milk Chocolate, regular:			
Plain/Nuts/Fruit, average, 1 oz	150	9	17
1.5oz Bar	230	13	25
2 oz Bar	305	17	34
4 oz Block	610	34	68
8 oz Block	1220	68	136
1 Pound, 16 oz	2440	136	272
Dark/White Chocolate, 1 oz	155	9	17
Sugar Free (Hershey's), 1 piece, 0.3 oz	40	2	5
Milk Chocolate-Coated:			
Almonds, 5-6, 1 oz	150	10	15
Clusters, Nut, 3 pieces, 1.2 oz	210	14	20
Coffee Beans, 1.4 oz	220	13	22
Cherry Cordial Centers, 2 pcs, 1 oz	145	6	21
Macadamias, 10 pieces, 1.4 oz	220	16	21
Mints, 1 medium, ½ oz	55	1	11
Nougat & Caramel, 1 oz	150	9	15
Peanuts, 12 medium, 1 oz	145	10	14
Raisins, 28 medium, 1 oz	110	4	19
Baking Chocolate:			
Bittersweet (Baker's), 1 oz	140	12	14
Semi-sweet (Baker's), 1 oz	140	9	16
Chips (Nestle): Dark, 1 T., ½ oz	70	5	3
Semi-Sweet, 1 Tbsp, ½ oz	70	4	9
Unsweetened, 1 oz	140	14	8
Carob, Plain, 1 oz	155	9	16

Brands & Generic

Per Piece/Serving	C	F	Cb
3 Musketeers: Orig., 1 bar, 2.15 oz	260	8	46
2 To Go, 1.65 oz Bar	200	6	35
Fun Size (3), 1.6 oz	190	6	34
Minis, 7 pieces, 1.4 oz	170	5	32
100 Grand: 1.5 oz bar	190	8	30
Super Size, 2.8 oz	360	14	58
Snack Size (1), ¾ oz	95	4	15
Abba Zabba, 2 oz bar	250	5	48
After Dinner Mints, 1 small	25	1.5	3
After Eight Mint (Nestlé), each	35	1.5	4
Airhead, 1 bar, ½ oz	60	1	14
Almond Joy: 2 bars, 1.6 oz	220	13	26
King Size, 3.25 oz	460	26	54
Snack, 0.6 oz bar	80	4.5	10
Pieces (46), 1.4 oz	200	10	27

Brands & Generic (Cont)

Per Piece/Serving	C	F	Cb
Almond Roca, 3 pieces, 1.25 oz	200	15	17
Almonds, sugar-coated (15), 1.4 oz	190	7	27
Almond Clusters:			
1 oz (True North)	170	12	9
1.2 oz (Trader Joe's)	190	14	13
Altoids (C & B), 3 pieces	10	0	2
Andes, Thins, av., all flav. (8), 1.4 oz	205	13	22
Anthon Berg:			
Creamy Mint (4), 1.4 oz	180	6	31
Marzipan with Plum, in Madeira	120	6	14
Atomic Fireball, 1 piece, 0.3 oz	35	0	9
Baby Ruth: King Size, 3.7 oz bar	500	24	66
2.1 oz bar	280	14	39
Fun size, 1.7 oz	170	8	24
Minis, 4 bars	210	11	28
Baci (Perugina),			
1 piece, ½ oz	75	6	7
Baskin-Robbins: Sugar Candy, 3 pcs	60	1	12
Sugar Free, 4 pieces, 0.6 oz av	40	1	15
Big Hunk, 2 oz Bar	230	3	47
Bit-O-Honey: 1.7 oz	180	3.5	39
Chews, 6 pieces, 1.4 oz	150	3	32
Bliss (Hershey's):			
Milk/Dark Choc./Caramel, 6 pcs	210	14	21
Meltaway Centers:			
Milk Choc, 6 pieces	220	15	24
Raspberry, 6 pieces	220	14	24
Blow Pops, each, 0.6 oz	60	0	17
Bon Bons, 3 pieces	65	0	15
Boston Baked Beans, (11), ½ oz	70	2	11
Brach's: Almond Supremes (10)	200	14	20
Bridge Mix (15), 1.4 oz	190	10	26
Double Dippers (15), 1.4 oz	210	14	22
Gummi Bears (14), 1.4 oz	130	0	30
Lemon Drops,			
Sugar Free, 4 pieces	35	0	17
(Note: Carbs include 16g Sugar Alcohols)			
Mandarin/Orange Slices (3), 1.6 oz	150	0	37
Maple Nut Goodies (8), 1.5 oz	190	9	27
Milk Maid Caramel (4), 1.4 oz	150	4	25
Peanut Butter Poppins (25), 1.5 oz	200	11	24
Peanut Cluster (3)	210	15	20
Breath Savers, all types, each	5	0	2
Bubble Gum ~ See 'Gum' Page 75			
Bulls Eyes, 3 pieces, 1.2 oz	130	3	23
Buncha Crunch, ⅓ cup, 1.4 oz	180	9	25
Movie Box, 3.2 oz	450	20	65
Burnt Peanuts, (31), 1.4 oz	170	6	29

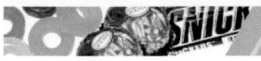

Brands & Generic (Cont)

Per Piece/Serving	C	F	Cb
Butterfinger: 2.1 oz bar	270	11	43
King Size (3 bars), 3.7 oz	480	18	75
Fun Size, (1), 0.75	100	4	15
Giant, (Pieces in Chocolate), ¼ bar, 1 oz	150	8	21
Miniatures:			
1 piece, 0.35 oz	45	2	7.5
4 pieces, 1.4 oz	180	8	29
Snack Pack, 4 pcs, 1.4 oz	180	7	29
Crisp Bar: Original, 2 oz bar	270	11	43
King Size, 3 pcs, 2 oz	310	17	38
Minis, 2 bars, 1.4 oz	210	11	25
Snackerz:			
Single, 1 pouch, 1.25 oz	170	8	23
Fun Size, 2 pcs, 1.2 oz	150	7	21
King Size, 10 pcs, 1.4 oz	190	8	25
Butter Mints, 7 pieces, 0.45 oz	50	0	12
Butterscotch: 3 pieces	60	0	15
Discs (Walgreens), 3 pieces, 0.63 oz	70	0	17
Cadbury: Caramello Bar, 1.6 oz	220	10	29
Caramel Egg, 1.2 oz	170	8	22
Dairy Milk Bar, 7 pieces, 1.4 oz	200	11	23
Mini Eggs (Candy), 12 pcs, 1.4 oz	190	8	28
Candy Apple, medium, 6.5 oz	280	0	60
Candy Cane, medium, 5", ½ oz	40	0	14
Candy Corn, 20 pieces, 1 oz	150	0	38
Candy Jar Mix (Jewel), (3), 0.6 oz	60	0	14
Candy Necklace (Smarties), (1), 0.75 oz	90	0.5	20
Caramels: Each, 0.35 oz	40	1	8
Chocolate, each, 0.23 oz	25	0.3	6
Creams (3), 1.25 oz	130	3	23
Caramel Popcorn, ⅔ cup	150	6	27
Cella's Cherries, 3 pieces, 1.5 oz	160	6	27
Certs, Breath Mints, 1 piece	5	0	2
Charleston Chew:			
Chocolate Bar (1), 1.4 oz	160	4.5	30
Mini, 1.5 oz	190	6	34
Charms: Blow Pop	60	0	17
Flat Pop, ½ oz	50	0	14
Chew-ets, Peanut Chews, Original (4), 1.65 oz	230	12	29
Chewz, 1 roll, 1 oz	120	1	28
Chick O Stick, 2 oz	240	9	42
Chocolate Parfait Nips, 2 pieces	60	2	11

Per Piece/Serving	C	F	Cb
Chunky Bar (Nestlé), King Size, 2.5 oz	340	19	44
Chupa Chups, 1 Pop	50	0	12
Cinn. Buttons (Walgreens), 3 pcs	60	0	18
Cinnamon Disks (Walmart), 3 pcs	70	0	18
Circus Peanuts (Spangler), 6 pieces, 1.35 oz	165	0	41
CocoaVia, Orig., 0.8 oz	100	6	12
Coconut Stacks, (8)	320	16	46
Coffee Go, Candy, (4)	60	1	12
Coffee Rio-Gold, Sugar Free, (4)	45	1.5	10
Conversation Hearts (Necco), 1 lge	10	0	3
Cookie Dough Bites, 1.4 oz	200	10	27
Cote d'Or: Dark 86% Coca, 3.5 oz	605	55	19
Dark, 70%, Orange, 3.5 oz	575	46	34
Dark, Raspberry, 3.5 oz	580	46	34
Milk, Intense, 3.5 oz	575	40	45
Cotton Candy, 1 oz	110	0	28
Cough Drops ~ See Page 75			
Cracker Jack, ½ cup, 1 oz	120	2	23
Creme Savers ~ See Lifesavers			
Crisped Rice, Choc Chip, 1 bar, 1 oz	115	4	20
Crows, 11 pieces, 1.4 oz	130	0	33
Dots, 11 dots, 1.4 oz	130	0	33
Double Dip Stick, 1 stick	16	0.5	3
Dove:			
Milk Choc: Singles Bar, 1.4 oz	220	13	24
Large Tablet Bar, 9 pcs, 1.48 oz	230	13	25
Choc. Covered Almonds, 13 pcs, 1.4 oz	220	15	19
Promises: Milk Choc., 1 pc, 0.3 oz	45	2.5	5
With Caramel, 1 piece, 0.3 oz	40	2	5
W/ Peanut Butter, 1 pc, 0.3 oz	45	3	4
Swirls, all varieties, 9 pieces 1.5 oz	230	14	25
Dark Choc: Singles Bar, 1.3 oz	220	13	24
Large Tablet Bar, 9 pcs, 1.5 oz	220	14	25
Choc. Covered. Almds, 13 pcs, 1.4 oz	210	15	19
Promises, Almond, 1 piece, 0.3 oz	40	3	4
Swirls, Raspberry, 9 pieces, 1.4 oz	220	14	24
Sugar Free, all flav., 5 pcs, 1.4 oz	195	15	21
Dum Dum Pops (Spangler), 1 pop	25	0	7
Drops (Hershey's):			
Milk Chocolate, 15 pieces, 1.4 oz	200	12	25
Cookies 'n' Creme, 14 pieces, 1.45 oz	210	11	26

Brands & Generic (Cont)

Per Piece/Serving	C	F	Cb
English Toffee, 1 piece, 0.4 oz	70	4	6
5th Avenue: 2 oz bar	260	12	38
King Size, 3.4 oz 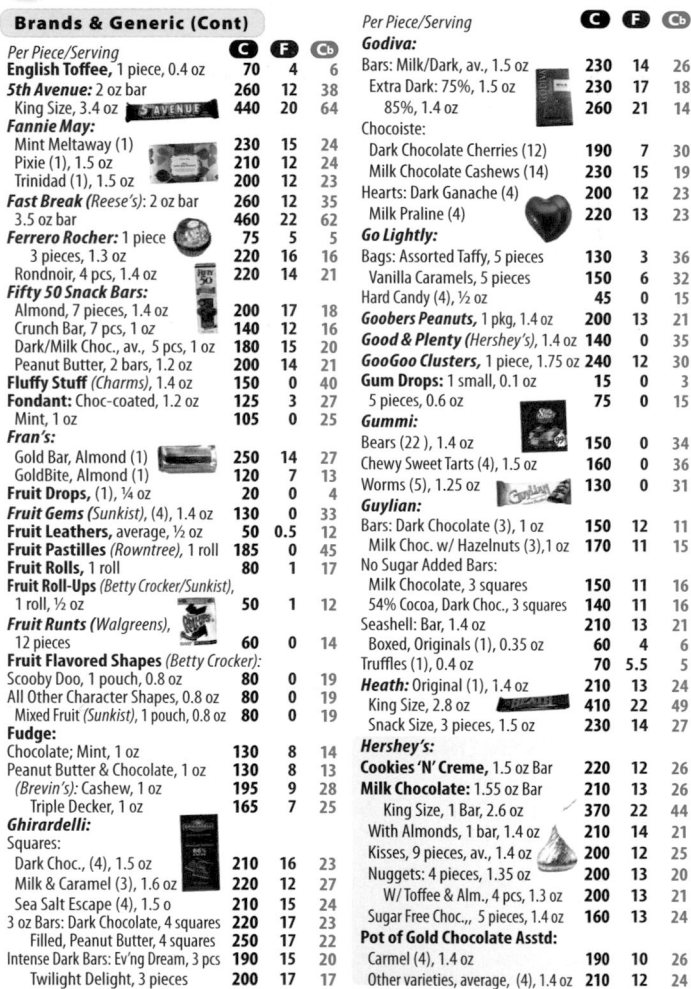	440	20	64
Fannie May:			
Mint Meltaway (1)	230	15	24
Pixie (1), 1.5 oz	210	12	24
Trinidad (1), 1.5 oz	200	12	23
***Fast Break** (Reese's):* 2 oz bar	260	12	35
3.5 oz bar	460	22	62
Ferrero Rocher: 1 piece	75	5	5
3 pieces, 1.3 oz	220	16	16
Rondnoir, 4 pcs, 1.4 oz	220	14	21
Fifty 50 Snack Bars:			
Almond, 7 pieces, 1.4 oz	200	17	18
Crunch Bar, 7 pcs, 1 oz	140	12	16
Dark/Milk Choc., av., 5 pcs, 1 oz	180	15	20
Peanut Butter, 2 bars, 1.2 oz	200	14	21
Fluffy Stuff (Charms), 1.4 oz	150	0	40
Fondant: Choc-coated, 1.2 oz	125	3	27
Mint, 1 oz	105	1	25
Fran's:			
Gold Bar, Almond (1)	250	14	27
GoldBite, Almond (1)	120	7	13
Fruit Drops, (1), ¼ oz	20	0	4
Fruit Gems (Sunkist), (4), 1.4 oz	130	0	33
Fruit Leathers, average, ½ oz	50	0.5	12
Fruit Pastilles (Rowntree), 1 roll	185	0	45
Fruit Rolls, 1 roll	80	1	17
Fruit Roll-Ups (Betty Crocker/Sunkist),			
1 roll, ½ oz	50	1	12
Fruit Runts (Walgreens),			
12 pieces	60	0	14
Fruit Flavored Shapes (Betty Crocker):			
Scooby Doo, 1 pouch, 0.8 oz	80	0	19
All Other Character Shapes, 0.8 oz	80	0	19
Mixed Fruit (Sunkist), 1 pouch, 0.8 oz	80	0	19
Fudge:			
Chocolate; Mint, 1 oz	130	8	14
Peanut Butter & Chocolate, 1 oz	130	8	13
(Brevin's): Cashew, 1 oz	195	9	28
Triple Decker, 1 oz	165	7	25
Ghirardelli:			
Squares:			
Dark Choc., (4), 1.5 oz	210	16	23
Milk & Caramel (3), 1.6 oz	220	12	27
Sea Salt Escape (4), 1.5 o	210	15	24
3 oz Bars: Dark Chocolate, 4 squares	220	17	23
Filled, Peanut Butter, 4 squares	250	17	22
Intense Dark Bars: Ev'ng Dream, 3 pcs	190	15	20
Twilight Delight, 3 pieces	200	17	17

Per Piece/Serving	C	F	Cb
Godiva:			
Bars: Milk/Dark, av., 1.5 oz	230	14	26
Extra Dark: 75%, 1.5 oz	230	17	18
85%, 1.4 oz	260	21	14
Chocoiste:			
Dark Chocolate Cherries (12)	190	7	30
Milk Chocolate Cashews (14)	230	15	19
Hearts: Dark Ganache (4)	200	12	23
Milk Praline (4)	220	13	23
Go Lightly:			
Bags: Assorted Taffy, 5 pieces	130	3	36
Vanilla Caramels, 5 pieces	150	6	32
Hard Candy (4), ½ oz	45	0	15
Goobers Peanuts, 1 pkg, 1.4 oz	200	13	20
Good & Plenty (Hershey's), 1.4 oz	140	0	35
GooGoo Clusters, 1 piece, 1.75 oz	240	12	30
Gum Drops: 1 small, 0.1 oz	15	0	3
5 pieces, 0.6 oz	75	0	15
Gummi:			
Bears (22), 1.4 oz	150	0	34
Chewy Sweet Tarts (4), 1.5 oz	160	0	36
Worms (5), 1.25 oz	130	0	31
Guylian:			
Bars: Dark Chocolate (3), 1 oz	150	12	11
Milk Choc. w/ Hazelnuts (3),1 oz	170	11	15
No Sugar Added Bars:			
Milk Chocolate, 3 squares	150	11	16
54% Cocoa, Dark Choc., 3 squares	140	11	16
Seashell: Bar, 1.4 oz	210	13	21
Boxed, Originals (1), 0.35 oz	60	4	6
Truffles (1), 0.4 oz	70	5.5	5
Heath: Original (1), 1.4 oz	210	13	24
King Size, 2.8 oz	410	22	49
Snack Size, 3 pieces, 1.5 oz	230	14	27
Hershey's:			
Cookies 'N' Creme, 1.5 oz Bar	220	12	26
Milk Chocolate: 1.55 oz Bar	210	13	26
King Size, 1 Bar, 2.6 oz	370	22	44
With Almonds, 1 bar, 1.4 oz	210	14	21
Kisses, 9 pieces, 1.4 oz	200	12	25
Nuggets: 4 pieces, 1.35 oz	200	13	20
W/ Toffee & Alm., 4 pcs, 1.3 oz	200	13	21
Sugar Free Choc.,, 5 pieces, 1.4 oz	160	13	24
Pot of Gold Chocolate Asstd:			
Carmel, 1.4 oz	190	10	26
Other varieties, average, (4), 1.4 oz	210	12	24

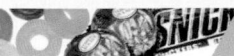

Brands & Generic (Cont)

Per Piece/Serving	C	F	Cb
Hershey's (Cont):			
Extra Dark Choc., 4 pieces, 1.4 oz	180	14	21
Simple Pleasures, 6 pieces, av.	180	8	29
Special Dark Choc.: 1.45 oz bar	190	12	25
Sugar Free, 5 pieces, 1.4 oz	190	15	23
Candy-Coated Eggs:			
Milk Chocolate: (8), 1.2 oz	170	8	27
With Almonds (8), 1.2 oz	200	12	18
Honeycomb: Plain, 1 oz	115	0	27
Choc-coated, 2 pieces	180	7	31
Hot Tamales,			
20 pieces, 1.4 oz	150	0	36
Hugs ~ See Kisses			
Jawbreakers (Sathers), (15), 0.6 oz	60	0	16
Jells (Joyva), Raspb., 3 pcs, 1.55 oz	160	0	38
Jelly Beans:			
Average all brands,			
Small Size (Jelly Belly): 1 bean	5	0	1
12 beans, ½ oz	50	0	13
Regular Size: 1 bean	10	0	2.5
10 beans, 1 oz	105	0	26
Large Size: 1 bean	15	0	38
10 beans, 1.5 oz	150	0	38
Sugar Free:			
Av. all brands, 25 beans, 1 oz	60	0	26
(Note: Carbs include sugar alcohol)			
Jelly Belly: 25 beans, 1 oz	105	0	26
3.5 oz package	360	0	90
Sugar Free,			
25 beans, 1 oz	60	0	26
(Note: Carbs include sugar alcohol)			
Chocolate Dips: 1 bean	4	0	1
10 beans	40	1	8
2.8 oz bag	300	8	62
Jelly Rings (Jewel), 5 pcs, 1.4 oz	110	0	26
Jolly Rancher:			
Crunch 'N Chew, 1.55 oz pkg	160	0.5	40
Gummies, 9 pieces	120	0	28
Hard Candy, 3 pieces	70	0	17
Jelly Beans/Sours, 1.4 oz	140	0	36
Lollipops (1), 0.55 oz	60	0	15
Jujubes, all types, (52), 1.4 oz	110	0	28
Juju Bears, 5 pieces	130	0	34
Juju Mix (Sathers), 11 pieces, 1.5 oz	150	0	36
Jujyfruits, 16 pieces, 1.4 oz	120	0	37
Junior Caramels: 13 pieces, 1.5 oz	190	6	33
Mini, 2 boxes, 1 oz	130	4	23

Per Piece/Serving	C	F	Cb
Junior Mints: 1.8 oz	220	4	45
16 pieces, 1.4 oz	170	3	35
Justin's, Peanut Butter Cups:			
Milk Choc, 2 cups, 1.4 oz pkg	200	14	18
Dark Choc, 2 cups, 1.4 oz pkg	200	16	20
Kisses:			
Air Delights, 11 pieces, 1.4 oz	200	12	24
Hugs, 9 pieces, 1.4 oz	210	12	24
Milk Choc.: 1 pc, 0.16 oz	25	1.5	3
9 pieces, 1.4oz	200	12	25
With Almonds (9), 1.4 oz	200	13	22
Caramel Filled 9 pieces, 1.5 oz	190	9	27
Special Dark, 9 pieces, 1.4 oz	180	12	25
Kit Kat:			
Milk Chocolate:			
4 piece bar, 1.5 oz	210	11	28
King Size, 8 pieces, 3 oz bar	420	22	56
Snack Size, 6 pieces, 1.48 oz	210	11	27
Extra Crispy, 1.58 oz bar	220	12	29
White Chocolate, 4 pieces, 1.5 oz	220	12	26
Kraft, Caramels (5), 1.4 oz	160	3.5	30
Lance, Peanut Bar, 2.2 oz package	340	19	29
Lemon Drops, (4), 0.6 oz	60	0	16
Sugar Free (Walgreens), (3), 0.6 oz	50	0	17
Lemonhead, (26), 1.4 oz	140	0	36
Licorice: Average all types, 1oz	100	0	25
Bites (Switzer), (1)	10	0	3
Chews (Panda), (1)	10	0	3
Tid Bits (1)	10	0	1.5
Twists: Black/Red, av., 1 pc	35	0	8
Sugar Free, 1 piece	13	0	2.5
American Licorice Co.:			
Natural Vines: Black, 9 pcs, 1.4 oz	140	1	33
Red, 9 pieces, 1.4 oz	150	1	34
Red Vines, 7 pieces, 1.4 oz	140	0	33
Sip-n-Chew, 1 package 1 oz	100	1	23
Snaps, 31 pieces, 1.4 oz	140	0.5	33
Sour Punch, 6 pieces, 1.4 oz	150	0	34
Super Ropes, 1 piece, 2 oz	200	0	46
Young & Smiley: Strawb. 11 pcs	150	1.5	33
Traditional Black, 11 pcs, 1.48 oz	140	1.5	32
Lifesavers: Large size, 1 candy	15	0	3
Regular: All flavors, 1 candy	10	0	2.5
1 Roll (14 candies), 1.15 oz	140	0	35
Creme Savers: 3 pieces, ½ oz	60	1	11
Sugar Free, 4 pieces	45	1.5	13
Pep-o-mint (3), 0.2 oz	20	0	5
Fruit Splosion (10), 1.4 oz	130	0	31
Sugar-Free Delites: Per Candy			
Orchard Fruits; Summer Blend	7	0	2.5
Butter Toffee; European Collection	10	1	2.5

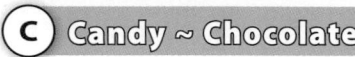
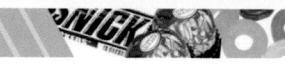

Brands & Generic (Cont)

Per Piece/Serving	C	F	Cb
Lik-m-aid (Wonka), Fun Dip, 1 pkg	50	0	13
Lindt: Lindor Truffles (1), average	75	6	5
Swiss Milk Chocolate Bars:			
70% Cocoa, 4 pieces	220	17	13
Classic, with Hazelnuts, 10 pieces	230	16	20
Raspberry filled, 7 pieces	200	10	25
Dark Choc. Truffles,			
w/ filling, 7 pieces	240	18	18
Lollipops: Mini, ¼ oz	25	0	6
Small, ½ oz	50	0	12
Medium, 1 oz	100	0	25
Giant (4" diam), 7 oz	790	0	198
M & M's:			
Milk Chocolate: 28 piece, 1 oz	145	6.5	21
1.5 oz package	210	9	30
1.7 oz package	240	10	34
Almond Choc., 1.5 oz	220	12	25
Minis, 1 tube, 1 oz	150	7	21
Peanut: 28 piece, 1 oz	155	8	17
1.75 oz pkg	250	13	30
Peanut Butter, 1.63 oz package	240	14	26
Dark Chocolate: 1.5 oz pkg	210	10	29
Peanuts, 1.5 oz	220	12	25
Premiums: Chocolate Trio, 1.5 oz	230	14	25
Mint Thrills, 1 oz	240	14	25
Pretzels, ½ pkg, 1.4 oz	180	6	29
Snack Mix, av. all var., ⅓ cup, 1.5 oz	200	9	25
Mamba Sour, Fruit Chews,			
6 pieces, 1 oz	100	1	22
Marshmallow Egg, 1 egg, 1 oz	120	3	22
Mary Jane (Necco), 5 pcs, 1.4 oz	160	3.5	32
Marshmallows: Firm/Soft, 1 oz	90	0	23
Regular size, 4 pieces, 1 oz	100	0	24
Mini-Marshmallow, ⅔ cup, 1 oz	95	0	24
Choc-coat. Twists (Joyva), each	95	2	10
Fluff, 2 Tbsp, 0.6 oz	60	0	15
Kraft: Mini, 1 oz	90	0	23
Creme, ½ oz	45	0	11
Jet-Puffed, 5 pieces, 1 oz	100	0	24
Funmallows, ⅔ cup, 1 oz	100	0	24
Marzipan, 2 Tbsp, 1.4 oz	160	4	29
Mauna Loa, Mountains, 4 pcs	230	17	21
Mexican Hats, (7), 1.34 oz	120	0	30
Mentos: Regular (1)	10	0	3
Sugar Free (1)	5	0	2.5
Mike & Ike:			
Original: 1 pkg, 2.1 oz	220	0	55
23 pieces, 1.4 oz	140	0	36
Milk Duds, 1 box, 1.8 oz	230	8	38

Per Piece/Serving	C	F	Cb
Milky Way:			
Bars: Single, 2 oz	260	10	41
Fun Size, 2 bars, 1.2 oz	150	6	24
To Go, 1.8 oz	230	9	36
Minis, 5 pieces, 1.5 oz	190	7	30
Midnight Bars: (1), 1.75 oz	220	8	36
Minis, 5 pieces, 1.4 oz	190	7	30
Simply Caramel, 2 oz	250	11	37
Mints: Uncoated, 3 pieces	70	0	17
1 mint	7	0	1
1 large mint	15	0	3
Mon Cheri (Ferrero), 4 pcs, 2 oz	260	18	20
Mounds: 1.75 oz bar	230	13	29
King Size, 4 pcs, 3.5 oz	460	26	58
Snack Size, 1 piece, 0.6 oz	80	4.5	10
Mr Goodbar: 1.75 oz bar	250	17	26
King Size, 2.6 oz bar	380	26	38
Munch Bar, 1.4 oz	220	15	18
Necco, Candy Wafers (40), 2 oz	220	0	56
Nestle Crunch: Orig.,1.55 oz bar	220	11	30
Fun Size, 3 bars, 1.34 oz	180	9	26
Miniatures, 4 bars, 1.4 oz	200	10	27
Buncha Crunch, ⅓ cup, 1.2 oz	180	9	25
Crunch Crisp, 1.72 oz	190	11	24
Newman's Own:			
Milk Chocolate: Caramel Cups (3)	160	8	21
Peanut Butter Cups (3)	180	12	17
Dark Chocolate: Caramel Cups (3)	160	9	20
Peanut Butter Cups (3)	180	13	16
Nips, all flavors, 2 pieces, ½ oz	60	2	11
Nougat: 3 pcs, 1.5 oz	170	1	39
Choc. Covered, 1 oz	125	4	22
Nuggets: Milk Chocolate, 4 pieces	200	12	25
W/ Toffee & Almonds, 4 pieces	200	12	25
Special Dark w/ Almonds, 4 pieces	200	13	20
Nutrageous Bar (Reese's), 1.8 oz	260	16	28
Oh Henry!, 2.2 oz bar	300	17	26
Orange Slices:			
Jewel, 3, 1.5 oz	140	0	35
Walgreens, 4 pieces, 1.6 oz	160	0	39
Pastel Mints (Walgreens), 20 pcs	60	0	14
PayDay Bar: 1.8 oz bar	240	13	27
King Size, 3.5 oz bar	440	24	50
Snack Size, 0.7 oz	90	5	10
Avalanche, 1.8 oz bar	250	13	29
Peanut Bar, 1.6 oz bar	235	15	21
Peanut Butter Cups ~ See Reese's; Newman's Own			
Peanut Brittle: 1 piece, 1.5 oz	190	5	32
Sugar Free (Russell Stover),			
4 pcs, 1.3 oz	140	10	24

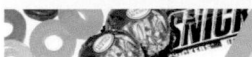

Candy ~ Chocolate C

Brands & Generic (Cont)

Per Piece/Serving	C	F	Cb
Peanuts, choc-covered, 14 pieces	230	14	23
Pearson's, Mint Patties, (5), 1.3 oz	150	2.5	31
Peppermints: 7 small, 0.5 oz	60	0	15
Brach's, 3 pieces	60	0	16
Pez, 1 roll	35	0	9
Planters: Choc. Peanuts, 1.4 oz	210	15	18
Double Peanut Bar, 1.6 oz	220	13	21
Pop Rocks, 0.34 oz package	35	0	9
Pot of Gold:			
Assortment: Caramel, 4 pieces	190	10	25
Nut, 4 pieces	210	13	23
Pretzels: Choc-covered, Mini (6)	200	9	25
White Choc Bites (23), 1.4 oz	200	9	25
Pretzel Flipz (Nestlé), 8 pcs, 1 oz	130	5	20
Raisinets: Milk Choc: 1 pkg, 1.6 oz	190	8	30
King Size, 2.8 oz	330	13	56
Movie Pack, 3.5 oz	380	16	64
Dark Chocolate, ¼ cup, 1.6 oz	180	8	32
Reese's:			
Clusters, 3 pieces, 1.5 oz	220	12	24
Crispy Crunchy Bar: 1.7 oz	260	18	22
2 pieces, 1.2 oz	170	10	19
King Size, 3 oz	480	32	40
Fast Break, 2 oz bar	260	12	35
Peanut Butter Chips, 1 Tbsp, ½ oz	80	4	8
Peanut Butter Cups: (2), 1.5 oz	210	13	24
Mini, 5 pieces, 1.55 oz	220	13	26
8-Pack, 1 piece, ½ oz	80	4.5	9
Snack Size, 1 piece, 0.75 oz	110	6.5	12
Dark Chocolate (2), 1.5 oz	210	14	23
Sugar Free: 5 pieces, av., 1.4 oz	180	13	27
Caramel Filled (2),1.4 oz	150	11	27
Big Cup, 1 cup, 1.4 oz	200	12	22
Pieces: Regular (51), 1.4 oz	190	9	25
Special Dark (50), 1.4 oz	180	8	29
Sticks: 1.5 oz	220	13	23
King Size (1), 3 oz	440	26	46
Snack Size (1), 0.6 oz	90	5	9
Snacksters, 1 package, ¾ oz	100	4	14
Whipps, 1.5 oz	230	9	37
Rice Krispies Treats (Kellogg's),			
1 bar, av. all varieties, 0.8 oz	95	2.5	17
Riesen, Choc. Chew, 4 pieces, 1.25 oz	170	6	28
Rocky Road, Milk/Dark, 1.8 oz bar	240	11	34
Roca Thins, all flavors, 3 pieces	200	15	23
Rolo: Regular, all var., 1.7 oz roll	220	10	33
Mini Chews, Caramel in milk choc. (11)	190	9	26
Root Beer Barrels, (3) 0.6 oz	60	0	17

Per Piece/Serving — C F Cb

Russell Stover Candy:	C	F	Cb
Boxed Chocolates: Chocolate Coated			
Assorted (2),1.15 oz	150	7	23
Cherry Cordials (3), 0.35 oz	150	5	25
Dairy Cream Caramels (2), 1.15 oz	150	7	22
Elegant Collection (3), 1.6 oz	210	10	29
French Choc. Mints (4), 1.35 oz	220	13	22
Nut, Chewy & Crisp Centers (2)	160	8	21
Sugar Free: Assort. Candies (3), 1.55 oz	180	12	26
Pecan Delights (2), 1.7 oz	220	17	26
Bags: Caramel (3), 1.3 oz	180	8	25
Coconut (3), 1.5 oz	200	10	26
Mint Patty (3), 1.5 oz	180	7	30
Pecan Delight (2), 1.2 oz	180	11	20
Salt Water Taffy (Brach's), (5)	170	2.5	36
Seashells (Guylian), 4 shells, 1.6 oz	260	17	24
See's Candies:			
Almond Royal (5), 1.3 oz	190	13	18
Butterscotch Chews (5), 1.5 oz	210	12	27
Krispy's: Caffe Latte (5),1.3 oz	180	8	27
Mint (5), 1.3 oz	170	8	27
Little Pops:			
Butterscotch (4), 0.5 oz	60	2	12
Chocolate (4), 0.5 oz	60	3	10
Vanilla (4), 0.5 oz	50	2	9
Lollypops, average, 0.7 oz	90	3	17
Milk Molasses Chips, 6 pcs, 1.4 oz	180	9	24
Milk Peppermints, 2 pieces, 1.25 oz	150	4	28
Peanut Brittle Bar, 1 oz	150	10	15
Peanut Butter Patties, 1.2 oz	170	10	16
Peppermint Twists (3), 0.5 oz	60	0	15
Toffee-ettes, 3 pieces, 1.6 oz	270	21	18
Sugar Free: Dark Bar, 1.5 oz	180	16	24
Dark Walnut Clusters, 1.5 oz	230	21	17
Peanut Brittle, 1.5 oz	170	14	17
Skinny Cow:			
Dreamy Clusters, all var. 1 pouch	120	6	20
Heavenly Crisps, all varieties, 1 bar	110	6	14
Skittles:			
Original, 2.15 oz	250	2.5	56
Sour, 1.8 oz	200	2	44
Tropical; Wild Berry, 2.15 oz	250	2.5	56
Fun Size, 1 bag, ½ oz	60	1	14
Tear & Share, 4 oz bag	420	4.5	93
Skor, Toffee Bar (1), 1.4 oz	200	12	25
Smarties: Candy Rolls (1), ¼ oz	25	0	6
Giant, 1 roll, 1 oz	100	0	25

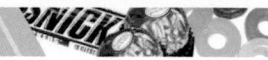

Brands & Generic (Cont)

Per Piece/Serving	C	F	Cb
Snickers: 2 oz bar	280	14	35
Fun Size, 2 bars, 1.2 oz	160	8	21
To Go Bar, 1.65 oz	220	11	28
Miniatures: 4 pieces, 1.25 oz	170	9	22
Sugar Free, 5 pieces	180	13	27
Dark Chocolate Bar, 1.85 oz	250	12	31
Almond Bar, 1.75 oz	230	11	32
P'nut Butter Squared, 2 bars, 1.8 oz	250	13	30
Sno Caps, ¼ cup, 1.4 oz	180	8	30
Soft 'N Chewy, Butter Toffee, each	30	0.5	5
Sorbee,			
Crystal Light Hard Candy, 4 pieces	25	0	13
(Note: Carb figures include Isomalt which has fewer calories than sugar.)			
Sour Patch: All types, 1.5 oz	150	0	37
1 straw	20	0	5
Spearmint Leaves: *Jewel,* (5), 1.4 oz	140	0	35
Walgreens, 4 pieces, 1.6 oz	160	0	39
Spree Candies: Original, 15 pieces	50	0	13
Chewy Spree, 8 pieces	60	0	13
Starburst: Candy Canes, ½ oz	70	0	18
Fruit Chews: Each	20	0.5	4
8 pieces, 1.4 oz	160	3.5	33
Gummibursts, 9 pieces, 1.4 oz	130	0	31
Jellybeans, 1.5 oz	150	0	37
Jellybean Egg, 2 oz	200	0	51
Tropical Fruit (8), 1.4 oz pack	160	3.5	34
Starlight Mints, 3 pieces, 0.55 oz	60	0	15
Suckers (Walgreens), (1), 0.4 oz	45	0	11
Sugar Babies, Original, 1.4 oz	160	1.5	37
Sugar Coated Peanuts, 1 oz	120	8	10
Sunbursts Sunflowers (Kimmie):			
Choco Rocks Milk, 1.4 oz	210	10	27
Kettle Corn Nuggets, 1.4 oz	200	9	29
Sunburst Milk, 1.4 oz	210	11	23
Swedish Fish, (7), 1.5 oz	140	0	36
SweeTARTS:			
Orig., 8 pieces, 0.5 oz	50	0	13
Mini Chewy, 23 pieces, 0.5 oz	50	0.5	12
Symphony:			
Milk Choc: 1.5 oz bar	220	14	23
Large Block: 5 pieces, 1.35 oz	200	12	22
W/ Alm. & Toffee, 5 pieces, 1.3 oz	200	13	21

Per Piece/Serving	C	F	Cb
Taffy:			
Fruit Chews (Starburst), 1 Piece	20	0.5	4
Laffy Taffy (Wonka),			
Original, 5 bars, 1.5 oz	160	2	36
Take 5 (Hershey's): Orig., 1.5oz	200	11	25
King Size, 2.25 oz	300	16	37
Snack Size, 2 pcs	210	11	26
3 Musketeers: Original, 2.15 oz	260	8	46
2 To Go, 1 bar, 1.6 oz	200	6	35
Fun Size, 3 bars, 1.6 oz	190	6	34
Minis, 7 pcs, 1.4 oz	170	5	32
Tang-a-Roos, 1 roll	25	0	6
Terry's: Choc. Orange (5), 1.5 oz	230	12	27
Dark Choc. Orange (5), 1.5 oz	240	13	28
Tic Tac, all varieties, each	2	0	5
Toblerone: 1.25 oz bar	180	9	23
1.4 oz bar	210	11	26
1.8 oz bar	260	13	32
Truffle Peaks (1), 1.45 oz	240	15	23
Toffees, Regular, 1 oz	160	9	18
Tootsie Pops, (1), 0.6 oz	60	0	15
Tootsie Roll: 2.25 oz roll	245	2	55
Mini Chews, 1.4 oz	140	3	28
Truffles: Reg., 1 pc, 0.4 oz	60	4	6
Large (Godiva), ¾ oz	110	6.5	12
Extra Large (J.Schmidt), 1.5 oz	220	13	24
Turtles: Original, 1 piece, 0.6 oz	85	5	10
Sugar Free, 1 piece, 0.4 oz	50	3.5	7
Twists, Licorice; Strawb., sugar free,			
7 pieces, 1.4 oz	90	0	25
Twix:			
Caramel: 2 cookies, 1.8 oz	250	12	33
Family Size, 1 cookie, 1 oz	130	6	17
King Size, 1 cookie, 0.8 oz	110	4	14
Minis, 3 pcs, 1 oz	150	8	20
Peanut Butter:			
Single, 2 cookies, 1.7 oz	250	15	26
King Size, 1 cookie, 0.7 oz	100	6	11
Twizzlers: Cherry Bites (17), 1.4 oz	140	0.5	32
Cherry Nibs, 29 pieces, 1.4 oz	140	1	32
Pull 'n' Peel, Cherry, 1 pc, 1.15 oz	110	0.5	26
Twists Strawb., 1.6 oz	160	0.5	36
U-No Bar, 1.5 oz	250	17	24
Weight Watchers (Whitman's):			
Butter Cream Caramel (3)	150	8	23
Caramel Medallions (3)	160	9	24
Coconut (3)	150	9	24
English Toffee Squares (3)	150	9	21
Mint Patties (3)	150	9	23
Peanut Butter Cups (4)	180	8	31
Pecan Crowns (3)	160	10	24

Brands & Generic (Cont)

Per Piece/Serving	C	F	Cb
Werther's: Original (3), 0.55 oz	70	1.5	14
Sugar-Free Original (5)	40	1	15
Chewy Caramel (6), 1.3 oz	170	6	28
Whatchamacallit: 1.6 oz Bar	230	12	28
King Size Bar, 2.6 oz	370	20	45
Whitman's, Boxed Chocolates:			
Sampler (4), 1.75 oz	240	11	34
12 oz Box, 2 pieces, 1.6 oz	230	12	27
Sugar Free, 10 oz Box, 3 pcs, 1.4 oz	180	13	25
Reserve, 7 oz Box, 2 pieces, 1.15 oz	160	9	21
Whoppers, av. all flav., 18 pieces	190	8	31
Wonka: Bar (1), 2.6 oz	360	19	49
Exceptional Bars, average all, 4 pcs	200	13	23
Gobstopper, ½ oz	60	0	14
Laffy Taffy: Original, 5 bars, 1.5 oz	160	2	36
Ropes, each	80	1.5	18
Stretchy & Tangy, all flav., 1.5 oz	150	3.5	29
Nerds, Giant, Chewy, 1.8 oz	170	0	44
Yogurt Candy,			
Coated Raisins, 27 pieces, 1.4 oz	180	8	28
York: Mints, (3)	10	0	3
Peppermint Pattie, reg, 1.4 oz	140	2.5	31
Pieces (50)	170	8	28
Zachary, Choc. Peanuts, 1.5 oz	240	15	21
Zagnut, 1.75 oz bar	220	9	35
Zero Bar: 1.8 oz bar	230	8	37
King Size, 3.5 oz	400	14	68

Gum

Per Piece	C	F	Cb
Bazooka	15	0	4
Beechies	6	0	2
Big League Chews	10	0	2
Bubble Yum: Regular	25	0	6
Sugarless	10	0	3
Candilicious	30	0	2
Carefree, Sugarless/Regular	5	0	2
Chiclet	5	0	1
Dentyne	5	0	0.5
Double Bubble Ball	20	0	5
Estee, bubble/regular	5	0	3
Extra (Wrigley's), Sugar-Free	5	0	2
Freshen-Up	10	0	3
Hubba Bubba: Reg.	25	0	6
Sugar-free, average	14	0	0.5
Ice Breakers	5	0	2
Jolt Gum	5	0	2
Super Bubble	15	0	4
Trident, Orig.; White	5	0	1
Wrigley's, all flavors	10	0	2

Carob Candy

Per Piece/Serving	C	F	Cb
Carob, Plain/Natural, 1 oz	155	9	15
Carob Coated: Raisins, 1 oz	130	8	15
Almonds/Peanuts, 1 oz	150	10	14
Malt Balls, 1 oz	135	8	15
Caramels, 1 oz	110	4	18
Dates, 1 oz	125	5	20
Soybeans	145	9	16
Trail/Party Mix, 1 oz	150	9	15

Cough Drops

Per Drop/Piece	C	F	Cb
Beech Nut, 1 drop	10	0	2
CVS, Sour Lemon Throat Drops			
Diabetic Tussin	0	0	0
Halls, Defense Vitamin C: Regular	15	0	4
Sugar Free	5	0	3
Fruit Breezers	15	0	4
Menthol Drops: Regular	15	0	4
Sugar Free	5	0	4
Plus	20	0	5
Listerine (Amer. Chicle), Lozenge	10	0	2
Luden's, Throat Drops: Reg., all flav.	110	0	2
Sugar Free	0	0	0
Pine Bros, Cough Drops	10	0	2
Ricola, Cough Drops:			
Regular	10	0	3
Sugar-Free Lemon Mint	0	0	1
Robitussin: Regular	15	0	3
Honey Cough	40	0	10
Sugar Free Throat	0	0	0
Sunny Orange Vitamin C	10	0	3
Rolaids, Sodium Free	5	0	1
Sathers, Peppermint Lozenges	15	0	3
Squibb, Cough/Throat Lozenges	10	0	4
Sucrets (Beecham), Lozenges	10	0	2
Wintergreen, Lozenges	15	0	3

Eat at least 5 servings of fruit and vegetables every day . . . and Enjoy Better Health!

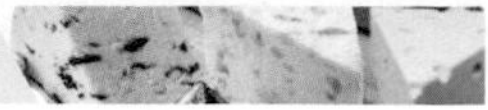

Quick Guide

	C	F	Cb
Firm/Hard Cheeses			
American, Cheddar, Jack, Swiss:			
Average All Brands			
Regular Cheese:			
Thin Deli slice, ¾ oz	80	6	0.5
1 oz slice/piece	110	9	0.5
8 oz package	870	72	2.5
Cubes: 1" cube, 0.6 oz	70	5.5	0.5
1¼" cube, 1 oz	115	9	0.5
Diced, 1 cup, 4.5 oz	510	41	3
Melted, ¼ cup, 2.1 oz	245	20	1
Shredded: ¼ cup, 1 oz	110	9	0.5
1 cup, 4 oz	440	36	2

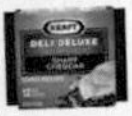

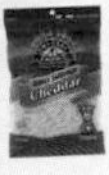

Cheese & Cheese Products

Per 1 oz Unless Indicated	C	F	Cb
Almond *(Lisanatti)*, Chunks, av.	50	1	3
American:			
Regular: 1 slice, 1 oz	105	9	0.5
Alpine Lace, Yellow/White,			
25% Red. Fat, 0.8 oz	90	6	1
Kraft: Regular, 0.67 oz slice	60	4.5	1
2% Milk, Deli Deluxe, 0.67 oz	60	4	1
Land O'Lakes: 1 oz slice	100	9	2
2% Milk, 1 oz	90	6	1
Soy Kaas, 0.67 oz slice	45	2	3
Borden, 1 slice, 0.7 oz	30	0	3
Babybel (Laughing Cow), Mini:			
Original (1), 0.75 oz	70	6	0
Light (1), 0.75 oz	50	3	0
Bonbel (1), 0.75 oz	70	6	0
Light Orig. (1), 0.75 oz	50	3	0
Gouda (1), 0.75 oz	80	6	0
Blue/Bleu: Average All Brands:			
Crumbled, ¼ cup, 1 oz	100	8	0
Light, 0.75 oz	35	1.5	2
Brie, average, 1 oz	95	8	0
Alouette,			
Baby Brie Wedge, 1 oz	110	10	1
Camembert, 1 oz	85	7	0
Caraway, 1 oz	105	8	1
Castello, 1 oz	120	12	0
Cheddar:			
Regular: Av., 1 oz	110	9	1
Shredded, ¼ cup, 1 oz	110	9	1
Extra Sharp *(Cracker Barrel)*:1 oz	120	10	0
Shredded, 1 oz	110	9	1
2% Milk, 1 oz	90	6	1
Kraft, Big Slice, 2% Milk, Red. Fat	60	4.5	0

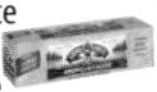

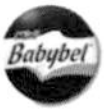

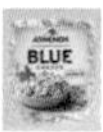

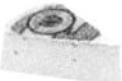

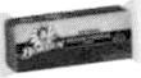

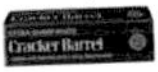

Cheese & Cheese Products (Cont)

Per 1 oz Unless Indicated	C	F	Cb
Cheddar (Cont):			
Reduced Fat:			
Borden, Shredded,			
¼ cup, 1 oz	110	9	1
Kaukauna:			
Cheese Balls, all varieties	100	6	4
Cheese Logs, all varieties	100	7	4
Cheese Curds:			
Fresh: ¼ cup, 1 oz	110	9	0
1 cup, 4 oz	440	36	0
Breaded & Fried:			
A&W, 5 oz	570	40	27
Culver's, Wisconsin, 6.7 oz	670	38	54
Cheese Logs *(Kaukauna)*, average	90	6	4
Cheese Whiz:			
Original, 2 Tbsp, 1 oz	90	7	4
Light, 2 Tbsp, 1 oz	80	3.5	6
Salsa Con Queso,			
2 Tbsp, 1 oz	90	7	4
Cheshire, 1 oz	110	9	1.5
Colby: Regular, 1 oz	110	8	1
Colby-Jack:			
Regular	110	9	1
Kraft, 2% Milk	60	4	0
Cottage Cheese: *Average All Brands*			
Creamed (4% milk fat):			
2 Tbsp, 1 oz	30	1	1.5
½ cup, 4 oz	120	5	6
With fruit, ½ cup, 4 oz	130	4	15
Reduced-Fat (2%): 2 Tbsp, 1 oz	25	0.5	1
½ cup, 4 oz	100	2	4
Low-Fat (1%): 2 Tbsp, 1 oz	20	0.5	1
½ cup, 4 oz	80	1	3
Fat-Free/Non-Fat: 2 T., 1 oz	20	0	1
½ cup, 4 oz	80	0	5
Cottage Cheese: *Brands*			
Fiber One, 1% Fat, ½ cup, 4 oz	80	2	8
Friendship:			
1% Low-Fat Pineapple, 4 oz	120	1	16
Nonfat w/ P'apple, ½ cup, 4 oz	110	0	17
Pot Style, 2%, ½ cup, 4 oz	90	2.5	3
Hood, with Chive/Onion, 4 oz	90	1	5
Knudsen/Breakstone's:			
Free, Non-Fat, ½ cup, 4.oz	70	0	7
2% Milk Fat, ½ cup, 4 oz	100	2.5	6
On the Go!:			
Low-Fat, 4 oz carton	90	2.5	6
Lactaid, Low-Fat, ½ cup, 4 oz	80	1	7
Light N' Lively:			
Fat-Free, ½ cup, 4.4 oz	80	0	8
Low-Fat, ½ cup, 4.4 oz	80	1.5	6

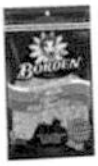

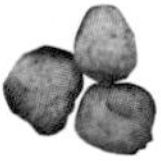

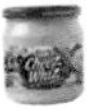

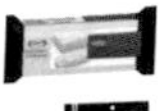

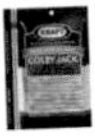

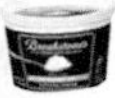

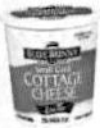

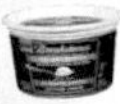

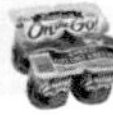

Cheese & Cheese Products (Cont)

Per 1 oz Unless Indicated — L, F, Cb

Item	L	F	Cb
Cream Cheese: *Average All Brands*			
Regular/Soft:			
2 Tbsp, 1 oz	90	9	2
3 oz package	300	27	3
8 oz package	720	72	13
Light, Plain, 1 oz 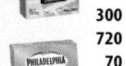	70	5	2
Fat-Free, Plain, 1 oz	30	0	2
Easy Cheese (Kraft),			
American, 2 Tbsp, 1.2 oz	90	6	2
Edam, 1 oz 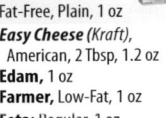	100	8	0.5
Farmer, Low-Fat, 1 oz	40	2.5	0
Feta: Regular, 1 oz	75	6	1
Crumbled, ½ cup, 2.5 oz	190	15	3
Reduced-Fat (Athenos), 1 oz	60	4	1
Fontina, 2 Tbsp, 1 oz	110	9	0.5
Galaxy: (Cheese Substitute):			
Grated Parmesan Flavor, 2 tsp, 0.2 oz	15	0	1
Rice, Mozzarella flavor, 1 sl., 0.6 oz	40	2.5	0.5
Veggy, all varieties, 1 slice, 0.5 oz	40	2.5	0.5
Goat's Milk Cheese:			
Chevre: Original, 2 Tbsp 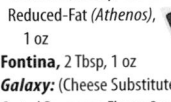	75	6	0.5
Semi-Soft, 1 oz	100	8.5	1
Hard, 1 oz	130	10	0.5
Chavrie: Original, 2 Tbsp, 1 oz	50	3.5	1
Caramelized Onion, 2 Tbsp	50	3	4
Logs, all varieties, average, 1 oz	80	7	3
Gjetost, fresh, 1 oz 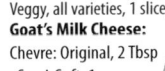	130	8	12
Myzithra, grated, 1 oz	80	4	2
Gorgonzola, 1 oz	100	8	0.5
Galbani, Dolcelatte, 1 oz	95	8	1
Gouda, 1 oz	100	8	0.5
Gruyere, 1 oz	115	9	1
Handi-Snacks (Kraft): 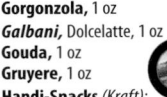			
Breadsticks 'n Cheez Single, 1 oz	110	4.5	14
Ritz Crackers 'n Cheez Dip, 0.95 oz	100	6	11
Havarti (Land O'Lakes), 0.75 oz	80	7	0
Italian Pasta Blend (Sargento), 1 oz	90	6	3
Jarlsberg: Average, 1 oz,	100	8	0
Reduced Fat, shredded, 1 oz	70	3.5	0
Labneh, (Lebanese Cream Chse) 1.8 oz	70	4	4

Cheese & Cheese Products (Cont)

Per 1 oz Unless Indicated — C, F, Cb

Item	C	F	Cb
Laughing Cow, Wedges: 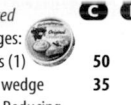			
Original Creamy Swiss (1)	50	4	1
Light Varieties, av., 1 wedge	35	2	2
Lifetime, Cholesterol Reducing,			
Low Fat, all varieties, 1 Slice, 1 oz	45	1.5	1
Limburger, 1 oz 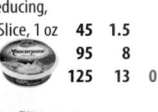	95	8	0
Mascarpone, av., 1 oz	125	13	0.5
Mexican: *Per 1 oz*			
Cacique: Cotija 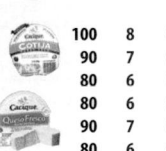	100	8	0
Enchilado; Manchego	90	7	0
Panela	80	6	0
Queso Fresco	80	6	1
Queso Quesadilla	90	7	0
Ranchero	80	6	0
Chi-Chi's, Salsa Con Quéso, Mild	45	3	4
Kraft, Mexican Four Cheese; Taco,			
Shredded	100	8	1
Sargento, 4 cheese, Shredded	110	9	1
Supremo: Quéso Chihuahua, 1 oz	100	8	0
Quéso Oaxaca	80	5	1
Monterey Jack: 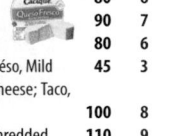			
Regular, shredded, 1 oz	100	8	1
Alpine Lace,			
Co-Jack, 1 oz	70	5	0
Kraft, 1 oz	100	8	1
Mozzarella: 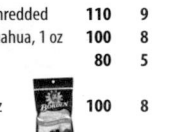			
Regular: Average 1 oz	85	6.5	0.5
Land O'Lakes/Polly-O:			
Slice, av., 1 oz	90	6	1
Shredded, 1 oz	90	6	1
Light: (Polly-O Lite), Shredded, 1 oz	60	2.5	1
2% Milk Fat (Kraft), Reduced Fat	70	4	1
Part Skim: (Alpine Lace), 25% Red.	60	4	1
Borden/Kraft, Shredded	80	5	1
Kraft, String	80	6	0
Fat-Free, (Kraft/Polly-O), 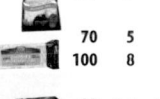			
Shredded, 1 oz	35	0	1
Muenster: 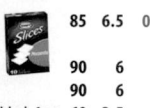			
Regular, 1 oz	105	9	0.5
Low-Fat, 1 oz	85	5	1

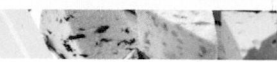

Cheese & Cheese Products (Cont)

Per 1 oz Unless Indicated **C** **F** **Cb**

	C	F	Cb
Parmesan:			
Fresh/Block, Dry, 1 oz	110	7.5	1
Grated (Packaged): 1 Tbsp	20	1.5	0
1 oz	120	8	1
½ cup, 1.75 oz	215	14	2
Kraft, Reduced-Fat Topping, 1 Tbsp	20	1	2
Philadelphia:			
Cream Cheese: Original, 2 T. 1 oz	100	9	1
3 oz package	300	27	3
Regular, 1 oz	90	9	2
Creme, Cooking, av. all flav., ¼ c.	110	9	4
Flavored:			
Blueberry, 1 oz	80	6	5
Honey Nut; Strawb., av., 1 oz	80	7	5
Garden Vegetable, 1 oz	80	7	2
Salmon, 1 oz	70	7	1
Light, Plain, 1 oz	70	5	2
⅓ Less Fat: Plain, 2 T., 1 oz	70	6	2
Garden Vege.; Chive & On., 1 oz	70	5	2
Neufchatel, 2 T., 1 oz	70	6	1
Fat-Free, Plain, 1 oz	30	0	2
Whipped:			
Reg., 0.7 oz	60	6	1
Mixed Berry, 0.7 oz	70	5	3
Indulgence:			
Dark/Milk Chocolate, 2 Tbsp., 1¼ oz tub	110	7	11
8 oz container	700	44	70
White Chocolate: 2 T., 1.25 oz	120	7	12
8 oz container	760	44	76
Pizza Four Cheese, shredded, Regular *(Kraft),* ¼ cup, 1 oz	90	7	1
Port de Salut, 1 oz	100	8	0
Port Wine *(Kaukauna/WisPride):*			
8 oz Tub: Average, 1 oz	85	7	3
Lite, 2 Tbsp, average, 1 oz	60	3	5
Ball, 1 oz	100	6	4
Log, 1 oz	100	7	4
Provolone: Regular, 1 oz	100	7.5	0.5
Reduced-Fat: *Alpine Lace,* 0.8 oz	60	4.5	0
Sargento, Deli Style, 1 sl., 0.67 oz	50	3	0
Pub *(Rondele),* average	95	7	1
Quark: 40% fat	47	3	1
20% fat	32	1.5	1
Skim/Non-Fat	22	0	1.5
Queso:			
Anejo/Asadero/Blanco, 1 oz	105	9	0
Chichuahua/De Papa, 1 oz	110	9	2
Rice Cheese Chunks *(Lisanatti),* average, 1 oz	60	3	2
Swiss *(Lifetime),* Fat Free, 1 oz	40	0	1

Cheese & Cheese Products (Cont)

Per 1 oz Unless Indicated **C** **F** **Cb**

	C	F	Cb
Ricotta Cheese:			
Whole Milk, 1 oz	50	3.5	1
½ cup, 4.5 oz	215	16	4
Part Skim, 1 oz	40	2	1.5
½ cup, 4.5 oz	170	10	6
Light/Low-Fat, 1 oz	25	1	1.5
½ cup, 4.5 oz	125	5	6
Fat-Free, ½ cup, 4.5 oz	100	0	10
Baked Ricotta, 2 oz	130	9	3
Romano: Block/Loaf	110	8	1
Grated: 1 oz	120	9	1
1 Tbsp, 0.2 oz	20	1.5	0
Roquefort, 1 oz	105	9	0.5
Sargento:			
Artisan Blends: Dble Cheddar, 1 oz	110	9	1
Authentic Mexican, 1 oz	100	8	2
Mozzarella & Provolone, 1 oz	90	7	1
Snacks: Cubes, Mild Chedd., (7), 1 oz	120	10	1
Sticks, Pepper Jack, (1), 0.75 oz	80	7	0
Sheep's Milk, 1 oz	45	3	1
Soy Cheese:			
Trader Joe's, Cheddar flavor, 0.7 oz	45	2	3
Soy Kaas: Cheddar, 1 oz	50	2	8
Monterey Jack, 1 oz	60	4	0
Soy Sation, Chunks, all var., 1 oz	60	3	2
Smoked Cheddar, average, 1 oz	110	10	0
Stilton, average, 1 oz	110	10	0
String:			
Regular, average all brands	80	6	0.5
(Kraft) Twist-Ums & String-ums, Super Long, 1 stick, 1.1 oz	90	6	1
Light/Lite:			
(Frigo), String	60	2.5	0.5
(Polly-O), String, 1 oz	80	6	0
(Sargento): 1 pce, 0.75 oz	50	2.5	1
Part Skim, 0.85 oz	70	4.5	1
Swiss: Regular, 1 oz	110	8	1.5
Reduced-Fat: *Alpine Lace,* 0.8 oz	70	4.5	1
Kraft, 2% Milk, 0.67 oz	45	2.5	2
Tilsit, 1 oz	100	7.5	0.5
Tybo, 1 oz	100	7	0.5
Tofutti, Better Than Cream Cheese, all varieties, 1 oz	85	5	9
Velveeta *(Kraft):*			
Original, 1 cup, 2.39 oz	220	8	29
Regular, 1 oz	80	6	3
Reduced Fat, 2% Milk, 1 oz	60	3	4
Extra Thick, 1.2 oz	100	7	3
Mexican: Hot, 1 oz	90	6	3
Mild, 1 oz	80	6	3

Dips/Spreads   C   F   Cb

Per 2 Tbsp, 1 oz, Unless Indicated

Average All Brands

	C	F	Cb
Avocado/Guacamole	45	4	2
Baba Ghanoush (Eggplant/Sesame)	70	6	2
Cheese Fondue, ½ cup, 4 oz	260	15	4
French Onion Dip	60	4.5	3
Hummus, 2 Tbsp	50	1	5
½ cup, 4.5 oz	220	4.5	23
Tzatziki (Cucumber/Yogurt)	30	2.5	2
Clearman's, Original Spread	150	16	0
De La Casa, 5 Layer Party Dip	45	2.5	4

Fritos: *Per 2 Tbsp*

Dips:

	C	F	Cb
Chili Cheese	45	3	3
Bean; Hot Bean w/ Jalap.	35	1	5
Jalapeno Cheddar Cheese	50	3.5	3

Guiltless Gourmet,

	C	F	Cb
Black Bean/Spicy Black Bean Dip	40	0	7

Heluva Good Cheese,

	C	F	Cb
French Onion Dip, 2 Tbsp	50	4.5	2

Hidden Valley,

	C	F	Cb
For Everything Topping, av.	130	14	3

Kaukauna *(Wisconsin):*

Spreadable Cheddar,

	C	F	Cb
Sharp/Smokey Cheddar	90	7	3

Kemps:

	C	F	Cb
Dips: French Onion	60	5	2
Ranch Style	60	5	2

Top The Tater,

	C	F	Cb
Taco Fiesta; Veggie Ranch	60	5	3
Kroger, Dips, all flavors	60	5	2

Kraft:

	C	F	Cb
Dips: Average all flavors	60	5	3
Cheez Whiz: Original	90	7	4
Light	80	3.5	6
Salsa Con Queso	90	7	4
Spreads: Olive & Pimento, 1.15 oz	70	6	3
Old English Sharp; Roka Blue, av.	85	8	2

Marzetti: *Per 2 Tbsp*

	C	F	Cb
Dips: Choc Fruit, 1.35 oz	110	1	25
Caramel Apple, fat free, 1.4 oz	100	0	25
Veggie: Dill, Light, 1 oz	60	5	2
Ranch, Singles, 1.5 oz	180	18	2.5
Ranch, Fat-Free, 1 oz	30	0	6

Dips/Spreads (Cont)   C   F   Cb

Per 2 Tbsp, 1 oz, Unless Indicated

Marie's: *Per 2 Tbsp*

	C	F	Cb
Dips: Buttermilk Ranch; Crmy Dill. av.	100	10	2
Guacamole	40	3	3
Nalley's, Ranch Chip Dip	100	10	2

Naturally Fresh:

	C	F	Cb
Dips: Chocolate	70	0	12
Cream Cheese Strawb.	90	3.5	14
Caramel	100	4	16
Old Dutch: French Onion, 1.1 oz	50	3	5
Mild Cheddar, 1.1 oz	40	3	2
Nacho Cheese, 1.1 oz	35	2.5	2

Old El Paso:

	C	F	Cb
Dips: Cheese & Red Pepper	35	2	3.5
Thick N' Chunky Salsa	10	0	2.5

Price's:

	C	F	Cb
Dips: Pimiento Cheese	85	7	3
Light Pimiento	55	3	3
Zesty Jalapeno	75	6	2.5

Stop & Shop:

	C	F	Cb
Dips: Veggie	100	10	3
Sour Cream French Onion	60	4.5	2

TGI Fridays,

	C	F	Cb
Spinach, Cheese & Artichoke Dip	30	1.5	2
Toby's: Tofu Pate	80	7	2
Ohr varieties	40	2.5	2

Tostitos:

	C	F	Cb
Dips: Creamy Spinach, 1.1 oz	50	4	2
Salsa Con Quéso	40	2.5	5
Smooth & Cheesy, 1.1 oz	50	3.5	4

Wise:

	C	F	Cb
Dips: French Onion, 1.15 oz	60	5	3
Ranch, 1.15 oz	50	4	3

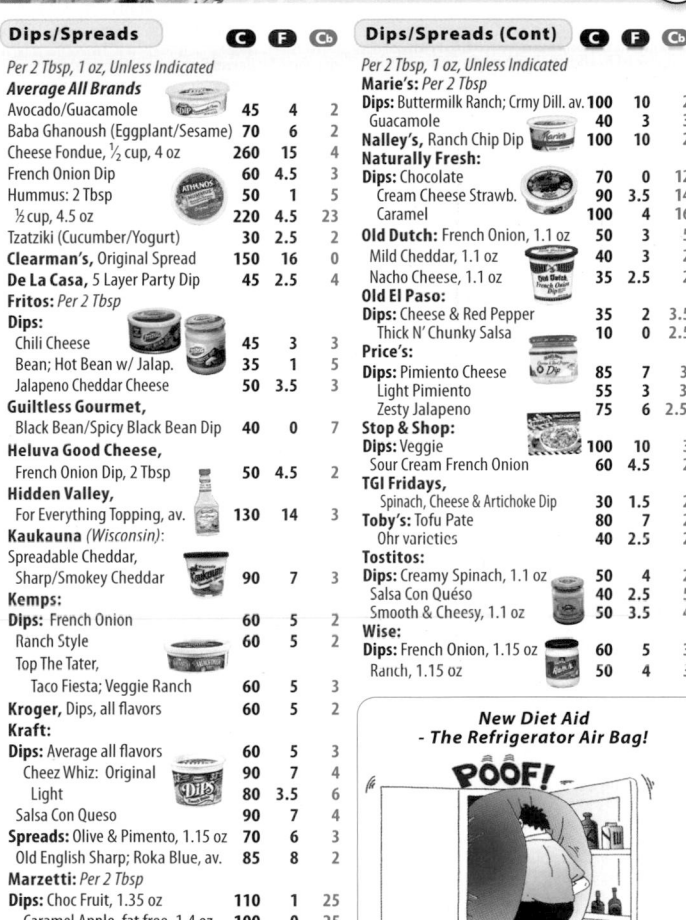

**New Diet Aid
- The Refrigerator Air Bag!**

POOF!

Condiments, Sauces   C   F   Cb

Average of Brands Also See Page 102

Item	C	F	Cb
Apple Sauce ~ *Also See Page 102*			
Sweetened, ¼ cup, 2.5 oz	55	0	13
Unsweetened, ¼ cup, 2 oz	25	0	7
Barbecue Sauce:			
Average, 2 Tbsp, 1 oz	40	0	10
Bull's Eye, Original, 1 oz	60	0	14
Bearnaise Sauce, ¼ cup, 2.5 oz	190	19	5
Buffalo Wing Sce: Hon. Mustard, 1 T.	40	3	2
Average other varieties, 1 Tbsp	25	2	2
Cheese, h/made, ¼ cup, 2.5 oz	150	10	12
Chef-Mate, Hot Dog, ¼ cup	70	2.5	9
Chili Sauce:			
Heinz, 1 T., ½ oz	20	0	5
Del Monte, 1 Tbsp, ½ oz	20	0	5
Cocktail Sauce, 2 Tbsp, 1 oz	110	0	15
Fat-Free *(Walden Farms)* 1 Tbsp	0	0	0
Cranberry Sce: Av all types, 2T., 1 oz	45	0	11
¼ cup, 2.5 oz	110	0	27
Demi Glaze Gold, 2 tsp	30	0.5	7
Honey Mustard *(French's)*, 2 Tbsp	60	0.5	12
Horseradish: 1 tsp	2	0	0
Kraft, 1 tsp	15	1.5	1
Ketchup: Regular, 1 T., ½ oz	15	0	4
Heinz, One-Carb, 1 Tbsp	5	0	1
Simply Heinz, 1 Tbsp	20	0	5
Mole:			
Dona Maria, 2 Tbsp, 1 oz	200	13	10
Rogelio Bueno, 2 Tbsp, 1 oz	160	11	12
Mushroom Sce, ½ cup, 2 oz	50	2	5
Mustard, average, 1 tsp	5	0	0.5
Pesto Sauce, ¼ cup, 2 oz	270	28	2
Pizza Sauce, cnd., ¼ cup, 2 oz	30	0	6
Seafood Cocktail Sce, ¼ cup	60	0	15
Soy Sauce: Av., 1 Tbsp	10	0	1
Kikkoman, Lite Soy, 1 Tbsp	10	0	1
Spaghetti Sce, ½ cup, 4.5 oz	135	6	19
Steak Sauce: A1, 1 Tbsp, ½ oz	15	0	3
Lea & Perrins, 1 Tbsp, ½ oz	20	0	5
Strawb. Puree Sce, Unsweet., 2 T.	10	0	2
Sweet & Sour Sauce:			
Contadina, 1 Tbsp	40	1	8
Kraft, 1 Tbsp	60	0	13
Tabasco Sauce, 1 tsp	2	0	0
Taco Sauce, average, 2 Tbsp, 1 oz	10	0	1
Tartar Sauce *(Heinz)*, 2 Tbsp, 1 oz	120	11	4
Hellmann's, Regular, 2 Tbsp, 1 oz	80	7	4
McCormick, Fat-Free, 2 Tbsp, 1 oz	30	0	7
Teriyaki Sauce *(Kikkoman)*, 1 T., ½ oz	15	0	2
Vinegar, White or Wine, 2 T.	4	0	1
White Sauce, ½ cup, 5 oz	130	7	10
Worcestershire Sauce, 1 tsp	5	0	1

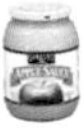

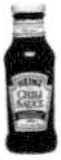

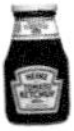

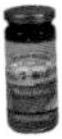

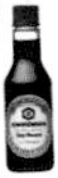

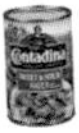

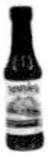

Pickles & Relish   C   F   Cb

Average All Brands

Item	C	F	Cb
Bread & Butter Pickles, 4 sl.,1 oz	25	0	6
Chutney, 2 Tbsp, 1.25 oz	50	0	11
Dill Pickles:			
Slices, 4 slices, 1 oz	4	0	1
1 large, (3¾"x 1¼" diam.), 2.25 oz	12	0	3
Extra lrg (4"x 1¾" diam.), 5 oz	30	0	6
Halves: Small, 1 oz	3	0	0.5
Large, 2.5 oz	8	0	2
Gherkins, sweet, 1 medium, 1 oz	30	0	7
Green Chiles, chopped, 2 Tbsp	5	0	1
Horseradish, 1 Tbsp	10	0	2
Jalapenos, pickled (2), 2 oz	10	0.5	2
Jalapeno Relish, 1 Tbsp, 0.5oz	5	0	1
Mustard, avg. all brands, 1 tsp	5	0	0.5
Peppers, Hot/Mild (1), 1.6 oz	20	0	4
Pickled: Beets, ½ cup, 4 oz	75	0	19
Onions, 1 medium, ¾ oz	10	0	2
Cocktail Onion, 1 onion	2	0	0
Red Cabbage, ½ cup, 3 oz	65	0	15
Pickles: Sweet, 2 Tbsp, 1 oz	35	0	8
Large (3" x ¾ diam.),1.25 oz	40	0	10
Pickle in a Pouch, 1 large	0	0	3
Relishes: S'wich Spread, 1 tsp	20	1	5
Cranberry-Orange, 1 Tbsp	30	0	7
Hot Dog *(Heinz)*, 1 Tbsp, ½ oz	17	0	3
Sweet Pickle, 1 Tbsp, ½ oz	20	0	5
Sweet Cauliflower, 1 oz	35	0	8
Sugar Free Relish, 1 tsp	5	0	1
Sweet Gherkins (2), 1 oz	5	0	1
Sauerkraut,			
Drained, 1 cup, 5 oz	25	0	6

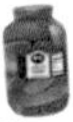

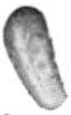

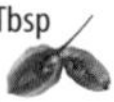

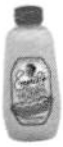

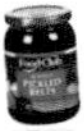

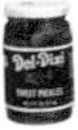

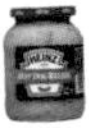

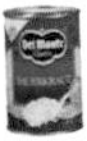

Salsa

Average all Types:

Item	C	F	Cb
Reg., w/out oil, 2 Tbsp, 1 oz	15	0	3.5
Made with oil, 2 Tbsp, 1 oz	40	3	4
La Victoria, 2 Tbsp, 1 oz	10	0	2
Old El Paso, 1 Tbsp, 1 oz	10	0	3
TGI Friday's, 1.2 oz	15	0	4

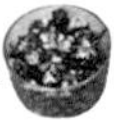

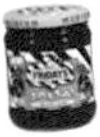

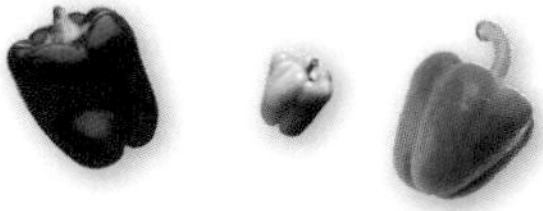

Quick Guide   C   F   Cb

Cookies
Average All Brands: *Per Cookie*

	C	F	Cb
Biscotti: Small, ½ oz	70	3	10
Regular, 1 oz	140	6.5	18
Chocolate Chip Cookies:			
Small/Thin, ½ oz	70	3.5	9
Regular, 1 oz	140	7	18
Large (Mrs Fields), 3 oz	350	17	45
Extra Large, 4 oz	555	28	73
Oatmeal/Oatmeal Raisin:			
Small/Thin, ½ oz	65	2.5	10
Regular, 1 oz	130	5	20
Large (Mrs Fields), 2.5 oz	330	14	44
Extra Large, 4 oz	510	20	78
Peanut Butter:			
Small/Thin, ½ oz	70	3.5	9
Regular, 1 oz	135	7	17
Large (Mrs Fields), 2.5 oz	330	17	41
Extra Large, 4 oz	540	27	67
Low-Fat Cookies:			
Choc Chip (Low-Fat), (1), ½ oz	65	2	10
Oatmeal Raisin (Fat-Free), (1),1 oz	95	0.5	22
Peanut Butter (Low-Fat), (1),1 oz	105	5	15

Quick Guide   C   F   Cb

Crackers
Average All Brands: *Per Cracker Unless Indicated*

	C	F	Cb
Cheese Crackers: Plain, 1" square	5	0	0.5
Bag, single serving, 1 oz	140	7	16
Sandwich:			
Cheese/P'nut Butter filled	30	1.5	4
Crispbread, Rye	35	0	8
Graham, 2½" square	30	0.5	5
Melba Toast, Plain, 1 piece	20	0	4
Matzo, Plain, 1 oz	110	0.5	23
Oyster/Soup, ½ cup	95	2	17
Rice Crackers: 1 small	10	0	1.5
Rice Snacks, Oriental-Style, 1 oz	130	2.5	23
Saltines, 5 crackers	65	2	11
Snack-type, 1 round cracker	15	1	2
Soda Crackers (Saltine), 2	25	1	4.5
Water Cracker (Carr's), Original	14	0.5	2.5
Wheat: Wheat Thin	10	0.5	1.5
Sandwich, Cheese/P'nut Butter filled	35	2	4

Brands   C   F   Cb
Per Cookie/Cracker, Unless indicated

	C	F	Cb
Albertsons:			
Animal Crackers (6), 1 oz	130	3.5	22
Chocolate Chip:			
Original (3), 1 oz	150	7	20
Chewy (2), 1 oz	130	6	18
Chunky, 0.6 oz	80	3.5	10
Chocolate Sandwich Cremes (3) 1 oz	150	6	25
Double Filled (2), 1 oz	140	6	21
Fudge Graham (3), 1 oz	140	7	19
Fudge Wafer (3), 1 oz	140	8	18
Graham Crackers: Cinnamon (3)	130	3	25
Honey (2), 1 oz	140	3	24
Low-Fat Honey (2), 1 oz	110	1	22
Marshmallow Ring (1)	120	5	19
Pinwheels, Choc. Marshmallow (1)	120	5	20
Vanilla Wafers (9), 1 oz	140	4	25
Annie's:			
Cheddar Bunnies:			
Regular: 1 oz Snack Pack	140	6	19
7.5 oz Box	1050	45	145
Sour Cream & Onion, 1 oz	150	7	19
White Cheddar, 1 oz	150	7	19
Whole Wheat, 1 oz	140	6	18
Bunny Grahams:			
Choc.; Choc Chip, 1 oz	130	4.5	21
Friends, 1 oz	130	4.5	22
Honey, 1 oz	140	4.5	22
Organic Bunny Classics:			
Buttery Rich, 1 oz	140	7	18
Cheddar, 1 oz	140	7	18
Saltine, 1 oz	140	3	22
Austin:			
Sandwich Cookies: *Per Package*			
Choco Cremes, 1.8 oz	240	10	37
Lemon OHs!; Vanilla Cremes, 1.8 oz	250	11	37
Sandwich Crackers: *Per Package*			
Cheese: With Cheddar Cheese	190	10	23
With Peanut Butter	190	10	23
Chocolatey Peanut Butter Flavored	190	8	26
Grilled Cheese Flavored, 1.4 oz	190	9	24
PB & J Flavored, 1.4 oz	190	8	26
Toasty Crackers w/ P'nut Butter, 1.3 oz	190	9	23
Zoo Animal Crackers, 1 oz	120	1.5	25

Per Cookie/Cracker, Unless Indicated	C	F	Cb
Barbara's Bakery:			
Cookies: Fig Bars, all var., 1.35 oz	110	0.5	26
Lowfat, all varieties, 1.35 oz	120	1	27
Snackimals: Double Choc., 1 oz	140	4.5	23
Choc. Chip; Snickerdoodle, 1 oz	120	4	19
Peanut Butter, 1 oz	150	7	20
Wheat Free, Oatmeal, 1 oz	120	5	17
Bear Naked:			
Soft Baked Cookies:			
Double Chocolate	130	5	20
Fruit & Nut	130	6	18
BelVita (Nabisco), Bkfast Biscuits,			
average, 1.75 oz package	230	8	36
Blue Diamond:			
Nut Chips			
all varieties, 14 chips, 1 oz	130	4	21
Nut Thins Crackers,			
all varieties average: 17 crackers, 1 oz	130	3	23
Brent & Sam's:			
Chocolate Chip Pecan (2)	130	8	14
Key Lime White Chocolate	130	7	16
Oatmeal Raisin, with Pecans	130	7	16
Triple Chocolate Bliss (2), 1 oz	110	5	14
White Chocolate Macadamia (2), 1 oz	130	7	14
Carr's:			
Cookies, Ginger Lem. Cremes (2)	140	6	21
Crackers: Poppy & Sesame (4)	80	5	9
Table Water (4)	60	1	10
Whole Wheat (2)	80	4	10
Cheez·It ~ See Sunshine, Page 87			
Chips Ahoy! ~ See Nabisco, Page 85			
Country Choice:			
Sandwich Cremes (2), all varieties	130	5	19
Snacking: Ginger Snaps (5)	140	5	22
Vanilla Wafers (7)	140	5	22
Soft Baked, all flavors, average	95	4	16
Dr. Kracker:			
Crispbreads, all varieties, average	100	4	11
Snacker Krackers (8), all var., av.	120	5	14
Erin Baker's:			
Original Breakfast Cookies: Per 3 oz			
Banana Walnut	300	8	53
Peanut Butter	320	11	49
Vegan Peanut Butter Choc. Chunk	320	11	48
Minis: Per 1 oz Cookie			
Peanut Butter	110	3.5	16
Other varieties, average	100	2	18
Organic Brownie Bites, average	95	2	18

Per Cookie/Cracker, Unless Indicated	C	F	Cb
Famous Amos:			
Bite Size Cookies:			
Chocolate Chip:			
4 Cookies, 1 oz	150	7	20
15 oz box	2250	105	300
Chocolate Chip & Pecans (4)	150	8	18
Sandwich, Creme Filled:			
Chocolate (3), 1 oz	160	7	25
Vanilla (3), 1 oz	170	7	25
Fig Newtons ~ See Nabisco, Page 85			
Fresh & Easy:			
Cookies:			
Chocolate Cremes (3), 1.3 oz	180	7	26
Iced Oatmeal (3), 1 oz	120	3	21
Peanut Sensation (1)	170	9	20
Pecan Shortbread (2)	150	9	20
Girl Scouts:			
Cookies: Caramel DeLites/Samoas (2)	140	7	19
Do-si-dos (3)	160	6	26
Peanut Butter Patties (2)	130	7	15
Savannah Smiles (5)	140	5	23
Thanks-A-Lot (2)	150	6	22
Thin Mints (4), average	160	8	22
Goldfish ~ See Pepperidge Farm, Page 86			
Grandma's: Per Cookie Unless Indicated			
Homestyle Cookies:			
Chocolate Chip	170	9	22
Oatmeal Raisin	150	6	23
Peanut Butter	170	9	19
Sandwich Cremes: P'nut Butter (5)	200	9	25
Vanilla (5)	190	9	27
Mini's, Vanilla (9)	150	7	22
Great American Cookies:			
Chewy Chocolate Supreme	180	7	27
Chewy Pecan Supreme	230	12	31
Double Fudge with Reese's	230	11	33
Original,			
with Reese's M&M's	240	12	31
Peanut Butter w/ M&M's	250	14	29
Snickerdoodles	240	11	33
White Chunk Macadamia	250	14	30
Double Doozies:			
Original, 5.3 oz	690	34	94
M&M Big Bite, 2.57 oz	340	17	46
Cookie Cakes: 16", 3.6 oz slice	460	22	67
16" M&M, 4 oz slice	500	24	73
Heart Shaped, 3.5 oz slice	440	21	64

Per Cookie/Cracker, Unless Indicated	Ⓒ	Ⓕ	Ⓒb
Great Value (Walmart):			
Cookies: Choc Chip (3)	150	7	21
Switch-A-Roos (2)	140	6	21
Twist & Shout (3)	170	6	26
Crackers: Buttery Rounds, Baked (5)	80	4.5	10
Reduced Fat (5)	70	2	11
Saltines (1)	60	1	12
Woven Squares (6)	120	4.5	19
Health Valley			
Cookies:			
Cremes Sandwich (2), all varietes	130	5	20
Oatmeal Raisin (1)	90	3.5	14
Mini: Choc. Chip (4)	140	6	18
Choc. Choc. Chip (4)	140	7	18
Crackers:			
Grahams: Amaranth (6)	120	3	22
Oat/Rice Bran (6)	120	3	22
Organic (4), all var., av.	70	3	10
Joseph's:			
Sugar Free Cookies: Per 4 Cookies			
Almond; Chocolate Walnut	95	3.5	13
Chocolate Chip; Pecan Choc. Chip	95	5	13
Other varieties, average	95	4	15
Each cookie contains 6 grams Malitol			
Kashi:			
Cookies: Per Cookie			
Chocolate Almond Butter	130	5	19
Happy Trail Mix, Chewy	140	5	21
Oatmeal: Dark Chocolate	130	5	20
Raisin Flax	130	4.5	20
Snack Crackers:			
Country Cheddar (18)	130	4.5	20
Fire Roasted Veggie., (15)	120	3.5	19
Honey Sesame (15)	120	3	22
Original 7 Grain (15)	120	3.5	19
Toasted Asiago (15)	130	4	21
Heart To Heart Whole Grain:			
Original (7)	120	3.5	22
Roasted Garlic (7)	120	3.5	22
Pita Crisps:			
Original 7 Grain with Salt (11)	120	3	22
Zesty Salsa (11)	120	3	22
Keebler:			
Cookies: Per 2 Cookies Unless Indicated			
Animals, Iced (6)	140	4.5	22
Cinnamon Roll, all varieties	150	6	23

Per Cookie/Cracker, Unless Indicated	Ⓒ	Ⓕ	Ⓒb
Keebler Cont:			
Cookies: Per 2 Cookies Unless Indicated			
Chips Deluxe: Original	160	8	19
Chocolate Lovers	160	9	20
Coconut	160	9	18
Dark Chocolate Chunk	170	9	20
Rainbow Choc Chip	160	8	20
Minis, 1.4 oz package	200	10	27
Soft & Chewy	140	6	21
Danish Wedding, (4)	140	7	19
E.L. Fudge: Original	170	7	25
Double Stuffed	180	9	24
Fudge Shoppe:			
Cheesecake Middles, Original (3)	130	7	17
Deluxe Grahams (3)	140	7	18
Fudge Sticks: Original (3)	150	8	20
Jumbo (1)	160	8	21
Fudge Stripes:			
Original (3)	150	7	21
Mini's, 1.4 oz pkg	200	9	27
Dark Chocolate; Oatmeal (3)	150	7	22
Grasshopper (4)	140	7	20
Mint Creme Middles (3)	130	7	17
100 Calorie Rite Bites:			
Mini Fudge Stripes, 1 pouch	100	3.5	16
Dark Chocolate, 0.75 oz pouch	100	4	15
Gripz, Chips Deluxe 0.88 oz pouch	120	5	18
Oatmeal:			
Original	140	6	20
Country Style w/ Raisins	130	6	19
Iced	140	5	20
Sandies Cookies:			
Dark Chocolate Almond	170	10	19
Pecan Shortbread	170	10	18
Vienna Fingers:			
Regular	150	6	23
Reduced Fat	140	4.5	24
Wafers: Vanilla (8)	140	5	22
Mini Vanilla (18)	140	5	22
Crackers:			
Club: Original (4)	70	3	9
Reduced Fat (5)	70	2	12
Grahams:			
Original (8)	120	3.5	22
Cinnamon (8)	130	3.5	23
Honey (8)	140	4.5	23
Town House:			
Original (5)	80	4.5	10
Reduced Fat (6)	60	1.5	11
Wheatables: Tsted Honey Wheat (17)	140	6	20
Other varieties (16), average	140	6	20

Per Cookie/Cracker, Unless Indicated   **C**   **F**   **Cb**

Kroger:
Cookies:
Chip Mates:

	C	F	Cb
Original (3), 1.5 oz	150	7	22
Chunky (2), 1 oz	120	6	17
Peanut Butter (2), 1 oz	120	7	15
White Chip (2), 1 oz	120	6	16

Kid-O's:

	C	F	Cb
Chocolate Lovers (2), 1 oz	140	6	21
Double Filled Sandwich (2) 1 oz	140	6	21
Chocolate Sandwich (3) 1.15 oz	150	6	25
Olde Sthrn Pecan Shortbread (2),1 oz	150	9	16
Vanilla Wafers (7), 1 oz	130	3.5	23

Crackers:

	C	F	Cb
Grahams, Original; Honey (4)	120	3	21
Saltines, Original, (5), ½ oz	60	1.5	10

Lance:
Cookies: *Per 6 Pack*

	C	F	Cb
Nekot, Peanut Butter	240	11	32
Choc-O-Lunch, Vanilla Cream	230	10	32
Van-O-Lunch, Vanilla Cream	230	10	33

Cracker Creations: *Per 2 Crackers*

	C	F	Cb
W/ Cream Cheese Filling, av., 1 oz	150	8	14
Granola: Chocolate Filling, 1.3 oz	190	9	24
Peanut Butter, 1.3 oz	190	9	23
Five Grain,			
Peanut Butter Filling	140	7	16

Sandwich:

	C	F	Cb
Malt, with Peanut Butter Filling	180	8	20
Nip Chee, Chedd. Chse	200	10	23

Toastchee:

	C	F	Cb
Peanut Butter	220	12	23
Peanut Butter Red. Fat	190	8	23
Toasty, Peanut Butter	180	8	21
Wholegrain, Cheddar Cheese	200	9	26

Little Debbie:
Cookies:

	C	F	Cb
Fig Bar	160	3	32
Marshmallow Pie, average	180	7	28
Marshmallow Treat	160	4	31
Oatmeal Creme Pie, 1.35 oz	170	7	26
Nutty Bar (2), 2 oz	310	18	33

Lu:
Cookies:

	C	F	Cb
Le Petit Beurre (4)	140	4	24
Le Petit Ecolier, average (2)	130	7	15
Pim's, Orange (2)	100	3	17

Macaroni & Cheese, *(Nabisco),*

	C	F	Cb
average all flavors	150	7	18

Manischewitz:

	C	F	Cb
Cookies: Dark Choc. Macaroon (1)	45	2	8

Crackers, Tam Tam Snack:

	C	F	Cb
Original (10)	110	4	16
Other varieties (10), av.	140	5	20

Mary's Gone Crackers:

	C	F	Cb
Cookies: Choc. Chip ; Dble Choc (2)	130	6	19
Ginger Snaps (3)	140	5	23
"N'Oatmeal" Raisin w/out Oats (2)	120	4	20
Crackers, all varieties (13)	140	5	21

Miss Meringue:
Madeleines:

	C	F	Cb
Tradt'nl Recipe (2), 1.2 oz	160	9	19
Traditional & Dipped (2), 1.2 oz	160	9	18

Meringue Classiques:

	C	F	Cb
Cappuccino (4), 1 oz	110	0	26
Mint Choc. Chip (4), 1 oz	120	1.5	25
Triple Chocolate (4), 1 oz	120	1.5	25
Vanilla Rainbow/Van. (4), 1 oz	110	0	27

Meringue Minis:

	C	F	Cb
Chocolate (13), 1 oz	110	0	26
Choc. Chip (12), 1 oz	130	1.5	27
Mint Chocolate Chip (12), 1 oz	120	1.5	25
Vanilla; Rainbow Van. (13), 1 oz	110	0	27
Sugar-Free: Chocolate (13), ½ oz	40	0	8
Vanilla (13), ½ oz	35	0	9

Mother's:

	C	F	Cb
Cookies: Choc. Chip (4), 1 oz	150	7	20
11.5 oz Tray (2), 1.1 oz	160	8	21
Circus Animal (6), 1 oz	150	7	20
Coconut Cocadas (5), 1.2 oz	160	8	21
Double Fudge (2), 1.3 oz	170	7	27
English Tea (2), 1.3 oz	180	7	27
Macaroons (2), 1 oz	170	11	17
Oatmeal (2), 1 oz	130	5	19
Taffy (2), 1.3 oz	180	8	27
Vanilla Creme (2), 1.3 oz	180	7	26
Iced: Lemonade (4), 1 oz	150	7	19
Oatmeal (4), 1.15 oz	150	6	23

Mrs Fields Cookies ~ *Fast-Foods Section, Page 219*

Murray:
Sugar Free Cookies:
Fudge-Dipped:

	C	F	Cb
Grahams (4)	140	8	19
Mint Cookies (4)	130	7	17
Vanilla Wafers (4)	150	10	19
Oatmeal (3)	140	7	21
Peanut Butter (3)	130	9	16
Sandwiches, Lemon; Creme (3), av	130	7	20
Shortbread (8)	130	5	21
Shortbread Pecan (3)	160	11	18
Vanilla Wafers (9)	130	5	24
Vanilla Creme Wafers (4)	130	8	19

Cookies ◆ Crackers C

Per Cookie/Cracker, Unless Indicated **C F Cb**

Nabisco:
Cookies:
Chips Ahoy!, Chocolate Chip:

	C	F	Cb
Original: 1.1 oz	160	8	22
1.4 oz	190	9	27
Mini Choc. Chips: Go-Pak (14)	150	7	21
Snak Saks (5)	150	7	21
Chewy, 0.95 oz	120	5	18
Chewy Gooey (2), all var., 1.1 oz	150	7	21
Chunky, Choc. Chunk (1), 0.6 oz	80	4	10
Ginger Snaps, (4)	120	2.5	23
Mallomars, 0.95 oz	120	5	18
Newtons: Fig (2), 1.1 oz	110	2	22
(4), 2.2 oz	220	4	44
Minis, 1.34 oz	130	3	26
Fat-Free (2), 1 oz	90	0	22
100% Whole Grain (2), 1 oz	110	2	22
Raspberry; Strawberry: (2), 1 oz	100	1.5	21
Mini Strawberry, 1.35 oz pkg	130	3	26
Fruit Crisps, all var., av., 1 pack	100	2	20
Fruit Thins, (3), all var., av., 1 oz	140	5	21
Nilla Wafers: (8), 1 oz	140	6	21
Reduced-Fat (8), 1 oz	120	2	24
Nutter Butter:			
P'nut Butter Sandwich:			
16 oz package, (2), 1 oz	130	5	20
1.9 oz package	250	10	37
Bites: 1.25 oz	170	7	24
Go-Pak, 4 oz pkg	540	22	80
Snak Sak, 1 oz	140	6	21
Oreo Sandwich Cookies:			
White Cream Filling:			
3 cookies, 1.2 oz	160	7	24
2 oz cookie	270	11	41
Choc. White Fudge Covered,			
3 cookies, 0.7 oz	100	5	13
Double Stuf (2), 1 oz	140	7	21
Mini Bite, Single Serve, 1.23 oz	170	7	25
Chocolate Creme Filling (2), 1.2 oz	150	7	21
Cool Mint; Peanut Butter (2), 1 oz	140	7	20
Fudge Cremes:			
Chocolate, 1.23 oz	170	9	24
Golden, 1.23 oz	180	9	25
Peanut Butter, 1.23 oz	170	9	23

Nabisco (Cont):
Oreo Sandwich Cookies Cont:

	C	F	Cb
Golden, White Creme Filling:			
3 cookies, 1.2 oz	170	7	25
1.8 oz Cookie	250	10	37
Double Stuf (2), 1 oz	150	7	21
Choc. Creme Filling, 1.2 oz	170	7	24
Triple Double, Chocolate, (1), 0.7 oz	100	4.5	15
Teddy Grahams:			
Snacks: Honey; Cinnamon (24)	130	4	23
Chocolate varieties (24), av.	130	4.5	22
Snak Saks, Mini Honey (47)	130	4	23
100 Calorie Packs:			
Thin Crisps/Cookie Crisps:			
Chips A'hoy, ¾ oz	100	3	18
Variety Pack, ¾ oz	100	3	16
Cookie Crisps, Lorna Doone , 0.7 oz	100	3	16
Toasted Chips,			
Baked Snack Crackers, 0.75 oz	100	3	16

Snackwells ~ See Page 87
Crackers:
	C	F	Cb
Barnum's: (8), 1 oz	120	3.5	22
Snak Saks 17), 1 oz	140	4	24
Flavor Originals:			
Chicken In A Biskit			
(12), 1 oz	160	8	19
Vegetable Thins (21), 1 oz	150	7	20
Honey Maid:			
Grahams: Original (8)	130	3.5	24
Low-Fat (8), av., 1.25 oz	140	2	28
Chocolate (8), 1.25 oz	140	3.5	27
Honey (8), 1. oz	130	3	24
Mini S'Mores, 1 oz	140	6	21
Premium:			
Original (5), ½ oz	70	1.5	12
Minis, ½ oz	70	2	11
Saltine, Original (5), ½ oz	70	1.5	12
Unsalted Tops (5), ½ oz	70	1.5	13
Triscuit: Per Serving			
Original (15), 1 oz	120	4.5	19
Roasted Garlic (8), 1 oz	120	4.5	20
Thin Crisps, all varieties, 1 oz	140	5	22
Wheat Thins:			
Original (16), 1 oz	140	5	22
Baked, Red.-Fat (16), 1 oz	130	3.5	22
Other varieties, av., (16), 1 oz	140	5	22
Fiber Selects (14),			
av. all varieties, 1.oz	120	4.5	22
Flatbread (2),			
av. all varieties, ½ oz	60	1.5	12
Multigrain (15), 1 oz	140	4.5	22
Wheatsworth,			
Stone Ground Wheat (5)	80	3.5	10

Updated Nutrition Data ~ www.CalorieKing.com
Persons with Diabetes ~ See Disclaimer (Page 22)

85

Per Cookie/Cracker, Unless Indicated **C F Cb**

Newman's Own Organics:
Cookies:

	C	F	Cb
Alphabet (10), average	120	3	21
Chocolate Cups:			
Milk/Dark Chocolate:			
Peanut Butter (3), average	180	13	17
Caramel (3), average	160	9	21
Dark Chocolate Peppermint (3)	190	11	18
Fig Newman's: Fat-Free, 2 bars	100	0	24
Low-Fat, 2 bars	110	1.5	23
Wheat/Dairy-Free, 2 bars	120	1.5	26
Newman-O's: Original (2)	130	5	19
Choc. Creme (2); Mint Creme (2)	120	5	19
Ginger-O's (2)	130	4.5	20

Nonni's:
Biscotti:

	C	F	Cb
Original, (1), 0.7 oz	90	3	14
Decadence (1), 0.85 oz	100	4	16
Av. other varieties (1), 0.85 oz	110	4	17
Bites: Classic Almond (4)	130	6	17
Almond Dark Chocolate (3)	120	6	16
Caramel Milk Chocolate (3)	110	4	18

Oreo Cookies ~ *See Nabisco, Page 85*

Peek Freans:
Cookies:

	C	F	Cb
Assorted Creme (3)	140	6	19
Nice Biscuits (1)	160	6	25
Shortcake (2)	140	7	18

Pepperidge Farm:
Cookies: *Per Cookie Unless Indicated*
American Collection:

	C	F	Cb
Chesapeake, Dark Chocolate Pecan	130	6	17
Lexington, Milk Chocolate, Toffee Almond	130	7	17
Nantucket: Dark Chocolate	130	6	18
Double	140	7	19
Sausalito, Milk Chocolate	130	6	17
Tahoe, White Choc. Macadamia	130	6	17
Brussels, (3)	150	7	20
Favorites, Chocolate (2)	130	7	16
Geneva, (3)	160	9	19
Milano: Original; Milk Choc (3), av.	175	10	21
Double Chocolate (2)	140	8	17
Orange; Raspberry (2)	130	7	16
Melts (2), all varieties	140	7	18
Slices (3), all varieties, average	150	8	18
Pirouettes, (2), all varieties, av.	120	4	19
Tahiti, Coconut (2)	170	10	17
Tim Tams:			
Caramel (2)	190	9	26
Choc. Creme (2)	190	10	24

100 Calorie Pouches,

	C	F	Cb
all varieties, average, 1 pouch	100	4.5	12

Per Cookie/Cracker, Unless Indicated **C F Cb**

Pepperidge Farm (Cont):
Crackers:

	C	F	Cb
Baked Naturals: 4 Cheese Crisps, (20), all varieties	140	6	19
Crackers (2), all varieties, average	135	4.5	23
Golden Butter (4)	70	2	10
Harvest Wheat (4)	100	4	14
Wheat Crisps (17)	140	5	21
Goldfish:			
Average all varieties: (55), 1 oz	140	5	23
1.5 oz pouch	210	8	37
2 oz carton	280	10	46
Jingos!, (23), all varieties, av.	135	4	22
Pretzel Thins:			
Baked Naturals (11)	110	0	21

Ritz:

	C	F	Cb
Crackers: Original, ½ oz	80	4.5	10
Reduced-Fat, ½ oz	70	2	10
Hint of Salt, ½ oz	80	4	10
Honey Butter (5), 0.6 oz	80	4	10
Roasted Vegetable, 0.6 oz	80	3.5	10
With Peanut Butter, 1.4 oz pkg	190	9	24
With Real Cheese, 1.4 oz package	200	12	22
Whole Wheat, ½ oz	70	2.5	11
100 Calorie Toasted Chips, Snack Mix, 0.78 oz	100	3	16
Crackerfuls, all varieties, 1 oz	130	7	17

Ritz Bits, Cracker Sandwiches:

	C	F	Cb
Cheese: Single Serve, 1.5 oz	220	13	24
3 oz Pack	450	25	50
Go-Pak (13), 1 oz	150	9	17
Cheddar Cheese, 1 oz pack	130	7	17
Four Cheese, 1 oz pack	130	7	17
P'nut Butter: Single Serve, 1.25 oz	170	10	20
Big Bag: (12), 1 oz	140	8	16
Whole Bag (36), 3 oz	420	23	48

Toasted Chips:

	C	F	Cb
Main Street Orig., 1 oz	130	4.5	21
All other Varieties, 1 oz	130	6	19

Safeway Select:

	C	F	Cb
Homestyle, Oatmeal Raisin, 1 oz	130	6	18
Indulgent: Dble Choc Chunk, 1 oz	130	7	18
Milk Choc. Macadamia Nut, 1 oz	140	8	17

Gourmet Sandwich Cremes:

	C	F	Cb
Maple Creme (2), 1 oz	170	7	25
Raspb. Swirl (2), 1 oz	130	5	20
Strawb. Swirl (2), 1 oz	130	6	19

Shar Gluten Free ~ *See CalorieKing.com*

Per Cookie/Cracker, Unless Indicated	C	F	Cb
Special K: Per 1 oz Serving			
Crackers: Multi/Herb, all var., av.	120	3	22
Cracker Chips (27), all varieties, av.	110	2.5	22
Popcorn Chips (28), all varieties, av.	120	2.5	23
Snackwell's:			
Creme S'wich (2) 1 oz	110	3	21
Devil's Food Cake, Fat-Free, ½ oz	50	0	12
100 Calorie Packs, all var., av., ¾ oz	100	4.5	17
Stella D'Oro:			
Biscotti, all varieties, av., ¾ oz	100	4.5	13
Breakfast Treats: Choc. Cookie	90	2.5	15
Original (1), 0.75 oz	90	3	14
Viennese Cinnamon	90	2.5	16
Margherite (2)	130	5	20
Roman Egg Biscuits, 1.1 oz	130	4	21
Swiss Fudge (2) 1.1 oz	170	9	22
Toast & Sponge:			
Almond Toast (2)	100	2	20
Anisette Sponge (2)	90	1	18
Anisette Toast, 1.1 oz	130	1	27
Streit's:			
Wafers: Chocolate (3)	160	9	19
Lemon (3)	170	10	19
Rolls, Chocolate (3)	105	6	12
Sunshine:			
Crackers:			
Krispy: Original; Whole Wheat (5)	60	1.5	11
Soup & Oyster, 16 crackers	60	1.5	11
Cheez-It, Snack Crackers:			
Original: 1.23 oz pkt	180	9	20
Red.-Fat (29), 1 oz	130	4.5	20
Big, Original (13), 1 oz	150	8	17
Cheddar Jack (25), 1 oz	140	7	17
Trader Joe's:			
100 Calorie Packs, average	100	2.5	18
Almond Windmill (2), 1 oz	140	6	18
Charmingly Chewy Choc Chip (2), 1 oz	130	5	20
Cherry Granola (2), 1 oz	110	4	19
Chocolate Almond Lacey's (1)	120	8	12
Chocolate Chip: Small (4), 1 oz	140	7	18
Large, singles, 1.7 oz	280	14	35
Vegan (1), 1 oz	130	6	18
Caramel Cashew (3), 1 oz	140	7	16
Crispy crunchy Choc Chip (12)	150	9	19
Crispy Oatmeal Choc Chip (12)	150	7	19
Dark ChocChunks w/ almonds (3)	140	7	17
Dunkers: Choc. Chip (2), 1.2 oz	160	7	21
Choc. Coated Choc. Chip (2), 1.3 oz	190	9	25
Ginger Snaps, Gluten Free, (5), 1 oz	140	6	21
Highbrow Chocolate (2)	140	7	19
Joe Joe's S'wich Cremes, Choc./Vanilla (2), 1 oz	130	6	19

Per Cookie/Cracker, Unless Indicated	C	F	Cb
Trader Joe's (Cont):			
Lemon Crisps (5)	150	7	19
Macarons A La Parisienne, 2 cookies, ¾ oz	90	3	10
Meringues, Fat-Free, Vanilla (4)	110	0	27
Oatmeal Raisin, 1.8 oz	270	12	35
Pecan Southern Style (4), 1 oz	150	9	15
Petite Cocoa Batons (17), 1 oz	140	5	22
Thins: Meyer Lemon (9), 1 oz	130	4.5	22
Toasted Coconut (8)	130	4.5	22
Triple Ginger (9), 1 oz	130	4	23
Triple Choc Chunk (4)	140	7	20
Ultimate Vanilla Wafers (5), 1 oz	120	6	15
Way More Chocolate Chip (3)	160	11	14
Crackers, Water (5)	60	1	12
Triscuits ~ See Page 85			
Voortman:			
Classics: Almond Krunch (2), 1 oz	140	6	20
Chunky Chip (1), 0.74 oz	100	4.5	14
Sugar Free, Choc. Chip (1), 0.7 oz	80	5	13
Wafers: All varieties (3), 1 oz	140	6	20
Sugar Free, Peanut Butter (4), 1 oz	150	7	17
Whole Foods (365 Organic):			
Choc Chip (2), 1 oz	150	7	21
Classic Fig Bars (2), 1.3 oz	140	2.5	27
Lemon Wafers (7), 1oz	110	3	19
Oatmeal (2), 1 oz	130	4.5	20
Sandwich Cremes (2), average	130	5	19
Sugar (2), 1 oz	130	4.5	21
WhoNu?:			
Chocolate/Vanilla Sandwich (3), av.	150	6	24
Crispy, Chocolate Chip (3)	160	7	22
Vanilla Wafers (8), 1 oz	130	5	20

Cookie ~ Mixes

Prepared as Directed			
Betty Crocker:	C	F	Cb
Pouch Mix: Per 2 Cookies			
Double Choc. Chunk; P'nut Butter, av.	140	6	21
Walnut Chocolate Chip	170	9	20
Other Varieties, average	145	6	22
Duncan Hines, Chocolate Chip, 2 cookies, 1.1 oz	180	9	23
Pillsbury:			
Chocolate; Oatmeal Choc. Chunk (2)	110	2.5	22
Funfetti: Chocolate (2)	110	2	22
Sugar, with Candy Bits (2)	110	2.5	23
Perfectly Pumpkin; Sugar (2)	110	2	23
Snickerdoodle (2)	110	1.5	23

Thaw, Bake & Serve | C | F | Cb

Pillsbury Cookies: *Per Cookie Unless Indicated*

Refrigerated Cookie Dough: *Per 1 oz cookie Dough*

Chocolate Chip Cookies	130	6	18
Peanut Butter	120	5	17
Sugar: Regular	120	5	18
Peppermint, 0.77 oz	100	4.5	14

Ready To Bake:

Chocolate Chip (2)	170	8	23
Chocolate Chunk & Chip (2)	170	8	23
Holiday Cookies, Sugar (2), all varieties, average	120	6	15
Sugar Cookie (2)	170	8	22

Big Deluxe Classics:

Chocolate Chip (1)	170	8	23
Oatmeal Raisin (1)	150	6	24
Peanut Butter Cup (1)	170	8	22
White Chunk Macadamia Nut	170	9	22
Simply Cookies: Chocolate Chip	150	7	20
Peanut Butter	140	6	19

Refrigerated Sweet Buns/Rolls~ *See Page 67*

Toll House (Nestle): *Per Cookie Unless Indicated*

Refrigerated Dough Bars:

Chocolate Chip (1)	90	4	11
Mini Brownie Bites (3)	160	8	20
Mini Choc. Chip (3)	160	8	20
Oatmeal Raisin (2)	160	6	24
P'B Chocolate Chip (1)	80	4.5	10
Sugar Cookie (1)	160	7	23

Ultimates Refrigerated Dough:

Chocolate Chip Lovers	180	9	23
Choc. Pecan Deluxe (1)	190	10	22
Choc P'nut Butter Deluxe (1)	180	9	23
Dark Choc. Delight (1)	160	8	21
Pecan Turtle Delight (1)	160	7	23

Crispbreads | C | F | Cb

Per Crispbread Unless Indicated

Finn Crisp:

Classic: Traditional, Rye	40	0.5	7
Hi-Fibre	40	0.5	6.5
Round: Original	45	0.5	7.5
Sesame	50	1	8

Kavli Norwegian:

Crispy Thin (3)	50	0	10
Golden Rye (1)	40	0	7
Hearty Thick (2)	60	0	12
Malsovit, Meal Wafers	75	4	7

New York Flatbread Crisps,

Everything, 0.4 oz	50	1.5	7
Ry-Krisp: Natural (2)	50	0	11
Seasoned (2)	60	1	11
Sesame (2)	60	1.5	10

Ryvita:

Crackerbreads: Orig.; Wholegrain	20	0	4
Crispbreads: Original; Dark	35	0	6.5
WASA: Crisp'n Light 7 Grain (3)	60	0	13
Fiber, 0.35 oz	35	0.5	8
Hearty, 0.5 oz	45	0	11
Light Rye (2), 0.5 oz	60	0	14
Multi Grain, 0.5 oz	45	0	10
Whole Wheat, 0.5 oz	50	1	10

Matzos

Manischewitz:

Matzos: Egg'n Onion, 1 oz	80	0.5	17
Thin Salted/Tea,av., 0.9 oz	95	0	20
Whole Wheat, 1 oz	110	1	21
Yolk Free, 1.2 oz	100	0	20

Crackers:

Tam Tam: Orig. (10), 1 oz	110	4	16
Everything; Onion (10), 1 oz	140	5	19
Sesame (10), 1 oz	140	6	19

Streit's:

Mediterranean Matzos, 1 Matzo, 1 oz	90	0.5	18
Unsalted Matzos, 1 Matzo, 1 oz	100	0	23

    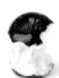

Quick Guide **C** **F** **Cb**

Cream
Average All Brands
Half & Half Cream:

	C	F	Cb
1 Tbsp, ½ oz	20	1.5	0.5
2 Tbsp, 1 oz	40	3	1
¼ cup, 2 oz	80	6	2
Single Serve Cup, ⅜ fl.oz	15	1.5	0.5
Light: Coffee/table (20% fat): 1 Tbsp	30	3	0.5
2 Tbsp, 1 oz	60	6	0.5

Sour Cream:

	C	F	Cb
Regular: 1 Tbsp, ½ oz	25	2.5	1
1 cup, 8 oz	445	45	7
Low-Fat/Light: 1 Tbsp, ½ oz	20	1.5	1
2 Tbsp, 1 oz	40	3	2
Fat-Free: Av., 2 Tbsp, 1 oz	20	0	4.5
Hood, 2 Tbsp, 1 oz	25	0	4
Kroger, 2 Tbsp, 1 oz	20	0	3
Naturally Yours; Oak Farm, 2 Tbsp	20	0	3
Knudsen, 2 Tbsp, 1 oz	30	0	5

Sour Cream Substitute:

	C	F	Cb
Albertson's, 2 Tbsp, 1 oz	60	5	2
Tofutti Sour Supreme, 2 Tbsp, 1 oz	85	5	9

Whipping Cream:
Heavy: (37% fat):

	C	F	Cb
1 T. fluid/2 T. whipped	50	5.5	0.5
¼ cup whipped	105	11	1
½ cup fluid/1 cup whipped	410	44	3.5

Light: (30% fat)

	C	F	Cb
1 Tbsp fluid/2 Tbsp whipped	45	4.5	0.5
½ cup fluid/1 cup whipped	350	37	3.5

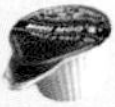

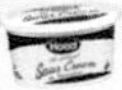

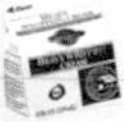

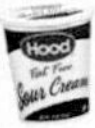

Coconut Cream/Milk

Coconut Cream: (Canned):

	C	F	Cb
Plain/unsweetened: 2 Tbsp, 1 oz	75	6.5	3
½ cup, 4 oz	285	26	12
Sweetened:			
Coco Lopez: 1 oz	130	5	21
½ cup, 4 oz	520	20	84

Coconut Milk: (Canned):

	C	F	Cb
Lite (Thai Kitchen), ¼ cup, 2 fl.oz	50	4.5	1
Premium (Thai Kitchen), 2 fl.oz	140	14	3
Coconut Water, (Center), 1 cup	45	0.5	9

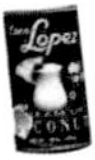

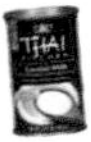

Whipped Toppings **C** **F** **Cb**

Average All Brands

	C	F	Cb
Cream (Pressurized): 2 T.	20	1.5	1
¼ cup	40	3.5	2
½ cup	75	6.5	4
Cream Topping, Lite, 2 T.	20	1	3
Cool Whip: Original, ⅓ oz	25	1.5	2
Extra Creamy, 2 Tbsp	25	2	2
Lite, 2 Tbsp, ¼ oz	20	1	3
Free, 2 Tbsp, 0.32 oz	15	0	3
Kraft, Dream Whip, 2 Tbsp	10	1	2
Reddi-Wip:			
Original, 2 T., 0.28 oz	15	1	1
Chocolate, 2 Tbsp, 0.28 oz	15	1	1
Extra Creamy, 2 Tbsp, 0.28 oz	15	1	1
Fat-Free, 2 Tbsp, 0.28 oz	5	0	1

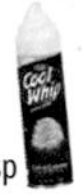

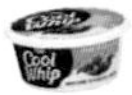

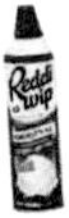

Creamers (Non-Dairy)

Powder:
Coffee-Mate/Cremora/N-Rich:

	C	F	Cb
Original: 1 tsp	10	0.5	1
1 heaping tsp	25	2	2
Lite, 1 tsp	10	0	2
Varieties: Av., 4 tsp	60	3	8
Fat-Free, average, 4 tsp	50	0	11

Liquid/Refrigerated: Per Tablespoon

	C	F	Cb
Bailey's: All varieties, av.,1 Tbsp	40	1.5	6
Fat Free, all varieties, 1 Tbsp	25	0	5
Coffee-Mate:			
Natural Bliss: All varieties,1 T.	35	1.5	5
Vanilla, Low-fat, 1 Tbsp	20	1	3
Unflavored: Original, 1 Tbsp	20	1	2
Fat-Free, 1 Tbsp	10	0	1
Low-Fat, 1 Tbsp	10	0.5	2
Varieties: All var., av.,1 Tbsp	35	1.5	5
Fat-Free, all varieties, 1 Tbsp	25	0	5
Hood, Country Creamer, 1 Tbsp	20	1.5	2
International Delight:			
American/Classic Varieties:			
Regular, all varieties, Tbsp	35	1.5	6
French Vanilla, fat free, 1 T.	30	0	7
CoffeeHouse Inspirations:			
All varieties, 1 Tbsp	35	1.5	6
Skinny, all varieties, 1 Tbsp	30	0	7
Kroger:			
Coffee, Fat-Free & Lactose Free:			
Caramel Vanilla, 1 Tbsp	25	1.5	6
Hazelnut, 1 Tbsp	35	1.5	6
Silk: Original, 1Tbsp	15	1	1
French Van.; Hazelnut, 1 Tbsp	20	1	3

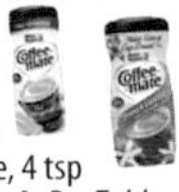

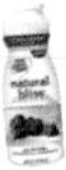

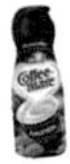

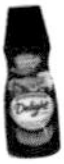

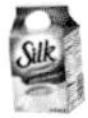

Ready-To-Serve   C F Cb

Hunt's: *Per 3.5oz Cup*

Snack Pack Puddings:

	C	F	Cb
Chocolate; Butterscotch, average	115	3	21
Tapioca	110	2.5	20
Vanilla	100	2.5	20
Chocolate, Fat Free	90	0	20
Sugar Free, all flavors, av.	65	3	11
Fruit Blasts: Lemon	120	2.5	24
Juicy Gels, all var., av.	100	0	25
Sugar Free, all var., av.	10	0	1

Jell-O *(Kraft):*

Cheesecake Snacks, (6 Pack),

Strawberry, 3.5 oz	130	2	25

Gelatin Snacks *(6 Pack):*

All varieties, 3.5 oz Cup	70	0	17
Sugar Free, 3.25 oz	10	0	0

Pudding Snacks: *Per 4 oz Cup*

Original: Chocolate	120	1.5	25
With Van. Swirls	110	1.5	24
Vanilla	110	1.5	23
Sundae Toppers, av.,	110	1.5	23
Tapioca, fat free	100	0	23

Smoothie Snacks, (6 Pack),

Mixed Berry; Strawb, Ban., 4 oz cup	100	2.5	18

Kozy Shack:

Puddings:

Choc., ½ cup, 4.6 oz	140	2.5	27
Butterscotch, 4 oz	120	2	24

Rice: *Per 1 Cup, 4 oz*

Original	130	2.5	24
Cinnamon Raisin	150	2.5	28
European Style	140	2.5	24

No Sugar Added:

Chocolate; Tapioca, av., 4 oz cup	70	1	14
Vanilla, 1/2 cup	90	3	10
Rice	70	1	14

Bread Pudding,

all varieties, av., 3.5 oz	145	2.5	26

Flan, Creme Caramel, 1 cup | 150 | 3.5 | 27 |

Kroger: *Per Container*

Butterscotch, 3.5 oz	110	2	22
Chocolate, 3.5 oz	110	2.5	21

Ready-To-Serve (Cont)   C F Cb

Swiss Miss:

Puddings: *Per 4 oz Cup*

	C	F	Cb
Classic Butterscotch	130	3.5	22
Creamy Vanilla	140	3.5	24
Triple Chocolate Dream	160	4	27

Pudding Snacks: *Per 4 oz Cup*

Banana Cream Pie	130	3	24
Vanilla	100	2.5	20
Chocolate	120	3	21
Fat Free	90	0	20

Homemade Puddings

Apple Tapioca, ½ cup	150	0	32
Bread Pudding, ½ cup	250	8	40
Blancmange, ½ cup	140	5	19
Chocolate, ½ cup	190	6	30
Crème Brûlée, ½ cup	400	35	16
Plum Pudding, 2 oz	170	3	32
Rice w/ Raisins, ½ cup	200	4	38
Sponge Pudding, 3.5 oz	340	16	45
Tapioca Cream, ½ cup	110	4	15
Trifle, ½ cup	180	7	26

Custards

Custard Mix *(Jello/Royal Flan), average:*

Dry, ¼ of 2.9 oz package, 0.73 oz,	80	0	19
Prepared: Whole milk, ½ cup	155	4	25
2% milk, ½ cup	140	2.5	24
Non-Fat milk, ½ cup	125	0	2

Home Made Egg Custard:

With Whole Milk, ½ cup	170	8	18
With 2% Milk, ½ cup	155	6.5	18

Gelatin • Parfait • Jell-O

Gelatin Dessert Mix: Prepared

Jell-O: Regular, all varieties, ¼ pkg	80	0	18
Sugar Free/Low Calorie, ¼ pkg	10	0	0

Creme Gelatin/Parfait: *Per ½ Cup*

Ida Mae	90	2	18
Reser's, Parfaits, all var., av., 3.88 oz	100	2	19

Meringues

Meringue Swirl, ½ oz	50	0	8
Meringue Shell, 1 oz shell	100	0	16

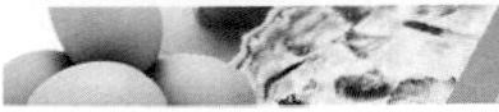

Chicken Eggs

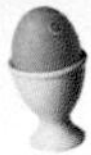

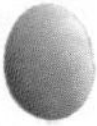

	C	F	Cb
Fresh Eggs:			
Raw (weight with shell):			
Small, 1.4 oz	65	4	0
Medium, 1.55 oz	70	4	0
Large, 1.76 oz	75	4.5	0
Extra Large, 1.98 oz	80	5	0
Jumbo, 2.22 oz	90	5.5	0
Egg Yolk, 1 extra large	63	5	0
Egg White, 1 extra large	16	0	0
Dried Egg Powder:			
Whole Egg: ¼ cup, 1 oz	170	12	0
1 Tbsp	30	2	0
Egg White, ¼ cup, 1 oz	105	0	0
Egg Yolk, ¼ cup, 1 oz	195	18	0

Egg Substitutes

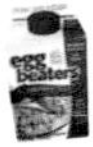

¼ Cup (Equivalent to 1 Egg) ~ Zero Cholesterol

	C	F	Cb
All Whites (Crystal Farms), 1.6 oz	25	0	0
Better 'n Eggs (Crystal Farms):			
Regular, ¼ cup, 2 oz	30	0	1
Plus, ¼ cup, 2 oz	35	0	1
Egg Beaters (Conagra):			
Original, 3 Tbsp, 1.6 oz	25	0	1
Southwestern Style, 3 Tbsp, 1.6 oz	20	0	1
Egg Replacer (Ener-g), 1.5 tsp,	15	0	4
Eggs (Second Nature),			
Fat-Free, ¼ cup, 2 fl.oz	35	0	0.5
Egg Substitute (Albertson's), ¼ cup	30	0	1
Naturegg (Burnbrae Farms),			
Simply Egg White, ¼ cup, 2 oz	30	0	1

Other Eggs

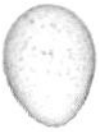

	C	F	Cb
Duck, 1 large, 2.5 oz	130	9.5	0
Goose, 1 large, 5 oz	280	19	0
Quail, 3 eggs, 1.6 oz	42	3	0
Turkey, 1 large, 3 oz	135	9.5	0
Turtle, 1 egg, 1.75 oz	75	5	0

Omega-3 Fat Enriched

	C	F	Cb
Eggland's Best, 1 large	70	4	0
Eggs Plus (Pilgrim's Pride), 1 large	70	4.5	1

Note: Cholesterol content same as regular eggs, but Omega-3 fats inhibit blood cholesterol increase.
Extra Notes ~ See Page 259

Cooked Eggs

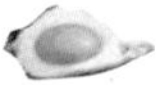

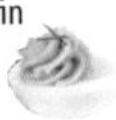

	C	F	Cb
Boiled Egg: *Same as Raw Egg*			
Hard-Cooked, Small, Peeled	65	4	0
Fried Egg:			
With fat: 1 large egg	105	9	0.5
2 small eggs	175	13	1
No fat/nonstick pan, 1 large	75	5	0.5
Deviled Egg, 2 halves	145	13	0.5
Eggs Benedict, (2)			
on Toast or English Muffin	860	56	25
Eggs Florentine, (2)			
on Toast or English Muffin	890	59	25
Pickled Egg, 1 large	80	5.5	0
Poached Egg, 1 large	65	4	0
Quiche (Homemade):			
Egg & Bacon, 1 slice, 5.3 oz	580	43	27
Ham & Cheese, 1 slice, 5.3 oz	475	33	29
Scotch Egg, 1 egg	300	21	16
Scrambled Eggs: 1 large egg:			
With 1 Tbsp milk + 1 tsp fat	120	9	1
With 1 Tbsp skim milk/no fat	85	5.5	1
2 large eggs:			
With 2 Tbsp milk + 2 tsp fat	260	20	2
With 2 Tbsp skim milk, w/o fat	180	11	2

Omelets

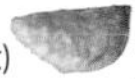

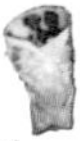

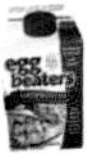

	C	F	Cb
1 Egg: Plain (with 1 tsp fat)	125	10	0.5
With: ½ oz cheese	175	15	0.5
½ oz cheese + ½ oz ham	200	16	0.5
2 Eggs: Plain (with 2 tsp fat)	250	20	1
With: 1 oz cheese	360	29	2
1 oz cheese + 1 oz ham	410	32	2
3 Eggs: Plain (with 1 Tbsp fat)	360	29	1.5
With: 2 oz cheese	580	47	2.5
2 oz cheese + 2 oz ham	680	53	2.5
Extras: Tomato/Onion/Veggies	20	0	4.5
Egg Substitute (EggBeaters):			
2 eggs (½ cup) + 1 tsp fat	100	4	2
3 eggs (¾ cup) + 2 tsp fat	160	8	3
Extras: 1 oz Cheese	110	9	1
1 oz Ham	50	3	1
Tomato/Onion/Veggies	20	0	4.5

Egg Nog

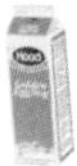

	C	F	Cb
Average all Brands,			
½ cup, 4 oz	170	9.5	17
Regular (Borden), ½ cup	160	9	17
Golden (Hood), ½ cup	180	9	22
Light/Low-Fat (Horizon; Hood),	140	4	22

Breakfast Sides

	C	F	Cb
Toast: Plain, 1 thick slice	85	1	13
With: 2 tsp butter/margarine	155	9	13
3 tsp/1 Tbsp fat	190	13	13
English Muffin: Plain, 2 oz	130	1	26
With 3 tsp fat	230	12	26
Bacon, 2 strips	70	5	0
Ham, Lean, 2 oz	100	3	0
Hash Browns:			
½ cup, 3 oz	125	6.5	14
1 cup serving, 6 oz	250	13	28
Sausages, 2 links (1 oz each)	180	16	1.5

Frozen Egg Breakfasts

Aunt Jemima:
Breakfast Sandwiches: *Per Sandwich*

	C	F	Cb
Biscuits: Sausage, Egg & Cheese	340	21	27
Croissant, Sausage, Egg & Cheese	350	23	23
Griddlecake, Ham, Egg & Cheese	240	8	33

Jimmy Dean:
Breakfast Sandwiches: *Per Sandwich*

	C	F	Cb
Biscuits: Chicken	330	16	35
Ham & Cheese	230	10	34
Sausage, Egg & Cheese	330	20	26
Croissant, Sausage, Egg & Cheese	420	28	30
Muffin, Sausage, Egg & Cheese	330	20	26
Omelets: *Per Omelet*			
Three Cheese	290	23	4
Ham & Cheese	250	19	4

Pillsbury,

	C	F	Cb
Egg Scrambles, Bacon/Ssg & Chse	280	16	26

Red Baron:
Scrambles: *Each*

	C	F	Cb
Bacon, 5 oz	390	19	38
Sausage; Western, 5 oz	360	17	38

Frozen Pancake/Waffles ~ *See Page 132*
Toaster Pastries ~ *See Page 64*

Frozen Egg Rolls

Kahiki: *Each*

	C	F	Cb
Chicken, 3 oz	90	3.5	12
Pork, 3 oz	110	6	11
Vegetable, 3 oz	80	3	12
La Choy,			
Chicken Mini (1), 3 oz	140	4.5	18
Lotus: Chicken; Pork (1)	160	7	25
Vegetarian, 3 oz	120	4.5	21
Pagoda Express: *Without Sauce*			
Chicken (1)	140	4.5	20
Vegetable (1)	130	4.5	20
Trader Joes,			
Vegetable (1), 3 oz	110	4	16

Fast-Foods/Restaurants

Arby's,

	C	F	Cb
Bacon, Egg & Cheese Croissant	380	24	24
Au Bon Pain, Egg on a Bagel	430	12	58

Bob Evans:
Omelets: Border Scramble

	C	F	Cb
Omelets: Border Scramble	630	45	15
Ham & Cheddar	485	36	4
Western	495	35	7
Bojangles: Egg & Cheese Biscuit	515	34	35
Bacon, Egg & Cheese Biscuit	550	37	35

Bruegger's:

	C	F	Cb
Bagels: With Egg & Cheese, 6.8 oz	430	18	63
With Egg, Chse & Sausage, 8.8 oz	500	24	64

Burger King:

	C	F	Cb
Croissan'wich's: Bacon, Egg & Chse	320	18	25
Ham, Egg & Cheese	320	16	25
Double, Sausage, Egg & Dble Chse	660	48	27
Carl's Jr, Bacon & Egg Burrito	560	32	37

Chick-Fil-A,

	C	F	Cb
Chkn, Egg & Chse on Multigr. Bagel	480	20	48
Del Taco, Egg & Cheese Burrito	400	17	22

Denny's: *Without Sides*

	C	F	Cb
T-Bone Steak & Eggs	790	36	4
Omelette: Fit Fare	390	18	25
Ultimate	605	48	8
Veggie-Cheese	440	33	9

Dunkin Donuts:

	C	F	Cb
Bacon, Egg & Cheese Croissant	550	34	31
Ham, Egg & Cheese Bagel	500	15	68

Eat 'N Park:
Omelettes:

	C	F	Cb
Ham & Cheese	535	35	4
Meat Lovers	725	55	3.5
Hardee's: Loaded Omelet Biscuit	610	42	36
Smoked Sausage, Egg & Cheese Bisc.	750	56	38
IHOP: T-Bone Steak & Eggs, 12 oz	1250	68	74
Spinach & Mushroom	910	70	24

Jack in the Box:

	C	F	Cb
Bacon, Egg & Cheese Biscuit	430	25	35
Sausage, Egg & Cheese Biscuit	570	38	36
McDonald's: Egg McMuffin	300	12	30
Bacon & Cheese Biscuit, regular	420	23	37

Whataburger,

	C	F	Cb
Breakfast Platter with Bacon	730	45	93

Quick Guide

Butter

Average All Brands

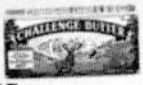

	C	F	Cb
Regular: 1 tsp, 0.18 oz	35	4	0
1 Pat/Single Portion, 0.18 oz	35	4	0
1 Tbsp, approximately, ½ oz	100	11	0
2 Tbsp, 1 oz	205	23	0
1 Stick, ½ cup, 4 oz	810	92	0
1 Pound, 2 cups, 16 oz	3255	368	0
Light: (Regular) 40% Fat:			
1 tsp, 0.18 oz	25	3	0
1 Tbsp,½ oz	75	8.5	0
2 Tbsp, 1 oz	145	16	0
Whipped Butter: (Regular):			
1 tsp, 0.14 oz	30	3	0
1 Tbsp, 0.35 oz	65	7.5	0
1 Stick, ½ cup, 2 .66 oz	545	62	0
Whipped Light Butter *(Land O Lakes):*			
1 tsp, 0.15 oz	15	1.5	0
1 Tbsp, 0.4 oz	45	5	0
2 Tbsp, 0.8 oz	90	10	0
Unsalted: Same as Salted			

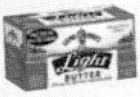
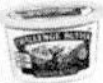
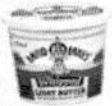

Flavored Butter/Spreads

Average All Brands

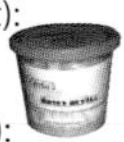
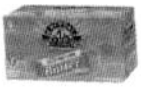

	C	F	Cb
Honey Butter: (60% Fat):			
1 Tbsp, ½ oz	90	8	4
Downey's, 1 Tbsp, 0.5 oz	60	1	11
Garlic Butter: (80% Fat):			
1 Tbsp, ½ oz	100	11	0
Sweet Cream Butter:			
Regular, 1 Tbsp	100	11	0
Stick *(Parkay)*, 60% Fat, 1 Tbsp	80	9	0
Tub *(Land O'Lakes)*, 50% Fat,1 Tbsp	70	8	0

Butter & Butter Blends

Per 1 Tablespoon

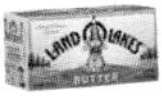

	C	F	Cb
Challenge: Stick, ½ oz	100	11	0
Tub, Whipped, 0.3 oz	70	7	0
Brummel & Brown,			
Butter Blended with Yogurt, ½ oz	45	5	0
Downey's, Honey Butter, ½ oz	60	1	11
Land O'Lakes:			
Sticks: Original, ½ oz	100	11	0
Light, ½oz	50	6	0
Tubs: Light, Whipped, 0.4 oz			
Butter With Olive Oil, ½ oz	90	10	0
Honey Butter Spread, 0.45 oz	70	6	4

Ghee (Clarified Butter)

(Example: *Purity Farms*)
Note: Ghee is 100% fat compared to regular butter (80% fat + 20% water)

	C	F	Cb
1 tsp, 0.18 oz	45	5	0
1 Tbsp, ½oz	120	14	0

Light & Reduced Fat Spreads

Per 1 Tablespoon

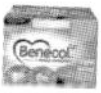
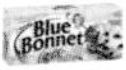

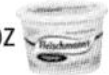
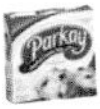

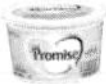
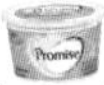
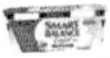
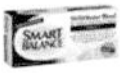

	C	F	Cb
Best Life, Buttery, 0.45 oz	60	6	0
Benecol: Reg., ½ oz	70	8	0
Light, ½ oz	50	5	0
Blue Bonnet:			
Stick, Light Spread, ½ oz	50	5	1
Tub, Original Soft Spread, ½ oz	60	6	0
Country Crock *(Shedd's):*			
Tubs: Regular Spread, ½ oz	70	7	0
Light Spread, ½ oz	50	5	0
Fleischmann's:			
Original Soft Spread, 0.4 oz	60	7	0
Light Spread, ½ oz	40	4.5	0
'I Can't Believe It's Not Butter':			
Tubs: Original Soft Spread, ½ oz	70	8	0
Light, ½ oz	5	5	0
Imperial, Stick, ½ oz	80	9	0
Parkay:			
Original Soft Spread, 0.4 oz	80	9	0
Spray, 5 sprays	0	0	0
Squeeze Bottle, ½ oz	70	8	0
Promise:			
Activ, Light Spread, ½ oz	45	5	0
Buttery Spread, ½ oz	80	8	0
Light Spread, ½ oz	45	5	0
Fat-Free Spread, ½ oz	45	0	0
Smart Balance:			
Spread, Omega 3, 1 tbsp, ½ oz	100	11	0
Tubs: Buttery Spread, Orig., ½ oz	80	9	0
Light Original, ½ oz	50	5	0
HeartRight, Light, ½ oz	45	5	0
Omega 3: Orig., 0.45 oz	80	8	0
Light, ½ oz	50	5	0
Whipped, low sodium, 0.4 oz	60	7	0

Butter Substitutes

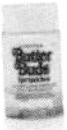

	C	F	Cb
Butter Buds:			
Butter Flavored Mix, 1 tsp	5	0	2
Butter Flavored Sprinkles, 1 tsp	5	0	2
Earth Balance,			
Non GMO, 1 T.	100	11	0
Molly McButter, ½ tsp	5	0	1
Shedd's Willow Run, Soy, 1 Tbsp	100	11	0
Sunsweet, (Butter/Oil Replacement),			
Lighter Bake, 1 Tbsp, 0.67 oz	35	0	9

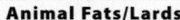
Animal Fats/Lards **C** **F** **Cb**

Average All Types
Beef Tallow/Drippings, Lard (Pork),
Chicken, Duck, Goose, Turkey:

1 Tbsp, 13g		**115**	**13**	0
2¼ Tbsp, 1 oz		**255**	**28**	0
1 cup, 7.25 oz		**1850**	**205**	0
½ pound, 8 oz		**2040**	**227**	0

Ghee/Butter/ Oil ~ *See Page 93*

Vegetable Shortening

Average All Types

1 Tbsp, 13g		**115**	**13**	0
2¼ Tbsp, 1 oz		**250**	**28**	0
1 cup, 7.25 oz		**1810**	**205**	0

Vegetable Oils

Includes almond, avocado, canola, corn, coconut, flaxseed, grapeseed, linseed, mustard, olive, palm, peanut, rice bran, safflower, sesame, sunflower, soybean, wheat germ.
Note: Oil is 100% fat.

1 tsp, 5g		**45**	**5**	0
1 Tbsp, ½ oz		**120**	**14**	0
2 Tbsp, 1 oz		**240**	**28**	0
1 cup, 7.25 oz		**1930**	**205**	0

Fish Oils

Average All Types
(Includes Cod Liver, Herring,
Salmon, Sardines): 1 Tbsp, ½ oz **125** **14** 0

Cooking Sprays/Squeezes

Cooking Sprays: (PAM, Mazola, I Can't Believe It's Not Butter, Weight Watchers, Wesson):

Pam: ¼ second spray	**2**	**0**	0
1-3 second spray	**6**	**1**	0
I Can't Believe It's Not Butter,			
Original Spray	**0**	**0**	0
Parkay, Buttery Spray	**0**	**0**	0

Olestra (Olean) **C** **F** **Cb**

Olestra *(Olean)* **0** **0** **0**
Note: Olean is Proctor & Gamble's brand name for Olestra – a no-calorie cooking oil that gives snacks (like potato chips, tortilla chips and crackers) taste and texture without adding fat or calories.
Examples:
• *Frito-Lay,* Light Products
  (Lays, Ruffles, Tostitos, Doritos)
• *Pringles,* Fat-Free Potato Crisps

Quick Guide

Mayonnaise
Regular: *Per 1 Tbsp, 0.5 oz Unless Indicated*

Average All Brands	**90**	**10**	0
Best Foods/Hellmans; Kraft:			
Original/Real	**90**	**10**	0
½ cup, 4 oz	**720**	**80**	0
Hain, Safflower Mayonnaise	**100**	**11**	0
Spectrum, Canola Mayo	**100**	**11**	0

Light/Reduced Fat: *Per 1 Tbsp, 0.5 oz*

Best Foods/Hellman's,	**35**	**3.5**	1
Kraft, Original/Olive Oil	**45**	**4**	2
Smart Balance, Omega Plus	**50**	**4.5**	2
Spectrum, Light Canola Mayo Eggless	**35**	**3.5**	2

Fat Free:

Kraft: Original, 1 Tbsp	**10**	**0**	2
½ cup, 4 oz	**80**	**0**	16
Sugar Free, Dukes Mayo, 1 Tbsp	**100**	**12**	0

Mayonnaise Style Dressing:
Per 1 Tbsp, 0.5 oz

Best Foods, Sandwich Spread	**60**	**5**	2
Kraft:			
Miracle Whip Dressing:			
Original	**40**	**3.5**	2
Light	**20**	**1.5**	2
Free	**15**	**0**	3
Sandwich Shop Mayo:			
Chipotle	**40**	**4**	2
Horseradish-Dijon	**40**	**3.5**	2
Hot & Spicy	**100**	**11**	2
Nasoya, Tofu Base/Dairy Free/Eggless:			
Original	**35**	**3.5**	1
Fat-Free	**10**	**0**	2

Quick Guide

Fresh Fish **C F Cb**

Low Oil (Less than 2.5% fat):
White/Lightly-colored flesh. Examples:
Cod, Flounder, Haddock, Halibut, Mahi Mahi,
Perch, Pike, Pollock, Snapper, Sole, Whiting.

Per 4 oz Edible Portion

	C	F	Cb
Raw, 4 oz (without bones)	100	1	0
Steamed, Broiled, Baked	140	1.5	0
Fried: Lightly Floured	210	8	3.5
Breaded	260	12	8
In Batter	320	16	27

Medium Oil (2.5-5% fat):
Lightly-colored flesh. Examples: **C F Cb**
Bluefin Tuna, Catfish, Kingfish, Orange Roughy,
Salmon (Pink), Swordfish, Rainbow Trout, Yellowtail.

Raw, 4 oz (without bones)	145	7	0
Baked, Broiled, 4 oz	195	8	0
Fried, 4 oz	230	11	8

High Oil (Over 5% fat):
Darker-colored flesh. Examples: **C F Cb**
Albacore Tuna, Mackerel, Salmon
(Atlantic/Chinook/Sockeye), Sardines, Trout.

Raw, 4 oz (without bones)	220	14	0
Baked, Broiled, 4 oz	275	17	0
Fried, 4 oz	340	23	12

> **Cooking Yields (Fin Fish):**
> 4 oz Raw wt. = 3.5 oz Cooked weight
> 4 oz Cooked wt. = 5 oz Raw weight
>
> **Calorie & Fat Variations:**
> The amount of fat/oil in fish varies with the species,
> season and locality. Within the same fish, fat/oil
> content is generally higher towards the head.

Fish & Shellfish **C F Cb**

Edible Weights: (no bones/shell)

	C	F	Cb
Abalone: Raw, 3 oz	90	0.5	5
Fried, 3 oz	160	6	9.5
Ahi Tuna, grilled, 6 oz fillet (w/o fat)	235	2	0
Anchovy: Paste, 1 Tbsp, 0.5 oz	45	3	1
Pickled, 1 oz	50	3	0
Canned in oil, drained, (5), 0.7 oz	40	2	0
Barracuda (Pacific), raw, 4 oz	130	3	0
Basa (Swai), raw, 4 oz fillet	70	2	0
Bass:			
Sea: Raw, 4.6 oz fillet	125	2.5	0
Baked, 3 oz	105	2	0
Striped: Raw, 1 fillet, 5.5 oz	150	3.5	0
Baked, 3 oz	105	3	0
Freshwater: Raw, 3 oz	95	3	0
Baked, 3 oz	125	4	0

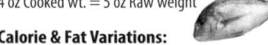

Fish & Shellfish **C F Cb**

Edible Weights: (no bones/shell)

	C	F	Cb
Calamari/Squid:			
Raw: 4 oz	100	1.5	3.5
Baked, 1 cup	190	6.5	5.5
Fried, 3 oz	150	6	7
Catfish:			
Farmed: Raw, 1 fillet 5.6 oz	190	9.5	0
Baked, 1 fillet 5 oz	205	10	0
Wild: Raw, 1 fillet, 5.6 oz	150	4.5	0
Baked, 1 fillet, 5 oz	150	4	0
Breaded, fried, 1 fillet, 3 oz	200	12	0
Caviar, black/red, 1 Tbsp, 16g	40	3	0.5
Clams: Raw, 3 oz (4 large/9 small)	70	1	3
Breaded, Fried, 6.6 oz (20 small)	380	21	20
Canned, drained, 1/2 cup, 2.8 oz	115	1	0
Steamed, 3.3 oz (10 small)	140	2	5
Clam Juice (*Snow's*), 1 Tbsp	0	0	0
Cod:			
Atlantic: Raw, 4 oz	95	1	0
Baked, 3 oz	90	1	0
Canned, solids & liquid	90	0.5	0
Pacific: Raw, 4 oz	80	0.5	0
Baked, 3 oz	70	0.5	0
Crab:			
Alaska King,			
1 leg, cooked, 4.7 oz	130	2	0
Blue: Raw, 1 crab, 6 oz	150	1	0
Steamed, 3 oz	70	0.5	0
Canned, drained, 6.5 oz can	105	0.5	0
Dungeness: Raw, 1 crab, 5.75 oz	140	1.5	0
Steamed, 4.45 oz	140	1.5	0
Crab Cakes (*Capt. D's*), (1), 2.8 oz	250	16	16
Crayfish:			
Farmed: Raw, 3 oz	60	1	0
Steamed, 3 oz	75	1	0
Wild: Raw 3 oz	65	1	0
Steamed, 3 oz	70	1	0
Cuttlefish, raw, 3 oz	70	1	1
Dolphinfish ~ *See Mahi-Mahi*			
Eel: Raw, 3 oz	155	10	0
Baked, 3 oz	200	13	0
Fish & Chips (*Red Lobster*),			
Battered, w/out condiments	630	26	54
Fish Sandwich (*Burger King*),			
w/o Tartar Sauce	410	12	53
Fish Oil, 1 Tbsp, 0.5 oz	125	14	0
Flounder/Sole:			
Raw, 4 oz	80	2	0
Baked, 3 oz	75	2	0
Frozen Fish ~ *See Pages 114-122*			

Fish & Shellfish (Cont)

Edible Weights: (no bones/shell)

	C	F	Cb
Haddock: Raw, 4 oz	85	0.5	0
Baked, 3 oz	75	0.5	0
Smoked, 3 oz	100	1	0
Halibut:			
Atlantic: Raw, 4 oz	105	1.5	0
Baked, ½ fillet, 5.6 oz	175	2.5	0
Herring:			
Atlantic, raw, 4 oz	180	10	0
Canned: Plain, drained, 3 oz	130	8	0
In Tomato Sauce, 3.5 oz	140	8	2
Pickled, 2 pieces, 1 oz	75	5	3
Smoked, kippered, 4 oz	245	14	0
Jellyfish: Raw, 4 oz	30	0	0
Dried, Salted, 1 cup, 2 oz	20	1	0
Ling, raw, 4 oz	100	0.5	0
Lobster, Northern:			
Whole Lobster, 1.5 lb:			
Edible portion: Raw, 6.25 oz	140	1.5	0
Boiled: 5 oz	140	1	0
Lobster Salads, average, ½ cup	220	13	5
Lobster Newberg, average, ¾ cup	360	20	9
Lobster Thermidor, av., 1 serving	370	22	15
Lobster Tail (Red Lobster), grilled/roasted	170	1	1
Lox, Regular/Nova, 2 oz	65	2.5	0
Mackerel, Atlantic: Raw, 4 oz	230	16	0
Baked, 3 oz fillet	225	15	0
Pacific/Jack: Raw, 4 oz	180	9	0
Baked, 3 oz	170	9	0
Spanish: Raw, 4 oz	160	7	0
Baked, 3 oz	135	5.5	0
Mahi-Mahi (Dolphinfish):			
Raw, 4 oz	95	1	0
Baked, 4 oz	125	1	0
Monkfish: Raw, **4 oz**	85	1.5	0
Baked, **3 oz**	80	2	0
Mullet, striped: Raw, 4 oz	135	4.5	0
Baked, 3 oz	130	4	0
Mussels:			
Raw: 4 oz (edible wt)	100	2.5	4
1 cup, 5.25 oz (edible wt)	130	3.5	5
Cooked, moist heat, 3 oz	150	4	6
Ocean Perch:			
Atlantic: Raw, 4 oz	90	2	0
Baked, 3 oz	80	1.5	0
Octopus:			
Common: Raw, 4 oz	95	1	2.5
Boiled, 4 oz	140	2	4
Orange Roughy: Raw, 4 oz	85	1	0
Baked, 3 oz	90	1	0

Fish & Shellfish (Cont)

Edible Weights: (no bones/shell)

	C	F	Cb
Oysters, Common: Raw, 3 oz	70	2	4
Eastern:			
Farmed: Raw, 6 medium, 3 oz	50	1.5	4.5
Cooked, dry heat, 6 med., 2 oz	45	1.5	4.5
Wild: Raw, 6 medium, 3 oz	45	1.5	2.5
Cooked, dry heat, 6 med., 2 oz	45	1.5	2.5
Breaded & Fried, 6 medium, 3 oz	175	11	10
Pacific: Raw, 1 medium, 1.75 oz	40	1	2.5
Steamed, 1 medium, 0.9 oz	40	1	2.5
Perch ~ *See Ocean Perch*			
Pike: Northern: Raw, 4 oz	100	1	0
Baked, 3 oz	95	1	0
Walleye: Raw, 4 oz	105	1.5	0
Baked, 3 oz	105	1.5	0
Pollock, Atlantic: Raw, 4 oz	105	1	0
Baked, 3 oz	100	1	0
Pompano, Florida, raw, 4 oz	185	11	0
Red Snapper ~ *See Snapper*			
Roe, raw, 2 Tbsp, 1 oz	40	2	0.5
Sablefish: Raw, 4 oz	220	17	0
Smoked, 3 oz	220	17	0
Salmon:			
Atlantic, Farmed: Raw, 4 oz	235	15	0
Baked, 3 oz	175	10	0
Steaks: Raw, 7 oz	410	27	0
Baked, 6 oz	365	22	0
Atlantic, Wild: Raw, 4 oz	160	7	0
Baked, 3 oz	155	7	0
Steaks: Raw, 7 oz	280	13	0
Baked, 6 oz	310	14	0
Chinook: Raw, 4 oz	205	12	0
Baked, 3 oz	195	11	0
Smoked, 3 oz,	100	3.5	0
King: Raw, 3.5 oz	185	12	0
Kippered, 3.5 oz piece	265	16	0
Smoked & canned, 3.5 oz	150	6	0
Coho:			
Farmed: Raw, 4 oz	180	8.5	0
Baked, 3 oz	150	7	0
Wild: Raw, 4 oz	165	6.5	0
Steamed, 3 oz	155	6.5	0
Pink/Chum: Raw, 4 oz	145	5	0
Baked, 3.5 oz	155	5.5	0
Canned: Drained solids, 11.1 oz	435	16	0
W/o skin & bones, 8.54 oz	330	10	0
Sockeye: Raw, 4 oz	160	6.5	0
Baked, 3 oz	145	5.5	0
Canned, Drained solids, 3 oz	140	6.5	0
Smoked, 3.5 oz	205	7.5	0
Salmon Cake (1), 3 oz	240	15	6

Fish (Cont)

	C	F	Cb
Sardines (Canned): *Average All Brands*			
Drained of Oil:			
¼ cup drained, 2.15 oz	130	9	0
3.75 oz can, drained, 3.25 oz	190	11	0
1 large/2 medium, ⅗", 0.8 oz	50	3	0
In Tomato Sauce, 3.75 oz	150	8	3
Sashimi ~ *See Japanese Foods, Page 171*			
Scallops: Raw, 6 large/15 small, 3 oz	65	0.5	3
Breaded, Fried, 6 pieces, 5 oz	385	20	39
Steamed, 3 oz	95	0.5	0
Sea Bass: Raw, 4 oz	110	2	0
Baked, 3 oz	105	2	0
Seafood Salad, Deli Style,			
½ cup, 3.5 oz	250	21	11
Shark: Raw, 4 oz	145	5	0
Baked, 3 oz	185	7	0
Batter-dipped, fried, 4 oz	260	16	7
Shrimp:			
Raw: Small/Medium (4), 0.75 oz	15	0	0
Large (4), 1 oz	20	0	0
3 oz	60	1	0
Breaded & Fried, 4.75 oz	395	24	27
Steamed, in shell, 3 oz	100	1.5	0
Canned, 1 can, 4.5 oz	130	2	0
Snapper: Raw, 4 oz	115	1.5	0
Baked, 3 oz	110	1.5	0
6 oz fillet	220	3	0
Sole: Raw, 4 oz	80	2	0
Baked, 3 oz	75	2	0
Squid ~ *see Calamari*			
Surimi, (Imitation Crab), 4 oz	110	0.5	17
Swai, (Basa), raw, 4 oz	70	2	0
Swordfish: Raw, 4 oz	165	7.5	0
Medium Steak, 6 oz	250	11	0
Baked: Small Steak, 4 oz	205	7	0
Medium Steak, 6 oz	290	13	0
Tilapia: Raw, 4 oz	110	2	0
Baked, 3 oz	110	2.5	0
Trout, Rainbow:			
Farmed: Raw, 4 oz	160	7	0
Baked, 3 oz	145	6.5	0
Wild: Raw, 4 oz	135	4	0
Baked, 3 oz	130	5	0
Tuna: *Average All Brands*			
Raw: Bluefin, 4 oz	165	5.5	0
Skipjack, Yellowfin, av., 4 oz	120	1	0
Baked: Bluefin, 3 oz	155	5.5	0
Skipjack, Yellowfin, av., 3 oz	110	1	0
Canned:			
In Water, drained:			
Chunk Light: 2 oz can	50	0.5	0
3 oz can	75	1	0
6 oz can	150	2	0

Tuna (Cont):	C	F	Cb
In Water, drained (Cont):			
Solid White: 2 oz can	75	1.5	0
3 oz can	110	2.5	0
6 oz can	220	5	0
In Oil, drained:			
Chunk Light: 2 oz can	110	4.5	0
6 oz can	315	14	0
Solid White: 2 oz can	105	4.5	0
6.3 oz can	330	14	0
Tuna Salad, Deli Style, ½ cup, 4oz	280	20	8
Whitefish: Raw, 4 oz	150	6.5	0
Baked, 3 oz	145	6.5	1
Smoked, 3 oz	90	1	0
Whiting: Raw, 4 oz	100	1.5	0
Baked, 3 oz	100	1.5	0
Yellowtail: Raw, 4 oz	165	6	0
Grilled, 3 oz	160	6	0

Other Canned/Packaged Fish

	C	F	Cb
Bumble Bee:			
Tuna Salad Kits: *With Crackers*			
Original: 3.5 oz pkg	300	22	18
With Mayo., 4.9 oz	560	39	34
Fat-Free, 3.5 oz	150	2	24
Lunch on the Run Kit, 8.2 oz	500	26	52
Seafood Salad, w/ Crackers, 3.3 oz pkg	150	5	24
Sensations Bowls:			
Lemon & Cracked Pepper Tuna, 3 oz	110	3	2
Spicy Thai Chili Tuna, 3 oz	160	7	9
Chicken of the Sea:			
Albacore Tuna in Water, 2.5 oz pouch	100	1.5	0
Pink Salmon, skinless/boneless, 2.6 oz pouch	90	3	0
Shrimp, medium, 4 oz can	90	1	2
Gorton's *(Frozen)* ~ Page 114			
Kroger *(Frozen)* ~ Page 116			
Starkist:			
Autentico, 2 oz drained, av.	85	5	3.5
Pouch: *Per 2.6 oz Pouch*			
Albacore Tuna in water	90	2	1
Chunk, Light, Tuna in water	80	0.5	1
Lunch-To-Go Kit: Chunk Light Tuna			
With Mayo & Crackers, 4 oz	240	9	20
Tuna Creations: *Per 2.6 oz package*			
Herb & Garlic	110	4	2
Lemon Pepper	80	0.5	0
Van De Kamp's *(Frozen)* ~ Page 122			

Restaurant Chains

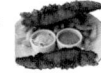

Captain D's Seafood ~ *Page 187*
Long John Silver's ~ *Page 213*
Southern Tsunami ~ *Page 242*

Flours & Grains	C	F	Cb
Amaranth Flour, ½ cup, 3.5 oz	365	6.5	65
Arrowroot Flour, ½ cup, 2.25 oz	230	0	56
Barley: Grain, reg., ½ cup, 2.6 oz	255	1	55
Pearled, raw, 3½ oz	350	1	78
Buckwheat: Grain, ½ cup, 3 oz	290	3	61
Flour, whole-groat, ½ cup, 2 oz	200	2	42
Groats: Roasted, dry, ½ cup, 2.9 oz	285	2	62
Roasted, cooked, 3.5 oz	80	0.5	17
Bulgur: Dry, ½ cup, 2.5 oz	240	1	53
Cooked, ½ cup, 3.2 oz	75	0.5	17
Carob Flour, ½ cup, 1.8 oz	115	0.5	46
Corn Kernels, av., ckd, ½ cup	80	0.5	18
Corn Bran, ½ cup, 1.3 oz	85	0.5	33
Corn Flour/Masa, ½ cup, 2 oz	215	2.5	43
Corn Grits: Dry, ½ cup, 2.75 oz	290	1	62
Cooked, ½ cup, 4¼ oz	70	0.5	15
Corn Germ, toasted, ½ cup, 4 oz	100	1.5	22
Cornmeal: Average all Types,			
3 Tbsp, 1 oz	105	0.5	22
½ cup, 2½ oz	255	1	54
Mixes: same as above	230	1	48
Cornstarch: 1 Tbsp, 0.3 oz	30	0	8
½ cup, 2¼ oz	245	0	58
Couscous: Dry, 1 oz (3 oz cooked)	110	0	22
1 cup cooked, 5.5 oz	175	0.5	37
Farina: Dry, ½ cup, 3.1 oz	325	0.5	69
Cooked, ½ cup, 4.1 oz	55	0	12
Flaxseed: Whole, 1 T., 0.3 oz	45	3.5	3
Ground, 2 Tbsp, 0.3 oz	60	4.5	4
Garbanzo (Chick Pea), ½ cup, 1.6 oz	180	3	27
Gluten Free (King Arthur), 3 Tbsp	110	0	24
Matzo Meal, ½ cup, 2.2 oz	230	0.5	48
Millet: Raw, ½ cup, 3.5 oz	380	4	73
Cooked, ½ cup, 3 oz	105	1	21
Oat Bran: Raw, ½ cup, 1.1 oz	75	2	21
Cooked, ½ cup, 3.75 oz	45	1	13
Oats, rolled/oatmeal:			
Dry/Groats, ½ cup, 1.5 oz	160	3	28
Cooked, ½ cup, 4.2 oz	75	1	13
Polenta ~ See Cornmeal			
Potato Flour, ½ cup, 2.8 oz	285	0.5	66
Psyllium Husks, 1 Tbsp, 0.15 oz	20	0	4
Quinoa: Dry ½ cup, 3 oz	320	5	59
Cooked, ½ cup, 3¾ oz	130	2	24
Rice Bran, ½ cup, 2 oz	180	12	28
Rice Flour, ½ cup, 2.75 oz	290	1	63

Flours & Grains (Cont)	C	F	Cb
Rice Polish, ½ cup, 3.5 oz	360	0.5	80
Rye Flour: Dark, ½ cup, 2.3 oz	210	2	44
Medium, ½ cup, 1.8 oz	180	1	40
Light, ½ cup, 1.8 oz	190	1	41
Rye Grain: ½ cup, 3 oz	280	2	59
Flakes, ¼ cup, 1 oz	100	0.5	21
Semolina, ½ cup, 3 oz	300	1	61
Sorghum, ½ cup, 3.4 oz	325	3	72
Soy Flour:			
Defatted, 1 cup, 3.5 oz	330	1	38
Low-Fat, 1 cup, 3 oz	325	6	33
Full-Fat, 1 cup, 3 oz	365	17	29
Soy Meal, defatted, 1 cup, 4.3 oz	415	3	49
Spelt Flour, ½ cup, 2 oz	190	1	41
Tapioca, Pearl:			
Dry, ½ cup, 2.7 oz	270	0	67
3 Tbsp, 1 oz	100	0	25
Teff (Seed) Flour, 2 oz	215	2	42
Tortilla Flour Mix, ½ cup, 2 oz	220	6	37
Triticale: ½ cup, 3.4 oz	325	2	70
Flour, wholegrain, ½ cup, 2.3 oz	220	1	48
Wheat Bran, unproc., ½ cup, 1 oz	65	1	19
Wheat Flakes, ½ cup, 1.5 oz	160	1	35
Wheat Germ:			
Raw, ¼ cup, 1 oz	105	3	15
Toasted, ¼ cup, 1 oz	110	3	14
Wheat Flour:			
White, All Purpose/Self-Rising:			
1 level Tbsp, 0.28 oz	30	0	6
½ cup, 2.2 oz	230	0.5	48
1 cup, 4.4 oz	455	1.5	95
Whole Wheat, 1 cup, 4.2 oz	405	2	87

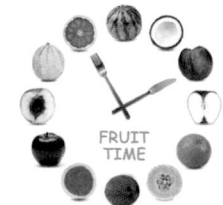

FRUIT TIME

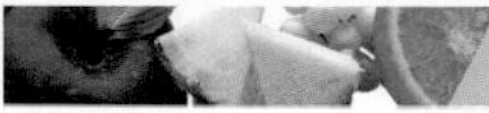

Weights As Purchased	C	F	Cb
Apples: Average all varieties,			
Whole (with skin):			
1 small (4 per lb), 4 oz	55	0	14
1 med., (3 per lb), 5.5 oz	75	0	19
1 large (2 per lb), 8 oz	110	0	28
1 extra large, 11 oz	145	0	36
Flesh only (no skin or core): 1 oz	15	0	3.5
1 cup slices, 4 oz	55	0	14
Candy/Caramel Apple, 1 med., 6.5 oz	245	4	54
Chiquita Apple Bites, 10 slices, 3.5 oz	50	0	12
Apricots: 1 small (12 per lb)	20	0	4
1 medium (8 per lb), 2 oz	25	0	6
1 large (5-6 per lb), 3 oz	40	0	10
Asian Pear, (Nashi Fruit), 1 med., 7 oz	85	0	21
Avocado, (Wt. without seed/skin):			
Average: ½ med., 3.5 oz	160	15	8
Salad slice, 0.5 oz	25	2	1
Mashed/Puree: 2 Tbsp, 1 oz	50	4.5	2
¼ cup, 2 oz	90	9	5
Californian, ½ medium, 3 oz	160	14	8
Mashed/Puree, ½ cup, 4 oz	190	18	10
Florida, ½ medium, 5.5 oz	180	15	12
Mashed/Puree, ½ cup, 4 oz	140	11	9
½ cup cubed, 3 oz	105	8	7
Banana, (weights with skin):			
1 small (6", 4 per lb), 4 oz	90	0	23
1 medium (7", 3 per lb), 5 oz	105	0	27
1 large (8"), 7 oz	120	0	30
1 extra large (9"), 9 oz	135	0	35
without skin, 1 oz	25	0	6
Black Raspberries, 1 cup, 5 oz	70	0	16
Blackberries, 1 cup, 5 oz	60	0.5	14
Blueberries: ¼ cup, 1 oz	15	0	4
1 cup, (½ pint)	80	0.5	20
Boysenberries, 1 cup, 4.5 oz	60	4.5	14
Breadfruit, ½ cup, 4 oz	115	0	30
Cactus Pear, 1 fruit, 3.5 oz	40	0	9
Cantaloupe: Flesh (without rind), 1 oz	10	0	2
1 cup pieces/balls, 5.5 oz	55	0	13
Slices, ½ Circle (no rind):			
1 thin (buffet), (⅛"), 0.5 oz	5	0	1
1 medium (¼"), 1 oz	10	0	2
1 thick (½"), 2 oz	20	0	5
Wedges (Length cut, w/o rind):			
1 thin, 1/16 medium, 2 oz	20	0	5
1 thick, ⅛ medium, 4 oz	40	0	9
Whole (Weights with seeds and rind):			
½ small, 20 oz	195	1	46
½ medium, 28 oz	270	1.5	65
½ large, 2.5 lb	370	2	90
Carambola, (Starfruit), 1 med., 3 oz	30	0	6

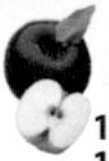

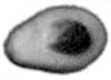
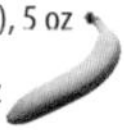

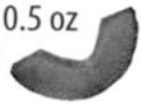
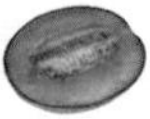

Weights As Purchased	C	F	Cb
Cassava, ⅓ cup, 2.5 oz	115	0	27
Cherimoya, 1 fruit, 11 oz,			
8¼ oz edible	175	1.5	41
Cherries: Sweet (Red/White), raw,			
8 cherries, 2 oz	30	0	8
1 cup, 4.5 oz	75	0	19
½ lb (30 cherries)	130	0.5	32
Sour, red, raw, 1 cup, 4 oz	50	0	12
Clementine, 1 medium, 2.6 oz	35	0	9
Coconut: Fresh,			
1 piece, 2"x2"x ½", 1 oz	100	10	4.5
Shredded, fresh, ½ cup, 1.4 oz	140	13	6
Sweetened, dried, ½ cup, 1.6 oz	235	16	22
Crabapples, ½ cup slices, 2 oz	40	0	11
Cranberries, ¼ cup, 1 oz	25	0	6.5
Currants, raw, ½ cup, 2 oz	35	0	8
Custard Apple ~ *See Cherimoya*			
Dragon Fruit, (Pitahaya),			
1 medium, 12 oz	145	0.5	39
Durian, flesh, 4 oz	165	6	31
Elderberries, ½ cup, 2.5 oz	55	0.5	13
Feijoa, (Pineapple Guava),			
1 medium, 2 oz	30	0.5	5.5
Figs, green/black:			
1 medium, 2 oz	40	0	10
1 large, 3 oz	60	0	15
Gooseberries, raw, ½ cup, 2.5 oz	35	0	7
Grapefruit: Av. all types,			
½ fruit, 10 oz (6 oz flesh)	55	0	13
1 cup sections w/ juice, 8 oz	75	0	18
Grapes: Average, 1 cup, 5.5 oz	105	0	28
1 small bunch, 4 oz	80	0	20
1 medium bunch, 7 oz	140	0	36
1 large bunch, 16 oz	315	0	82
Granadilla, flesh, 3.5 oz	95	0	23
Guava, 1 medium, 4 oz	80	1	16
Honeydew: 1 slice, ¾" thick, 3 oz	30	0	7
1 wedge (⅛ of 7" diam.),			
12 oz (with rind)	80	0	20
1 cup cubes/balls, 6 oz	60	0	14
½ small (4½ lb whole)	180	0.5	42
½ medium (6lb whole)	230	1	56
Honey Murcots, 1 only, 5 oz	45	0	11
Jaboticaba, flesh, 4 oz	75	2	15
Jackfruit, flesh, ⅛ average, 4 oz	105	0	27
Java-Plum, 4 plums, 0.5 oz	10	0	2
Kiwifruit,: 1 Medium, 2.7 oz	45	0	11
1 Large, 3.2 oz	55	0.5	13
Kumquats, 5 medium, 3.5 oz	65	1	15
Kiwano, ½ medium, 5 oz	35	0	8
Langsat, Duku, 1 medium, 2 oz	25	0	5
Lemon: 1 medium, 3 oz	25	0	8
1 wedge, 1 oz	5	0	1.5
Peel, grated, 1 Tbsp	5	0	1

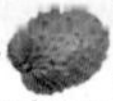
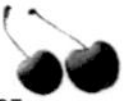
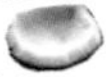

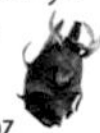
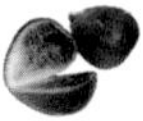

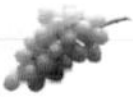

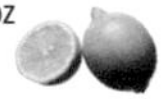

Updated Nutrition Data ~ www.CalorieKing.com
Persons with Diabetes ~ See Disclaimer (Page 22)

Weights As Purchased	C	F	Cb
Limes, 1 medium (2" diam.), 2.4 oz	20	0	7
Loganberries, frozen, ½ cup, 2.5 oz	40	0	9
Longans, 5 fruit, 0.5oz	10	0	2.5
Loquats, 4 fruit, 2.25 oz	30	0	8
Lychees, 4 fruit, 2.25oz	30	0	7
Mamey Apple, ¼ fruit, 7 oz	100	1	25
Mandarin Orange:			
1 small, 3 oz	35	0	9
1 medium, 4 oz	45	0	11
1 large, 6 oz	50	0	13
Mango: Flesh, ½ cup slices, 3 oz	55	0	14
1 small mango, 7 oz	90	0.5	24
1 medium: 10 oz	130	0.5	34
1 cheek, 4 oz	60	0	14
1 large, 17 oz	220	1	58
1 extra large mango, 24 oz	310	1.5	82
Marionberries, 1 cup, 5 oz	75	1	15
Melon, av., 1 c., cubes/balls, 6 oz	60	0	14
Monstera Deliciosa,			
Edible part, 4 oz	50	0	11
Mulberries, 20 fruit, 1 oz	15	0	3
Nashi Fruit, (Asian Pear), 1 med. 7 oz	85	0	21
Nectarines: 1 medium, 4 oz	50	0	12
1 large, 5.5 oz	70	0	16
Oheloberries, ½ cup, 2.5 oz	20	0	5
Olives, (Pickled): Green, 10 lge, 1.5 oz	60	6.5	1.5
Ripe, Greek Style, 10 medium, 1 oz	70	6	4
Ripe (Black) Californian:			
1 small/medium	5	0	0.2
1 large/extra large	6	0.5	0.5
1 jumbo	7	0.5	0.5
1 colossal	11	0.5	0.5
Oranges: Average all varieties (weights with skin)			
1 small, 5 oz	45	0	11
1 medium (3" diam.), 7 oz	85	0	21
1 large, 10 oz	130	0	33
Californian Valencia,			
1 medium (2¾" diam.), 6 oz	60	0	14
Calif. Navels (3" diameter), 7 oz	70	0	17
Sunkist, Navel, large, 14 oz	130	0	30
Florida Orange, 1 med, 7 oz	70	0	17
Flesh only, 1 cup, 6 oz	85	0	21
Peel, 1 Tbsp	0	0	0
Papaya: 1 cup, 1" pieces, 5 oz	60	0	15
1 medium, (5"x3" diam.), 16 oz	120	0	30
Green (unripe), ½ cup, 3.5 oz	20	0	5
Passionfruit,			
1 medium, 1.25 oz	35	0	8
Peaches: 1 small/donut, 3 oz	30	0	7.5
1 medium (4 per lb), 4 oz	45	0	11
1 large, 6 oz	65	0	16
1 extra large, 10 oz	110	0	27

Weights As Purchased	C	F	Cb
Pears: Average all types:			
1 mini, 2.5oz	35	0	8
1 small, 5 oz	75	0	18
1 medium, 7 oz	105	0	25
1 large, 9 oz	135	0	33
1 extra large, 12 oz	175	0	42
Pepino, ½ medium, 4 oz	20	0	4
Persimmons: Native, 1 oz	35	0	9
Japanese (2½"d. x 2½"h), 7 oz	120	0	30
Seedless (Maui), 1 medium, 5 oz	100	0	25
Pineapple, (wts w/out skin):			
1 thin slice (½"), 2 oz	25	0	6
1 thick slice (¾"), 3 oz	40	0	10
1 cup, diced, 5.5 oz	75	0	19
1 medium, 1½ lb (peeled)	325	0	86
Wedges (Del Monte), 12 oz pkg	195	0	47
Canned ~ See Page 102			
Pitanga, (Surinam-Cherry) (5), 1.2 oz	10	0	2
Plantains: ½ cup slices, 2.5oz	90	0	22
Plums: Average all types,			
Mini/Damson, (1" diameter), 0.5 oz	10	0	1.5
Small (2" diameter), 2.25oz	30	0	7
Med. (2½" diam.), 3.5 oz	45	0	10
Large (3" diameter), 5 oz	60	0	14
Pluot, (Plum-Apricot), 1 med. 5 oz	80	0	19
Pomegranate, 1 medium, 10 oz	105	0.5	25
Pomelo, flesh, ½ cup, 3.5 oz	35	0	9
Prickly Pear, (Nopal):			
1 small, 2.5 oz	20	0	5
1 medium, 5 oz	40	0	10
Quince, 1 medium, 3.5 oz	55	0	14
Rambutan, (Rambotang),			
Red/Yellow, 1 medium, 2 oz	15	0	4
Raspberries: ½ cup, 2 oz	30	0	7
10 Raspberries, 0.75 oz	10	0	2
1 Cup, 4.25 oz	65	1	15
1 Pint, 11 oz	160	2	37
Sapodilla, (Chico), 1 med., 7.5 oz	140	2	34
Sapote, ½ medium, 8 oz	150	0.5	38
Satsuma Tangerine, 1 med., 3 oz	45	0	11
Soursop, 1 cup pulp, 8 oz	150	0.5	38
Starfruit, 1 medium, 3 oz	30	0	6
Strawberries: 1 cup, 5.5 oz	50	0.5	12
6 medium/3 large, 2 oz	20	0	4
1 pint, 13 oz	115	1	27
Chocolate Dipped, 1 large	45	2.5	6
Sugar Apple, (Custard Apple)			
½ cup pulp, 4 oz	120	0	30
Tamarillo, 1 medium, 3 oz	20	0	3
Tamarind: 1 fruit (3"x1")	5	0	1.5
Pulp, ½ cup, 2 oz	140	0.5	37

Weights as Purchased	C	F	Cb
Tangelo: 1 small, 4 oz	55	0	13
1 medium, 5 oz	70	0	17
1 large, 7 oz	95	0	23
Tangerine, 1 med., (2½" diam.), 4 oz	50	0	13
Tangor, 1 medium, 4 oz	35	0	7
Tomatillos: 3 med., 3.5 oz	35	0.5	6
1lb (16 oz)	160	2	27
Tomatoes:			
1 small (2¼" diameter), 3 oz	15	0	3
1 medium (2¾" diameter), 5 oz	25	0	5
1 large (3½" diameter), 8 oz	40	0.5	9
1 extra large (3" diameter), 12 oz	60	0.5	14
Grape, 5 medium, 2 oz	10	0	2
Yellow Tear Drop, 3 medium, 1 oz	5	0	2
Cherry: 4 medium, 2 oz	10	0	2
1 cup, 5 oz	25	0	6
Slices (Medium Tomato):			
2 thin slices, 1 oz	5	0	1
2 thick (⅜"), 2 oz	10	0	2
Wedge, ¼ med. tomato, 1.25 oz	6	0	1
Fried Green Tomato, 2 sl., 2.5 oz	140	11	9
Canned Tomatoes/Products ~ *See Page 144*			
Tree Tomato, (Tamarillo), 3 oz	20	0	5
Ugli Fruit, Tangelo type, 5 oz	40	0	8
Watermelon: Flesh only, 1 oz	8	0	2
1 thin slice, (¼ circle, ⅜"), 2 oz	15	0	4
1 cup cubes or balls, 5½ oz	45	0	11
10 balls, 4.3 oz	35	0	9
Buffet Slice, thin, 1 oz	8	0	2
Regular, (Long Shape):			
1 thick (1") slice (¼ circle, 4½" radius)			
9 oz w. skin (5½ oz no rind)	50	0	12
1 thin (½") slice (¼ circle)	25	0	6
1 thick (1") slice (½ circle)			
18 oz with rind	100	1	22
1 whole melon (15" long, 7½"diameter)			
20 lb w/ rind, 10 lb w/o rind	1360	7	330
Seedless, (Round Shape):			
Medium size (13 lb, 8¼" diameter)			
1 whole, 8½ lb without rind	1160	5	280
Wedge (⅛ whole melon),			
26 oz with rind	145	1	35
Flesh only, without rind, 8 oz	70	0.5	17
Mini size (6 lb, 6½" diameter):			
1 whole, 3½ lb without rind	480	2.5	110
Wedge (⅛ whole),			
1.5 lb, with rind	60	0.5	14

FRUIT & VEGETABLE JUICES
~ See Page 41

Dried Fruit

	C	F	Cb
Apples, 5 rings, 1 oz	80	0	19
Apricots, 8 halves, 1 oz	65	0	16
Banana Chips, ½ cup, 1.5 oz	220	14	25
Banana Flakes, 4 Tbsp, 1 oz	80	0	20
Cranberries *(Craisins):*			
Sweetened, ¼ cup, 1 oz	100	0	24
Unsweetened, ¼ cup, 1 oz	80	0	19
Choc-coated, 1 oz	135	7.5	18
Currants, ¼ cup, 1.25 oz	100	0	25
Dates: 5 medium dates, 1.5 oz	120	0	29
Large Californian: 1 date, 0.7 oz	55	0	13
3 dates, 2 oz	170	0	39
½ cup, chopped, 3 oz	240	0	58
Pecan Date Rolls, 1 oz	100	2.5	19
Date Crumbles *(Bob's Redmill),*			
¼ cup, 1 oz	90	0	22
Figs, 3 medium figs, 1 oz	90	0	23
Goji Berries, 3 Tbsp, 1 oz	100	1	20
Longans; Lychees, 1 oz	80	0	20
Mango Slices, 5 pieces, 1.4 oz	25	0	6
Papaya Spears, 2 pieces, 1.4 oz	120	0	30
Peaches, 2 halves, 1 oz	60	0	15
Pears, 3 halves, 2 oz	140	0.5	34
Plums *(Sunsweet),* (5), 1.4 oz	100	0	24
Prunes, (dried Plums): With pits, 1 oz	70	0	17
1 medium (60/lb)	16	0	4
1 large (50/lb)	22	0	5
1extra large (40/lb)	25	0	6
Without pits, 4 medium, 1 oz	70	0	17
Cooked: With sugar, ½ cup, 5 oz	155	0	38
Without sugar, ½ cup, 4.5 oz	135	0	33
Raisins: 2 Tbsp, 1 oz pack	85	0	20
½ cup, 2.8 oz	220	0.5	56

Candied/Glazed Fruit

	C	F	Cb
Apricot, 1 medium, 1 oz	70	0	17
Cherry, (Maraschino) (1)	8	0	2
Citron/Fruit Peel, 1 oz	85	0	20
Ginger, 1 oz	90	0	21
Pineapple, 1 slice, 1.25 oz	120	0	29

Fruit Leather/Rolls

	C	F	Cb
Average All Brands, 1 oz	105	1	24
Betty Crocker: Fruit By The Foot,			
1 roll, ¾ oz	80	0	17
Fruit Gushers 1 oz	90	1	20
Fruit Roll-Ups, 1 roll	50	1	12
Stretch Island, Leathers, 2 pcs, 1 oz	90	0	24

Canned/Bottled Fruit

Solids & Liquids:
Per ½ Cup, 4½ oz Unless indicated

	C	F	Cb
Apricots: In water/diet	35	0	8
In juice/lite	60	0	15
In syrup	105	0	28
Black/Blueberries:			
Heavy syrup	120	0	30
In light syrup	110	0	26
Cherries, pitted: In water	55	0	15
In light syrup	85	0	22
In heavy syrup	105	0	27
In extra heavy syrup	135	0	34
Maraschino, 1 oz	50	0	12
Pie Cherries, ⅔ cup, 5 oz	90	0	23
Fruit Salad: In water/diet	35	0	10
In light juice	60	0	16
In heavy syrup	95	0	25
Gooseberries, Light syrup	90	0	24
Grapefruit: Juice pack	45	0	12
In light syrup	75	0	20
Lychees, ½ cup, 4.5 oz	105	0	26
Mixed Fruit: In water/diet	40	0	10
In fruit juices/light syrup	70	0	18
In heavy syrup	90	0	24
Peaches (halves/slices): In water/diet	30	0	7
In juice/light	55	0	14
In light syrup	70	0	18
Drained, ½ peach	55	0	14
In heavy syrup	100	0	26
Pears: In water/diet	35	0	10
In light juice	60	0	16
In heavy syrup	100	0	26
Pineapple: All types			
In own juice	75	0	20
In heavy syrup	100	0	26
1 slice (ring), drained, 1.5 oz	15	0	4
Prunes: In heavy syrup	125	0	33
In Liqueur, 4.4 oz	280	0	70
Stewed in Water, ½ cup	135	0	35
Tropical Fruit Salad: In light syrup	80	0	21
In heavy syrup	110	0	29

Fruit Snack Cups

	C	F	Cb
Deli/Take-Out: Small, 6 oz	70	0	16
Large, 12 oz	140	0	32
Yogurt & Fruit Cup, 15 oz	380	4.5	75
Del Monte:			
Bowls: *Approx. ¼ of 20.5 oz Container, 4.4 oz*			
Cherry Mixed Fruit	70	0	17
Citrus Salad; Grapefrt Duo	60	0	16
Red Grapefruit	60	0	14
Fruit Naturals: *Per ½ of 7 oz cup, 3.5 oz*			
Cherry Mixed Fruit; Peach Chunks, av.	60	0	16
Mandarin Orange Segments	70	0	17
Pineapple Chunks	70	0	18
Red Grapefruit	60	0	16
Average others	70	0	18
Pull Top Cans: In 100% Juice, ½ c.	65	0	17
Lite varieties, ½ cup	60	0	15
Snack Cups: *Per 4 oz Cup*			
Cherry Mix	70	0	18
Average other varieties	70	0	17
No Sugar Added, av. all varieties	35	0	11
Super Fruits: *Per 6 .oz Cup*			
Mixed Fruit Chunks in Juice	120	0	29
Peaches/Pears in Juice, av	110	0	29
Dole Fruit Bowls:			
4 oz Bowls: Diced Peaches	80	0	19
Mixed Fruit	80	0	19
Pineapple; Tropical Fruit, average	60	0	15
Fruit-n-Gel Bowls, av. all, 4.3 oz	95	0	23
Safeway (Vons):			
Fruit Cocktail: *Per ½ Cup, 4.5 oz*			
In heavy syrup	100	0	25
Lite in Pear Juice	60	0	14

Apple & Fruit Sauces

	C	F	Cb
Apple Sauce:			
Regular/sweetened, 2 Tbsp, 1 oz	20	0	6
4 oz package	85	0	22
¼ cup	50	0	13
Fruit Sauces & Purees:			
Average all fruit types: 2 Tbsp, 1 oz	25	0	6
½ cup, 4 oz	100	0	24
Mott's:			
Apple Sauce: Original, 4 oz	90	0	24
Fruit Flavored, average, 4 oz	90	0	23
Healthy Harvest, 3.92 oz	50	0	13
Ocean Spray: *Per ¼ Cup*			
Jellied Cranberry Sauce	110	0	25
Whole Berry Cranberry Sauce	110	0	25

Pie Fillings ~ *See Page 134*

Quick Guide · C · F · Cb

Ice Cream

Vanilla: *Average All Brands*
Other flavors ~ *See Brand Listings.*
Counts per USDA food database unless specified

Regular (10% fat):

	C	F	Cb
1 scoop, 3 fl.oz	175	9	20
½ cup, 4 fl.oz	235	13	27
1 Pint, 16 fl.oz	940	50	107
½ Gallon (4 pints, 64 fl.oz)	3755	200	428

Rich/Premium (16-17% fat):
Examples: Baskin Robbins, Haagen-Dazs

	C	F	Cb
1 scoop, 3 fl.oz	210	14	19
½ cup, 4 fl.oz	285	19	25
1 Pint, 16 fl.oz	1130	74	100
½ Gallon (4 pints, 64 fl.oz)	4525	295	400

Super Rich (20-21% fat):
Example: Haagen-Dazs Butter Pecan

	C	F	Cb
1 scoop, 3 fl.oz	235	17	16
½ cup, 4 fl.oz	310	23	21
1 Pint, 16 fl.oz	1240	92	84

Reduced-Fat/Light (5% fat):
Examples: Breyers Half The Fat, Friendly's Light

	C	F	Cb
1 scoop, 3 fl.oz	105	4	15
½ cup, 4 fl.oz	140	5	21
1 Pint, 16 fl.oz	560	25	84

Fat-Free:
Example: Dreyers Fat-Free

	C	F	Cb
1 scoop, 3 fl.oz	70	0	16
½ cup, 4 fl.oz	90	0	21
1 Pint, 16 fl.oz	360	0	84

Soft Serve:

	C	F	Cb
Regular: ½ cup, 4 fl.oz	255	15	25
1 cup, 8 fl.oz	510	30	50
Light: ½ cup, 4 fl.oz	145	3	25
1 cup, 8 fl.oz	290	6	50

Quick Guide · C · F · Cb

Frozen Yogurt
Average All Brands

	C	F	Cb
Hard: Low-Fat, ½ cup	110	3	19
Non-Fat, ½ cup	110	0	24
Soft: Low-Fat, ½ cup	120	4	17
Non-Fat, ½ cup	100	0	30

Brands ~ *See Ice Cream & Ices Section*

Quick Guide · C · F · Cb

Gelato/Ices/Frozen Custard

Gelato: *Per ½ Cup*

	C	F	Cb
Milk base: Vanilla	160	6	25
Chocolate Hazelnut	230	15	21
Water base, ½ cup	100	0	26

Frozen Custard: *Per ½ Cup*

	C	F	Cb
Chocolate	140	6	18
Orange Sherbet	105	2	21
Vanilla	130	6	16

Ice (Milk base): *Average all flavors*

	C	F	Cb
Hard (4% fat), ½ cup	100	3	15
Soft Serve (3% fat), ½ cup	110	2	19
Shaved Ice, average, 12 fl.oz	160	0	40
Sherbet, average, ½ cup	110	1.5	22
Sorbet, Fruit (without fat), ½ cup	70	0	19
Fruit Ice Pops	80	0	20

Sundaes · C · F · Cb

Baskin Robbins:

Classic:	C	F	Cb
Banana Royale	620	28	87
Banana Split	1010	34	173
Brownie	920	47	119

Premium:	C	F	Cb
Chocolate Chip Cookie Dough	990	43	138
Made With Snickers	1000	46	138
Reeses Peanut Butter Cup	1220	80	109

Denny's:

	C	F	Cb
Banana Split, 15 oz	810	31	125

Toppings ~ See Page 195

McDonald's:

	C	F	Cb
Hot Caramel Sundae	340	8	60
Hot Fudge Sundae	330	10	54
Strawberry Sundae	280	6	49
Toppings, Peanuts, ¼ oz	45	3.5	2

Ice Cream Cones & Cups

Average All Brands	C	F	Cb
Wafer Cone/Cup, average	20	0	4
Sugar Cone, average	50	0	14
Waffle Cone:			
Small	50	1	10
Large	90	0.5	19
Brands:			
Oreo, Chocolate Cone	50	1	10
Comet, Sugar Cone	50	0	11
Keebler, Sugar Cone	50	0	10

103

Ice Cream & Frozen Yogurt

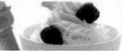

Brands C F Cb

Baskin-Robbins ~ *See Fast-Foods Section*

Ben & Jerry's:

Scoop Shop: *Hand Scooped, Per ½ Cup*

	C	F	Cb
Americone Dream, 3.27 oz	240	12	30
Bonnaroo Buzz, 3.27 oz	250	13	28
Butter Pecan, 3.16 oz	260	18	20
Choc. Chip Cookie Dough, 3.24 oz	240	12	29
Chocolate Fudge Brownie, 3.24 oz	220	10	28
Chocolate Nougat Crunch, 3.27 oz	240	12	29
Chocolate Therapy, 3.2 oz	220	12	27
Chunky Monkey, 3.24 oz	250	15	27
Coconut Seven Layer Bar, 3.27 oz	270	16	28
Late Night Snack, 3.27 oz	250	13	29
Mint Chocolate Chunk, 3.1 oz	230	14	23
NY Super Fudge Chunk, 3.24 oz	270	16	28
Strawberry Cheesecake, 3 oz	220	12	23
Sweet Cream & Cookies, 3.1 oz	220	13	24
Vanilla Heath Bar Crunch, 3.24 oz	260	16	27

1 Pint Tubs: *Per ½ Cup*

	C	F	Cb
Banana Split, 3.85 oz	250	15	27
Boston Cream Pie, 3.65 oz	250	13	29
Cake Batter, 3.7 oz	260	16	27
Cherry Garcia, 3.7 oz	240	13	28
Choc. Chip Cookie Dough, 3.7 oz	270	14	33
Chubby Hubby, 3.9 oz	340	20	33
Everything But The... ,3.85 oz	290	17	31
Imagine Whirled Peace	270	16	27
Karamel Sutra, 3.75 oz	260	14	31
Milk & Cookies, 3.55 oz	270	15	30
Peanut Brittle, 3.65 oz	260	15	29
Peanut Butter Cup, 4 oz	360	26	27
Phish Food, 3.75 oz	280	13	39
Red Velvet Cake, 3.56 oz	250	13	30
S'mores, 3.73 oz	280	16	35
Triple Caramel Chunk, 3.75 oz	280	16	32
What a Cluster, 3.66 oz	320	19	31

Frozen Yogurt: *Per ½ Cup*

	C	F	Cb
Fro Yo: Cherry Garcia, 3.8 oz	200	3	37
Chocolate Fudge Brownie, 3.65 oz	180	2.5	35
Pfish Food, 3.6 oz	240	6	41
Greek: Strawb. Shortcake, 3.5 oz	180	5	28
Other flavors, average, 3.48 oz	205	7	29
Sorbet, average all flavors, 3.3 oz	120	0	27

Blue Bunny: *Per ½ Cup* C F Cb

Ice Cream:

Premium Ice Cream: *Per ½ Cup of Pint Container*

	C	F	Cb
Banana Split, 2.96 oz	180	9	23
Bunny Tracks, 2.92 oz	220	13	23
Choc. Champion, 2.57 oz	150	8	19
Cookies 'n Cream, 2.71 oz	190	10	18

Fat Free, No Sugar Added: *Per ½ Cup*

(Carbs include 2-8 g sugar alcohol)

	C	F	Cb
Brownie Sundae	90	0	23
Caramel Toffee Crunch	90	0	23
Vanilla	80	0	20

Hi Lite: Chocolate, 2.3 oz | 110 | 3 | 17 |

	C	F	Cb
Fudge Nut Sundae, 2.3 oz	120	4	19
Homemade Van., 2.35 oz	110	3.5	18

Personals, Frozen Yogurt: *Per Container*

	C	F	Cb
All Natural: Double Raspb., 3.7 oz	160	3.5	32
Caramel Praline Crunch, 3.7 oz	190	6	31

Bars/Pops ~ *See Page 108*

Breyers: *Per ½ Cup*

	C	F	Cb
Original: Butter Pecan	150	10	14
Cherry Vanilla	130	6	18
Cookies & Cream; Rocky Road, av.	155	7	20
Vanilla, Chocolate	130	7	16
Half The Fat: Butter Pecan	130	6	16
Choc. Chocolate Chip	140	5	21
Cookies & Cream	130	4	20
Creamy, Chocolate/Vanilla, av.	120	3.5	17
Mint Chocolate Chip	130	4.5	18
Strawberry Cheesecake	130	3.5	20
Vanilla, Chocolate, Strawb.	110	3.5	17
Fat Free, all flavors	90	0	21

No Added Sugar:

(Carbs include 5g sugar alcohol and 4g fiber)

	C	F	Cb
Butter Pecan	110	6	15
Vanilla; Chocolate; Strawberry	90	4	15

	C	F	Cb
Blasts!: Chips Ahoy	140	5	22
Mrs Field's Mint Fudge Brownie	140	4	17
Oreo Cookies and Cream	140	6	21
Snickers	170	8	21
Whoppers	140	6	14
CarbSmart, all varieties	90	6	13

(Carbs include 5g sugar alcohol and 4g fiber)

Brands (Cont)

	C	F	Cb
Bruster's:			
Ice Cream, Choc./Van., 3.53 fl. oz	210	12	24
Fat Free, No Added Sugar: *Per ½ Cup*			
Chocolate	100	0	26
Chocolate Caramel Swirl	120	0	31
Cinnamon; Coffee; Vanilla, av.	100	0	23
Fudge Ripple	120	0	31
Frozen Yogurt,			
Chocolate; Vanilla, average	150	4.5	24
Carvel Ice Cream ~ *See Fast-Foods Section*			
Clemmy's, Sugar Free: *Per ½ Cup*			
Butter Pecan	200	15	20
Chocolate: Chocolate Chip	175	13	21
Coffee; Vanilla Bean, av.	160	11	21
Orange Cream	120	6	23
Toasted Almond	170	11	26
Note: Carbs include 13-15g sugar alcohols			
Coldstone Creamery ~ *See Fast-Foods Section*			
Dairy Queen/Brazier ~ *See Fast-Foods Section*			
Dippin' Dots:			
Dots 'n Cream Ice Cream: *Per ½ Cup*			
Banana Split	190	9	23
Caramel Cappuccino	170	7	30
Mint Chocolate	230	14	25
Vanilla Bean	190	9	22
Vanilla Over The Rainbow	170	7	24
Wild About Chocolate	240	14	26
Dove: *Per ½ Cup*			
Ice Cream:			
Mint Chocolate Chunk	180	11	17
Unconditional Chocolate	200	12	23
Vanilla Chocolate Chunk	180	11	17
Dreyers/Edys: *Per ½ Cup*			
Ice Cream:			
Grand: Chocolate	140	7	17
Mint Chocolate Chip	150	8	18
Neapolitan; Vanilla Bean	140	7	16
Real Strawberry	120	5	16
Vanilla	140	7	16
Slow Churned: ½ The Fat:			
Chocolate	100	3.5	15
Double Fudge Brownie	120	3	19
Snack Cups: Chocolate, 1 cup	170	6	25
Mint Chocolate Chip, 1 cup	210	8	29
Yogurt Blends, av. all flavors	110	4	19

	C	F	Cb
FitFreeze,			
Chocolate; Vanilla, ½ cup	150	5	17
Friendly's: *Per ½ Cup*			
Ice Cream: Rich & Creamy			
Butter Crunch	150	7	19
Chocolate Almond Chip	160	9	17
Classic Chocolate	150	8	16
Coffee	130	7	15
Strawberry	140	6	18
Vanilla	140	8	15
Vienna Mocha Chunk	170	9	19
Smooth Churned: *Per ½ Cup*			
Light: Black Raspberry, 2.15 oz	110	3	18
Choc. Chip Cookie Dough, 2.2 oz	140	5	21
Fudge Swirl, 2.36 oz	130	4	21
Mint Chocolate Chip, 2.2 oz	120	4.5	19
Purely Pistachio, 2.2 oz	130	5	18
Vanilla, 2.15 oz	110	3.5	17
Frozen Yogurt,			
average all flavors, ½ cup, 2.6 oz	145	5	24
Sherbet, all flavors	130	1.5	28
Sundaes To Go: *Per Single Container*			
Original Fudge	300	14	39
Choc. Chip Cookie Dough	330	15	46
Reese's P'nut Butter Cup	430	25	42
Gelati-da:			
Gelato: *Per ½ Cup, 4 oz*			
Amaretto Chocolate	150	4.5	23
Choc Mint Milano	120	2.5	22
Coffee Fudge Latte	130	2	22
Limoncello; Vanilla Marsala, av.	120	3	21
Red Raspberry	130	1.5	25
Great Value *(Walmart):* *Per ½ Cup*			
Ice Cream: Chocolate; Vanilla, av	170	9	21
Choc. Chip Cookie Dough	180	10	22
Sherbet, all flavors	110	0	26
Haagen-Dazs: *Tubs, Per ½ Cup*			
Regular: Banana Split	280	16	31
Butter Pecan	310	23	21
Chocolate Peanut Butter	360	24	27
Cookies & Cream	270	17	23
White Chocolate Raspb. Truffle	310	18	32
Five: Caramel	240	11	29
Coffee; Milk Choc., av.	220	12	23
Lemon; Mint, average	215	12	24
Healthy Choice:			
Greek Yogurt,			
⅓ carton, all flavors, av., 2.5 oz	100	1.5	18
Ice Cream, Sorbet, Frozen Yogurt ~ *See Fast-Foods Section*			
Bars ~ *See Page 109*			

Ice Cream & Frozen Yogurt

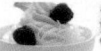 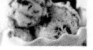

Brands (Cont) — C F Cb

Hood: *Per ½ Cup*

Frozen Fat-Free Yogurt:

	C	F	Cb
Choc Chip Cookie Dough	130	3	23
Maine Blueberry & Sweet Cream	90	0	19
Mocha Fudge	100	0	22
Strawberry	80	0	18
Strawberry Banana	90	0	20
Tangy, average all flavors	110	1	24

Ice Cream: *Per ½ Cup*

	C	F	Cb
Cookies 'N Cream	150	8	19
Chocolate	140	6	18
Classic Trio	140	7	17
Cookie Dough Delight	160	8	19
Creamy Coffee	140	7	16
Fudge Twister	140	6	20
Golden/Natural Vanilla; Patchwork	140	7	17
Maple Walnut	150	9	17

New England Creamery ~ www.CalorieKing.com

Bar ~ *See Page 109*

Jerseymaid (Vons): *Per ½ Cup*

Ice Cream:

	C	F	Cb
Cookies & Crm	160	8	18
Choc Chip; Mint Choc Chip	150	9	16
Heavenly Hash	165	9	19
Mocha Almond Fudge; Chocolate	150	9	16
Neapolitan; Real Vanilla	140	8	15
Strawberry	130	6	17

Oberweis: *Per 6 oz Scoop*

Super Premium Ice Cream:

	C	F	Cb
Chocolate	480	31	43
Chocolate Peanut Butter	550	39	42
Cookie Dough	500	28	56
Vanilla	460	31	40

Pinkberry:

Frozen Yogurt: *Without Toppings*

	C	F	Cb
Original: Mini, 3.2 oz	90	0	19
Small, 4.9 oz	140	0	29
Medium, 8 oz	230	0	48
Large, 12.95 oz	370	0	78

Other Flavors: *Per Medium Serving*

	C	F	Cb
Chocolate	275	3.5	53
Coconut	320	1	69
Mango; Psn'fruit, av.	230	0	53
Cone, with 3 oz Frozen Yogurt	105	0	23

Purely Decadent (Non Dairy):

Coconut Based: *1 Pint Carton, Per 1 Cup, 3 oz*

	C	F	Cb
Chocolate	150	9	20
Coconut; Mint Chip, av	170	10	20
Vanilla Bean	150	8	19
Gluten Free, Cookie Dough, 3 oz	190	9	24

Soy Based: *1 Pint Carton, Per ½ Cup*

	C	F	Cb
Belgian Chocolate, 3.5 oz	180	7	30
Chocolate Obsession, 3.1 oz	210	7	27
Gluten Free, Cookie Dough, 3.53 oz	230	8	36

Red Mango:

Frozen Yogurt: *No Toppings Included*

	C	F	Cb
Original/Tangomonium: 3.28 oz	80	0	19
Small, 4.6 oz	110	0	27
Regular, 7.54 oz	185	0	43
Large, 11.48 oz	280	0	67
Pomegranate: 3.28 oz	90	0	21
Small, 4.6 oz	125	0	29
Regular, 7.54 oz	205	0	48
Large, 11.48 oz	315	0	74

Rice Dream (Non-Dairy):

Frozen Dessert: *Per ½ Cup, 2.82 oz*

	C	F	Cb
Carob Almond	180	10	26
Cocoa Marble Fudge	170	6	31
Cookies & Dream	170	8	27
Neapolitan; Orange Van. Swirl	160	6	26
Strawberry	160	8	25
Vanilla	160	8	26

Bars ~ *See Page 110*

Skinny Cow: *Per Single Serve Cup*

	C	F	Cb
Choc Fudge; Cookies 'N Cream, av.	150	2	29
Caramel Cone	160	2.5	33
Dulce de Leche; Strawb. Cheesecake, av.	150	1	32

Bars/Sandwiches/Cones ~ *See Page 110*

So Delicious (Non Dairy): *Per ½ Cup, 3 oz*

Coconut Based:

	C	F	Cb
Cherry Amaretto	130	6	22
Chocolate	150	9	20
Coconut Almond Chip	180	12	20
Turtle Trails	160	8	26

Soy Based:

	C	F	Cb
Butter Pecan	160	7	22
Chocolate Velvet	130	3.5	24
Creamy Vanilla	130	3	24
Dulce de Leche	140	3	26
Mint Marble Fudge	140	3	27
Mocha Fudge	130	3	26
Neapolitan; Strawberry, average	120	3.5	23

Brands (Cont) — C F Cb

Soy Dream (Non-Dairy):
Frozen Dessert: *Per ½ Cup, 2.47 oz*

	C	F	Cb
Butter Pecan	190	11	23
Choc. Fudge Brownie	170	9	21
French Vanilla; Vanilla	140	8	17
Mocha Fudge	140	9	23
Vanilla Fudge	170	9	23

Starbucks: *Per ½ Cup*
Ice Cream:

	C	F	Cb
Caramel Macchiato	240	13	27
Coffee	210	13	21
Java Chip Frappuccino	250	15	25
Mocha Frappuccino	220	13	23

Stonyfield Farm (Organic):
Premium Ice Cream: *Per ½ Cup, 100g*

	C	F	Cb
After Dark Chocolate	240	16	22
Creme Caramel	260	14	28
Gotta Have Vanilla	250	16	21

Stop & Shop: *Per ½ Cup*
Ice Cream:

	C	F	Cb
Chocolate	150	8	18
Neapolitan; Vanilla, av.	140	7.5	17
Vanilla Fudge Swirl	140	7	18
Light: Moose Tracks	130	5	18
Vanilla, 2 oz	100	3	17
Premium: Cookies & Cream	170	9	21
Mint Chocolate Chip	160	9	18
Simply Enjoy: Chocolate	210	12	22
Strawberry	220	11	26
Vanilla	230	14	23

Tasti D-Lite:
Soft Serve: *Per 4 fl.oz*
Calories will vary with density (air in product) and serving size. Best to weigh product and calculate on 25 cals per 1 oz weight.

	C	F	Cb
Banana	70	1	13
Blueberry Cheesecake	70	1.5	14
Brownie Batter	70	1.5	13
Buttercrunch Mania	90	3.5	13
Chocolate Cookie Dough	70	1.5	12
Vanilla Marshmallow	80	1	14

TCBY ~ *See Page 250*
Tofutti, Non-Dairy: *Per ½ Cup*
Premium Pints: Better Pecan

	C	F	Cb
Better Pecan	210	13	21
Chocolate Cookie Crunch	210	11	26
Chocolate Supreme	180	11	18
Vanilla	210	13	21
Vanilla Almond Bark	240	15	24
Vanilla Fudge; Wild Berry, average	190	9	25

Turkey Hill: *Per ½ Cup*
Premium Ice Cream:

	C	F	Cb
Black Cherry	130	6	18
Butter Pecan	160	10	15
Choco Mint Chip	160	9	17
Choc. P'Nut Butter Cup	180	11	18
Cookies 'n Cream	150	8	19
Rocky Road	170	8	23
Tin Roof Sundae	150	8	19
Vanilla Bean	140	7	16
Light: Moose Tracks	130	6	19
Vanilla Bean	100	2	17
Average other flav.	130	4	19
All Natural, av. all flavors	150	8	17

No Sugar Added:

	C	F	Cb
Cherry Fudge Ripple	80	0	22
Dutch Chocolate; Vanilla Bean, av.	70	0	20
Moose Tracks	120	5	22

Frozen Yogurt:

	C	F	Cb
Choc. Chip Cookie Dough	120	2	23
Fat-Free: Chocolate Marshmallow	110	0	24
Average other flavors	100	0	19
Sherbet, all flavors	120	1	26

Walgreens:
Premium Ice Cream: *1 Pint Container, Per ½ Cup*

	C	F	Cb
Homemade Vanilla	130	7	16
Strawberry Cheesecake	130	6	18
Toasted Butter Pecan	170	10	18
Waffle Cone	150	7	19
Premium: 1.75 Quarts Container:			
Homemade Vanilla, ½ cup	150	8	17
Moose Tracks	170	10	19
Old Fashioned: 1.75 Quarts (Square), average all flavors, ½ cup	140	7	16
Sherbet: Orange Citrus	120	1	16
Rainbow Sherbet	120	1	27

Wawa:
Premium Ice Cream: *1 Pint Container, Per ½ cup*

	C	F	Cb
Butter Pecan; Mint Choc Chip, av	180	10	20
Chocolate; Vanilla Bean, av	160	8	20
Cookies & Cream	180	9	21
Strawberry Shortcake	160	7	22

Wegmans: *Per ½ Cup, 2.3 oz*

	C	F	Cb
Chocolate/Choc. Marshmallow, av.	130	7	17
Chocolate Chip	160	8	20
Chocolate Peanut Butter Swirl	150	10	15
Cookies & Cream	160	8	21
French Vanilla; Vanilla	140	7	18
Neapolitan	130	7	17
Peanut Butter Sundae	220	14	20
Premium, Vanilla, ½ Cup, 3.7 oz	270	18	22

1 Ice Cream Bars & Pops

Bars & Pops

C **F** **Cb**

Per Bar/Serving Unless Indicated

	C	F	Cb
Ben & Jerry's:			
Bars: Cherry Garcia	260	16	23
Fudgy Brownies	350	20	38
Half Baked	360	22	37
Big Bear ~ *See Klondike*			
Blue Bunny:			
Pops, Banana, 1.87 oz	35	0	9
Bars: Big Fudge, 2.5 oz	100	1	20
Big Star, 1.48 oz	110	7	11
Caramel Crunch, 1.69 oz	150	10	14
Choc. Ice Cream Sundae Crunch	170	9	21
Chocolate Raspberry, 2.82 oz	270	18	26
English Toffee, 1.38 oz	130	9	12
Milk Choc. with Almonds, 3.14 oz	320	23	25
Orange Dream, 1.86 oz	70	1	15
Root Beer Float, 2.22 oz	90	2.5	15
Strawberry Sundae Crunch, 2.19 oz	170	9	20
King Size: Chocolate Eclair, 2.82 oz	220	12	27
Crunch with Candy Center, 3 oz	340	28	24
Strawberry Shortcake, 2.78 oz	210	11	26
Champ Cones: Banana Split	220	8	33
Caramel Lovers	320	19	34
Caramel Nut	320	19	34
Chocolate Lovers	290	15	37
Vanilla	310	19	31
King Size, Strawberry Shortcake	400	18	54
Mini Swirls, Birthday Party, 1.66 oz	160	8	22
FrozFruit:			
Banana; Strawberry & Cream, av.	160	6	27
Creamy Pina Colada, 4.3 oz	190	3.5	34
Creamy Coconut	200	14	19
Jolly Rancher: Cool Tubes, 3 oz	110	1	25
Ice Pop, 3.9 oz	120	0	24
Sandwiches:			
Big: Bopper, 5.01 oz	460	23	60
Double Strawberry, 3.84 oz	270	10	41
Mississippi Mud, 3.75 oz	280	12	39
Neapolitan, 3.67 oz	260	11	37
Chips Galore, 3.42 oz	310	16	40
Mississippi Mud, 2 oz	150	4	25

Per Bar/Serving

C **F** **Cb**

	C	F	Cb
Breyers:			
Pure Fruit Bars:			
Regular, all flavors	40	0	10
No Sugar Added, all flavors	25	0	5
(Carbs include 2g sugar alcohol)			
Carb Smart:			
Almond Bar	180	15	9
(Carbs incl. 2g sugar alcohol)			
Fudge Bar	100	7	9
(Carbs include 5g sugar alcohol)			
Vanilla Ice Cream Bar	170	15	9
(Carbs include 2g sugar alcohol)			
Smooth & Dreamy: Bars, av. all	125	5	18
Sandwiches, all flavors	160	4	30
Butterfinger *(Nestle):*			
1.6 oz bar	150	10	15
King Size, 4 oz	280	18	27
Cool Classics:			
Arctic Blasters: Crispy Bar	160	11	15
Fudge Bar	100	1	21
Ice Cream Bar	150	10	13
Orange Cream	100	2.5	18
Strawberry Shortcake	210	11	28
Toffee Bar	160	11	14
Icepix: Grape; Cherry; Orange	35	0	8
Honeydew; Watermelon; Cantelope	35	0	9
Swirl Pops, Mango-Cherry	80	0	20
Creamsicles: 100 Calorie Bar	100	2	20
Low Fat	70	13	20
Sugar-Free, all flavors	40	0.5	12
Dove: *Per 2.6 oz Bar*			
Caramel Swirl w/ Milk Choc. & Cashews	250	16	23
Milk Chocolate with Vanilla	250	16	24
Milk Chocolate with Almonds	250	17	24
Dark Chocolate with Vanilla	250	17	24
70 Calorie Miniatures, Vanilla w/ Milk Choc.,	70	4.5	6.5
Dreyer's/Edy's:			
Real Fruit Bars:			
Acai Blueb.; Lime, Strawb., Wildb.	60	0	15
Creamy Coconut	120	3	21
Grape; Lemonade; Lime	80	0	20
Peach	100	0	24
Pomegranate	70	0	17
Average other flavors	80	0	20

Bars & Pops (Cont)

Per Bar/Serving   **C**   **F**   **Cb**

	C	F	Cb
Drumstick *(Nestlé)*: Classic Choc.	310	16	37
Classic Vanilla	290	16	33
Vanilla Caramel/Fudge	310	16	37
King Size, Triple Choc.	350	16	48
Simply Dipped: Mint	290	14	38
Vanilla	270	13	37
Lil' Drums, average all flavors	120	6	16
Super Nugget, (1)	310	18	33
Edy's ~ *See Dreyer's*			
Fat Boy:			
Sundae On A Stick:			
Casco Vanilla Nut, 3 oz	270	20	22
Peppermint, 3 oz	280	20	26
Vanilla, Milk Choc. Dipped	270	20	21
Sandwiches: Chocolate, 3 oz	210	9	31
Cookies n' Cream 3 oz	220	9	33
Mint Chocolate Chip, 3 oz	230	10	32
Rasp. Cheesecake, 3 oz	220	8	35
Strawberry, 3 oz	210	9	30
Vanilla, 3 oz	210	9	30
Fresh & Easy, Vanilla Sundae Cone	260	15	29
Fudge Bar *(Nestle)*:			
Regular, 2.8 oz	110	2.5	21
Super, 5 oz	230	6	42
Fudgesicle:			
Fudge Bar	100	2	17
Fat-Free	60	0	14
No Added Sugar	40	1	10
Good Humor:			
Bars:			
Orig. Vanilla, 285 oz	250	15	27
Oreo Bar, 2.75 oz	240	13	31
Candy Center Crunch	300	21	27
Chocolate Eclair	210	9	30
Reese's Peanut Butter Cups, 3 oz	300	18	31
Toasted Almond, 2.7 oz	210	10	27
King Cones:			
Vanilla, 2.96 oz	240	12	32
Giant:			
Triple Choc. Brownie, 5.5 oz	380	14	57
Vanilla Chocolate, 5 oz	360	17	48
Sandwiches: Choc. Chip Cookie	270	10	44
Giant Neapolitan, 3.35 oz	220	5	40
Giant Vanilla, 3.35 oz	220	5	40
Great Value *(Walmart)*:			
Chocolate Fudge Sticks (2), 3.45 oz	130	1.5	28
Ice Cream Cone, Van., Choc Dipped	270	14	34
Sandwiches: Vanilla, 2.1 oz	160	5	25
Minis, Vanilla, 1.4 oz	100	3.5	16
Ice Pops, Assorted, 1.85 oz	45	0	11

Per Bar/Serving   **C**   **F**   **Cb**

Haagen-Dazs:

	C	F	Cb
Milk Chocolate Bars:			
Vanilla & Almonds	310	22	22
Vanilla	280	20	21
Snack Size: Coffee & Alm. Crunch	190	13	15
Vanilla & Almonds	190	14	14
Dark Chocolate: Chocolate	290	20	24
Vanilla	280	20	21
Sundae Cones: Vanilla Caramel	170	9	18
Vanilla Chocolate	170	10	17
Healthy Choice: Fudge Bar	80	1.5	13
Mocha Swirl	90	1	17
Sorbet & Cream Bar	80	0.5	18
Vanilla Sandwich	150	1.5	30
Hershey's:			
Cones: Candy Bar Overload	320	12	48
Crazy	120	2	24
Incredible	250	13	28
Moose Tracks	430	27	43
P-Nutty	210	13	20
Low Fat, Cookies & Cream	120	1.5	25
Pops, all varieties	35	0	10
Sandwiches:			
Chocolate	230	10	30
Strawberry	220	8	33
Vanilla	210	9	30
Signature Bars: Choc. Eclair	230	10	30
Cotton Candy	280	15	33
Strawberry Cheesecake	230	9	34
Hood: Ice Cream Bar	150	11	12
Fudge Stix	70	0	14
Orange Cream	90	1.5	19
Hoodsie Cups: Vanilla; Chocolate Pops	100	5	12
	60	0	16
Red Sox Choc Dipped Sundae Cone, 1 cone 3.17 oz	240	16	21
Sandwiches, Vanilla	170	6	28
Klondike:			
Bars: Original Vanilla, 3 fl.oz	250	14	29
Dark Chocolate	250	14	29
Double Chocolate	240	14	27
Heath, English Toffee	230	15	25
Krunch	250	14	30
Neapolitan	250	14	29
Oreo Cookies & Cream	250	15	29
Reese's	260	16	26
Sandwiches:			
Choco Taco	290	15	38
Classic Vanilla	180	4.5	31
Oreo	200	7	34
Slim-a-Bear S'wich, Vanilla, no sugar added	170	9	21

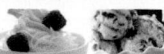

Bars & Pops (Cont) C F Cb

Per Bar/Serving

Luigi's Real Italian Ice:

	C	F	Cb
Cups: Lemon; Cherry; Mango, 6 fl.oz	100	0	26
Watermelon; Blue Rasp., 6 fl.oz	160	0	39
Swirls, av. all flavors, 6 fl.oz	150	0	38
M&M's: Cone, Single, 2.8 oz	250	12	33
Cookie Ice Cream Sandwich, 3 oz	260	12	34
Magnum: Almond, 2.8 oz	270	18	24
Classic, 2.7 oz	240	16	22
Dark, 2.7 oz	240	17	20
Double Choc., 2.9 oz	340	21	34
Mint; Mochaccino, 2.7 oz	250	16	24
White, 2.7 oz	250	16	23
Minis (2), av. all varieties, 3 oz	310	21	27
Minute Maid:			
Juice Bars	60	0	15
Soft Frozen Lemonade	70	0	19
Nestlé:			
Bars: Crunch Van., 3 oz	210	15	20
Eskimo Pie	150	10	15
Toll House, Choc. Chip, 1.7 oz	150	9	18
Crunch, Vanilla	200	13	19
Dibs, Mint/Vanilla, 4 oz	340	24	30
Drumsticks: Chocolate	310	17	34
Vanilla Fudge	310	16	37
Push Up Pops, av.	70	1	16
Sandwiches: *6 Packs*			
Caramel Trio	160	4	29
Vanilla	160	4	29
Popsicle:			
Firecracker	35	0	9
Rainbow	45	0	11
Scribblers	30	0	8
SpongeBob Pop-Ups	80	1	16
Super Heroes	40	0	11
Sugar Free: Orange Cherry Grape	15	0	4
Tropicals	15	0	4
Slow Melts: Dora The Explorer	30	0	7
Mighty Minis, 3 pcs	40	0	10
Reese's, Peanut Butter Ice Cream	310	21	27
Rice Dream, Van. Nutty Bar, 3.35 oz	320	24	27
Skinny Cow:			
Bars: Fudge Bars, low fat	100	1	22
Minis Fudge Pops (2)	100	2	19
Truffle Bars, av. all flavors	105	2	19
Sandwiches, average all flavors	145	3	30
Snickers:			
Bars: Regular, 2 oz	180	11	18
Mini Bar, 4 pieces	370	23	36
Cone, 3.7 oz	280	15	33
Ice Cream Brownie, 4.5 oz	300	14	42
Snow Cone *(Wonder)*, av. all, 7 fl.oz	60	0	15

Per Bar/Serving C F Cb

So Delicious *(Turtle Mtn):*

Coconut Based Bars:

	C	F	Cb
Mini: Almond	170	10	15
Vanilla	150	7	14
Soy Based Bars, av.	85	2	18
Soy Dream *(Non-Dairy):*			
Creamy Fudge Bar, 2.25 oz	90	2	18
Sandwiches, Choc./Vanilla, 2.25 oz	150	3	27
Stop&Shop, Ice Cream Sandwich	160	6	23
Sweet Nothings *(Turtle Mtn),*			
Bars, all flavors	100	0	23
Tampico, Freezer Pops, all var., 1.35 oz	30	0	7
Tofutti: *(Non-Dairy)*			
Cuties: Cookies 'N Cream	130	6	11
Mint Chocolate Chip; Vanilla, av	130	6	18
Vanilla	130	6	17
Sticks:			
Choc. Fudge Treats	30	1.5	6
Marry Me Bar	170	8	22
Mint By Mintz	170	7	17
Totally Fudge Pops	95	1.5	19
Trader Joe's:			
Fruit Floes: Caribbean	80	0	21
Lime	60	0	16
Strawberry	100	0	24
Bars:			
Coffee Latte & Cream, 1.4 oz	90	6	9
Mango & Cream, 1.4 oz	60	2	10
Mini Mint S'wich, 1.4 oz	120	6	18
Peach Pops, 1.75 oz	45	0	11
Turkey Hill:			
Sandwiches: Double Decker	190	7	30
Vanilla Bean	190	7	30
Sundae Cone, Van. Fdge	320	18	33
Twix Bar, 2.65 oz	280	16	31
Wegmans:			
Bars: Fudge, low fat	100	1.5	20
Vanilla, Choc Coated, 1.9 oz	160	11	14
Cones: Nutty Sundae, 2.47 oz	210	11	25
Sundae Nut, 3 oz	260	15	29
Weight Watchers:			
Bars: Choc. Dipped Strawberry	100	4	18
Dark Chocolate:			
Dulce de leche	110	4	18
Rasp. Cheesecake	110	4	18
Giant: Chocolate/Cookies & Cream	130	5	24
Fudge/Latte Bar, av.	100	1	23
Cones, Choc./Vanilla, av.	140	4	27
Cups: Chocolate Chip Cookie Dough	150	1.5	32
Mint Chocolate Chip	140	2.5	29
Sandwiches: Vanilla	120	2	28
Round, Vanilla	140	1.5	31
Yosicle: Duos!, average all var.,	55	1	11
Torpedoes!, 2 oz	90	2	16

Canned & Packaged Meals

Amy's (Frozen): *Per Serve* — Ⓒ Ⓕ Ⓒb

Asian Meals:

	C	F	Cb
Stir-Fry: Thai, 9.5 oz	310	11	45
Asian Noodle, 10 oz	300	7	50

Bowls:

Baked Ziti, 9.5 oz	390	12	62
Broccoli & Cheddar Bake, 9.5 oz	430	19	45
Cheese Ravioli with Sauce, 9.5 oz	380	12	55
Pesto Tortellini, 9.5 oz	430	19	45

Burritos:

Bean & Cheese, 6 oz	310	9	46
Bean & Rice, 6 oz	300	8	48
Breakfast Burrito, 6 oz	270	8	38

Entrees:

Cheese Enchilada, 4.5 oz	240	14	18
Cheese Lasagna, 10.3 oz	380	14	44
Macaroni & Cheese, 9 oz	410	16	47
Macaroni & Soy Cheese, 9 oz	370	15	42
Roasted Vegetable Lasagna, 10 oz	350	11	47
Vegetable Lasagna, 9.5 oz	310	12	35

Light & Lean: *Per 8 oz Serve*

Black Bean & Cheese Enchilada	240	4.5	44
Pasta & Veggies	210	5	33
Soft Taco Fiesta	220	4.5	40

Pot Pies:

Broccoli, 7.5 oz	460	24	50
Mex. Tamale; Shepherd's Pie, av., 8 oz	155	3.5	27
Vegetable, 7.5 oz	420	19	54

Snacks: Nacho, Chse & Bean, 5-6 pcs 220 8 25

Cheese Pizza, 5-6 pieces	210	7	25

Veggie Burgers,

All American (1), 2.5 oz	140	3.5	14

Whole Meals: Cheese Enchilada, 9 oz 370 15 41

Black Bean Enchilada, 10 oz	330	8	53
Black Bean Tamale Verde, 10.5 oz	330	10	55
Enchilada Verde, 10 oz	400	13	54
Veggie Loaf, 10 oz	290	8	47

Wraps:

Indian Samosa, 5 oz	250	9	35
Indian Spinach Tofu, 5.5 oz	270	13	28
Teriyaki, 5.5 oz	310	7	51

Extra Product Listings ~ *www.CalorieKing.com*

B & M:

Baked Beans: *Per ½ Cup, 4.6 oz*

Original	170	2	31
Barbeque	190	0.5	39
Vegetarian	160	1	28

Raisin Brown Bread,

½" slice, 2 oz	130	0.5	29

Bagel Bites:

Three Cheese, 4 pcs, 3 oz	190	5	28
Cheese, Ssge & Pepp., 4 pcs	200	7	26

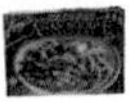

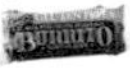

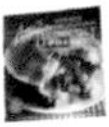

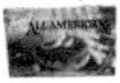

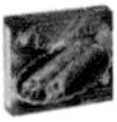

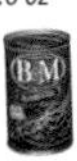

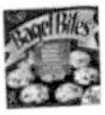

Banquet: — Ⓒ Ⓕ Ⓒb

Homestyle Bakes: *Includes Topping*

	C	F	Cb
Asian Style Fried Rice, ½ filling & ¼ cup rice	240	1.5	47
Cheesy Chicken Alfredo, ¾ cup filling & ½ cup pasta	410	21	40
Cheesy Ham & Hashbrowns ½ cup filling & ⅓ cup potato	290	15	30
Chicken & Dumplings, ¾ cup filling & ¼ cup dumplings	220	6	30
Country chicken, ½ cup filling, ¼ cup biscuit mix & ¼ cup potato mix	360	17	43
Lasagna, ¾ c. meat sauce, ⅓ c. pasta	330	13	39
Pasta & Meatballs, ¾ cup filling & ⅓ c pasta	310	10	42

Frozen:

Dinners: Boneless Pork Rib, 10 oz 320 11 42

Cheesy Smothered Meat Patty, 7 oz	280	16	21
Chicken Fingers, 7 oz	480	21	56
Chicken Pasta Marinara, 6.5 oz	290	14	29
Fettuccine Alfredo, 8 oz	280	11	35
Fish Sticks, 7.5 oz	310	10	44
Fried Beef Steak, 10 oz	390	18	43
Lasagna w/ Meat Sce, 8 oz	250	7	34
Mac & Cheese, 8 oz	260	6	39
Macaroni & Beef, 8 oz	210	4.5	32
Meat Balls in Tom. Sauce (5), 5 oz	200	13	9
Meatloaf, 9.5 oz	280	17	28
Mex. Beef Enchil. & Tamale, 8.5 oz	310	10	45
Mex. Style Chkn Enchiladas, 8.5 oz	280	8	45
Pepperoni Pizza, 5.75	340	12	47
Salisbury Steak, 9.5 oz	250	12	25
Savory Pork Patty, 8 oz	300	17	26
Spaghetti & Meatballs, 9 oz	330	14	35
Swedish Meatballs, 10.25 oz	440	18	51
Turkey , 9.25 oz	250	7	32

Pot Pies: Beef, 7 oz 390 22 36

Chicken; Turkey, av., 7 oz	375	21	35
Chicken & Brocolli, 7 oz	360	20	34

Select Recipe Dinners:

Chkn Parmigian, 10 oz	350	15	37
Corn Dog Meal, 7.5 oz	460	16	68
Homestyle Pot Roast Meal, 9.5 oz	170	5	19
Original Fried Chicken Meal, 9 oz	440	26	30
Spag. with Popcorn Chicken, 7 oz	270	8	37
Sweet & Sour Chicken, 8 oz	390	14	56

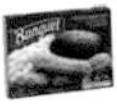

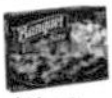

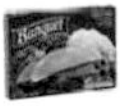

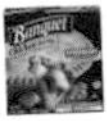

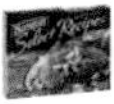

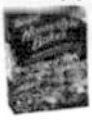

Betty Crocker:

	C	F	Cb
Helpers: *Per 1 Cup, Prepared*			
Asian, Chicken Fried Rice	280	11	21
Chicken: Italian Fettuc. Alfredo	330	11	31
Mexican Cheesy Chkn Enchilada	350	7	42
Helper Complete Meals: *Per 1 Cup, Prepared*			
Cheesy Beef Taco	220	5	35
Chicken & Buttermilk Biscuits	260	9	37
Chicken Cheesy Rice & Broccoli	230	6	36
Stroganoff	230	8	33
Hamburger Helper: *Per 1 Cup, Prepared*			
Beef Pasta	280	12	24
Cheeseburger Macaroni	320	13	27
Cheesy Baked Potatoes	310	12	30
Cheesy Jambalaya	320	13	30
Cheesy Nachos	330	12	36
Crunchy Taco	330	14	33
Salisbury	280	11	27
Tuna Helper: *Per 1 Cup, Prepared*			
Creamy Parmesan	270	10	30
Average all varieties	270	10	30
Side Dishes/Casseroles: *Per Serving, Prepared*			
Casseroles: Au Gratin, ½ cup	150	5	24
Cheddar & Bacon; Cheesy Scalloped	145	5	23
Roasted Garlic, ½ cup	120	3.5	21
Scalloped Potatoes, ⅔ cup	130	3	23
Sour Cream and Chives, ⅔ cup	140	6	18
Flavored Potatoes, prepared, average all flavors, ⅔ cup	145	6	18
Seasoned Skillets: *Prepared*			
Hash Brown, ½ cup	120	4	18
Roasted Garlic & Herb, ⅔ cup	170	9	21
Traditional, ½ cup	180	9	22
Bowl Appetit: *Per Bowl, Prepared*			
Cheddar Broccoli Rice	290	6	52
Homestyle Chicken Pasta	250	5	44
Pasta Alfredo	350	9	55
Teriyaki Rice	250	1	57
Three-Cheese Rotini	340	7	59

Biggest Loser:

	C	F	Cb
Simply Sensible: *Per ½ Package*			
Beef Pot Roast & Gravy	220	5	16
Beef Tips & Gravy	200	3.5	21
Lasagna	200	5	28
Medit.-Style Chicken	250	6	36
Zing Chicken	230	1.5	38

Bird's Eye (Frozen):

	C	F	Cb
Voila!: *Per 1 Cup Prepared Unless Indicated*			
Heat and Serve:			
Alfredo Chicken, 1½ cups	280	12	37
Beef & Broccoli Stir Fry	160	6	13
Beef Lo Mein	230	3	37
Chicken Florentine	230	6	27
Chicken Parmesan	360	11	50
Garlic Chicken	240	8	29
Garlic Shrimp	230	9	30
Shrimp Scampi	190	2.5	31
Sweet & Sour Chicken	200	1	38
Three Cheese Chicken	210	8	31

Boca (Frozen):

	C	F	Cb
Burger:			
Cheeseburger, 2.5 oz	100	4.5	6
All American Classic, 2.5 oz	140	5	9
Grilled Vegetables, 2.5 oz	80	1	7
Original Vegan, 3.5 oz	100	1	8
Chik'n: Orig. Nuggets, 3 oz	180	7	17
Patties (1), 2.5 oz	160	6	15
Veggie Patties, Bruschetta	90	1.5	9

Boston Market (Frozen):

	C	F	Cb
Dinners: Beef Steak & Ndles, 14 oz	460	14	51
Chicken Parmesan, 16 oz	570	18	74
Oven Roasted Chicken, 16 oz	330	8	36
Salisbury Steak, 16 oz	670	36	57
Swedish Meatballs	720	37	61

Buitoni (Frozen): *Per ½ Package Unless Indicated*

	C	F	Cb
Butternut Squash Ravioli, 12 oz	490	14	76
Five Cheese Cannelloni, 13 oz	560	27	52
Lobster Ravioli, 1/4 pkg., 8.5 oz	420	20	47
Shrimp & Lobster Ravioli, 11 oz	500	16	68

Bush's Best: *Per ½ Cup, 4.6 oz*

	C	F	Cb
Black Beans	105	0.5	23
Chili Beans, Pinto w/ sauce	110	1	20
Dark Red Kidney Beans	100	0	22
Garbanzo Beans	105	2	20
Refried Beans: Traditional	150	3	24
Fat Free	130	0	24
Baked Beans: Original	140	1	29
Vegetarian	130	0	29
Other varieties, average	150	1	32
Grillin' Beans:			
Black Bean Fiesta	110	1	21
Sweet Mesquite	160	1	32
Texas Ranchero	120	2	20
Other varieties, average	170	0.5	35

Campbell's:	C	F	Cb
Beans: *Per ½ Cup*			
Baked Beans,			
Sugar & Bacon Flav	160	2.5	30
Pork & Beans	140	1.5	25
Chunky Microwavable Bowls: *Per Cup*			
Firehouse; Roadhouse,			
Beef & Beans Chili	220	5	27
Sirloin Burger w/ Country Veggies	120	2	18
Spaghetti O's: *Per Cup*			
Original	170	1	35
With Meatballs	240	7	32
With Sliced Franks	220	6	32
Chef Boyardee:			
15 oz Cans: *Per Cup*			
Beef Ravioli in Tomato			
& Meat Sauce	220	7	31
99% Fat Free	180	12	33
Cheese Ravioli	230	6	34
Pepperoni Pizza Raviol,i in Zesty Sce	250	7	38
Mini Varieties:			
Beef Ravioli, & Meatballs in Sauce	280	12	32
Beef Ravioli, in Tom. & Meat Sce	230	8	32
15 oz Cans (Cont): *Per Cup*			
Overstuffed:			
Beef Ravioli,			
in Tom. & Meat Sauce	250	6	38
Ital. Sausage Ravioli in Sauce	240	5	39
Microwaveable:			
14.25 oz Bowls, (40% More): *Per cup*			
Beef Rav. in Tom. & Meat Sce	230	7	34
Mini Beef Ravioli,			
in Tomato & Meat Sauce, 1 c.	240	7	35
7.5 oz Cups: *Per Cup*			
Beef Ravioli in Tom. & Meat Sce	200	6	29
Mini Micro Beef Ravioli,			
in Tomato & Meat Sauce	160	4	26
Mini Beef Ravioli & M'balls,			
in Sce	240	9	31
Cheese Ravioli, in Tomato Sauce	190	5	29
Boxed Kits:			
Cheese Pizza Maker,			
⅛ package, 4 oz	260	4	47
Pepperoni Pizza Maker,			
⅛ package, 4.5 oz	280	7	45
Pizza Sauce, ¼ cup, 2 oz	35	1.5	4

Contessa (Frozen):	C	F	Cb
On The Stove: *Per Serving w/ Sauce, Prepared*			
Chicken Fried Rice, 8 oz	250	3.5	40
Jambalaya, 8 oz	240	7	29
Mongolian Beef, 8 oz	310	7	48
Shrimp Stir-Fry, 10 oz	180	0.5	29
Microsteam: *Per 1 Cup Prepared*			
Chicken Alfredo	260	13	24
Italian Sausage Rigatoni	300	11	41
Spaghetti Bolognese	300	13	34
Dennison's Chili: *Per Cup*			
Chili Con Carne:			
Original: With Beans, 9 oz	350	15	31
Without Beans, 8.75 oz	310	16	20
Chili: Original, with Beans, 9 oz	360	14	38
Chunky, with Beans, 8.8 oz	300	10	32
Hot, with Beans, 9 oz	350	14	36
Vegetarian, 99% fat free, 9 oz	190	1.5	34
Dinty Moore: *(Hormel Foods)*			
Cans: Chicken & Noodles, 7.5 oz can	190	9	19
Beef Stew, 15 oz can, 1 cup, 8.5 oz	200	10	17
Big Bowl (15 oz):			
Chicken & Dumplings, 8.5 oz	220	7	29
Scalloped Potatoes & Ham, 8.5 oz	280	16	23
Microwave Ready:			
Beef Stew, 10 oz tray	250	11	22
Noodles & Chkn, 7.5 oz	190	9	20
Scalloped Pot. & Ham, 7.5 oz cup	240	13	20
Dr. McDougall's: *Per 2 oz Package*			
Noodles: Thai Peanut	220	3	40
Average other varieties	200	1	43
Eden Organics: *Per ½ Cup (4.6 oz)*			
Baked Navy Beans w/ Sorghum, Mstrd	150	0	27
Black Eyed Peas	90	1	16
Black Soy Beans	120	6	8
Refried: Black Beans	110	1.5	18
Pinto; Kidney Beans, av.	85	1	17
Farmhouse:			
Pasta: *Per 1 Cup, Prepared*			
Herb & Butter, 4.7 oz	440	22	48
White Cheddar, 6.2 oz	380	14	51
Rice: *Per 1 Cup, Prepared*			
Chicken Flavor, 6 oz	230	5	43
Long Grain & Wild Herb & Butter	250	7	43
Mexican, 6 oz	230	5	42

	C	F	Cb
French's:			
French Fried Onions:			
Original; Cheddar:			
2 Tbsp, 0.25 oz	45	3.5	3
¼ cup, 0.5 oz	90	7	6
1 cup, 2 oz	360	28	24
Fresh & Easy (Refrigerated):			
Family Package: *Per 1 Cup Serving:*			
Cheese Tortellini Caprese	300	11	34
Lemon Rosemary Chkn	190	6	24
Linguini Carbonara	400	19	42
Ravioli Bolognese	310	14	26
Single Serve: *Per 9-10 oz Package*			
Beef & Broccoli	270	6	40
Sweet & Sour Chkn	270	2	51
Teriyaki Chicken	350	6	52
Turkey with Stuffing	230	4.5	37
GardenBurger (Frozen),			
Veggie Burgers, average all var.	100	3	18
garden lites (Frozen): *Per 7 oz Serving*			
Butternut Squash Souffle	180	2	35
Zucchini Marinara/Portabella	110	4	19
Gorton's (Frozen):			
Battered Pollock Fillets:			
Beer Battered (2), 3.7 oz	250	18	16
Crispy Battered (2), 3.8	240	3	20
Lemon Pepp. Battered (2), 2.7 oz	270	18	20
Breaded Pollock Fillets:			
Classic Crunchy Golden (2), 3.8 oz	240	12	23
Garlic & Herb (2), 3.5 oz	230	12	22
Lemon Herb Peppered (2), 3.5 oz	240	13	21
Grilled Fillets:			
Classic Salmon (1), 3.2 oz	100	3	2
Garlic Butter Pollock (1), 3.8 oz	90	3	0
Signature Tilapia (1), 3.2 oz	80	2	2
Shrimp:			
Butterfly (5), 3.5 oz	250	11	27
Shrimp Scampi, 4 oz	120	6	8
Grilled: Classic, 4 oz	110	1.5	5
Shrimp Scampi, 4oz	130	4.5	4
Great Value *(Walmart):*			
Dirty Rice Mix, 1 cup, prep'd	130	0	29
Rice & Vermicelli,			
average all flavors, 1 cup, prep'd	320	9	54
Frozen:			
Breakfast Bowls: *Per 8 oz*			
Bacon/Sausage, Eggs & Pot., av.	490	34	21
Maple P'cakes & Ssg Griddle S'wch	380	22	36

Great Value (Cont):	C	F	Cb
Complete Skillet Meals: *Per ½ Package*			
Chkn Florentine & Farfalle	570	32	40
Italian Ssg & Rigatoni	500	26	46
Lean Cafe: *Per Container*			
Cheese Ravioli, 8.5 oz	220	5	32
Chicken Fettuccini, 9.25 oz	265	6	33
Salisbury Steak, 9.5 oz	260	9	21
Meals: *Per ¼ of 32 oz Package, 8 oz*			
Cheese Manicotti	320	16	24
Lasagna	280	9	36
Healthy Choice (Frozen):			
All Natural Entrees:			
Asian Potstickers, 10 oz	340	4.5	66
Portabella Spin. Parm., 9.4 oz	270	7	39
Ravioli: Lobster Cheese, 9 oz	260	5	41
Pumpkin Squash, 9.2 oz	310	6	52
Tortellini Primavera Parm., 9 oz	230	5	37
Asian/Cafe/Mediterranean Steamers:			
Beef Teriyaki, 10 oz	300	6	44
Lem. Garlic Chkn & Shrimp, 10 oz	280	4	42
Roasted Beef Merlot, 10 oz	210	6	23
Baked:: 4 Cheese Ziti Marin., 9.2 oz	310	5	46
Italian Sausage Pasta, 8.5 oz	270	6	40
Roasted Chicken & Potatoes, 9.7 oz	180	3.5	21
Complete Meals:			
Beef Pot Roast, 11 oz	250	6	32
Chkn Parmigiana, 11.5 oz	350	10	49
H'mestyle Salisbury Steak, 12.5 oz	310	6	46
Select Entrees:			
Bacon & Smokey Cheddar Chicken	250	6	31
Ravioli Florentine Marinara, 8.5 oz	230	4	34
Spicy Caribbean Chicken, 8.5 oz	300	2.5	52
Extra Product Listings ~ *www.CalorieKing.com*			
Health Valley:			
Vegetarian Chili: *Per 8.65 oz Cup*			
3 Bean Chipotle	200	3	37
Black Bean Mango	210	3	41
Other varities, average			
Heinz,			
Vegetarian Beans,			
½ cup, 4 oz	140	0.5	27
Hormel:			
Compleats: *Per 10 oz Serving*			
Beef Steak Tips	260	9	29
Chicken & Dumplings	230	6	32
Chicken & Noodles	240	8	27
Chicken Alfredo	330	18	28
Chkn Breast & Gravy	210	3.5	26
Hm'style Beef Pot Roast	230	6	22

Hormel (Cont):	C	F	Cb
Compleats (Cont): *Per 10 oz Serving*			
Lasagne with Meat Sce	280	7	42
Meatloaf with Potatoes & Gravy	300	11	34
Salisbury Steak	280	11	30
Santa Fe Style Chkn	250	4	36
Sesame Chicken	290	6	41
Spaghetti with Meat Sauce	290	9	36
Teriyaki Chicken with Rice	250	1.5	50
Turkey & Dressing	290	9	31
Turkey & Hearty Vegetables	180	3.5	24
Chili with Beans: *Per 8.7 oz Serving*			
Regular; Hot; Chunky	260	7	33
Turkey	210	3	28
Vegetarian	190	1	35
Without Beans: *Per 8.3 oz*			
Regular; Hot Chili	220	9	18
Turkey	190	3	16
Kid's Kitchen: *Per 7.5 oz Microwave Cup*			
Beans & Wieners	310	13	37
Cheesy Mac 'N Cheese	270	14	24
Mini Beef Ravioli	240	6	38
Noodle Rings & Chicken	140	4	18
Hot Pockets (Frozen):			
Calzones: *Per ½ Calzone, 4.2 oz*			
4 Meat & 4 Cheese	300	13	34
Pepperoni & 3 Cheese	320	16	34
Supreme	280	12	33
Mexican Style: *Per Sandwich*			
Three Cheese & Chkn Quesadilla	270	9	36
Average other varieties	285	12	34
Paninis: *Per ½ Panini*			
Bruschetta Chicken	190	6	25
Steak & Cheddar	260	11	26
Pizzeria: Four Cheese	320	12	40
Pepperoni	340	17	37
Sausage	340	16	39
Sandwiches: *Per 4 oz Sandwich*			
Barbeque Recipe Beef	340	13	44
Cheeseburger	310	12	39
Meatballs & Mozzarella	340	15	39
Philly Steak & Cheese	310	13	37
Snackers: *Per 4 Pieces*			
Fiesta Nacho Bites	220	8	28
Grilled Italian Style Bites	210	6	28
Loaded Potato Skins Bites	230	10	25
Toasted Five Cheese Ravioli	220	6	33
Hungry Jack, Mashed Potatoes, average all varieties, 2 Tbsp dry mix	80	0	19

Hungry Man (Frozen):	C	F	Cb
Dinners:			
Boneless Fried Chkn	860	39	85
Boneless Pork Ribs	810	36	98
Classic Fried Chkn	1030	62	63
Country Fried Chkn	570	27	53
Homestyle Meatloaf	660	35	61
Mexican Style Fiesta	570	21	83
Pub Favorites:			
Beer Battered Chicken	760	34	74
Bourbon Steak Strips	480	11	70
Grilled Beef Patty	540	34	35
Honey Bourbon Chicken Strips	620	24	69
XXL Sandwiches: *Per 1 Box Serving*			
Angus Beef Charbroil	740	47	52
BBQ Chicken	490	14	64
Buffalo Fried Chicken	650	27	73
Chicken Parmesan	610	29	63
Crispy Fried Chicken	670	32	64
Hunt's, Manwich Sloppy Joe, Original, ¼ cup, 2.25 oz	40	0	9
José Olé (Frozen):			
Breakfast Burritos:			
Egg & Bacon, 4 oz	260	9	33
Egg & Ham, 4 oz	250	8	34
Egg & Sausage, 4 oz	270	10	34
Premium Burritos:			
Chicken Monterey (1)	270	6	41
Steak & Cheese (1)	300	10	40
Premium Chimichangas:			
Chicken & Cheese (1), 5 oz	330	11	45
Steak & Cheese (1), 5 oz	350	14	41
Snacks:			
Mini Chimichangas, Steak & Cheddar (3)	370	20	37
Quesadillas:			
Gr. Chicken & 3 Cheese (1)	270	9	31
Grilled Steak & 3 Cheese (1)	260	9	32
Tacos, Beef & Cheese Mini, (4)	230	12	23
Taquitos: Chkn, Corn Tortillas, (3)	200	8	26
Steak & Cheese, Flour Tortillas, (2)	250	12	26
Kids Cuisine (Frozen): *Per Meal*			
Chicken Breast Nuggets, 8.78 oz	430	18	54
Cheese Stuffed Crust Mini Pizza	330	7	54
Fish Stix, 7.58 oz	320	11	45
Fried Chicken, 10 oz	530	22	53
Hot Dog, 7.2 oz	320	5	55
Mac & Cheese, 10.6 oz	420	11	69
Pancakes, 7.23 oz	400	15	59
Popcorn Chicken, 8,64 oz	370	12	53
Spaghetti & Mini Meatballs,10.2 oz	290	6	45

Knorr: *Sides, Prepared As Directed*

Asian: Chicken Fried Rice	280	7	48
Teriyaki Noodles	280	9	45
Teriyaki Rice	280	7	48
Cajun: Garlic Butter Rice	260	4	48
Red Beans & Rice	290	1.5	63
Fiesta: Mexican Rice	280	6	51
Spanish Rice	280	6	48
Taco Rice	250	1.5	51
Pasta: Alfredo	290	10	39
Alfredo Broccoli	300	10	39
Butter	260	8	39
Butter & Herb	260	7	39
Cheesy Cheddar	270	7	39
Parmesan	290	10	39
Stroganoff	260	7	39
Rice: Cheddar Broccoli	280	6	48
Chicken Broccoli	270	5	48
Chicken Flavor	280	6	48

Kraft:

Macaroni & Cheese Dinner: *Per 1 Cup Prepared*

Original, family size, 2.5 oz	400	12	48
Alfredo, 2.5 oz	400	17	51
Easy Mac. av. all varieties, 2 oz	230	4.5	42
Premium White Cheddar, 2.5 oz	400	18	51
The Cheesiest, Original flavor, 2.5 oz	400	19	47
Thick 'N Creamy, 2.5 oz	410	17	50
Deluxe: Four Cheese, 3.5 oz	320	10	46
Sharp Cheddar, 3.5 oz	320	9	46

Velveeta Potatoes: *Per ½ Cup, Prepared*

Cheesy: Au Gratin	190	7	24
Bacon Scalloped	200	7	24
Cheesy Mashed, Twin Pack	180	9	21
Shells & Cheese, Orig., 4 oz	360	12	49

Kroger:

Kitchen Creation Skillet Dinners: *1 Cup Prepared*

Creamy Broccoli	300	12	33
Creamy Pasta	300	13	33
Double Cheeseburger	320	13	30
Lasagna	280	12	26
Stroganoff	320	14	27

Frozen:

Healthy Meals Made Simple: *Refrigerated, Per Cup*

Braised Beef Pot Roast & Gravy	220	5	15
Lean Beef Tips & Gravy	210	4	20
Lemon Herb Chicken	170	1.5	23
Sweet & Spicy Chicken	270	1.5	48

Kroger (Cont):

C F Cb

Frozen (Cont):

Meals Made Simple:

Beef Stir Fry, 1¾ cups	180	4	23
Chicken Florentine, 2¼ cups, 6.9 oz	320	18	22
Chicken Stir Fry, 1½ cups	180	2	25
Shrimp Fried Rice, 1¼ cups, 8 oz	240	0	44

Oven Ready:

Breaded Calamari Rings (10), 3 oz	200	10	21
Coconut Shrimp (5), with 4 tsp Dipping Sauce, 4 oz	310	16	31

La Choy:

Beef Chow Mein, 1 cup	80	1	11
Chicken Chow Mein, 1 cup	100	4	11
Chop Suey Vegetables, ½ cup	15	0	3
Chow Mein Noodles, ½ cup	130	5	19

Creations: *Per Cup, Prepared*

Sweet & Sour Chicken	320	4.5	46
Sweet Sesame Chicken	340	9	38
Teriyaki Chicken	310	6	40

Lean Cuisine (Frozen):

Culinary Collection: *Per Complete Meal*

Baked Chicken	240	7	30
Beef & Broccoli	270	5	43
Beef Chow Fun	320	5	54
Beef Portabello	200	6	24
Beef Pot Roast	210	6	26
Chicken with Almonds	250	4	38
Chicken Fettuccini	330	6	42
Chicken Parmesan	300	8	39
Lemon Garlic Shrimp	280	6	43
Lemon Pepper/Parmesan Fish, av.	290	8	42
Roasted Turkey & Veggies	200	7	18
Salisbury Steak	270	8	32
Shrimp Alfredo	210	4	28
Thai Style Chicken	260	4	35

Sandwiches & Snacks: *Per Each, Unless Indicated*

Dips w/ Pita Bread, av. all, 8 oz	195	5	29
Flatbread Melts:			
Chicken Ranch Club	370	9	52
Sun-Dried Tom. Basil Chicken	360	8	49
Paninis: Chicken Club Panini	360	9	45
Chicken, Spinach & Mushroom	310	7	42
Philly-Style Steak & Cheese	320	9	39
Steak, Cheddar & Mushroom	340	9	43

Lean Cuisine (Cont):

	C	F	Cb
S'wiches & Snacks (Cont): *Per Each, Unless Indicated*			
Spring Rolls:			
Fajita Style Chicken (2)	200	7	20
Garlic/Thai Chicken (2), av.	200	8	24
Market Collections:			
Asiago Cheese Tortellini	270	7	39
Chicken Margherita	300	8	38
Shanghai Style Shrimp	250	3	41
Sweet & Spicy Ginger Chicken	280	2	43
Simple Favorites:			
Asian Style Pot Stickers	260	4	49
Cheese Ravioli	220	5	33
Macaroni and Cheese	280	6	43
Spa Collection:			
Butternut Squash Ravioli	260	7	40
Lemongrass Chicken	260	6	33
Salmon with Basil	210	6	25
Pizzas ~ See Page 136			
Extra Product Listings ~ www.CalorieKing.com			
Lean Pockets (Frozen): *Per Single Pocket*			
Sandwiches:			
Breakfast, Bacon, Egg & Cheese	260	9	37
Culinary Creations:			
Garlic Chicken White Pizza	270	8	38
Grilled Chicken, Mshrm & Rice	250	7	39
Originals: Cheeseburger	290	9	42
Italian Style Meatballs & Mozz.	300	9	40
Other varieties, av.	270	6	41
Pretzel Bread, average	275	9	35
Stuffed Quesadillas:			
Grilled Chkn & Three Chse	180	4	24
Grilled Chicken Fajita	170	4	24
Lightlife (Vegetarian):			
Smart Cutlets: Original (1), 3 oz	110	0.5	8
Classic Marinara (1), 5 oz	150	1.5	15
Spicy Sweet & Sour (1), 5 oz	230	1	36
Smart Wings: Buffalo (4), 3 oz	110	3	6
Honey BBQ (4), 3 oz	120	0	16
Smart Tenders:			
Lemon Pepper (3), 3 oz	110	0.5	9
Savory Chick'n (3), 3 oz	110	1	7
Lunchables *(Oscar Mayer):* Per Package, w/out Drink			
Bologna & American Crackers Stackers	390	22	34
Extra Cheesy Pizza	280	9	31
Ham & Cheddar/Swiss w/ Crackers, av.	340	19	23
Nachos, Cheese Dip & Salsa	380	21	40

Lunchables (Cont):

	C	F	Cb
Per Package without Drink			
Pepperoni Pizza	310	13	31
Turkey & American Cracker Stackers	390	20	41
Turkey & Cheddar with Crackers	350	19	28
Lunchmakers *(Armour):*			
Loco Nachos	400	14	69
Cheese Pizza	360	9	53
Macaroni Grill: *Prepared*			
Restaurant Favorites: Per 1 Cup, Prepared			
Chicken Alfredo with Linguine	310	11	27
Chicken Marsala	330	13	30
Classic Lasagna	390	19	27
Creamy Basil Parm. Chkn	300	10	27
Frozen:			
Basil Parmesan Chicken, 1½ cups	480	21	45
Grilled Chicken Florentine, 1 cup	420	14	39
Marie Callender's (Frozen):			
Bakes: Per 1 Cup			
Chicken, Spinach & Mshrm Lasagna	290	11	32
Scallop Potatoes & Ham	320	18	23
Southwest Chipotle Chicken	280	11	33
Complete Dinners: Per Meal			
Country Fried Chicken & Gravy	570	27	60
Golden Battered Fish Fillet	400	13	50
Grilled Chicken Bake	500	26	34
Honey Roasted Chicken	320	10	38
Honey Roasted Turkey	320	11	31
Old Fashioned Beef Pot Roast	260	6	31
Pasta Al Dente:			
Cavatappi Genovese, 11 oz	410	15	44
Fettuccine Chkn Balsamic, 10.5 oz	440	18	46
Penne Chicken Modesto, 10 oz	410	17	43
Pot Pies: Per Pie			
Beef, 16.5 oz	1020	58	96
Chicken, 16.5 oz pie	1040	62	90
Creamy Mshrm & Chicken, 16.5 oz	1080	66	96
Honey Roasted Chicken, 16.5 oz	1040	60	96
Turkey, 10 oz	630	36	58
Salisbury Steak Dinner, 14 oz	370	15	35
Spaghetti with Meat Sauce, 15 oz	490	14	67
Maruchan:			
Ramen, Noodle Soup, 3 oz block/pkg., av.	380	16	52
Instant Lunch Noodles, average, 1 package	290	11	39

continued next page...

	C	F	Cb
Maruchan (Cont):			
Yakisoba: *Per 4 oz Package*			
Chicken/Teriyaki Beef Flavor, av.	520	21	72
Sweet & Sour Chicken	560	22	78
Michael Angelo's: *Per Cup, Prepared*			
Chicken Alfredo, 11 oz	480	17	57
Chicken Piccata, 10 oz	510	24	52
Eggplant Parmesan, 11oz	430	28	26
Lasagna: 4 Cheese/Ssg & Egg, 11 oz	480	18	51
Manicotti with Sauce, 11 oz	410	18	39
Shrimp Scampi, 10 oz	540	28	46
Veggie Lasagna, 11 oz	390	15	44
Minute Rice:			
Ready To Serve: *Per 4.4 oz Container, Prepared*			
Brown/Chicken Rice Mix, av.	230	3.5	40
White/Yellow Rice	195	4	38
Steamers: *Per 1 Cup*			
Broccoli & Cheese Rice, 6.5 oz	200	3.5	37
Spanish Rice, 6.5 oz	280	6	51
Morningstar Farms (Frozen):			
Biscuits:			
Bacon, Egg & Cheese	270	8	40
Sausage & Egg	270	8	39
Burgers: *Per Patty*			
Grillers Original (1)	130	6	5
Mushroom Lovers (1)	110	6	8
Spicy Black Bean (1)	120	4	13
Entrees: *Per Entree*			
Chik'n Enchilada (1), 9.5 oz	280	7	47
Sesame Chik'n, 9.5 oz	310	9	46
Sweet & Sour Chk'n, 10 oz	340	6	56
Chik'n: Buffalo Wings (5)	200	8	20
Chik'n Nuggets (4)	190	9	19
Patties: Breakfast (1)	80	3	4
Hot & Spicy Veggie Sausage (1)	70	3	3
Newman's Own:			
Skillets: *Per ½ Package, 12 oz*			
Chicken: Fettuc, Alfredo	350	7	46
Florentine & Farfalle	370	10	42
Parmigiana & Penne	490	25	47
Garlic Chkn , Veggie & Farfalle	300	8	40
Italian Sausage & Rigatoni	510	28	28
Nissin:			
Chow Mein: *Per 4 oz Package*			
Chicken Flavor	480	18	70
Spicy Chicken Flavor	520	22	72
Teriyaki Beef/Thai P'nut	540	24	72
With Shrimp	560	28	64
Cup Noodles,			
Beef/Chicken/Shrimp, 1 cup	300	13	38
Top Ramen, average, 3 oz pkg	380	14	54

	C	F	Cb
Old El Paso:			
Dinner Kits: *Per Serving, Prepared with Chicken*			
Chicken Soft Taco	300	10	30
Enchilada	390	16	27
Refried Beans,			
Traditional, 4.25 oz	90	0.5	16
Tortilla Stuffers: *Per ⅓ Cup, Includes Meat*			
Carne Asada Steak; Mesq. Chkn, 1.95 oz	90	2	14
Garlic Chili Chicken, 1.75 oz	80	2	11
Pasta Roni: *Per Cup, Prepared*			
Angel Hair Pasta varieties, average	310	14	40
Butter & Herb Italiano	300	11	41
Chicken & Broccoli	360	15	49
Chicken Flavor	300	12	40
Fettuccine Alfredo	450	24	44
Four Cheese Corkscrew	370	15	49
Shells & White Cheddar	290	12	38
Tomato Parmesan	270	9	40
Nature's Way:			
Creamy Parmesano	270	7	43
Mushroom in Cream Sce	280	9	41
Olive Oil & Italian Herb	250	8	38
P.F. Chang's (Frozen): *Per ½ Package, 11 oz*			
Beef with Broccoli	350	17	26
General Chang's Chicken	400	13	51
Ginger Chicken & Broccoli	330	12	33
Orange Chicken	440	16	58
Shrimp in Garlic Sauce	280	8	32
Sweet & Sour Chicken	380	10	58
Rice-A-Roni:			
Classic Favorites: *Per Cup, Prepared*			
Beef; Herb & Butter; Rice Pilaf, av.	310	9	52
Broccoli Au Gratin	350	16	46
Chicken Flavor	300	9	50
Chicken & Broccoli	220	5	40
Spanish Rice	260	8	44
(Reduced Fat Recipe: If only 1 Tbsp fat is used instead of 2 Tbsp, deduct 35 calories and 4g fat.)			

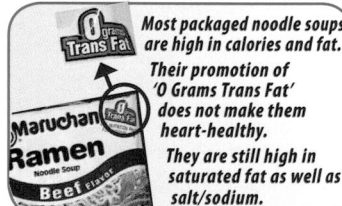

Most packaged noodle soups are high in calories and fat.

Their promotion of '0 Grams Trans Fat' does not make them heart-healthy.

They are still high in saturated fat as well as salt/sodium.

Rice-A-Roni (Cont):	C	F	Cb
Nature's Way: Ital. Cheese & Herb	340	12	52
Long Grain & Wild Rice	250	7	43
Parmesan & Romano Cheese	280	9	42

Whole Grain Blends:

	C	F	Cb
Chicken & Herb Classico	260	8	41
Roasted Garlic Italiano	270	9	41
Spanish	250	8	42

Rosarita:
Refried Beans: *Per ½ Cup*

	C	F	Cb
Traditional; Spicy	120	2	18
Vegetarian	120	2	19
Non-Fat: Refried Beans	100	0	18
Black Beans	110	0	19

Safeway Select (Frozen):

	C	F	Cb
Beef Salisbury Steak, 9.35 oz	410	28	23
Chicken Cacciatore, 8.75 oz	290	10	34
Fettucini Alfredo, 11.5 oz	380	12	55
Five Vegetable Lasagna, 10.6 oz	330	8	48
Homestyle Baked Chicken, 9 oz	260	11	31
Orange Chicken, 9 oz	360	7	61
Penne Pasta, 8 oz	300	11	42
Pot Roast, 9 oz	270	11	23
Spaghetti with Meat Sauce, 12 oz	450	16	61
Swedish Meat Balls, 11.5 oz	470	24	43
Three Cheese Tortellini, 7.5 oz	350	16	38
Triple Cheese Enchilada, 9 oz	410	14	57

S & W: *Per ½ Cup*

	C	F	Cb
Black Beans, 4.5 oz	100	1	17
Chili Beans.			
in Zesty Tom. 5ce, 4.55 oz	110	1	23
Kidney Beans, 4.65 oz	100	0.5	23
White Beans, 4.5 oz	110	0.5	19

Seapak ~ *See www.calorieking.com*

Shedd's:
Country Crock Side Dishes:

	C	F	Cb
Cheddar Rice & Broccoli, 7 oz	260	11	32
Elbow Macaroni & Cheese, 8 oz	330	14	38
Garlic Mashed Potato, 5 oz	140	7	18
Loaded Mashed Potatoes, 5 oz	190	11	18

Simply Asia:
Noodle Bowls: *Per 8.5oz Bowl*

	C	F	Cb
Roasted Peanut	490	10	87
Sesame Teriyaki	410	1	91
Soy Ginger	420	5	79
Spicy Mongolian	450	1	101

Noodles & Sauce: *Per ⅓ package*

	C	F	Cb
Sesame Teriyaki	300	3	60
Soy Ginger	320	4.5	60
Spicy Kung Pao	350	7	63

Simply Asia (Cont):	C	F	Cb
Quick Noodles: *Per 8.8 oz Tray*			
Honey Teriyaki	430	3.5	85
Pad Thai	460	3	93
Szechwan Chow Mein	460	7	83
Average other varieties	430	3	86

Smart Ones (Frozen):
Classics: *Per Meal*

	C	F	Cb
Angel Hair Marinara	230	4	40
Chicken Enchiladas Suiza	290	5	49
Chicken Oriental	230	1.5	41
Lasagna Bake w/ Meat Sauce	270	4	46
Lasagna Florentine	310	11	41
Lemon Herb Chicken Piccata	230	1.5	41
Macaroni Cheese	270	2	52
Pasta Primavera	250	4	41
Pasta with Ricotta & Spinach	280	6	43
Ravioli Florentine	270	5	43
Salisbry Steak, 9.5 oz	280	9	33
Sesame Chicken	360	7	49
Spaghetti with Meat Sauce	290	5	44
Spicy Szechuan Style, Vegetable & Chkn	240	5	38
Swedish Meatballs	270	6	35
Three Cheese Macaroni	300	6	48
Three Cheese Ziti Marinara	300	8	44
Traditional Lasagna w/ Meat Sce	300	7	41
Tuna Noodle Gratin	240	4.5	39

Satisfying Selections: *Per Meal*

	C	F	Cb
Chicken & Broccoli Alfredo	300	4	39
Chicken Broccoli with Cheese	340	6	37
Chicken Teriyaki Stir Fry	340	6	49
Sesame Chicken	360	7	49
Ziti w/ M'balls & Cheese	390	9	52

Smart Beginnings: *Per Meal*

	C	F	Cb
Breakfast Quesadilla	230	7	29
Canad. Bacon Eng. Muffin	210	6	27
English Muffin S'wich	210	5	28
Stuffed Breakfast Sandwich	240	7	30

Smart Creations: *Per Meal*

	C	F	Cb
Chicken Carbonara	260	5	32
Chicken Fettucini	290	6	40
Chicken Parmesan	290	5	35
Cranberry Turkey Medallions	250	2	43
Homestyle Turkey Brst w/ Stuffing	260	9	39
Meatloaf	240	8	22
Teriyaki Chicken & Vegetables	230	2.5	39

So Yah!:

	C	F	Cb
Creamy Coconut Curry	180	9	20
Red Vindaloo Curry	150	4	24

Stagg Chili:	C	F	Cb
Chili with Beans: *14.3 oz Can*			
Classic; Dynamite Hot, 1 cup	335	17	29
Chunkero, 1 cup	320	16	28
Country Brand, 1 cup	320	16	28
Fiesta Griller, 1 cup	250	10	25
Ranch House Chkn, 1 cup	240	8	26
Silverado Beef, 1 cup	250	7	30
White Chili, 1 cup	260	12	20
Low-Fat:			
Turkey Ranchero, 1 cup	240	3	31
Vegetable Garden Four-Bean 1 cup	200	1	37
No Beans,			
Steakhouse, 1 cup	320	22	14

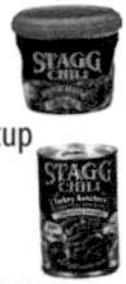

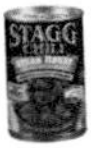

Stouffer's:	C	F	Cb
Frozen:			
Easy Express Skillets: *Per Serving*			
Broccoli & Beef, 12.5 oz	350	6	57
Teriyaki Chicken, 12.5 oz	270	4	41
Yankee Pot Roast, 12 oz	300	8	38
Farmers' Harvest: *Per Single Serve Package*			
Chicken Fettuccini Alfredo, 12 oz	510	29	44
Chicken-Parm. Pasta Bake, 12 oz	310	8	39
Rstd Chicken & Bow Tie Pasta w/ Veg	430	18	46
Made With Whole Grain Pasta:			
Lasagna w/ Meat & Sce, 10 oz	360	12	40
Spag. & M'balls w/ Veggies, 12 oz	320	9	41
Vegetable Lasagna, 10.5 oz	400	19	43
Satisfying Servings: *Per Single Serve Package*			
Bourbon Steak Tips, 14 oz	490	17	61
Macaroni & Cheese, 20 oz	680	32	72
Monterey Chkn, 14.5 oz	530	21	54
Sesame Chicken, 15 oz	590	16	87
Shrimp Scampi, 14 oz	400	12	56
Saute's For Two: *Per ½ Package*			
Braised Beef & Portabello Tortellini	370	15	36
Cajun Style Shrimp Alfredo	400	16	46
Steak Gorgonzola	730	26	90
Signature Classics: *Per Single Serve Package*			
Baked Chkn Breast, 8⅞ oz	240	8	17
Beef Pot Roast, 8⅞ oz	240	8	27
Beef Strog., 9.75 oz	380	17	34
Chkn Fettuccini, 0.5 oz	570	27	55
Chicken Parmigiana, 12 oz	410	14	47
Fettuccini Alfredo, 11.5 oz	630	35	63
Five Cheese Lasagna, 10.75 oz	370	14	39
Lasagna, with Meat & Sauce, 10.5 oz	350	11	38
Meatloaf, 9⅞ oz	320	16	23

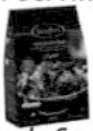

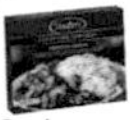

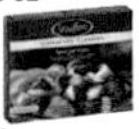

Stouffer's:	C	F	Cb
Frozen:			
Signature Classics (Cont): *Per Single serve Package*			
Salisbury Steak, 9⅝ oz	360	19	22
Swedish M'balls, 11.5 oz	560	27	47
Stromboli:			
Chicken Broccoli Cheddar, 6 oz	360	11	45
Italian-Style, 6 oz	430	19	47
Pepperoni & Provolone, 6 oz	430	17	47
Toasted Subs:			
M'ball Italiano, 6⅞ oz	400	18	42
Phill-Style, Steak & Cheese, 6 oz	370	16	39
Simple Dishes: *Per Serving*			
Cheddar Potato Bake, 10 oz	540	34	42
Creamed Spinach, 9 oz	460	38	20
Mac. & Cheese, 12 oz	680	32	66
Swanson's:			
Frozen:			
Pot Pies: Beef (1), 7 oz	390	24	33
Chicken/Turkey (1), 7 oz	380	22	34
Taco Bell:			
Taco Dinners: *Per Serving, Prep'd as Directed*			
Cheesy Dble Decker, ⅙ pkg., 2.5 oz	340	16	30
Soft Taco Dinner, ⅕ pkg., 3.5 oz	370	13	40
Taco Shells, Salsa & Seasoning (1)	250	11	20
Refried Beans:			
Fat-Free, 4.5 oz	100	0	18
Vegetarian Blend, 4.5 oz	120	1	20
Tasty Bite:			
Vegetarian Entrees: *Per ½ Package, 5 oz*			
Agra Peas & Greens	150	8	13
Bengal Lentils	160	6	20
Bombay Potatoes	130	4	19
Jaipur Vegetables	180	11	12
Jodhpur Lentils	110	2.5	16
Madras Lentils	150	6	18
Punjab Eggplant	150	9	13
TGI Friday's:			
Frozen:			
Beer Battered Onion Rings (3)	180	8	26
Buffalo Popcorn Chicken & Sauce	230	7	15
Buffalo Wings (3)	180	11	4
Honey BBQ Wings (3)	200	11	10
Mozzarella Sticks, with Marinara Sauce, 1 stick	110	5	9
Potato Skins, Chedd. & Bacon (3)	210	12	17
Complete Skillet Meals:			
Sizzling Chicken Fajitas, 1¼ cups	360	14	34
Sizzling Shrimp Stir Fry, 1⅓ cups	300	6	54

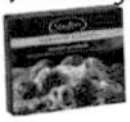

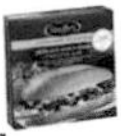

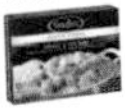

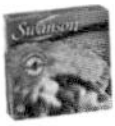

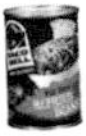

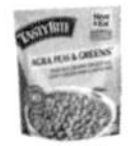

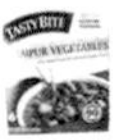

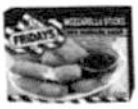

Thai Kitchen:	C	F	Cb
Microwaveable Take-Out Meals: *Per ½ Package*			
Original Pad Thai	250	2	54
Thai Basil & Chili	250	3	50
Thai Peanut	270	5	51
Noodle Carts: *Per 9 oz Tray*			
Pad Thai	460	2	104
Thai Peanut	510	9	96
Rice Noodle Soup Bowls,			
average all flavors, 2.5 oz	240	2	50
Stir-Fry Rice Noodles: *Per ½ Package*			
Original Pad Thai	390	3.5	84
Thai Peanut	390	2	87

Tofurky *(Vegetarian):*	C	F	Cb
Deli Slices: Pepperoni, 8 slices, 1 oz	60	0.5	6
Roast Beef; Bologna, 3 slices, 1.8 oz	100	3	5
Holidays: Tofky Rst & Gravy, ⅓ pkt	250	6	13
Tofurky Feast, ⅓ package, 5 oz	300	7	16
Sausages: Beer Brats (1), 3.5 oz	260	13	12
Italian Ssg (1), 3.5 oz	270	13	11
Kielbasa (1), 3.5 oz	240	12	12

Trader Joe's:	C	F	Cb
Chicken Chili with Beans, 1 cup	290	9	32
Pasta, Shells & White Cheddar, 1 cup	280	6	47
Organic Baked Beans, av., ½ cup	140	0	29
Turkey Chili w/ Beans, 1 cup	240	4.5	30
Black Beans: Reg., ½ cup	110	0	19
Cuban Style, ½ cup	100	0.5	19
Potatoes: Garlic Mashed, ½ cup	150	7	19
Cheddar Cheese Au Gratin, ½ cup	140	5	21
Frozen:			
Meals: *Per Serving*			
Butter Chkn w/ Basmati Rice, 1 cup	270	8	33
Chicken Chow Mein, ⅓ pkg, 6.7 oz	210	2	35
Chicken Quesadilla (1), 6 oz	320	16	26
Citrus Glazed Chicken w/ Rice, 8 oz	270	5	40
Mac & Cheese: Reg., 1 cup, 7 oz	360	15	40
Reduced Guilt, 7 oz	270	6	40
Shrimp Stir Fry, 6.4 oz	70	0.5	6
Spag. & Beef Meatballs, 1 cup, 9 oz	380	13	48
Spicy Beef & Broccoli, 1.75 cups	430	13	64
Thai Vegetable Kao Soi, 12.6 oz	430	20	55
Vegetable Pad Thai, 10.5 oz tray	520	21	74
Pies: Chicken Pot Pie, ½ pie, 8 oz	360	22	28
Shepherd's Pie, 1 cup, 8 oz	170	3	22

Tyson:	C	F	Cb
Frozen:			
Beef: *Per 5 oz Serving Unless Indicated*			
Heat & Serve: Pot Roast in Gravy	180	8	4
Steak Tips: In Bourbon Sauce	190	5	17
In Burgundy Sauce	170	9	7
Grilled & Ready, Beef Strips, 3 oz	140	6	1
Chicken Any'tizers:			
Chicken Fries,			
Homestyle (7), 3.17 oz	230	13	14
Empanitas, Chkn Bacon Ranchero (3)	200	8	20
Fajita Quesa Dippers,w/ Lime Salsa	200	0	19
Wings: Buffalo Style, Hot, 3 oz	190	13	3
Honey BBQ, 3 oz	190	12	8
Hot & Spicy, 3 pcs	220	15	1
Stuffed Chkn Cordon Bleu,			
Minis, 3 pieces	180	10	9
Deli Market, Pasta Entrees: *Per 11.8oz Package*			
Bacon, Vege. & Chicken Alfredo	620	40	43
Cajun-Style Sausage Tortellini	660	37	57
Italian Mixed Grill	400	11	56
Meaty Mac & Cheese	620	31	55
Grilled & Ready: *Per 3 oz*			
Fajita Chkn Strips, 3 oz	110	4	1
Sthwstrn Chkn Breast Strips	120	3	3
Nuggets: Breast, 5 pieces	220	13	15
Fun Shaped, 5 pieces	280	18	16
Southern Style, 6 pcs	270	21	11
Pork: *Per 5 oz Serving*			
Maple & Brown Sugar Glazed Ham	180	3.5	18
Pork Loin,			
in Sweet & Tangy Sce	190	7	15
Pork Roast in Gravy	190	10	5

Uncle Ben's:	C	F	Cb
Country Inn: *Per Cup, Prepared with Water Only*			
Broccoli Rice Au Gratin	210	2.5	41
Chicken & Vegetable Rice	210	1.5	44
Mexican Fiesta Rice	190	1	42
Oriental Fried Rice	210	1	45
Long Grain & Wild Rice: *Per Cup, Prep'd w/ Water Only*			
Original	200	0.5	44
Herb Roasted Chicken	210	1.5	43
Roasted Garlic & Olive Oil	210	1	43
Ready Rice: *Per Package, Heat & Serve*			
Butter & Garlic Flavored Rice	220	4	41
Garden Vegetable	200	2.5	41
Roasted Chicken	210	3	42
Teriyaki Style	220	3	42

continued next page...

Uncle Ben's (Cont):

Ready Whole Grain Medley: *Per Pkg., Heat & Serve*

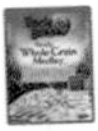

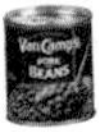

Brown & Wild	220	3.5	42
Chicken Medley	210	2.5	41
Garden Vegetable	200	2.5	41
Roasted Garlic	200	3	38
Santa Fe	220	3	42
Vegetable Harvest	220	3	44

Van Camp's:

Baked Beans, Orig., ½ cup, 4.75 oz	160	1	30
Beanee Weenees, Orig./Smoked, 7.75 oz	240	8	29
Pork & Beans, 28 oz can, ½ cup, 4.6 oz	110	1	23

Van De Kamp's (Frozen):

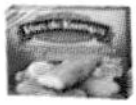

Crispy Halibut Fillets (3)	280	13	24
Crunchy Fish Sticks (6)	240	11	22
Fish Shaped Nuggets, 4 nuggets, 4.25 oz	280	13	25
Fried, Beer Battered Fillets (2)	240	13	18
Breaded: Butterfly Shrimp, 7 pcs	330	16	31
Popcorn Fish, 8 pieces, 4.13 oz	270	13	25

Worthington/Loma Linda:

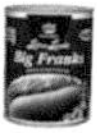

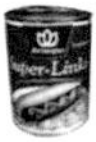

Big Franks: 1 link, 1.8 oz	110	6	3
Low-fat, 1 link, 1.8 oz	80	2.5	3
Chili, 1 cup, 8.10 oz	280	10	25
Choplets, 2 slices, 3.2 oz	90	1	4
Diced Chik, 2 oz	50	0	2
FriChik, Original, low fat, 2 pcs, 3 oz	80	2.5	4
Linketts, (1), 1¼ oz	70	4	1
Little Links (1), 1.6 oz	90	5	3
Redi-Burger, ⅝" slice, 3 oz	120	2.5	7
Saucettes (1), 1 oz	90	6	1
Super Links (1), 1.5 oz	110	8	2
Tender Bits/Rounds (6), av., 2.8 oz	120	4.5	7
Vegetable Skallops, ½ cup, 3 oz	90	1	4
Vegetarian Burger, ¼ cup, 1.9 oz	70	1.5	3
Veja-Links (1), 1 oz	50	3	1
Low-Fat Veja-Links (1), 1 oz	45	1.5	2

Frozen:

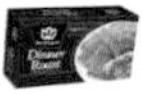

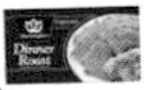

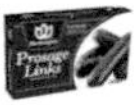

Chic-ketts, 2 slices	110	5	3
Dinner Roast, ¾" slice	180	11	6
Fried Chik'n w/ Gravy, 2 pcs	150	10	5
FriPats, 1 pattie, 2.25 oz	130	6	5
Leanies, 1 link, 1.4 oz	100	7	2
Meatless:			
Chicken Style Roll, ⅜" slice	90	4.5	2
Smoked Turkey Roll, ⅜" slice	130	8	4
Prosage Links (2), 1.6 oz	80	3	3
Stakelets, 2.5 oz piece	150	7	7
Stripples, 2 strips, 0.56 oz	60	4.5	2
Swiss Stake, with Gravy, 1 piece	130	6	9

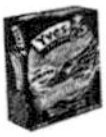

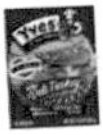

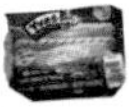

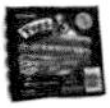

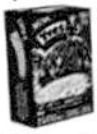

Yves Veggie Cuisine:

	C	F	Cb
Breakfast: Patties (2), 1.8 oz	80	2	4
Canadian Bacon, 3 slices	80	0.5	2
Burgers: Meatless Beef Burger (1)	110	4	8
Meatless Chicken (1)	100	3	5
Deli Slices:			
Meatless: Ham, 4 slices	80	2.5	2
Bologna, 4 slices	100	2	5
Pepperoni, 6 slices	80	2.5	2
Roast w/out the Beef, 4 slices	110	2.5	4
Salami, 4 slices	80	0	4
Smoked Chicken, 4 sl.	100	1.5	5
Turkey, 4 slices	100	1.5	5
Ground Rounds:			
Meatless: Turkey, ⅓ cup, 1.95 oz	60	1	4
Taco Stuffers, ⅓ cup, 1.95 oz	90	2.5	5
Heart's Desire:			
Meatless Beef Strips, 3 oz	120	1	4
Meatless Chicken Strips, 3 oz	110	1	3
Hot Dog:			
Good Dog (1), 2 oz	70	3.5	1
Hot Dog (1), 1.5 oz	50	0.5	2
Jumbo Hot Dog (1), 2.75 oz	110	3	5
Tofu Dog (1), 1.5 oz	45	1	2
Brats:			
Veggie Classic (1), 3.5 oz	160	5	9
Zesty Italian (1), 3.5 oz	150	5	9
Skewers,			
Lemon Herb Chicken (1), 3 oz	100	1	7
Veggie: Breasts,			
in Curry Flav. Vindaloo Sce, 5.5 oz	170	3	13
Chorizo, 1/3 link, 2 oz	80	4.5	56
Meatballs (4), 2 oz	80	2	8

Zatarain's:

New Orleans Style: *Per ⅓ Cup Dry Mix Only*

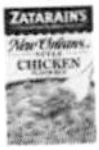

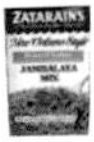

Black Beans & Rice	220	0.5	47
Caribbean Rice	160	1.5	34
Chicken Creole Rice	130	0.5	28
Chicken Flavor Rice	210	1	44
Garlic & Herb & Rice	150	0	33
Gravy & Rice	200	0.5	45
Rice Pilaf	200	0	45
Smothered Chicken Rice			
Yellow Rice	190	0	43

Frozen:

Meals: *Per 10.5 oz Serve Unless Indicated*

Blackened Chicken Alfredo	510	24	50
Jambalaya Flavored w/ Ssge, 12 oz	500	14	79
Jambalaya Pasta w/ Chkn & Ssge	380	10	56
Red Beans & Rice w/ Sausage, 12 oz	510	20	68

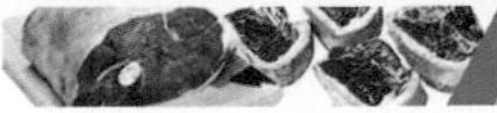

Note: Cooking reduces weight of meat by 20-45% due to water and fat losses. Average weight loss is 30%. Actual loss depends on cooking method and cooking time.

Examples:

4 oz raw weight = approx. 3 oz cooked weight
4 oz cooked weight = approx. 5½ oz raw weight

What 3 oz Cooked Meat Looks Like:

• Rectangular piece (4" x 2½" x ½" thick)
• Deck of cards (3½" x 2½" x ⅝" thick)

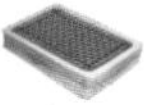

STEAK QUICK GUIDE

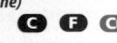

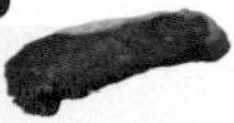

Sirloin (Choice Grade):
External fat trimmed to ⅛"
Broiled, Edible Portion (no bone)

	C	F	Cb
Small/Regular Serving, 3 oz (cooked):			
(from 4-4½ oz raw)			
Lean + external fat (⅛"), 3 oz	220	13	0
Lean + marbling, 3 oz	185	9	0
Lean only, 3 oz	160	6	0
(No external fat or marbling)			
Medium Serving, 5 oz (cooked wt):			
(from approximately 7 oz raw)			
Lean + external fat (⅛"), 5 oz	365	22	0
Lean + marbling, 5 oz	310	15	0
Lean only, 5 oz	265	10	0
Large Serving, 8 oz (cooked wt):			
(from 11-12 oz raw)			
Lean + external fat (⅛"), 8 oz	585	36	0
Lean + marbling, 8 oz	500	24	0
Lean only, 8 oz	425	15	0
Extra Large Serving, 12 oz (cooked wt):			
(from approximately 16-17 oz raw)			
Lean + external fat (⅛"), 12 oz	875	54	0
Lean + marbling, 12 oz	745	36	0
Lean only, 12 oz	640	22	0
Pan Fried:			
Sirloin (Choice), medium serving,			
Lean + external fat (⅛"), 5 oz	445	30	0

Other Steaks

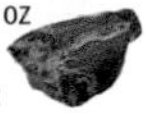

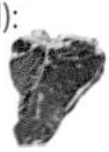

	C	F	Cb
Filet Mignon (Tenderloin):			
1 Medium steak (6 oz raw weight):			
Broiled, with ¼" fat trim:			
Lean + fat (¼"), 4 oz	360	27	0
Lean only, 3½ oz	230	12	0
New York/Club Steak:			
Top Loin/Short Loin:			
1 steak, regular (9¼ oz raw, ¼" fat):			
Broiled: Lean + fat (¼"), 6.25 oz	580	43	0
Lean + marbling, 5.5 oz	400	25	0
Lean only, 5.25 oz	360	20	0
Porterhouse Steak:			
1 Medium, 6 oz raw weight (no bone), broiled:			
Lean + fat (¼"), 4.25 oz	410	33	0
Lean only, 3.5 oz	210	11	0
1 Large ,12 oz raw weight (no bone), broiled:			
Lean + fat (¼") 8.5 oz cooked	820	66	0
Lean only, 7 oz cooked	420	22	0
T-Bone Steak: *Broiled or Grilled*			
Medium Size: *8 oz raw weight, no bone*			
(Approximately 6 oz cooked):			
Lean + Fat (¼"), 5 oz	400	28	0
Lean only, 4 oz	265	12	0
Large Size: *12 oz raw wt*			
(Approximately 9 oz cooked):			
Lean + fat (¼"), 7 oz (no bone)	560	39	0
Lean only, 6 oz (no bone)	400	18	0
Extra Large Size: *20 oz raw weight*			
(Approximately 16 oz cooked):			
Lean + Fat (¼"), 12 oz (no bone)	960	66	0
Lean Only, 10 oz (no bone)	660	30	0

Also See Fast-Foods & Restaurants Section ~
Lone Star Steakhouse ; Outback Steakhouse

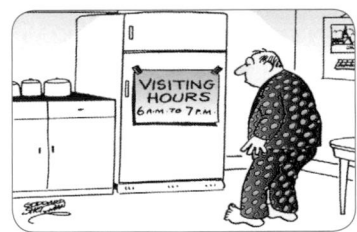

Beef – Individual Cuts

Average All Grades
Edible Weight (no bone)

	C	F	Cb
Brisket, whole, braised:			
Lean + fat (¼" trim), 3 oz	330	27	0
Lean + marbling, 3 oz	250	17	0
Lean only, 3 oz	185	9	0
Chuck blade, braised:			
Lean + fat (¼"), 3 oz	310	24	0
Lean + marbling, 3 oz	295	22	0
Lean only, 3 oz	245	13	0
Flank: Raw, 4 oz	175	8	0
Braised, 3 oz	225	14	0
Broiled, 3 oz	155	6	0
Round, bottom, braised:			
Lean + marbling, 3 oz	190	7.5	0
Lean only, 3 oz	185	6.5	0
Round, eye/tip, rstd:			
Lean + fat (¼"), 3 oz	205	11	0
Lean (w/ marbling), 3 oz	150	5	0
Round, top: Per 3 oz (cooked wt)			
Braised, Lean + fat	210	10	0
Lean only	170	4	0
Broiled, Lean + fat	180	8	0
Lean only	160	5	0
Pan-fried, Lean + fat	235	13	0
Lean only	195	7	0

Beef Ribs

	C	F	Cb
Back Ribs: 7" long, visible fat trimmed to ¼"			
10.3 oz raw w/ bone or 3.5 oz cooked, braised, w/o bone			
1 average rib	410	34	0
3 ribs	1230	102	0
Short Ribs: 2½" long, visible fat trimmed to ¼"			
6 oz raw with bone or 2.5² oz cooked, braised, w/o bone			
1 average rib	320	28	0
3 ribs	960	85	0

Ground Beef

	C	F	Cb
Ground Beef, Raw: Per 4 oz			
70% lean (30% fat)	380	34	0
75% lean (25% fat)	335	29	0
80% lean (20% fat)	290	23	0
85% lean (15% fat)	245	17	0
90% lean (10% fat)	200	12	0
95% lean (5% fat)	155	6	0
Baked/Broiled: Reg. (70%), 3 oz	230	16	0
Lean (80%), 3 oz	215	14	0
Extra lean (90%), 3 oz	185	10	0
Pan-Broiled:			
Reg. (70%), 3 oz	230	15	0
Lean (80%), 3 oz	210	14	0
Extra lean (90%), 3 oz	195	10	0
Ground Beef Patties: Average, 23% Fat			
Raw, 4 oz	330	25	0
Broiled, 3 oz (from 4 oz raw)	250	19	0

Quick Guide

Roast Beef

	C	F	Cb
Round (Eye/Tip, average): Average All Cuts			
Small/Regular Serving: 3 oz			
(2 thin slices/1 thick slice)			
Lean + fat (⅛" fat trim)	180	9	0
Lean only	145	4	0
Medium Serving: 5 oz			
(3-4 thin slices)			
Lean + fat (⅛" fat trim)	300	15	0
Lean only	245	6.5	0
Large Serving, 8 oz: 3 thick slices			
Lean + fat (⅛" fat trim)	480	24	0
Lean only	385	11	0

Roast Dinner Extras

	C	F	Cb
Gravy: Thin, 2 Tbsp	20	0.5	3.5
Thick, 2 Tbsp	50	2	0.5
1 Ladle/4 Tbsp	100	4	1
Veggies: Beans, green, ½ cup	20	0	5
Cauliflower w/ chse sauce, 4 oz	135	9	15
Corn, kernels, ¼ cup	35	0	9
Carrots, ¼ cup	20	0	3
Peas, ¼ cup	35	0	6
Potato: Rstd w/ fat, 1 small	155	8	30
Baked in Jacket, 1 large	280	0	63
with 1 Tbsp whipped butter	350	8	63
with Sour Cream, 2 Tbsp	270	5	64
Sweet Potato/Yam, 1 medium	105	1	24
Beef Kebab: Cooked			
Beef & Veggies, 2 oz	160	10	4
If very lean meat	100	4	4

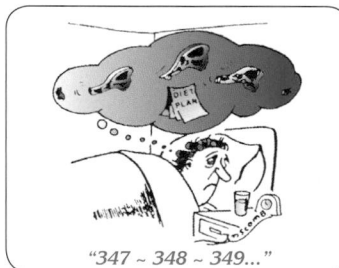

"347 ~ 348 ~ 349..."

Lamb

	C	F	Cb
Choice Grade:			
Leg (Whole), roasted:			
Lean + fat, 3 oz	220	14	0
Lean only, 3 oz	160	7	0
Leg (Sirloin Half), roasted:			
Lean + fat, 3 oz	250	18	0
Lean only, 3 oz	175	8	0
Leg (Shank Half), roasted:			
Lean + fat, 3 oz	190	11	0
Lean only, 3 oz	155	6	0
Loin Chop, broiled:			
1 chop (raw weight, 4.25 oz):	250	17	0
Lean + fat (2.25 oz edible)	180	12	0
Lean only (1.6 oz edible)	85	3.5	0
Rib Chop, broiled:			
1 chop (raw wt., 3.5 oz)			
Lean + fat (2.5 oz edible)	255	21	0
Lean only (1.75 oz edible)	105	6	0
Shoulder (Arm/Blade):			
Braised: Lean + fat, 3 oz	295	21	0
Lean only, 3 oz	240	12	0
Broiled: Lean + fat, 3 oz	240	17	0
Lean only, 3 oz	170	8	0
Roasted: Similar to Broiled			
Cubed Lamb (Leg/Shoulder):			
For stew or kebab			
Braised, lean only, 3 oz	190	8	0
Broiled, lean only, 3 oz	160	6	0

Veal

	C	F	Cb
Edible Weights:			
Leg (Top Round):			
Braised: Lean + fat, 3 oz	180	6	0
Lean only, 3 oz	175	5	0
Pan-fried, breaded:			
Lean + fat, 3 oz	195	8	9
Lean only, 3 oz	185	6	9
Pan-fried, not breaded:			
Lean + fat, 3 oz	180	7	0
Lean only, 3 oz	155	4	0
Roasted: Lean + fat, 3 oz	135	4	0
Lean only, 3 oz	130	3	0

Veal (Cont)

	C	F	Cb
Loin Chop: *1 chop, 7 oz raw weight*			
Braised: Lean + fat, 3 oz	240	15	0
Lean only, 3 oz	190	8	0
Roasted: Lean + fat, 3 oz	185	11	0
Lean only, 3 oz	150	6	0
Rib, roasted: *Lean + fat, 3 oz*	195	12	0
Lean only, 3 oz	150	7	0
Shoulder, Arm/Blade, roasted:			
Lean + fat, 3 oz	155	7	0
Lean only, 3 oz	140	5	0
Sirloin, roasted:			
Lean + fat, 3 oz	170	9	0
Lean only, 3 oz	145	6	0
Cubed for Stew, braised:			
Leg/Shoulder, lean only, 3 oz	160	4	0
(1 lb raw yields approx. 9.25 oz cooked)			

Pork

Fresh Pork: *Cooked Weight, without bone):*
4 oz raw weight = approx. 3 oz cooked weight

	C	F	Cb
Blade Steak, broiled:			
Lean + fat, 3 oz	220	15	0
Lean only, 3 oz	190	11	0
Country Style Ribs, broiled/roasted:			
Lean + fat, 3 oz	280	22	0
Lean only, 3 oz	210	13	0
Spareribs, braised: *lean & fat, 6 oz*	675	52	0
(from 1 lb raw weight)			
Leg (Ham), whole, roasted:			
Lean + fat, 3 oz	230	15	0
Lean only, 3 oz	180	8	0
Loin Chops, broiled: *Average*			
(From 1 chop: 5 oz raw weight with bone			
or 4 oz raw weight, without bone)			
Lean + fat, 3 oz	200	11	0
Lean only, 3 oz	165	7	0
Loin Roast, roasted:			
Lean + fat, 3 oz	210	13	0
Lean only, 3 oz	180	8	0
Rib Chops, (Boneless), broiled:			
Lean + fat, 3 oz	220	14	0
Lean only, 3 oz	185	9	0
Rib Roast:			
Lean + fat, 3 oz	215	13	0
Lean only, 3 oz	180	9	0

Pork (Cont)

	C	F	Cb
Sirloin Chop, broiled:			
Lean + fat, 3 oz	180	8	0
Lean only, 3 oz	165	6	0
Sirloin Roast, roasted:			
Lean + fat, 3 oz	175	8	0
Lean only, 3 oz	170	7	0
Tenderloin (Boneless), roasted:			
Lean + fat, 3 oz	125	4	0
Lean only, 3 oz	120	3	0
Ground Pork:			
Raw: Average, ¼ lb, 4 oz	300	24	0
Broiled, 3 oz	250	18	0
Pan-fried, drained, 3 oz	260	19	0

Bacon

	C	F	Cb
Raw: 1 med. slice, 0.75 oz	95	9	0
1 thick slice, 1⅓ oz	175	17	0
(1 lb raw yields approximately 5 oz cooked)			
Broiled/Pan-Fried:			
1 medium slice, 0.3 oz	40	3	0
3 medium slices, 0.8	125	10	0
2 thin slices, 0.5 oz	75	6	0
1 thick slice, 0.85 oz	65	5	0
Canadian Bacon:			
Cooked, 1 slice, 1 oz	45	2	0.5
Pkg, 3 slices, 2 oz	90	4	1
Bacon Bits, 1 T., 0.25 oz	35	2	0
Breakfast Strips, Broiled, 1 sl.,, 0.42 oz	50	4	0

Ham

	C	F	Cb
Boneless Ham, cooked:			
Regular, (approximately 13% fat):			
Roasted, 3 oz	150	8	0
Extra Lean (5% fat),			
Roasted, 3 oz	125	5	0
Whole Ham, cooked:			
Lean + fat (as purchased)			
Roasted, 3 oz	210	15	0
Lean only, Roasted, 3 oz	135	5	0
Canned Ham: *Similar to boneless ham*			
Chopped, canned, 3 oz	200	16	0
Ham Patties, cooked, 1 pattie, 2.25 oz	220	20	1
Ham Steak, extra lean, 2 oz	70	2.5	0
Lunch Slices ~ *See Deli Meats, Page 128*			

Game & Other Meats

	C	F	Cb
Bison Steak,	205	4	0
lean, 6 oz (raw)			
Boar (wild), roasted, 3 oz	140	4	0
Buffalo Steak: *New West Foods,* 4 oz	70	3	0
Trader Joe's, 1 pattie	430	30	1
Caribou, roasted, 3 oz	140	4	0
Deer/Venison, roasted 3 oz	135	3	0
Goat (Capretto):			
Raw, 3 oz	95	2	0
Roasted, 3 oz	120	2.5	0
Ostrich: *Blackwing Ostrich Meats,*			
Sport Jerky, 0.5 oz piece	25	0	0
Sausage Patties (2) 2 oz	60	0.5	0
New West Foods:			
Ground Ostrich, 4 oz	165	7	0
Ostrich Steak, 4 oz steak	130	2.5	0
Rabbit: Roasted, 3 oz	165	7	0
Stewed, 1 cup, diced, 5 oz	290	12	0

Variety & Organ Meats

	C	F	Cb
Brain (Lamb): Braised, 3 oz	125	9	0
Pan-fried, 3 oz	230	19	0
Chitterlings, pork, simmered, 3 oz	260	25	0
Ears, pork, simmered, 1 ear, 4 oz	185	12	0
Feet, pork: Simmered, 3 oz	200	14	0
Cured, pickled, 3 oz	170	14	0
Hormel, 2 oz	80	6	0
Head Cheese (Pork Snouts/Ears/Vinegar/Spices):			
1 oz slice	50	4	0
Heart, Beef, braised, 3 oz	140	4	0
Jowl, pork, raw, 4 oz	750	80	0
Kidneys, braised, 3 oz	140	5	0
Liver (beef): Raw, 4 oz	150	4	4
Braised, 3 oz	140	4	3
Pan-fried, 3 oz	185	7	7
Pancreas, pork, braised, 3 oz	185	8	0
Pork Cracklins, 0.5 oz	80	6	0
Pork Hocks, 1 piece, 6 oz	340	23	0
Scrapple, pork, 2 oz	120	8	8
Spleen, pork, braised, 3 oz	130	3	0
Stomach, pork, raw, 4 oz	185	12	0
Sweetbreads:			
Beef, cooked, 3 oz	125	9	0
Lamb, cooked, 3 oz	125	9	0
Tail, pork, simmered, 3 oz	340	31	0
Tongue, raised, Veal, 3 oz	170	9	0
Beef/Lamb, av., 3 oz	235	17	0
Tripe, beef, raw, 3 oz	85	3.5	0

Quick Guide

Franks & Weiners
Average All Brands | **C** | **F** | **Cb**

Regular (Pork Mix): *Per Frank*

	C	F	Cb
Regular (10/16 oz package), 1.5 oz	140	13	1
Bun Length/Jumbo, 2 oz	185	17	2
Extra Long, 2.75 oz	255	24	2
Small/Cocktail (50/lb), each	30	3	0.5

Beef Franks: *Per Frank*

	C	F	Cb
Regular (10/16 oz package), 1.5 oz	140	13	1
Bun Length/Jumbo, 2 oz	175	17	2.5
¼ lb Dog, 4 oz	375	33	5

Franks & Weiners C F Cb

Ball Park: *Per 2 oz Frank Unless Indicated*

Angus Beef:

	C	F	Cb
Original; Bun Size	170	15	3
Lower Fat, 1.87 oz	130	10	2

Beef: Original

	C	F	Cb
Fat Free, 1.75 oz	190	16	4
Lite, 1.75 oz	50	0	5
Deli Style	110	7	5
GrillMaster, Hearty Beef, 2.9 oz	140	12	2
Jumbo, 2.5 oz	250	21	3
Singles, 1.6 oz	240	20	5
	150	13	3

Cheese, with Turkey, Beef & Pork | 190 | 16 | 5

Meat: Original; Bun Size | 180 | 15 | 5

	C	F	Cb
Lite, 1.75 oz	100	7	4
Singles, 1.6 oz	140	12	3

Turkey: Original | 110 | 7 | 6
Smoked White, Bun Size, 1.75 oz | 45 | 0 | 5

Foster Farms, Chicken; Turkey, 2 oz | 140 | 12 | 1

Hebrew National: *Per Frank*

Beef: Regular, 1.72 oz

	C	F	Cb
Beef: Regular, 1.72 oz	150	14	1
¼ Pounder (4 oz)	360	33	3
Jumbo, 3 oz	270	25	2
97% Fat-Free, 1.6 oz	40	1	1
Beef Frank in a Blanket, 5 pcs, 3 oz	300	24	12

Jennie-O: *Per Frank*

	C	F	Cb
Turkey Franks: 1.2 oz	70	5	1
Jumbo, 2 oz	120	9	2

Oscar Mayer: *Per Frank*

Beef: Classic, 2 oz

	C	F	Cb
Beef: Classic, 2 oz	170	15	1
XXL Premium, 2.68 oz	230	22	1
Cheese Dogs, 1.6 oz	140	13	1

Turkey: Classic, 1.6 oz | 100 | 8 | 2
Classic Bun Length, 2 oz | 120 | 10 | 3

Shelton's: *Per Frank*

	C	F	Cb
Uncured: Chicken, 1.2 oz	70	6	0
Smoked Chicken, 3 oz	245	20	0
Turkey, 1.2 oz	70	6	0

Zacky Farms, Chkn; Turkey, av, 2 oz | 115 | 10 | 4

Quick Guide

Fresh Sausages
Pork/Beef: *Average All Types* | **C** | **F** | **Cb**

	C	F	Cb
Small: Raw, 4" link, 1 oz	85	7.5	0
Broiled/Pan-fried	80	7	0
Medium: Raw, 2 oz	170	15	0
Broiled/Pan-fried	165	14	0
Large: Raw, 3 oz	255	22	0
Broiled/Pan-fried	245	21	0
Italian: Raw, 3.2 oz	315	28	1
Cooked, 2.4 oz	230	18	3
Chorizo: Beef Chorizo, 2.5 oz piece	250	23	5
Pork Chorizo, 2 oz piece	250	23	5

Note: Fat is lost in broiling/pan frying.
(Cooked weight = approx. 60-70% raw weight)

Smoked Sausage C F Cb

Per Link:

Butterball,
Turkey, 2.8 oz | 150 | 8 | 7

Eckrich, Grillers, av., 2 oz | 180 | 15 | 4

Hillshire Farm:

	C	F	Cb
Beef & Pork, skinless, 2 oz	180	15	3
Cheddar Wurst, 2 oz	180	16	2
Hardwood Chicken, 2 oz	100	7	3
Turkey, 2 oz	90	5	3

Johnsonville ~ *See CalorieKing.Com*

Breakfast Sausages/Patties

Butterball:
Turkey: B'fast Ssg Links, cooked (3) | 110 | 6 | 2
Sausage Patties (2), cooked | 110 | 6 | 2

Jennie-O:
Breakfast Sausages, uncooked,
Turkey (1), 2 oz | 90 | 5 | 0

Breakfast Lovers,
Turkey Sausage, 3.95 oz | 250 | 20 | 1

Jimmy Dean:

	C	F	Cb
Heat 'N Serve: Sausage Links (3)	210	19	2
Maple Sausage Links (3)	170	14	2
Sausage Patties (2)	200	17	2

Breakfast Sandwiches ~ *See Page 92*

Jones Golden Brown:

	C	F	Cb
All Natural: Beef Sausage Links (3)	200	18	2
Maple Sausage (3)	240	22	2
Sausage Patties, All Natural (1)	120	11	0

Vegetarian Patties:
Boca ~ *See Page 117*
Garden Burger ~ *See Page 118*

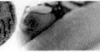

Meat ~ Hot Dogs ◆ Deli Meats

Bagel, Corn & Hot Dogs

Hot Dogs, Ready-To-Go:
(Includes Ketchup/Relish; w/o Mayo)

	C	F	Cb
Regular, 1.5 oz frank, 1.5 oz bun	260	15	22
Bun Length, 2 oz frank, 1.5 oz bun	290	18	21
Jumbo Dog, 2 oz frank, 2 oz bun	360	20	36
¼ lb Beef Dog, 2 oz bun	480	15	36
Mile Long Dog, 2.6 oz dog, 1.5 oz bun	360	24	23

Corn Dogs:
Beef/Pork Frank, average, 2.6 oz	170	10	16

Foster Farms
Corn Dogs:
Chili Cheese: (1), 2.7 oz	190	9	21
Extreme (1), 2.65 oz	200	10	22
Honey Crunchy: Reg. (1), 2.7 oz	180	9	19
Jumbo (1), 3.95 oz	280	15	26
Mini (4), 2.7 oz	210	12	18

State Fair with Ball Park Franks:
Beef Corn Dog (1), 2.7 oz	220	10	25
Classic Corn Dog (1), 2.7 oz	210	10	23

Bagel Dogs:
Einstein Bros,
Asiago/Original with Cheddar, av	545	28	56
Vienna Beef: Bageldog (1), 5 oz	420	17	33
Mini (1), 2.8 oz	150	4	20

Hot Dog Toppings/Extras:
	C	F	Cb
American Cheese, 1 slice, 1 oz	110	9	1
Chili Con Carne, ¼ cup	50	2	5.5
Ketchup, 1 Tbsp	15	0	4
Mustard, 1 Tbsp	20	0	1
Onions, chopped, 1 Tbsp	5	0	1
Pickle Relish, 1 Tbsp	20	0	5
Sauerkraut, ½ cup	20	0	5

Deli/Lunch Meats & Sausage

	C	F	Cb
Beef Jerky/Meat Snacks, Berliner (pork/beef), 1 oz	65	5	1
Beerwurst (Beef):			
Small (2¾"diam), ¹⁄₁₆" sl.	20	2	0
Large (4" diam), ⅛" slice	75	7	0.5
Beerwurst (Pork):			
Small (2.75"diameter), ¹⁄₁₆" slice	15	1	0
Large (4"diameter), ⅛" Slice	55	4	0.5
Blood Sausage, 1 oz	100	9	0.5

Deli/Lunch Meats & Sausages (Cont)

	C	F	Cb
Bologna:			
1 Slice, 1 oz	65	6	1
Fat-Free, 1 slice, 1 oz	20	0	2
Beef Bologna: 1 slice, 1 oz	90	8	1
Light, 1 slice, 1 oz	60	4	2
Light *(Oscar Mayer)*, 1 slice, 1 oz	60	4	2
98% Fat Free *(Oscar Mayer)*, 1 oz	25	0.5	3
Ring *(Boar's Head)*, 2 oz	150	13	1
Turkey, average, 1 oz	60	5	0.5
Bratwurst: Average, 1 oz	80	7	1
Beer *(Bob Evan's)*, 2.6 oz link	270	21	1
Braunschweiger, (Pork/Liver/Sausage), 2 oz slice *(Oscar Mayer)*	190	17	1
Chicken: *Average All Brands*			
1 thick or 2 thin slices, 1 oz	30	1	1
Oven Roasted *(Hillshire Farm)*, Ultra Thin, 2 oz	60	1	2
Corned Beef, average, full fat, 1 oz	60	5	0.5
Ham, Sliced:			
Baked/Broiled, 1 oz slice	30	1	0.5
1 oz slice *(Oscar Mayer)*,	60	2	0.5
Honey/Brown Sugar, av., 1 oz	35	1	1
Prosciutto, average, 1 oz	70	5	0
Ham & Cheese Loaf, average, 1 oz	70	5	1
Italian Sausage, 2.6 oz	250	20	3
Kielbasa, Polish Sausage, 2 oz	65	5	1
Beef, 2 oz link	190	17	1
1 oz *(Boar's Head)*	60	5	1
2.68 oz *(Hillshire Farm)*	250	22	4
Knockwurst, av., 1 oz	90	8	0.5
Linguica *(Gaspar's)*, 2 oz	130	9	1
Liverwurst, 1 oz	65	5	2
Liver Pate, fresh, average, 1 oz	90	8	1
Mortadella, 1 oz	105	9	0
Olive Loaf: Average, 1 oz	70	5	3
1 oz *(Oscar Mayer)*	80	6	3
Pancetta, *(Boars Head)*, 1 slice	50	4.5	0

Deli/Lunch Meats & Sausages (Cont)

	C	F	Cb
Pastrami (Beef):			
(Boar's Head), 2 oz	80	3.5	1
(Healthy Deli), 2 oz	70	2	1
(Hillshire), Deli Select, 6 slice, 2 oz	60	1	0.5
Peppered Beef, 1 oz slice	40	2	1
Pepperoni, 5 slices, 1 oz	140	13	0
Pickle Loaf, av., 1 oz	70	5	5
Pickle & Pepper Loaf,			
(Boars Head), 2 oz	150	13	2
Proscuitto/Proscuitti, av., 1 oz	70	5	1
Roast Beef, Lean, 1 oz	40	2	0
Salami: Beef, av., 1 oz	80	7	1
Hard (Oscar Mayer), 1 slice, 1.76 oz	100	8	1
Beer Salami, average, 1 oz	50	4	0.5
Cotto (Oscar Mayer), 1 slice, 1 oz	60	5	1
Dry, Hard, av., 4 slices, 1 oz	100	8	1
Genoa: Average, 1 oz	100	8	1
Stick, 1.75 oz	175	14	2
Italian (Bridgford), 1 oz	120	11	0
SPAM (Hormel): Per 2 oz Serving			
Classic: 2 oz serving	180	16	1
7 oz can	630	56	3.5
12 oz can	1080	96	6
Spam Lite: 2 oz	110	8	1
12 oz can	660	48	6
Other Spam Products:			
Hickory Smoked, 2 oz	170	15	2
Hot & Spicy, 2 oz	180	16	2
Oven Roastd Turkey, 2 oz	80	4	2
Spam with Bacon, 2 oz	180	16	2
Spam with Cheese, 2 oz	170	15	2
Spam Spread, 2 oz	140	12	2
25% Less Sodium	180	16	1
Spam Singles:			
Classic, 3 oz package	250	22	2
Lite, 3 oz package	160	11	2

Deli/Lunch Meats & Sausages (Cont)

	C	F	Cb
Summer Sausage:			
(Armour), 2 oz	190	17	2
(Hillshire Farm), 2 oz	190	16	0.5
Treet (Armour),			
canned, 2 oz	140	11	4
Turkey: Average, 1 oz slice	30	1	0.5
¾ oz slice	22	0.5	0.5
Turkey Breast:			
(Butterball), Roasted, 1 sl, 1.1 oz	30	0.5	1
(Hillshire Deli Select), 6 slices, 2 oz	50	0.5	2
Turkey Ham, 1 slice, 1 oz	35	1.5	0.5
Turkey Pastrami, 1 oz	35	1.5	1
Turkey Roll, 1 oz	40	2	0.5
Turkey Loaf, 1 oz	30	1	0.5
Vegetarian Deli ~ See Page 118			

Meat Spreads

	C	F	Cb
Average All Brands: Per ¼ Cup, 2 oz			
Chicken, white meat	130	10	2
Ham, Deviled	140	11	0
Liverwurst	190	16	2
Roast Beef	130	10	2
Sandwich Spread	140	10	9
Turkey	110	7	2
Underwood: Per 2 oz			
Chicken, White Meat	130	10	2
Deviled Ham	180	15	1
Liverwurst	160	13	4
Roast Beef	130	10	2

Paté

	C	F	Cb
Boar's Head:			
Strassburger Liverwurst, 2 oz	170	15	1
Braunschweiger, Light, 2 oz	120	8	1
Les Trois Petit Cochons: Per 2 oz			
Black Peppercorn	200	19	1
Chicken & Pork Livers with Truffle	140	11	2
Country Pate	200	22	1
Smoked Salmon	110	9	2
Marcel Henri:			
Pate de Champagne	210	19	1
Chicken Liver with Port Wine, 2 oz	200	19	1
Duck Truffle with Port Wine, 2 oz	240	24	1
Old Wisconsin Pate,			
Braunschweiger, 2 oz	210	18	3

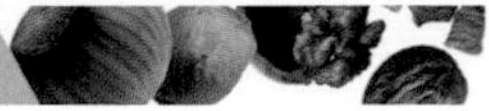

Nuts

Per 1 oz Unless Indicated

	C	F	Cb
Acorns, raw 1 oz	110	7	12
Almonds: Dried/Dry Roasted:			
Whole: 12 medium size, ½ oz	85	7.5	3
23-25 medium size, 1 oz	170	15	6
½ cup, 2½ oz	420	37	13
Ground, 1 cup, 3.4 oz	545	47	20
Sliced, ½ cup, 1.6 oz	260	22	10
Slivered, ½ cup, 2 oz	310	27	12
Chocolate Coated (5-6), 1 oz	150	10	15
Honey Roasted, 1 oz	170	14	8
Oil Roasted *(Blue Diamond)*, 1 oz	170	16	5
Brazil Nuts, 8 medium, 1 oz	185	19	3.5
Cashews, dry or oil roasted:			
14 large/18 med./26 small: 1 oz	165	14	9
½ cup, 2.4 oz	375	31	20
Honey Roasted, 1 oz	165	13	10
Chestnuts, av. all: Dried, 1 oz	105	1	22
Raw/Fresh, 5-6 nuts, 1 oz	60	0	13
Canned, water chestnuts,			
sliced/whole/drained, 1 oz	30	0	7
Coconut: Fresh:			
1 piece, 2"x2"x ½", 1 oz	100	10	4.5
Shredded, fresh, ½ cup, 1.4 oz	140	13	6
Dried (Desiccated):			
Unsweetened, 1 oz	185	18	7
Sweetened: Shredded, 1 oz	140	10	13
Grated, ½ cup, 1.3 oz	185	12	18
Cream (canned), ½ cup, 5.2 oz	285	26	12
Milk (canned), ½ cup, 4 oz	225	24	3
Water (center liquid), ½ cup, 4.25 oz	25	0	4.5
Filberts or Hazelnuts:			
Shelled, 18-20 nuts	180	17	4.5
Chopped, ¼ cup, 1 oz	180	18	5
Ground, ¼ cup, 0.6 oz	120	12	3
Ginkgo Nuts, canned, 14 med., 1 oz	32	0.5	6.5
Hickory, 30 small nuts, 1 oz	200	18	5
Macadamia Nuts: Shelled:			
Raw, 7 medium/14 small, 1 oz	200	21	4
½ cup, 2.3 oz	480	51	10
Dry Roasted, 1 oz	205	22	4
½ cup, 2.3 oz	480	51	9
Choc. coated, 2-3 pieces, 1 oz	170	12	14
Mixed Nuts: 18-22 nuts, 1 oz	170	15	7
Dry Roasted/Honey *(Planters)*	160	12	9
Oil Roasted, all types	170	16	6
Sweet Roasts, 26 pieces, 1 oz	160	12	10
Nut Toppings, chopped, 1 Tbsp, 0.25 oz	40	4	1.5

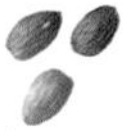

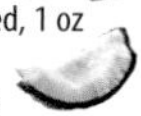

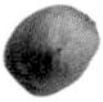

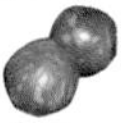

Per 1 oz Unless Indicated

	C	F	Cb
Peanuts, Dry or Oil Roasted, average:			
Small handful, ½ oz	85	7	3
⅕ cup, 1 oz	165	14	6
½ cup, 2.5 o	415	35	15
3 oz bag	500	42	18
7 oz bag	1160	98	42
Raw: Shelled, 1 oz	160	14	4.5
In shell, 1 oz	115	110	3
Cocktail (Planters):			
Regular; Lightly Salted, 1 oz	170	14	5
Dry Roasted	160	13	6
Other Flavors (Planters):			
Honey Roasted, 1 oz	160	12	8
Spanish Redskins, 1 oz	170	15	4
Sweet N' Crunchy, 1 oz	140	8	15
Japanese Style Peanuts,			
Coated in Crunchy Shell,			
¼ cup, 1 oz	150	8	13
Pecans: roasted:			
10 halves, 0.5 oz	95	10	2
20 Halves, 1 oz	195	20	4
1 cup, halves, 3.5 oz	680	71	14
Pilinuts, dried, ¼ cup, 1 oz	215	24	1
Pine Nuts, dried, 1 Tbsp, 0.3 oz	70	7	1.5
Pistachios: Unshelled (raw),			
½ cup, 2 oz	165	14	7
Shelled, raw, ½cup, 45 nuts, 1 oz	160	13	8
Roasted *(Lance)*, 1.5 oz	120	9	6
Sesame Nut Mix, 1 oz	160	13	9
Soy Nuts: Dry Roasted	130	6	9
½ cup, 3.3 oz	390	18	28
Chocolate coated *(Dr Soy)*, 1 oz pkg	140	7	13
Trail Mix (Planters):			
Daybreak, Berry Almond, 1.5 oz	180	7	27
Energy Mix, 1.5 oz	250	20	14
Fruit & Nut	140	9	14
Mixed Nuts & Raisins	160	12	11
Nut & Chocolate, 1.25 oz	180	12	16
Nuts, Seeds & Raisins, 1.1 oz	160	11	11
Spicy Nuts & Cajun Sticks	150	11	10
Sweet & Nutty, 1.1 oz	160	10	15
Walnuts, average all types:			
7-10 halves, 1/2 oz	90	9	2
15-20 halves, 1 oz	175	17	3
Chopped, 1/2 cup, 2.2 oz	380	36	6
Ground, ¼ cup, 0.7 oz	130	13	3

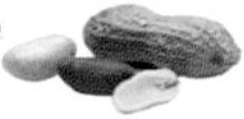

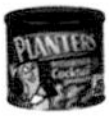

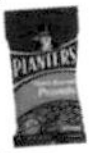

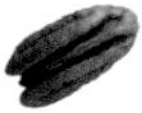

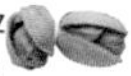

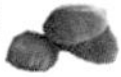

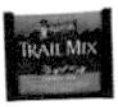

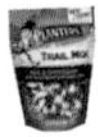

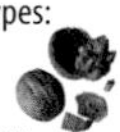

Quick Guide

	C	F	Cb
Peanut Butter: *Average All Brands*			
1 level tsp, 0.2 oz	35	3	1
1 level Tbsp, 0.6 oz	100	8.5	3.5
2 level Tbsp, 1.2 oz	200	17	7
1 oz Quantity	165	14	6
½ cup, 5 oz	835	72	29
Jif: Reduced Fat, all ar., 2 Tbsp	190	12	15
Natural, all varieties, 2 T.	190	16	8
Peanut Butter & Honey, 2 T	180	14	10
Laura Scudder's,			
Smooth; Nutty, 2 Tbsp	200	16	6
Peanut Wonder, Original, 2 T.	100	2	13
Peter Pan:			
Natural, Creamy/Crunchy, av., 2 Tbsp	210	17	6
Creamy/Crunchy, Red.-Fat, 2 Tbsp	200	13	14
Creamy, Whipped, 2 Tbsp	150	12	5
Planters: Creamy/Crunchy, 2 Tbsp	180	15	8
NUT-rition, all var., av. 2 Tbsp	185	14	11
Smucker's:			
Goober: Chocolate, 3 Tbsp	230	11	27
Grape/Strawb., 3 Tbsp	240	13	24
Skippy: Natural Crmy w/ Honey, 2 T.	190	16	9
Reduced Fat, all var., 2 T.	180	12	15
Roasted Honey Nut, all var., 2 Tbsp	190	16	7

Peanut Butter & Jelly Sandwich

	C	F	Cb
1 sandwich, with 2 oz Bread:			
Light Spread:	310	10	48
(1 Tbsp Peanut Butter + 1 Tbsp Jelly)			
Thick Spread:	480	19	67
(2 T. Peanut Butter + 2 Tbsp Jelly)			
With Goober Grape, 3 Tbsp, 2 oz	380	15	52

Nutella

	C	F	Cb
Nut & Chocolate Spread:			
1 Tbsp, 0.7 oz	100	5.5	11
2 Tbsp, 1.3 oz	200	11	22

Note: *Nutella* contains approximately 50% sugar and only 13% hazelnuts.

Other Nut & Seed Butters

Per 1 Tbsp, 0.5 oz

	C	F	Cb
Almond Butter	100	10	3.5
Almond Butter, Honey Roasted	90	7	5.5
Cashew Butter	95	8	4.5
Hazelnut Butter	105	10	2.5
Pecan Butter	110	10	2
Pistachio Butter	90	6.5	4.5
Sesame Butter (Tahini)	90	8	3
Soy Nut Butter	75	5	4
Tahini ~ See Sesame Butter			

Seeds

	C	F	Cb
Alfalfa Seeds,			
sprouted, ½ cup, 0.5 oz	5	0	1
Caraway/Fennel, 1 tsp	7	0.5	1
Chia Seeds: 1 Tbsp, 0.35 oz	45	3	4
3 Tbsp, 1 oz	140	8.5	12
Cottonseed Kernels,			
roasted, 1 Tbsp	50	3.5	2
Flax Seeds,			
3 Tbsp, 1 oz	140	9	9
Lotus Seeds,			
dried, ½ cup, 0.5 oz	55	0.5	10
Poppy Seeds, 1 tsp	15	1	1
Pumpkin/Pepita Seeds, whole:			
Roasted/Tamari, 1 oz	150	12	4
½ cup, 4 oz	590	48	15
Dried, (hulled), ¼ cup, 1 oz	155	13	5
Safflower Kernels, dried, 1 oz	150	11	10
Sesame Seeds:			
Dried, 1 Tbsp, 0.3 oz	50	4.5	2
Roasted/Toasted, 1 oz	160	14	7.5
Sunflower Kernels/Seeds:			
Dried, ¼ cup w/out hulls, 0.25 oz	200	18	7
Dry Roasted: 1 Tbsp, 0.3 oz	45	4	2
¼ cup, 1 oz	165	14	7
Oil Roasted, ⅓ cup, 1 oz	170	14	6.5
Watermelon Seeds,			
dried, ¼ cup, 1 oz	150	13	4

*N*ut eaters are healthier and live longer, say scientists.

Nuts are a nutritious source of protein, vitamins, minerals, fiber, healthy fats, and antioxidants.

The fat and fiber of nuts can help reduce blood cholesterol. Their protein and fiber also promotes meal satiety (fullness) and reduces hunger levels – of benefit in weight control.

Eat nuts instead of high-sugar snacks, candy and soft drinks. Add chopped nuts to breakfast cereals.

Updated Nutrition Data ~ www.CalorieKing.com
Persons with Diabetes ~ See Disclaimer (Page 22)

Quick Guide | C | F | Cb

Pancakes:

Plain: *Average All Types*

	C	F	Cb
Small (3" diameter), 0.75 oz	50	2	6
Medium (4" diameter), 1.25 oz	85	3.5	11
Large (6" diameter), 2.5 oz	175	7.5	22

Add Extra for Syrups/Butter

	C	F	Cb
Pancake Syrup: Regular, 1 Tbsp	50	0	12
¼ cup, 4 Tbsp	185	0	49
Lite, 1 Tbsp	25	0	6.5
¼ cup, 4 Tbsp	100	0	27
Butter/Margarine:			
Regular, 1 Tbsp	100	11	0
Whipped, 1 Tbsp	65	7.5	0

Waffles:

	C	F	Cb
Homemade, 7" waffle, 2.5 oz	220	11	25
Frozen + Toasted, (4" diam.), 1 oz	105	3	16

Frozen Breakfasts

Aunt Jemima:

Pancakes:

	C	F	Cb
Blueberry (3)	260	6	44
Buttermilk (3)	250	6	41
Low-Fat (3)	200	2	41
Homestyle (3)	250	6	41
Whole Grain (3)	240	6	42
Mini Pancakes (10)	280	8	45

Frozen Breakfasts:

	C	F	Cb
French Toast: Cinnamon, 2 slices	220	4.5	37
Homestyle, 2 slices	220	4.5	37
Sticks, Cinn., (4)	270	10	41

Eggo *(Kellogg's):*

	C	F	Cb
French Toaster Sticks, (2), av	220	6	35
Pancakes: Blueberry (3)	260	8	42
Buttermilk Minis (11)	280	9	44
Wafflers, average all varieties (2)	245	9	39

Jimmy D's *(Jimmy Dean):*

	C	F	Cb
French Toast Griddlers, 1 sandwich	210	8	27
Griddle Sticks, 1 stick	160	6	21
Pancake Griddlers, 1 sandwich	230	8	33

Krusteaz:

Pancakes:

	C	F	Cb
Premium Mini (4)	80	1	15
Buttermilk (3)	270	4	52
French Toast, Cinnamon, 4 sticks	230	5	41

Pillsbury:

Pancakes:

	C	F	Cb
Buttermilk (3)	230	4	45
Mini Buttermilk (11)	240	4	45
Toaster Strudels, w/ Icing, av. all (1)	180	9	24

Special K:

Breakfast Sandwiches:

	C	F	Cb
Egg, Veg's & Cheese, 3.3 oz	180	7	19
Ham/Ssg, Egg & Cheese, av., 3.6 oz	220	10	20

Pancake Brands | C | F | Cb

Aunt Jemima Mixes: *Prepared as Directed*

	C	F	Cb
Original, 4 - 4"	250	8	36
Original Complete, 2 - 4"	160	1.5	32
Buttermilk, 4 - 4"	180	6.5	23
Whole Wheat Blend, 3 - 4"	200	6.5	30

Betty Crocker Pancake Mixes: *Just Add Water*

	C	F	Cb
Complete Orig./Buttermilk (3)	200	2.5	40
Bisquick (Shake 'N Pour), (3)	220	3	43

Hungry Jack Pancakes:

Mixes: *Per ⅓ Cup, Prepared as Directed*

	C	F	Cb
Complete: Buttermilk, 3 - 4"	150	1.5	31
Extra Light & Fluffy, 3 - 4"	150	2	31
Traditional: Original,			
with 2% Milk, Oil, Egg, 3 - 4"	250	8	37
W/ Skim Milk, Oil, Egg Whites, 3 - 4"	180	1	37

Easy Packs: *Per ⅓ Cup Dry Mix, Prepared*

	C	F	Cb
Blueberry Wheat	160	2.5	32
Buttermilk	150	1.5	31
Northern Pines,			
3 - 4", 3.5 oz	200	3.5	38

Frozen Waffles

	C	F	Cb
Aunt Jemima: Buttermilk (2)	190	5	29
Homestyle; Blueberry (2)	165	5	26
Low-Fat (2)	160	3	27

Eggo *(Kellogg's):*

	C	F	Cb
Blueberry (2)	180	5	31
Chocolate Chip (2)	200	7	31
French Toast (1)	140	6	20
Homestyle (2)	190	7	27

Nutri-Grain:

	C	F	Cb
Wholewheat; Blueberry (2), av.	175	6	29
Low-Fat (2)	140	2.5	27
Kashi, Go-Lean, average (1)	150	5	25
Nature's Path: Flax Plus (2), av.	200	8	30
Homestyle (2)	180	7	26
Mesa Sunrise (2)	200	7	34
Smucker's,			
Snack'nWaffles, av. all var., (1)	215	8	32
Van's: Belgian Homestyle (2)	210	9	29
Mini: Chocolate Chip (8)	150	4	27
Totally Natural (8)	140	3.5	25
Sticks: Chocolate (1)	80	2	14
Vanilla (1)	70	1	14

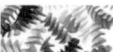

- Pasta includes all shapes and sizes; (e.q. spaghetti, fettuccini, elbows, shells, twists, sheets, cannelloni, linguini, tubes, ziti).
- All regular pasta products have the same cals/fat/carbs on a weight basis.
- 1 oz Dry = approximately 2.5 -3 oz cooked.

Dry Spaghetti/Pasta

	C	F	Cb
1 oz quantity	105	0.5	21
1lb box/pkg, 16 oz	1685	7	339
Elbows, 1 cup, 3.75 oz	380	2	80
Shells, small, 1 cup, 3¼ oz	330	1.5	69
Spirals, 1 cup, 3 oz	305	1.5	64

Cooked Spaghetti/Pasta

Plain, All Types (no added fat):

	C	F	Cb
Firm/Al Dente (8-10 minutes), 1 oz	42	0.5	8.5
Medium (11-13 minutes), 1 oz	37	0.5	7.5
Tender (14-20 minutes), 1 oz	32	0.5	7
(Longer cooking increases water absorbed)			
Spaghetti: ½ cup, 2.5 oz	90	0.5	18
Medium serving, 1 cup, 5 oz	225	1.5	44
Large serving, 2 cups, 10 oz	450	3	88
Extra Large, 3 cups, 15 oz	675	5	132
Elbows/Spirals, 1 cup, 5 oz	220	1.5	43
Small Shells, 1 cup, 4 oz	180	1	36
Protein-fortified: Dry, 1 c., 3.35 oz	350	2	63
Cooked, 1 cup, 5 oz	230	1	45
Spinach/Vegetable: Dry, 1 cup, 3 oz	310	1	61
Cooked, 1 cup, 5 oz	180	0.5	38
Whole-wheat: Dry, 1 cup, 3.75 oz	365	1.5	79
Cooked, 1 cup, 5 oz	175	1	37

Fresh Pasta (Refrigerated)

Plain/Spinach/Tomato: *Average:*

	C	F	Cb
As purchased, 4.5 oz	370	3	70
Cooked, 1 cup, 5 oz	185	1.5	35
Home-made, without egg,			
Cooked, 1 cup, 5 oz	175	1	35
Buitoni:			
Cut Pasta: *Per ⅓ of 9 oz Pkg*			
Angel Hair	230	3	43
Fettuccine	240	2	45
Linguine	240	2	46
Shirataki:			
Skinny Noodles: With Spinach, 4 oz	15	0	2.5
Other varieties, 4 oz	0	0	0.5

Pasta Meals (Refrigerated)

Buitoni:	C	F	Cb
Ravioli: Four Cheese,1¼ cups, 3.7 oz	340	12	42
Light Four Cheese, 1¼ cups, 3.3 oz	260	6	39
Whole Wheat Four Cheese, 3.7 oz	330	12	40
Tortellini: Herb Chicken, 1 cup, 4 oz	330	8	52
Spinach Cheese, 1 cup, 3.7 oz	320	7	49
Three Cheese, 1 cup, 3.7 oz	330	9	46
Tortellini:			
Chicken & Proscuitto, 1 cup, 3.85 oz	330	9	46
Cheese & Roasted Garlic, 1 c., 3.15 oz	310	9	43
Spinach & Ricotta, 1½ cups, 3.7 oz	270	7	39
Sweet Italian Sausage, 1 cup, 4 oz	350	10	51
Frozen Meals ~ *See Page 118*			
Pasta Sauces ~ *See Page 148*			

Macaroni & Cheese

Packaged (Hormel/Kraft) ~ *See Page 112*

Restaurant: *Average*	C	F	Cb
Side,	265	13	26
Medium serve, 1 cup, 9 oz	350	17	34
Large serve, 2 cups, 18 oz	700	34	68

Noodles

Plain/Egg: Dry, 1 oz	C	F	Cb
Plain/Egg: Dry, 1 oz	110	1.5	20
1 cup, 1.35 oz	145	1.5	27
Cooked: 1 oz	40	0.5	7
½ cup, 2.75 oz	110	1.5	20
1 cup, 5.5 oz	220	3.5	40
Stir-Fried: 1 cup, 5.5 oz	270	9	40
2 cup serving, 11 oz	540	18	80
Yolk Free (Cooked):			
'No Yolks' *(Foulds)*, 2 oz	210	0.5	41
Yolk Free *(Manischewitz)*, 2 oz	200	1	41
Chinese: Cellophane/Rice, dry, 1 oz	100	0	25
Chow Mein/hard, dry, 1 oz	150	9	16
Japanese: Soba: Dry, 1 oz	95	0.5	21
Cooked, 1 cup, 4 oz	115	0.5	24
Somen: Dry, 1 oz	100	0.5	21
Cooked, 1 cup, 6 oz	230	0.5	49
Japanese Style Pan Fried,			
Yaki-Soba *(Maruchan's)*, av., 5.6 oz	260	3	50
Ramen Noodles ~ *See Page 114*			
Rice Noodles: Dry, 3.5 oz	365	0.5	83
Cooked, 1 cup, 6.2 oz	190	0.5	44
Stir Fry *(Yakisoba)*, 3.5 oz	430	6	52
Tofu Shirataki *(House Foods)*, 4 oz	20	0.5	3
Udon *(Chikara)*, average, 7.5 oz pkt	250	1	52
Simply Asia/Thai Kitchen ~ *Page 115*			

Egg Roll/Won Ton Wrappers

	C	F	Cb
Egg/Spring Roll (1), 0.8 oz	65	0	15
Won Ton Wrapper (1), 0.25 oz	20	0	4

Quick Guide   C F Cb

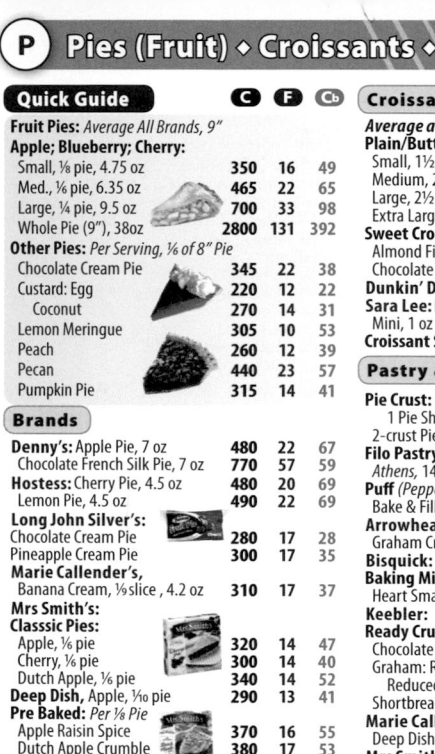

Fruit Pies: *Average All Brands, 9"*
Apple; Blueberry; Cherry:

	C	F	Cb
Small, ⅛ pie, 4.75 oz	350	16	49
Med., ⅙ pie, 6.35 oz	465	22	65
Large, ¼ pie, 9.5 oz	700	33	98
Whole Pie (9"), 38oz	2800	131	392

Other Pies: *Per Serving, ⅙ of 8" Pie*

Chocolate Cream Pie	345	22	38
Custard: Egg	220	12	24
Coconut	270	14	31
Lemon Meringue	305	10	53
Peach	260	12	39
Pecan	440	23	57
Pumpkin Pie	315	14	41

Brands

	C	F	Cb
Denny's: Apple Pie, 7 oz	480	22	67
Chocolate French Silk Pie, 7 oz	770	57	59
Hostess: Cherry Pie, 4.5 oz	480	20	69
Lemon Pie, 4.5 oz	490	22	69
Long John Silver's:			
Chocolate Cream Pie	280	17	28
Pineapple Cream Pie	300	17	35
Marie Callender's,			
Banana Cream, ⅑ slice , 4.2 oz	310	17	37
Mrs Smith's:			
Classsic Pies:			
Apple, ⅙ pie	320	14	47
Cherry, ⅙ pie	300	14	40
Dutch Apple, ⅙ pie	340	14	52
Deep Dish, Apple, ⅒ pie	290	13	41
Pre Baked: *Per ⅛ Pie*			
Apple Raisin Spice	370	16	55
Dutch Apple Crumble	380	17	53
Sara Lee:			
Creme Pies:			
Chocolate, ⅕ pie, 3.9 oz	450	27	50
Coconut, ⅙ pie, 4.5 oz	370	20	44
Key West Lime, ⅕ pie	410	17	60
Lemon Meringue, ⅕ pie, 4.6 oz	390	13	64
Tropical Coconut Cream, ⅕ pie	450	27	49
Oven Fresh Pies (9", 37 oz Box): *Per Slice, 4.6 oz*			
Apple, ⅛ pie	340	16	43
Cherry, ⅛ pie	340	17	44
Mince, ⅛ pie	380	17	53
Peach, ⅛ pie	320	15	42
Pumpkin, ⅛ pie	270	10	41
Tastykake: Apple	270	11	40
Coconut Cream	370	20	42
Lemon	300	14	44
Strawberry	340	12	55

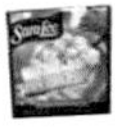

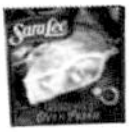

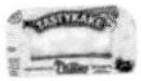

Croissants   C F Cb

Average all Brands
Plain/Butter/Cheese: Mini, 1 oz

	C	F	Cb
Mini, 1 oz	115	6	13
Small, 1½ oz	170	9	19
Medium, 2 oz	230	12	26
Large, 2½ oz	290	15	32
Extra Large, 3 oz	330	19	37
Sweet Croissants:			
Almond Filled, 3 oz	330	18	39
Chocolate Filled, 3 oz	360	19	43
Dunkin' Donuts, Plain Croissant	310	16	35
Sara Lee: French Style: Orig, 1¾ oz	185	9	21
Mini, 1 oz	230	11	26
Croissant Sandwiches ~ *See Page 165*			

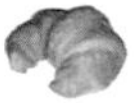

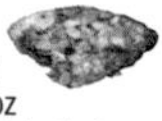

Pastry & Pie Crust   C F Cb

Pie Crust: Baked, 9" diameter shell

	C	F	Cb
1 Pie Shell, 6½ oz	970	64	87
2-crust Pie, 9", 11¼ oz	1660	109	150
Filo Pastry: 4 sheets, 2½ oz	210	2.5	40
Athens, 14"x18", 2½ sheets, 2 oz	180	1.5	37
Puff *(Pepperidge Farm),* ½ sheet	480	30	48
Bake & Fill Shell (1)	180	11	18
Arrowhead Mills,			
Graham Cracker Pie Crust, ⅛ of 9"	110	5	14
Bisquick:			
Baking Mix: Orig., ⅓ cup, 1.4 oz	160	4.5	26
Heart Smart, ⅓ cup, 1.4 oz	140	2.5	27
Keebler:			
Ready Crust: *Per ⅛ of 9" Crust*			
Chocolate	100	4.5	14
Graham: Regular	110	5	14
Reduced Fat	100	3.5	15
Shortbread Crust	110	5	14
Marie Callenders,			
Deep Dish Pie Crust, ⅛ pie, 1 oz	140	10	11
Mrs Smith's,			
Homestyle, Deep Dish, 9", ⅛	130	7	15
Nabisco:			
Honey Maid, Graham, ⅙ of 9", 1 oz	150	8	18
Nilla, Pie Crust, ⅙ of 9", 1 oz	140	8	18
Pillsbury, Rolled, ⅛, 0.9 oz	100	6	12
Trader Joe's, Pie Crust, ⅛ pie, 1.2 oz	190	13	17

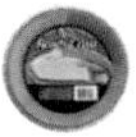

Pie Fillings (Canned)

Fruit: *Average all Fruits*
(Apple/Blueberry/Cherry/Strawberry)

	C	F	Cb
Sweetened: ⅓ cup, 3.2oz	90	0	22
1 cup, 9½ oz	270	0	66
1 can, 21 oz	600	0	150
Light/Lite, ⅓ cup, 3.2 oz	60	0	15
Unsweetened, ⅓ cup, 3.2 oz	35	0	8
Lemon Cream/Creme, ⅓ cup, 3.2 oz	130	1.5	28

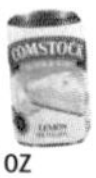

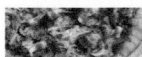

Figures Based On Pizza Hut **C** **F** **Cb**

Cheese Pizza ~ See Pizza Hut, Page 227

Ham & Pineapple:
Medium Size (12"):

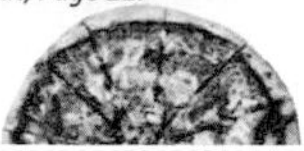

Deep Dish:

⅛ Pizza (1 slice)	230	9	28
½ Pizza (4 slices)	920	36	112
Whole Pizza (8 slices)	1840	72	224

Hand Tossed/Classic Crust:

⅛ Pizza (1 slice)	200	6	27
½ Pizza (4 slices)	800	24	108
Whole Pizza (8 slices)	1600	48	216

Thin Crust:

⅛ Pizza (1 slice)	180	6	23
½ Pizza (4 slices)	720	24	92
Whole Pizza (8 slices)	1440	48	184

Meat Lovers:
Medium Size (12"):

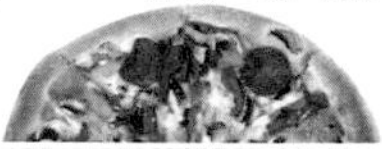

Deep Dish/Pan:

⅛ Pizza (1 slice)	330	18	27
½ Pizza (4 slices)	1320	72	108
Whole Pizza (8 slices)	2640	144	216

Hand Tossed/Classic Crust:

⅛ Pizza (1 slice)	300	16	26
½ Pizza (4 slices)	1200	64	104
Whole Pizza (8 slices)	2400	1088	208

Thin Crust:

⅛ Pizza (1 slice)	280	16	22
½ Pizza (4 slices)	1120	64	88
Whole Pizza (8 slice			

Pepperoni:
Medium Size (12"):

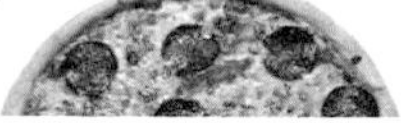

Deep Dish/Pan:

⅛ Pizza (1 slice)	290	14	27
½ Pizza (4 slices)	1160	56	108
Whole Pizza (8 slices)	2320	112	216

Hand Tossed/Classic Crust:

⅛ Pizza (1 slice)	230	9	25
½ Pizza (4 slices)	920	36	100
Whole Pizza (8 slice	1840	72	200

Thin Crust:

⅛ Pizza (1 slice)	200	9	21
½ Pizza (4 slices)	800	36	84
Whole Pizza (8 slices)	1600	72	168

Supreme:
Medium Size (12").

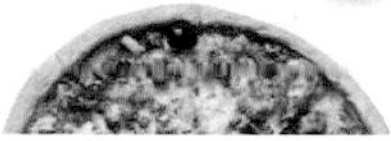

Deep Dish/Pan:

⅛ Pizza (1 slice)	290	14	27
½ Pizza (4 slices)	1160	56	108
Whole Pizza (8 slices)	2320	112	216

Hand Tossed/Classic Crust:

⅛ Pizza (1 slice)	260	12	26
½ Pizza (4 slices)	1040	48	104
Whole Pizza (8 slices	2080	96	208

Thin Crust:

⅛ Pizza (1 slice)	240	12	23
½ Pizza (4 slices)	960	48	92
Whole Pizza (8 slices)	1920	96	184

Veggie ~ *Same as Ham & Pineapple*

Individual Personal Pizzas (6"):
Deep Dish/Pan:

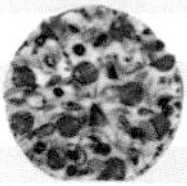

Cheese	600	24	69
Hawaiian	570	21	70
Meat Deluxe	900	50	70
Pepperoni	650	30	67
Supreme	720	36	69
Veggie	560	22	70

Large (14"):
Hand Tossed:

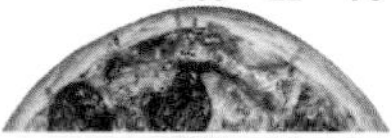

Cheese: ⅛ Pizza	320	12	38
½ Pizza	1280	48	152
Ham & Pineapple: ⅛ Pizza	290	9	40
½ Pizza	1160	36	160
Meat Lovers: ⅛ Pizza	440	23	38
½ Pizza	1760	92	152
Pepperoni: ⅛ Pizza	330	14	38
½ Pizza	1320	56	152
Supreme: ⅛ Pizza	380	17	39
½ Pizza	1520	68	156
Veggie Lover's: ⅛ Pizza	290	9	39
½ Pizza	1160	36	156

Extra Large, Single Slices:
(Example: Sbarro's)

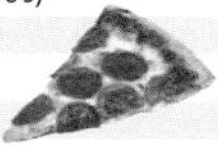

Cheese	460	13	60
Pepperoni	730	37	61
Sausage	670	31	60
Supreme	630	27	63

Frozen Pizzas

	C	F	Cb
Amy's: *Per ⅓ Pizza*			
Cheese Pizza	290	12	33
Mushroom & Olive	260	10	33
Pesto	310	12	39
Roasted Vegetable	280	9	42
Whole Wheat Crust, Cheese & Pesto	360	18	37

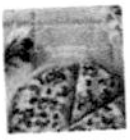

	C	F	Cb
California Pizza Kitchen:			
Crispy Thin Crust: *Per ⅓ Pizza*			
Margherita	290	13	31
Sicilian Recipe	310	14	30
Spinach & Artichoke	350	19	34
White	290	12	31
Self Rising Crust: *Per ⅓ Pizza*			
BBQ Chicken, 4.3 oz	270	9	33
Five Cheese & Tomato, 4.3 oz	390	17	41
Garlic Chicken, 4.3 oz	280	11	30
Traditional Crust: *Per Small Pizza*			
Four Cheese, 6.9 oz	510	17	69
Margherita, 6 oz	420	18	45
Sicilian, 5.5 oz	440	21	43

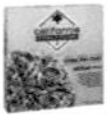

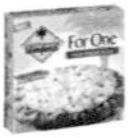

	C	F	Cb
Celeste:			
Pizza For One: Original, 1 pizza	340	16	39
Deluxe; Pepperoni	365	18	39
Meatball	420	22	40
Sausage & Pepperoni	420	23	40
Suprema	420	23	40
Zesty 4 Cheese; Four Cheese	350	16	38

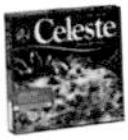

	C	F	Cb
DiGiorno: *Per Slice, Unless Indicated*			
Cheese Stuffed Crust: *Per ½ Pizza*			
Four Cheese, 4.23 oz	330	15	33
Pepperoni, 4.23 oz	340	16	33
Three Meat, 5 oz	360	18	34
Classic Thin Crust, av. all, ⅕ pizza	340	16	35
Crispy Flatbread Pizza: *Per ⅓ Pizza*			
Italian Sausage & Onion, 5.46 oz	400	26	27
Pepperoni & Rstd Peppers, 4½ oz	340	20	26
Tuscan Style Chicken, 4.65 oz	280	14	25
Deep Dish: *Per ½ Pizza, 3¾ oz*			
Four Cheese; Pepperoni	300	17	26
Italian Sausage	310	18	26
Flatbread Melts: *Per Whole Pizza, 6 oz*			
Chicken & Bacon Ranch	420	18	44
Chicken Parm.; Steak & Veges, av	380	14	45
Italian Meatballs & Four Cheese	400	17	46

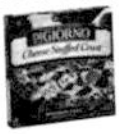

	C	F	Cb
DiGiorno (Cont):			
Garlic Bread: *Per ⅙ Pizza*			
Four Cheese, 5 oz	350	14	41
Pepperoni, 5 oz	380	17	40
Supreme, 4.25 oz	300	14	31
Traditional Crust: *Per Whole Pizza*			
Four Cheese, 9.2 oz	720	30	84
Pepperoni, 9.3 oz	770	35	83
Supreme, 10 oz	790	36	85
Ultimate Toppings: *Per ⅕ Pizza*			
Cheese, 4.6 oz	320	13	34
Four Meat, 5 oz	380	19	34
Pepperoni, 4.8 oz	370	19	34
Supreme 5.3 oz	360	18	35
Wyngz: *Per 4 oz Serving*			
Buffalo	190	7	20
Honey BBQ	230	6	32

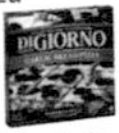

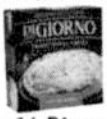

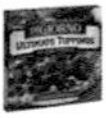

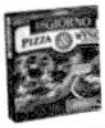

	C	F	Cb
Freschetta:			
Naturally Rising: *Per ⅕ of Large Pizza Unless Indicated*			
4 Cheese Medley	360	13	43
Can. Bacon P'apple	310	9	44
Meat Medley	380	15	44
Pepperoni	360	14	44
Supreme, ⅙ pizza	320	13	37
Simply Inspired: *Per ⅓ Pizza*			
Chicken Bianco	360	19	30
Classic Bruschetta	380	23	32
Harvest Supreme	350	18	32
Rustic Pepp. Pomodoro	390	22	30
Tuscan Farmhouse	300	15	31

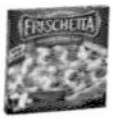

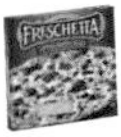

	C	F	Cb
Jeno's: *Per Pizza*			
Crispy 'N Tasty: Cheese, 6.85 oz	460	22	50
Pepperoni, 6.8 oz	490	26	48
Kashi:			
Thin Crust: *Per ⅓ Pizza*			
Four Cheese	260	8	36
Mediterranean	290	9	37
Mushroom Trio & Spin.	250	9	28

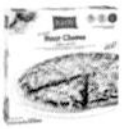

	C	F	Cb
Kroger:			
3 Minute Microwave: *Per 8 oz Pizza*			
3-Meat	500	17	64
Cheese	490	16	66
Combination	520	20	64
Pepperoni	530	20	65
Supreme	490	18	63
French Bread, Pepperoni, 5 oz	380	17	42

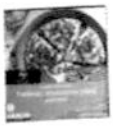

	C	F	Cb
Lean Cuisine:			
Casual Cuisine: *Per Pizza*			
Deep Dish:			
Roasted Vegetable	320	5	52
Spinach & Mushroom	340	7	52
Three Meat	390	9	55

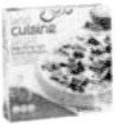

Frozen Pizzas (Cont)

	C	F	Cb
Lean Cuisine (Cont):			
Traditional: Four Chse	350	6	55
Mushroom	300	5	50
Pepperoni	380	9	55
Wood Fired: BBQ Recipe Chicken	340	7	48
Margherita	310	7	46
Rstd Garlic Chicken	350	8	47
Red Baron:			
Classic Crust: *Per ¼ Pizza Unless Indicated*			
4 Cheese, 5.15 oz	380	16	40
Pepperoni, 5 oz	370	16	40
Sausage & Pepp.,5.3 oz	400	19	41
Supreme, ⅕, 4.5 oz	310	14	34
Original Crust, Fire Baked: *Per ¼ Pizza*			
4-Cheese, 4.95 oz,	360	15	40
Pepperoni, 4.95 oz	370	17	40
Thin Crust: *Per ⅓ Pizza*			
5 Cheese, 4.9 oz	360	16	40
Pepperoni, 5.25 oz	400	19	40
Pan: *Per ⅕ Pizza Unless Indicated*			
4 Cheese, 5.25 oz	390	18	40
Meat Trio; Suprme, av., ⅙	355	18	35
Pepperoni, 5.25 oz	400	19	41
Pizza By The Slice:			
4 Cheese, 4.95 oz	340	13	41
Meat Trio, 5.3 oz	380	17	41
Pepp.; Supreme, av.	355	15	41
Singles: *Per Pizza*			
Deep Dish: 4 Chse; Meat Trio, av	405	18	46
Pepperoni; Supreme, average	420	19	46
French Bread: Extra Cheese	360	12	43
5 Cheese & Garlic	430	23	41
Pepperoni	380	15	43
Supreme	380	15	44
Safeway Select:			
Pizzeria Crust:			
Cheese Trio, ¼ pizza	340	15	34
Fajita Chicken Ole, ⅕ pizza	250	10	29
Pepperoni & Sausage, ⅕ pizza	320	17	30
Self Rising: *Per ⅙ Pizza*			
Four Cheese	300	9	41
Pepperoni	350	14	41
Sausage & Pepperoni	340	13	41
Ultra Thin Crust: *Per ⅓ Pizza Unless Indicated*			
BBQ Chicken, ¼ pizza	250	10	23
Garlic Chicken	320	12	31
Margherita	330	17	28
Primo Italiano Meat	330	16	27

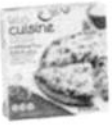
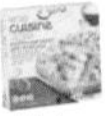
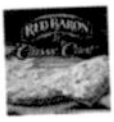
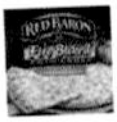
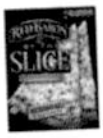
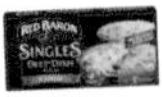
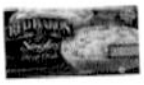

Updated Nutrition Data ~ www.CalorieKing.com
Persons with Diabetes ~ See Disclaimer (Page 22)

	C	F	Cb
Stouffer's: *Each*			
French Bread Pizzas:			
Two Per Box: Deluxe (1), 6 .19 oz	430	21	44
Sausage & Pepp. (1), 6.25 oz	460	24	43
Nine Per Box: Cheese (1), 5.88 oz	380	16	43
Pepperoni, 5.68 oz	430	21	44
Tombstone:			
Original: *Per ⅕ of Large 12" Pizza Unless Indicated*			
4 Meat	310	14	30
Canadian Style Bacon, ¼ pizza	320	12	37
Deluxe	290	12	31
Extra Cheese, ¼ pizza	350	15	36
Pepperoni, ⅓ pizza	280	14	28
Pepperoni & Sausage, ¼ pizza	370	17	37
Sausage & Mushroom	290	13	30
Supreme	300	14	31
Thin Crust: Three Cheese, ¼ pizza	310	15	28
Pepperoni; Sausage, av., ¼ pizza	315	16	28
Brick Oven Style: Cheese, ⅓ pizza	350	15	37
Pepperoni; Supreme, av., ¼ pizza	315	16	29
Tony's:			
Original Crust: Cheese, ⅓ pizza	290	12	37
Pepperoni, ⅓ pizza	310	14	36
Ssg & Pepperoni; Supreme, av., ⅓	340	17	37
Pizza For One: *Microwavable*			
Cheese (1)	380	14	50
Pepperoni (1)	410	18	48
Totino's:			
Crisp Crust Party Pizza: *Per ½ Pizza*			
Cheese	330	16	35
Classic Pepperoni	370	20	35
Pizza Rolls: Cheese (6), 3 oz	200	8	26
Pepperoni (6), 3 oz	210	10	24
Stuffers, average all, 1 piece	260	12	32
Trader Joe's:			
3 Cheese, ⅓ pizza	310	9	42
Parlanno, ¼ pizza	340	16	34
Pizza 4 Formaggi, ⅓ pizza	310	9	42
Spinach, ⅓ pizza	300	12	38
VitaPizza: *Per Single Serve Pizza*			
Cheese & Tomato	190	3	38
Meatless Pepperoni Supreme	190	2.5	38
Weight Watchers (Smart Ones): *Per Pizza*			
Fajita Chicken	380	7	58
Four Cheese	370	7	57
Pepperoni	390	8	58

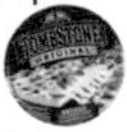
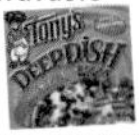
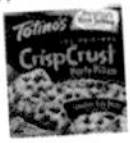
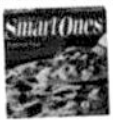

Quick Guide

Chicken
From 3lb ready-to-cook chicken

		C	F	Cb
Breast/Wing Quarter:				
Roasted: With skin		300	15	0
Without skin		185	5	0
Fried, batter dipped		530	30	17
Leg Quarter:				
Thigh & Drumstick:				
Roasted: With skin		270	16	0
Without skin		185	8	0
Fried, batter dipped		435	25	15
KFC ~ See Fast-Foods Section				

Per 4 oz Edible Portion

	C	F	Cb
Average of Light Meat: *Per 4 oz (no bone)*			
Roasted: With skin	250	12	0
Without skin	175	4.5	0
Stewed: With skin	230	12	0
Without skin	180	4.5	0
Fried: Batter-dipped, w/ skin, 4 oz	315	17	11
Flour-coated, w/ skin, 4 oz	280	14	2
Average of Dark Meat: *Per 4 oz (no bone)*			
Roasted: With skin	290	18	0
Without skin	235	11	0
Stewed: With skin	265	17	0
Without skin	220	10	0
Fried: Batter-dipped, w/ skin, 4 oz	340	21	11
Flour-coated, w/ skin, 4 oz	325	19	5

Chicken Parts

	C	F	Cb
Broilers or Fryers: *Edible Weights (no bone)*			
Breast: *Per ½ Breast*			
Raw: With skin, 5 oz	250	14	0
Without skin, 4.25 oz	130	1.5	0
Roasted: With skin, 3.5 oz	195	8	0
Without skin, 3 oz	140	3	0
Stewed: With skin, 4 oz	200	8	0
Without skin, 3.25 oz	145	3	0
Fried: Batter-dipped, w/ skin, 5 oz	365	19	13
Flour-coated, with skin, 3.5 oz	220	9	2
Drumstick: *Per Drumstick*			
Roasted: With skin, 2 oz	115	6	0
Without skin, 1.5 oz	75	2.5	0
Stewed: With skin, 2 oz	115	6	0
Without skin, 1.5 oz	80	3	0
Fried: Batter-dipped, 2.5 oz	195	11	6
Flour-coated, 1.75 oz	120	7	1

Chicken Parts (Cont)

	C	F	Cb
Broilers or Fryers (Cont): *Edible Weights (no bone)*			
Thigh Portion: *Edible Weight (no bone)*			
Raw: With skin, 3.3 oz (4¼ oz with bone)	200	14	0
Without skin, 2.4 oz	80	3	0
Roasted: With skin, 2¼ oz	155	10	0
Without skin, 2 oz	110	6	0
Stewed: With skin, 2.5 oz	160	10	0
Without skin, 2 oz	105	5	0
Fried: Batter-dipped, w/ skin 3 oz	240	14	8
Flour-coated, w/ skin, 2.25 oz	165	9	2
Wing: *Per Wing*			
Raw Weight, 3.2 oz, (with bone)			
Raw: With skin	110	8	0
Without skin	35	1	0
Roasted: With skin	100	7	0
Without skin	45	2	0
Fried: Batter-dipped, w/ skin	160	11	5
Flour-coated, w/ skin	105	7	1
Stewed: With skin, 4 oz	100	7	0
Buffalo Wings ~ *See Fast-Foods Section*			
Neck: Simmered, with skin	95	7	0
Without skin	30	2	0
Skin Only: *Skin from ½ Chicken*			
Raw skin, 2.75 oz	275	26	0
Roasted skin, 2 oz	255	23	0
Stewed skin, 2.52 oz	260	24	0
Fried, flour-coated, 2 oz	280	24	5
Fried, batter-dipped, 6.75 oz	750	55	44
Roasters: *Average of Light & Dark Meat*			
Roasted: With skin, 4 oz	250	15	0
Without skin, 4 oz	190	8	0
Light Meat, without skin, roasted	175	5	0
Dark Meat, without skin, roasted	200	10	0
Stewing Chicken:			
Average of Light & Dark Meat: Per 4 oz			
Stewed: With skin	325	22	0
Without skin	270	14	0
Light Meat, without skin	240	9	0
Dark Meat, without skin	290	17	0
Capon Chicken:			
Roasted: With skin, 4 oz	260	13	0
½ Chicken, w/ skin, 22.5 oz	1460	74	0
Chicken Offal & Stuffing:			
Giblets: Simmered, 1 cup	230	7	0.5
Fried, flour-coated, 1 cup	400	20	6
Gizzard, simmered, 1 cup	210	4	0
Heart, simmered, 1 cup	270	12	0.2
Liver: Raw, 4 oz	130	5.5	4
Simmered, 1 cup	215	8.5	1
Liver Pate, Fresh, 1 Tbsp, 0.5 oz	30	2	1
Stuffing, average, ½ cup	180	9	22

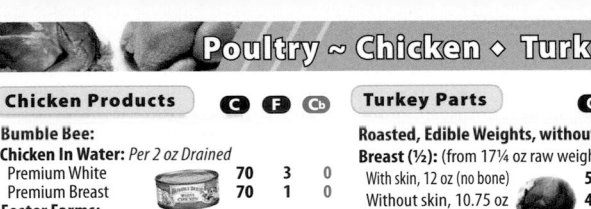

Chicken Products C F Cb

Bumble Bee:

Chicken In Water: *Per 2 oz Drained*

	C	F	Cb
Premium White	70	3	0
Premium Breast	70	1	0

Foster Farms:

	C	F	Cb
Grilled Chicken Breast Strips, 3 oz	100	1.5	2
Wings: Chipotle, 4 wings, 3 oz	190	14	1
Honey BBQ Glazed, 4 wings, 2.9 oz	170	10	5
Hot'n'Spicy, 4 wings, 2.9 oz	170	13	1

Tyson:

Any'tizers:

	C	F	Cb
Bites: Buffalo Style Popcorn, 8 pcs	190	9	12
Honey BBQ Boneless, 3 pieces	200	8	20
Popcorn, 7 pieces	180	9	11
Wings: Buffalo Style Hot (3)	190	13	3
Honey BBQ (3)	190	12	8
Canned, Premium Chunk, 2 oz	60	1	0
Pouch, Chunk Breast, 2 oz	70	1.5	0

Duck, Goose, Quail

	C	F	Cb
Duck: Roasted,			
With skin, 3 oz	290	24	0
Without skin, 3 oz	170	10	0
½ duck, with skin, 13.5 oz	1290	108	0
Goose: Roast, with skin, 3 oz	260	19	0
Without skin, 3 oz	200	11	0
Pheasant, cooked, 3 oz	210	10	0
Quail, cooked 1 whole, 6 oz	385	24	0

Turkey

Fryer-Roasters: *Per 3 oz Serving*

Roasted:

	C	F	Cb
Light Meat: With skin	140	4	0
Without skin	120	1	0
Dark Meat: With skin	155	6	0
Without skin	140	4	0

½ of Whole Turkey: (Approx. 3.25 lbs raw weight without neck and giblets; 1.8 lbs cooked weight)

	C	F	Cb
Roasted: With skin	1650	74	0
Without skin	1125	31	0

Ground Turkey, Raw: (4 oz raw wt. = 3 oz ckd wt.)

	C	F	Cb
Regular (85% lean), 4 oz	170	10	0
Lean (93% lean), average, 4 oz	160	8	0
94% lean *(Foster Farms)*, 4 oz	150	7	0
93% lean *(Jennie-O)*, 4 oz	170	8	0
93% lean *(Trader Joe's)*, 4 oz	150	8	0
Breast, no skin, 4 oz	115	1	0
Patties: Small, 3 oz	130	7	0
Medium, 4 oz	170	10	0
Large, 5.3 oz	225	13	0

Turkey Parts C F Cb

Roasted, Edible Weights, without bone:

	C	F	Cb
Breast (½): (from 17¼ oz raw weight with bone)			
With skin, 12 oz (no bone)	525	11	0
Without skin, 10.75 oz	415	2	0
Back (½): With skin, 4.5 oz	265	13	0
Without skin, 3.5 oz	165	6	0
Leg (Thigh & Drumstick):			
(from 1 lb raw weight with bone)			
With skin, 8.5oz (without bone)	410	13	0
Without skin, 7.75 oz	355	8.5	0
Wing: (From 7.25 oz raw weight)			
With skin, 3 oz (without bone)	185	9	0
Without skin, 2 oz (with bone)	100	2	0
Neck: Simmered, 1 neck,			
(9 oz with bone)	275	11	0
Giblets, simmered, 1 cup, 5 oz	240	7	3

Young Hens (Roasted)

	C	F	Cb
Light Meat:			
With skin, 3 oz	175	8	0
Without skin, 3 oz	135	3	0
Dark Meat: With skin, 3 oz	200	11	0
Without skin, 3 oz	165	7	0

Young Toms ~ *Similar to Young Hens*

Turkey Products

Foster Farms: *Cooked, Frozen*

	C	F	Cb
Meatballs: Homestyle (3)	160	9	3
Italian Style (3)	160	8	5
Hormel, Turkey Chunks, cooked, 2 oz	70	2.5	0

Jennie-O:

	C	F	Cb
Bacon, 1 slice	35	3	1
Bratwurst, lean,			
1 link, 3.85 oz	170	10	2
Burgers,			
All Natural, White Meat, 5.25 oz	160	5	0
Meatballs, Fully Cooked: Italian, 3 oz	190	12	3
Home Style, 3 oz	190	11	5
Spam, Oven Roasted Turkey, 2 oz	80	4	2
Trader Joe's,			
Italian Turkey Meatloaf, 3 oz	140	8	5
Valley Fresh, Premium White, 2 oz	50	1	0

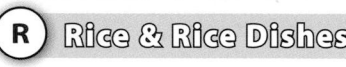

White Rice

	C	F	Cb
Raw: Short Grain, 1 cup, 7 oz	715	1	158
Long Grain, 1 cup, 6.5 oz	675	1	148
Glutinous, 1 cup, 6.5 oz	685	1	151
Cooked Rice: *(Boiled/Steamed):*			
Short/Medium Grain:			
½ cup, 3.25 oz	140	0	30
1 cup (½ Pint), 7.2 oz	265	0.5	59
2 cups (1 Pint), 13 oz	480	1	106
Long Grain: ½ cup, 2.75 oz	100	0	22
1 cup, 5.5 oz	205	0.5	44
Glutinous/Sticky, cooked, 1 c., 6 oz	170	0.5	37
Parboiled, cooked, ½ cup, 3 oz	105	0.5	22
Precook./Instant: Dry, ½ cup, 3.5 oz	380	1	82
Cooked, ½ cup, 3 oz	95	0.5	21
Wild Rice: Raw, 1 cup, 5.5 oz	570	2	120
Cooked, 1 cup, 5.75 oz	165	0.5	35

Brown Rice

	C	F	Cb
Average of Short or Long Grain			
Raw/Dry: ½ cup, 3.25 oz	340	2.5	71
1 cup, 6.5 oz	685	5.5	143
Cooked: ½ cup, 3.5 oz	110	1	22
1 cup, 7 oz	220	2	46

Rice Dishes

	C	F	Cb
Chinese Fried Rice:			
½ cup, 2.5 oz	140	4.5	21
1 cup, (½ Pint), 5 oz	280	9	42
2 cups, (1 Pint), 10 oz	565	18	84
Mexican Rice: 1 cup	500	12	90
6 oz, *(Taco John's)*	250	6	45
Seasoned, 4.6 oz, *(Taco Time)*	135	0	29
Rice-A-Roni ~ *See Page 114*			
Rice with Raisins/Pinenuts, 1 cup	400	11	60
Rice Pilaf: Restaurant, 1 cup	275	7.5	46
A La Carte *(O'Charley's),* 1 order	190	5	30
Rice Pudding *(Kozy Shack),*			
Original, 1 pudding cup	130	3	22
Risotto, 1 cup	420	12	70
Saffron Rice, 4 oz	175	7	25
Spanish Rice: 1 cup, 5 oz	390	9	72
Small *(El Pollo Loco),* 4.5 oz	170	2.5	32
Small *(Taco Cabana)*	120	0	25
Sticky Rice, 1 cup, 5 oz	155	0.5	34
Sushi Rice: 1 Tbsp	25	0	5
1 cup, 5.2 oz	390	0	77
Other Packaged Rice Products:			
Uncle Ben's / Zatarain's ~ *See Page 116*			

CalorieKing.com Recipes

See the CalorieKing website for a salubrious selection of healthy recipes – all analyzed for calories, fat, protein, carbohydrate, fiber and sodium.

Choose from:
- *Starters/Appetizers*
- *Salads*
- *Entrees: Meat, Fish and Chicken*
- *Vegetarian*
- *Desserts*
- *Cakes, Cookies*
- *Drinks*

www.CalorieKing.com/recipes

HEALTHY RECIPE TIPS

- **Use non-fat milk** in place of whole or 2% milk

- **Use low-fat yogurt** in place of sour cream
- **Skim fat** from surface of soups and casseroles after cooling
- **Add extra vegetables** to soups and hot entrees
- **Cakes/cookies/muffins:** Replace most or all the fat/oil with applesauce and/or prune puree (Example: *Sunsweet Lighter Bake*)
- **Drinks:** Replace sugar with no-calorie sweeteners such as *Equal, Stevia, Splenda* and *Sweet 'N Low*

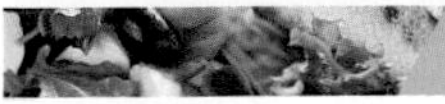

Deli Salads

Average All Outlets	C	F	Cb
Antipasto Salad, ½ cup	135	8	13
3-Bean Salad, ½ cup	90	4.5	12
Bulgur Salad, ½ cup	70	2	12
Caesar Salad, Classic, 1 cup	200	14	15
Side Salad, without Dressing	25	0	6
Carrot Raisin: With Dressing, ½ cup	135	12	6
Without Dressing, ½ cup	20	0	5
Chef's Salad: Regular, w/o Dressing	620	37	8
With 2 oz 1000 Island	860	61	8
Chicken Salad, ½ cup/scoop, 4 oz	280	21	2
Coleslaw: Traditional, ½ cup	150	8	18
W/ Low Cal Dressing, ½ c.	50	2	8
Corn, Mexican, ½ cup	240	12	33
Cucumber: Non-Oil Dressing, ½ c.	60	0	14
With Oil Dressing, ½ cup	140	12	8
Eggplant Salad, ½ cup	75	5	7
Fettucini, with veges, ½ cup	135	6	16
Garden Salad, without Dressing, 1 c.	10	0	2
Greek Salad, 1 cup	105	8	7
Greek Vegetables, 1 cup	110	8	6
Lobster Salad, ½ cup, 4 oz	250	21	11
Macaroni Salad, ½ cup, 5 oz	360	26	26
Nicoise, 1 cup	450	32	18
Pasta Salad, ½ cup	200	11	19
Potato Salad: Dijon, 3 oz	120	7	13
With Mayonnaise, ½ cup, 4 oz	215	15	17
Lowfat, ½ cup	110	1.5	21
Rice Salad, ½ cup	150	10	13
Saffron Rice, 4 oz	175	7	25
Spinach Salad, 1 cup	180	13	13
Tabouli, ½ cup	125	7	13
Three Bean Salad, ½ cup	90	4.5	12
Tomato & Mozzarella, ½ cup	180	14	10
Tortellini, with Basil Pesto, ½ cup	150	9	15
Waldorf, with Mayo, ½ cup	110	7	12
Signature Salads: *Per 6 oz Serving*			
(Supplied to Deli's and Institutions)			
Antipasto Salad	510	50	4
Artichoke Salad, marinated	400	41	8
California Medley	120	7	15
Cheese Agnolotti	250	8	23
Chicken Salad	420	33	11
Crabmeat Flavored	450	38	20
Signature Salads (Cont): *Per 6 oz Serving*			
Egg Salad	300	23	14
Fresh Button Mushroom	190	16	6
Garden Olive	630	67	3
Ham Salad	400	32	14
Prima Pasta Salad	360	30	18
Seafood Pasta Del Mar	170	10	21
Seafood with Crab & Shrimp	420	34	20
Shrimp Salad	360	32	8
Tuna Salad	450	36	14

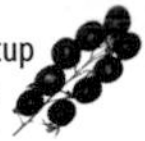

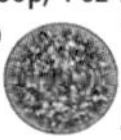

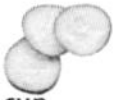

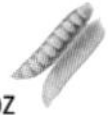

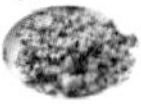

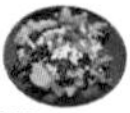

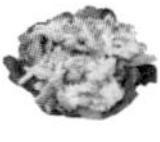

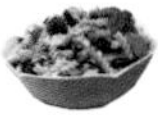

~ *Also See Fast-Foods & Restaurants Section*

Fresh Salad Packs

Pre-Packaged (Supermarkets):	C	F	Cb
Dole:			
Kits: *Per 3½ oz, Includes Dressing*			
Asian Island Crunch	130	7	15
Caesar	150	12	8
Perfect Harvest	160	12	11
Southwest	140	10	10
Salad Blends: *Without Dressing*			
American; Mediterranean, 3 oz	15	0	3
Arugula; Baby Spinach, 3 oz	20	0	3
Fresh Express:			
Complete Salad Kits: *Per 3½ oz, Prepared*			
Asian	120	5	17
Caesar: Regular	120	11	7
Lite	90	7	7
Supreme	140	12	6
Harvest Peach	170	12	14
Pear Gorganzola	130	6	17
Strawberry Fields	200	13	17
Gourmet Cafe: Tuscan Pesto Chkn	140	9	8
Waldorf Chicken	170	9	19

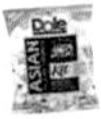

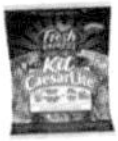

Salad Toppings

	C	F	Cb
Bac'n Pieces *(McCormick)*, 1T, ¼ oz	30	1	2
Bacon Bits *(Hormel)*, 1T.	25	1.5	0
Bac-os *(Betty Crocker)*, 1 Tbsp	30	1.5	2
Chow Mein Noodles, dry, ½ cup	120	7	13
Croutons, 2 Tbsp, 0.3 oz	40	1	7
Olives, 5 medium	25	2	0
Salad Toppins, 4 tsp *(McCormick)*	35	1.5	3
Sunflower Seeds, 1 T., 0.3 oz	45	4	1.5
Toasted Sliced Almonds, 2 T., 0.5 oz	85	7	3
Tortilla Chips, 12 chips, 1 oz	140	7	19

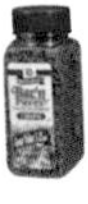

S — Salad Dressings

Quick Guide — C F Cb

Salad Dressings
Average All Brands: *Per 2 Tbsp, Approx 1 fl.oz*

Salad Dressings	C	F	Cb
Balsamic Vinaigrette:			
Regular	90	9	3
Light, 2 Tbsp	45	4	2
Fat Free, 2 Tbsp	25	0	5
Blue Cheese: Reg., 2 Tbsp	145	15	1.5
Regular, ¼ cup, 2 oz	280	30	3
Light, 2 Tbsp	30	1	4
Caesar: Regular, 2 Tbsp	165	17	1
Regular, ¼ cup, 2 oz	310	34	2
Light, 2 Tbsp	35	1.5	5.5
Coleslaw: Regular, 2 Tbsp	125	11	8
Regular, ¼ cup, 2 oz	245	21	15
Light, 2 Tbsp	110	7	14
French: Regular	145	14	5
Regular, ¼ cup, 2 oz	260	25	9
Light, 2 Tbsp	65	4	9
Fat/Oil-Free, 2 Tbsp	40	0	10
Italian: Regular, 2 Tbsp	85	8.5	3
Regular, ¼ cup, 2 oz	165	16	6
Light, 2 Tbsp	55	5.5	2
Fat/Oil-Free, 2 Tbas	15	0	2.5
Ranch: Regular, 2 Tbsp	145	16	2
Regular, ¼ cup, 2 oz	290	30	4
Light, 2 Tbsp	60	4	6.5
Fat-Free, 2 Tbsp	35	0.5	8
Thousand Island: Reg.	115	11	4.5
Regular, ¼ cup, 2 oz	210	20	9
Light, 2 Tbsp	60	3.5	7
Fat-Free, 2 Tbsp	40	0.5	10

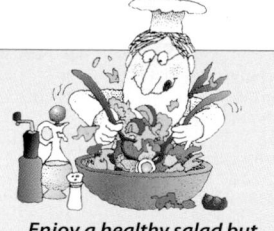

Enjoy a healthy salad but don't drown it in high-fat salad dressings. Use 'light' dressings to halve the fat and calories.

Brands ~ Salad Dressings

	C	F	Cb
Annie's Naturals: *Per 2 Tbsp*			
Organic: Buttermilk	70	6	1
French	110	11	3
Oil & Vinegar	120	13	1
Papaya & Poppy Seed	90	8	5
Thousand Island	90	8	5
Vinaigrettes: Pomegranate	70	7	2
Red Wine & Olive Oil	130	14	0
Sesame Ginger	90	8	4
Shitake Sesame	120	13	1
Bernstein's: *Per 2 Tbsp*			
Creamy Caesar	120	13	1
Herb Garden French	130	12	6
Italian	110	12	1
Restaurant Recipe Italian	120	12	1
Sweet Herb Italian	130	11	8
Fat-Free, Cheese & Garlic Italian	10	0	2
Light Fantastic: Cheese Fantastico	25	1.5	3
Roasted Garlic Balsamic	45	3.5	3
Best Foods: *Per 1 Tbsp Unless Indicated*			
Dijonnaise, 1 tsp	5	0	0.5
Mayonnaise: Canola	45	4.5	0.5
Low-Fat	15	1	2
Light	35	3.5	1
Mayonesa, Lemom-Lime	90	10	0
Olive Oil, 2 Tbsp	50	5	0.5
Real Mayonnaise	90	10	0
Tartar Sauce, 2Tbsp	80	7	4
Cardini's: *Per 2 Tbsp*			
Aged Parmesan Ranch	150	16	1
Caesar Original	160	17	1
Fat-Free Caesar	40	0	9
Light Caesar	80	7	5
Honey Mustard	140	13	5
Italian	100	8	7
Roasted Asian Sesame	120	10	7
Vinaigrette Dressing:			
Balsamic	100	8	5
Lite Balsamic	50	3	5
Great Value: *Per 2 Tbsp*			
Buttermilk Ranch; Caesar, av.	115	12	2
Thousand Island	90	7	6
Light: Buttermilk Ranch	80	7	3
Balsamic/Raspberry Vinaig., av.	50	3.5	4
Hidden Valley: *Per 2 Tbsp*			
Cole Slaw	150	15	5
Old-Fashioned Buttermilk	130	14	2
Ranch: Original	140	14	2
Light Original	80	7	3

Brands ~ Salad Dressings (Cont)

Hidden Valley (Cont):	C	F	Cb
Ranch, other flavors, av.	130	13	2
Farmhouse Originals:			
Dijon;Italian, average	80	8	4
Homestyle Italian	100	10	3
Pomegranate	60	6	3
Kraft: Per 2 Tbsp			
Regular Dressings:			
Caesar Vinaigrette with Parmesan	70	5	3
Catalina	130	11	7
Classic Caesar	130	12	2
Creamy Italian	100	11	2
Greek Vinaigrette	110	12	2
Honey Dijon Vinaigrette	90	7	6
Ranch	120	12	3
Roka Blue Cheese	120	13	1
Sweet Honey Catalina	130	10	8
Tangy Tomato Bacon	100	6	10
Thousand Island	110	10	5
Tuscan House Italian	130	13	3
Kraft Free (Fat-Free): Italian	20	0	4
Classic Caesar; Honey Dijon	50	0	11
Light: Asian Tst'd Sesame	50	2.5	7
Balsamic Vinaigrette	25	1	3
Creamy Caesar	35	2	4
Zesty Italian	25	1.5	3
Seven Seas:			
Green Goddess	130	13	2
Red Wine Vinaig.; Viva Robust Ital.	90	9	2
Reduced Fat: Viva Italian	45	4	3
Red Wine Vinaigrette	45	4	3
Special Collection,			
Parmesan Romano	140	14	2
Marie's: Per 2 Tbsp			
Caesar; Creamy Ranch	170	19	1
Chunky Blue Cheese	160	17	0
Honey Dijon	130	12	5
Poppy Seed	150	13	8
Potato Salad Dressing:			
Classic	170	19	0
Dijon Herb	140	15	1
German Style	110	11	3
Sesame Ginger	100	8	7
Spinach Salad	60	1.5	11
Thousand Island	150	15	4
Marzetti's:			
Organic: Caesar	150	16	1
Blue Cheese	130	14	1
Raspberry Cranberry	100	8	8
Chunky Blue Cheese	150	15	0
Classic Ranch	160	17	1

Marzetti's (Cont):	C	F	Cb
Thousand Island	150	15	5
Simply Dressed: Champagne	80	8	2
Greek Feta	110	12	2
Newman's Own: Per 2 Tbsp			
Regular: Balsamic Vinaigrette	90	9	3
Creamy Caesar	170	18	1
Family Recipe Italian	130	13	1
Olive Oil & Vinegar	150	16	1
Parmesan Roasted Garlic	110	11	2
Ranch	150	16	2
Light: Italian	60	6	1
Raspberry & Walnut	70	5	7
Organic: Light Bals. Vinaig.	45	4	3
Low Fat Asian	35	2	5
Tuscan Italian	100	11	2
Spectrum: Per 2 Tbsp			
Organic Omega-3:			
Asian Ginger	130	13	2
Creamy Garlic Ranch	120	13	1
Golden Balsamic Vin.	110	11	3
Pomegranate Chipotle	130	13	2
Vegan Caesar	90	9	2
Wish-Bone:			
Creamy: Chunky Blue Cheese	150	15	1
Creamy Caesar	180	18	1
Creamy Italian	110	10	4
Deluxe French	120	11	5
Ranch	130	13	2
Russian	110	6	14
Sweet 'n Spicy	140	12	7
Thousand Island	130	12	5
Light: Blue Cheese	70	6	2
Creamy Caesar	70	6	2
Honey Dijon	70	5	6
Italian	35	2.5	3
Parm. Peppercorn Ranch	60	5	2
Ranch	70	5	4
Thousand Island	60	5	4
Fat-Free:			
Chunky Blue Cheese	30	0	7
Italian	15	0	3
Ranch	30	0	6
Oil & Vinegar: Bals. Vinaig.	60	5	3
House Italian	110	10	3
Red Wine Vinaigrette	70	5	6
Robusto Italian	80	7	4
Light Vinaigrette: Balsamic & Basil	60	5	3
Asian with Sesame & Ginger	70	5	5
Raspberry Walnut	80	5	7
Salad Spritzers,			
10 sprays (¼ fl.oz), av all flav.	10	1	1

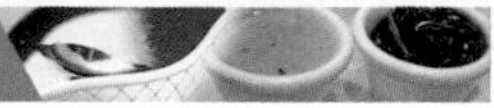

Gravy

	C	F	Cb
Homemade Gravy, average:			
Thin, little fat, 2 Tbsp, 1 oz	20	1	3
Thick: 2 Tbsp, 1.25 oz	50	2	9
¼ cup, 2.5 oz	100	4	18
McCormick Gravy Mix:			
Brown, 1 Tbsp	15	0.5	3
Turkey, 1 Tbsp	20	0.5	4

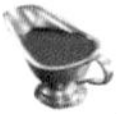

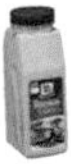

Gravy-In-Jars

	C	F	Cb
Boston Market,			
Classic Beef, ¼ cup, 2 oz	30	1	4
Campbell's, Slow Roast,			
Beef/Chicken/Turkey, ¼ cup, 2 oz	25	1	4
Heinz: *Per ¼ Cup, 2 oz*			
Homestyle: Chicken	30	1	4
Savory Beef	30	1	4
Sausage	45	1.5	1
Other flavors, average	20	0.5	3
Fat-Free, all flavors	10	0	3
Safeway, all flavors, ¼ cup, 2 oz	20	0.5	4

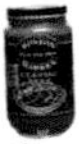

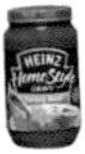

Tomato Products

	C	F	Cb
Whole/Chopped/Crushed/Diced:			
Regular, 1 cup, 8.5 oz	50	0	10
In Aspic, ½ cup	50	0	12
With Green Chili, 1 cup, 8.5 oz	60	0	16
Stewed, ½ cup, 1.7 oz	40	1.5	7
Wedges in Tomato Juice, 1 cup	70	0.5	18
Salsa, average, 2 Tbsp, 1 oz	25	0	6
Tomato Ketchup:			
Regular, 1 Tbsp, 0.5 oz	15	0	4
Single Serve, 1 packet	10	0	3
One-Carb *(Heinz)*, 1 Tbsp, 0.5 oz	5	0	1
Tomato Paste:			
Regular, 2 Tbsp, 1 oz	25	0	6
¾ cup, 6 oz	140	1	32
Tomato Puree, ½ cup, 4.5 oz	50	0	10
Tomato Sauce:			
Regular, ½ cup, 4.4 oz	50	0	11
Spanish Style, ½ cup, 4.3 oz	40	0	9
With Mushr., ½ cup, 4.3 oz	45	0	10
With Onions, ½ cup, 4.3 oz	50	0	12
Tomato Seasoning, 3 tsp	20	0	4
Sundried Tomatoes:			
Natural, 5-6 pieces, 0.4 oz	22	0	5
In Oil, drained, 6 pieces, 0.5 oz	40	2.5	4

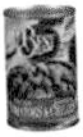

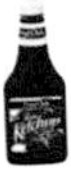

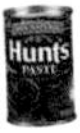

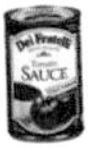

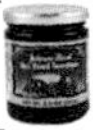

Sauces ~ Brands

	C	F	Cb
A-1:			
Marinades: *Per Tablespoon, ½ oz*			
Chicago Steakhouse	20	1	3
Ginger Teriyaki	25	0	5
New York Steakhouse	25	0	4
Steak Sauce: Bold & Spicy	20	0	5
Cracked Peppercorn	15	0	3
Kobe Sesame Teriyaki	25	0	4
Smokey Mesquite	30	0	8
Steak Sauce	15	0	3
Supreme Garlic	25	0	5
Thick & Hearty	25	0	6
Barilla:			
Pasta Sauces: *Per ½ Cup*			
Arrabbiata, Spicy Marinara	60	1.5	11
Basilico, Tomato & Basil	80	3	11
Calabrese, Sweet Peppers	70	1.5	11
Formaggi, Three Cheese	70	1.5	11
Marinara, Traditional	90	3.5	12
Montanara, Mushroom & Garlic	70	2.5	11
Napolentana, Roasted Garlic	80	3	13
Bertolli:			
Pasta Sauces: *Per ½ Cup*			
Traditional: Italian Sausage	90	3	14
Olive Oil & Garlic	80	3	14
Tomato & Basil	70	2	13
Vineyard Collection: Marinara	80	2	14
Portobello Mushroom, with Merlot	80	2.5	12
Best Foods/Hellmann's,			
Tartar Sauce, 2 Tbsp	80	7	4
Buitoni:			
Pasta Sauces:			
Alfredo, ¼ cup	140	12	6
Light Alfredo, ¼ cup	90	6	4
Marinara, ½ cup	70	3	10
W/ Roasted Garlic, ½ cup	60	1	10
Pesto: With Basil, ¼ cup	270	26	4
Reduced Fat, ¼ cup	230	17	6
Tomato Herb Parm., ½ cup	120	8	10
Bull's Eye: *Per 2 Tbsp*			
Original BBQ Sauce	60	0	14
Sweet & Tangy	60	0	13
Texas Style	45	0	10
Catelli: *Per ½ Cup*			
Sauces: Pizza, average	60	1.5	11
Meat Sauce	80	2.5	11
Garden Select 6 Vege Sauces:			
Country Mushroom	70	1.5	11
Diced Tomato & Basil	70	1	12

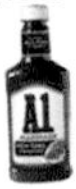

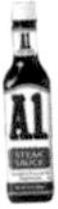

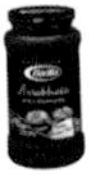

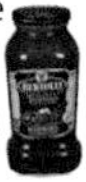

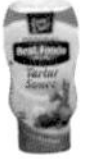

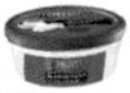

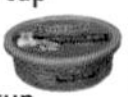

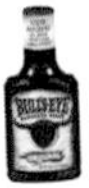

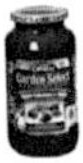

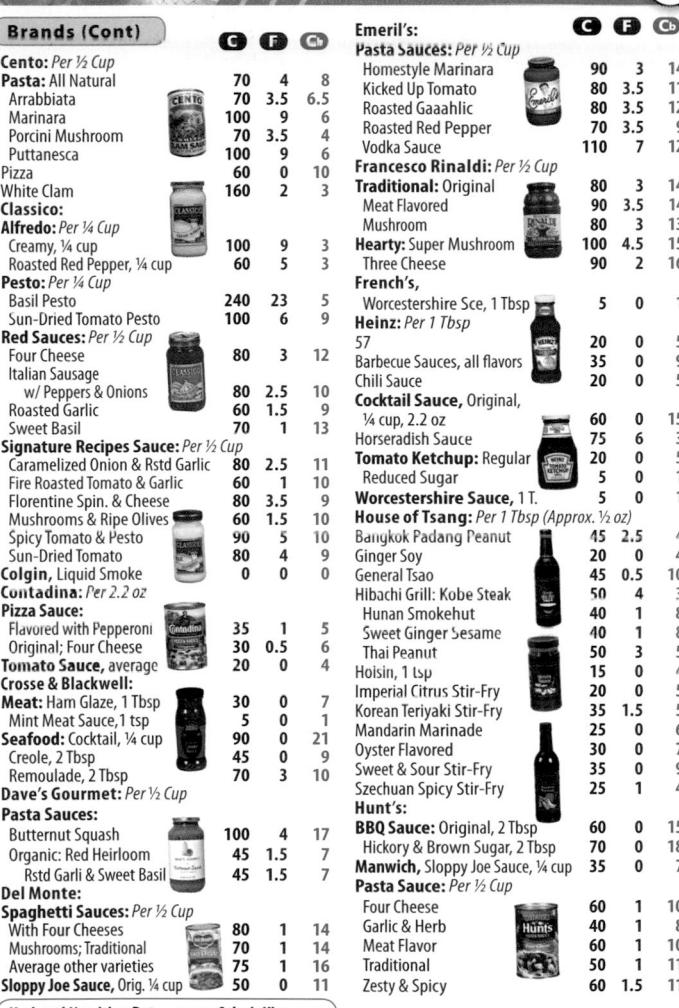

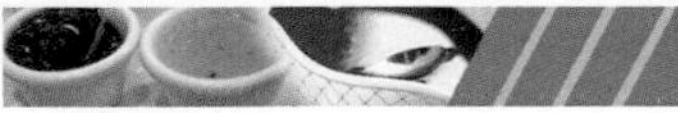

Brands (Cont)

	C	F	Cb
Cento: Per ½ Cup			
Pasta: All Natural	70	4	8
Arrabbiata	70	3.5	6.5
Marinara	100	9	6
Porcini Mushroom	70	3.5	4
Puttanesca	100	9	6
Pizza	60	0	10
White Clam	160	2	3
Classico:			
Alfredo: Per ¼ Cup			
Creamy, ¼ cup	100	9	3
Roasted Red Pepper, ¼ cup	60	5	3
Pesto: Per ¼ Cup			
Basil Pesto	240	23	5
Sun-Dried Tomato Pesto	100	6	9
Red Sauces: Per ½ Cup			
Four Cheese	80	3	12
Italian Sausage w/ Peppers & Onions	80	2.5	10
Roasted Garlic	60	1.5	9
Sweet Basil	70	1	13
Signature Recipes Sauce: Per ½ Cup			
Caramelized Onion & Rstd Garlic	80	2.5	11
Fire Roasted Tomato & Garlic	60	1	10
Florentine Spin. & Cheese	80	3.5	9
Mushrooms & Ripe Olives	60	1.5	10
Spicy Tomato & Pesto	90	5	10
Sun-Dried Tomato	80	4	9
Colgin, Liquid Smoke	0	0	0
Contadina: Per 2.2 oz			
Pizza Sauce:			
Flavored with Pepperoni	35	1	5
Original; Four Cheese	30	0.5	6
Tomato Sauce, average	20	0	4
Crosse & Blackwell:			
Meat: Ham Glaze, 1 Tbsp	30	0	7
Mint Meat Sauce, 1 tsp	5	0	1
Seafood: Cocktail, ¼ cup	90	0	21
Creole, 2 Tbsp	45	0	9
Remoulade, 2 Tbsp	70	3	10
Dave's Gourmet: Per ½ Cup			
Pasta Sauces:			
Butternut Squash	100	4	17
Organic: Red Heirloom	45	1.5	7
Rstd Garli & Sweet Basil	45	1.5	7
Del Monte:			
Spaghetti Sauces: Per ½ Cup			
With Four Cheeses	80	1	14
Mushrooms; Traditional	70	1	14
Average other varieties	75	1	16
Sloppy Joe Sauce, Orig. ¼ cup	50	0	11

	C	F	Cb
Emeril's:			
Pasta Sauces: Per ½ Cup			
Homestyle Marinara	90	3	14
Kicked Up Tomato	80	3.5	11
Roasted Gaaahlic	80	3.5	12
Roasted Red Pepper	70	3.5	9
Vodka Sauce	110	7	12
Francesco Rinaldi: Per ½ Cup			
Traditional: Original	80	3	14
Meat Flavored	90	3.5	14
Mushroom	80	3	13
Hearty: Super Mushroom	100	4.5	15
Three Cheese	90	2	16
French's,			
Worcestershire Sce, 1 Tbsp	5	0	1
Heinz: Per 1 Tbsp			
57	20	0	5
Barbecue Sauces, all flavors	35	0	9
Chili Sauce	20	0	5
Cocktail Sauce, Original, ¼ cup, 2.2 oz	60	0	15
Horseradish Sauce	75	6	3
Tomato Ketchup: Regular	20	0	5
Reduced Sugar	5	0	1
Worcestershire Sauce, 1 T.	5	0	1
House of Tsang: Per 1 Tbsp (Approx. ½ oz)			
Bangkok Padang Peanut	45	2.5	4
Ginger Soy	20	0	4
General Tsao	45	0.5	10
Hibachi Grill: Kobe Steak	50	4	3
Hunan Smokehut	40	1	8
Sweet Ginger Sesame	40	1	8
Thai Peanut	50	3	5
Hoisin, 1 tsp	15	0	4
Imperial Citrus Stir-Fry	20	0	5
Korean Teriyaki Stir-Fry	35	1.5	5
Mandarin Marinade	25	0	6
Oyster Flavored	30	0	7
Sweet & Sour Stir-Fry	35	0	9
Szechuan Spicy Stir-Fry	25	1	4
Hunt's:			
BBQ Sauce: Original, 2 Tbsp	60	0	15
Hickory & Brown Sugar, 2 Tbsp	70	0	18
Manwich, Sloppy Joe Sauce, ¼ cup	35	0	7
Pasta Sauces: Per ½ Cup			
Four Cheese	60	1	10
Garlic & Herb	40	1	8
Meat Flavor	60	1	10
Traditional	50	1	11
Zesty & Spicy	60	1.5	11

Brands (Cont)

	C	F	Cb
Kikkoman:			
Black Bean Sauce, w/ Garlic 2 T.	50	1	6
Hoisin Sauce, 2 Tbsp	80	1.5	17
Honey Mustard, 1Tbsp	30	0	6
Roasted Garlic & Herbs, 1 Tbsp	20	0	4
Teriyaki, 1 Tbsp	15	0	2
Teriyaki Roasted Garlic, 1 Tbsp	25	0	4
Knorr:			
Classic Sauce: *Per Whole Package*			
Bernaise, dry mix only	100	0	20
Hollandaise, dry mix only	100	0	20
Kraft:			
Barbecue Sauces, average, 2 Tbsp	65	0	15
Specialty Sauce: Cocktail, 2 Tbsp	60	0.5	13
Coleslaw Dressing, 1.2 oz	120	9	9
Horseradish, ½ oz	40	3	4
Sandwich Spread, 1 Tbsp	35	2.5	3
Sweet'n Sour, 2 Tbsp	60	0	14
Tartar, Original, 1 Tbsp	60	4.5	4
Las Palmas:			
Red Chile Sauce, ¼ cup, 2 oz	15	0.5	2
Enchilada Sauce:			
Green Chili, 2oz	25	1.5	3
Red Chili, hot, 2 oz	15	0.5	2
La Victoria,			
Red/Green Enchilada Sauce, av., 2 oz	25	1	3.5
Lawry's:			
30 Minute Marinade: *Per Tbsp*			
Caribbean Jerk; Mexican Chile & Lime	25	0	5
Herb & Garlic; Lemon Pepper	10	0	2
Mesquite; Steak & Chop	5	0	1
Sesame Ginger	30	0	7
Packet Seasonings: *Dry*			
Fajitas; Taco, average, 2 tsp	15	0	3
Average other flavors, 2 tsp	20	0	4
Lea & Perrins:			
Worcestershire Sauce: 1 tsp	5	0	1
Thick, Classic, 2 Tbsp	30	0	8
McCormicks:			
Seafood Sauces:			
Cajun Style, 2 T., 1.1 oz	15	0	3
Cocktail, Original/Extra Hot, ¼ cup	90	0.5	19
Tartar: Original, 2 Tbsp	140	14	3
Fat Free, 2 T., 1 oz	30	0	7
Scampi, 2 T., 1 oz	160	17	2

Mrs. Dash:	C	F	Cb
Marinades (Salt-Free): *Per 1 Tbsp*			
Garlic Lime	30	1.5	4
Lemon Herb Peppercorn	25	2	3
Southwestern Chipotle	25	1.5	2
Spicy Teriyaki	25	0.5	4
Newman's Own: *Per ½ Cup*			
Regular: Five Cheese	80	3	10
Fra Diavolo	70	3	10
Marinara; Sockarooni	70	2	12
Roasted Garlic & Peppers	70	2.5	11
Tomato & Basil Bombolina	90	4.5	13
Vodka	110	5	11
O Organics *(Von's): Per ½ Cup*			
Marinara; Roasted Garlic, av.	60	1.5	9
Mushroom; Tomato Basil	50	1.5	8
Roasted Garlic	60	1.5	8
Old El Paso:			
Enchilada Sauce:			
Green Chile, ¼ cup	25	1.5	4
Other varieties, ¼ cup	20	0	4
Salsas, Thick & Chunky, all var., 2 T.	10	0	2
Taco Sauce, all varieties, 1 Tbsp	5	0	1
Pace: *Per 2 Tbsp*			
Chunky Salsa	10	0	3
Picante Sauce	10	0	3
Mexican Four Cheese,			
Salsa Con Queso	90	7	5
Prego: *Per ½ Cup*			
100% Natural: Marinara	80	3	10
Flavored with Meat	80	2.5	13
Fresh Mushroom; Traditional	70	3	13
Italian Sausage & Garlic	90	3	13
Mini Meatball	100	3	13
Pizza Sauce, Pizzeria Style	80	3	10
Roasted Garlic & Herb	90	3	13
Three Cheese; Tom. Basil & Garlic, av.	80	2	13
Chunky Garden:			
Combo	70	1.5	13
Mushroom Supreme			
with Baby Portobellos	90	3	13
Other varieties	90	3	13
Heart Smart: Trad.; Mushroom	70	1.5	13
Premier Japan: *Per 1 Tbsp*			
Hoisin; Teriyaki	15	0	3
Ginger Tamari	5	0	1
Progresso: *Per ½ Cup*			
Recipe Starters: Roasted Tomato	50	1.5	9
Roasted Garlic	70	5	5
Other flavors, average	90	7	5

Brands (Cont)

Ragu:	C	F	Cb
Pizza Quick Sauce,			
Traditional, ¼ cup	45	2	6
Pizza Sauce,			
Homemade Style, ¼ cup	30	1	5
White: *Per ¼ Cup*			
Classic Alfredo	90	8	2
Light Parmesan	60	4	2
Roasted Garlic Parmesan	100	9	3
Red, Chunky: *Per ½ Cup*			
Mushroom & Green Pepper	80	2.5	13
Average other varieties	90	2.5	14
Light varieties, average	55	1	10
Old World Style: *Per ½ Cup*			
Flavored with Meat	70	3	9
Marinara	80	3	10
Mushroom	70	2.5	10
Traditional	80	2.5	11
Robusto!: *Per ½ Cup*			
7-Herb Tomato	80	3	12
Chopped Tomato, Olive Oil & Garlic	90	4	12
Roasted Garlic	80	2.5	13
Sauteed Onion & Garlic	90	3.5	12
Six Cheese	90	3	12
Safeway Select:			
Salsa, av. all flavors, 2 Tbsp	15	0	3
Select Sauces: *Per ½ Cup*			
Arrabbiata	110	8	10
Artichoke Pesto	60	2	9
Four Cheese	80	3.5	11
Marinara	60	2	10
Spicy Red Bell Pepper	50	1	9
Sundried Tomato & Olive	60	1.5	11
Tomato Alfredo; Vodka	130	10	9
Sophia's: *Per 2 Tbsp*			
Greek Island Dressing :			
W/ Feta Cheese & Calamata Olives	70	7	3
Average other varieties	60	6	3
Oil Free, Cilantro & Lime	10	0	3
Steel's, Spiced Cranberry Sauce,			
no sugar added, 2 Tbsp	30	0	8
Taco Bell, Jalapeno Sce, 2 Tbsp	110	11	3
Tony Roma's:			
Bold & Spicy, 2 Tbsp	50	0	12
Wing Sauce, 1 Tbsp	15	1	0
Trader Joe's:			
BBQ Sauce,			
Kansas City Style, 2 Tbsp	60	0	15
Tomato & Basil, ½ cup, 4.4 oz	80	4.5	10
Walnut Acres:			
Organic Pasta Sauces,			
All varieties, average, ½ cup, 4.5 oz	50	1	9

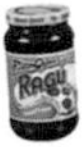

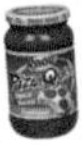

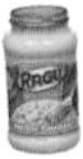

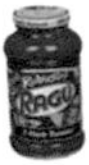

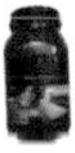

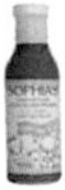

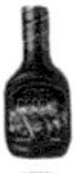

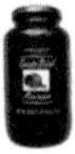

Seasonings & Flavorings

	C	F	Cb
Auromatic Bitters *(Angostua)*, 1 tsp	15	0	4
Bacon Bits, average, 1 Tbsp	35	2	2
Bacon Chips *(Durkee)*, 1 Tbsp	30	1	2
Bac-Os *(Betty Crocker)*,			
1Tbsp	30	1.5	2
Blends *(Mrs Dash)*, 1 tsp	0	0	0
Butter Buds, 1 tsp	5	0	2
Flavor Enhancer *(Accent)*, 1 tsp	0	0	0
Flavor Sprinkles *(Molly McButter)*,			
Natural/Cheese, 1 tsp	5	0	1
Garlic Bread Sprinkle, 1 tsp	8	0.5	1
Garlic Salt, 1 tsp	2	0	0
Italian Seasoning, 1 tsp	4	0	1
Lemon Pepper Seasoning,			
1 tsp	7	0	1
Meat Tenderizer, av., 1 tsp	7	0	1
Salad Crunchies *(McCormick)*,			
1 tsp	10	0.5	2
Salt, Reg., Sea Salt, Lite Salt	0	0	0
Seasoning *(Old Bay)*, ¼ tsp	0	0	0
Seasoning Mix *(Vegit)*, ¼ tsp	0	0	0
Seasoning Mixes, av., ¼ pkg	70	1	9
Taco Seasoning, av., ¼ pkg	30	0.5	4
Bragg's, Liquid Aminos	0	0	0
Old El Paso: Chili Season. Mix, 1 T.	8	0.5	1.5
Cheesy Taco Seasoning Mix, 1 Tbsp	10	0.5	2
Taco/Burrito Seasoning Mix, 2 tsp	15	0	4
Fajita Seasoning Mix, 1 tsp	5	0	1.5

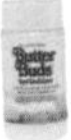

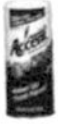

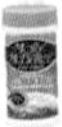

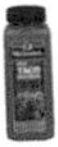

Spices & Herbs

Per Teaspoon: Average all types	5	0	1
All Purpose, 1 tsp	0	0	0
Allspice, ground	5	0	1
Chili Powder	8	0	1
Cinnamon, ground	6	0	2
Curry Powder	6	0	1
Garlic Powder	9	0	2
Nutmeg, ground	12	0	1
Onion Powder	7	0	2
Parsley, dried	4	0	1
Pepper, average	6	0	1
Saffron	2	0	0
Salt-Free Blends, 1 tsp	0	0	0
Tumeric, ground	8	0	1
Seeds: Fenugreek	12	1	2
Mustard, Poppyseed	15	1	0
Other types, average	7	0	1

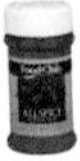

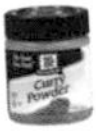

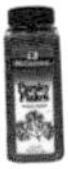

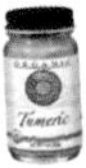

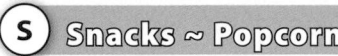

Home-Popped Popcorn

	C	F	Cb
Popping Corn Kernels, 2 Tbsp, 1 oz	110	1	26
(makes approximately 5 cups)			
Air-popped, w/o oil: Plain, 1 oz	110	1	22
1 cup, 0.2 oz	20	0	5
Oil-popped: Plain, 1 oz	145	8	16
1 cup, 0.4 oz	55	3	11
Popcorn Oil, 1 Tbsp	120	14	0

Microwave Popcorn

Average all Brands: *Per 1 Cup Popped, Unless Indicated*

	C	F	Cb
Butter: Regular	35	2	4
Light	25	1	4
Act II Popcorn:			
Butter: 1 cup	35	2	4
4½ cups, 1 oz	160	9	18
94% Fat-Free Butter: 1 cup	20	0.5	4
7 cups, 1 oz	130	2.5	28
Butter Lovers: 1 cup	40	2	4
4 cups, 1 oz	160	9	19
Xreme Butter: 1 cup	45	3	4.5
4 cups	180	12	18
American Fare (K-Mart):			
Smart Sense: Butter: 0.3 oz	40	2	5
3½ cups, 1 oz	130	4.5	19
Kettle Corn;Theater Butter: 1 cup	40	2	5
3½ cups	130	6	18
Jolly Time:			
American's Best	20	0	4
Blast O Butter: Regular	35	2	4
Light	30	1.5	4
Healthy Pop: Butter Flavor	20	0	4
Caramel Apple	20	0	6
Newman's Own:			
Butter Flavor:			
Regular, 3½ cups	130	5	18
Light, 3½ cups	120	5	19
Orville Redenbacher's:			
Family Favorites:			
Butter: 4 cups	170	12	17
Light, 5½ cups	120	5	19
Movie Theater Butter, 4 c.	170	12	16
Ultimate Butter, 5 cups	170	12	16
Sweet & Savory,			
Cheddar Cheese; Spicy Nacho, average, 4½ cups	180	14	15
Pop Secret: *Per 1 Cup Popped*			
1-Step, Cheddar, 1 cup	30	2	33
94% Fat-Free, Butter	15	0	3
100 Calorie Pop, Butter	15	0.5	3
Butter; Extra Butter, av.	30	2	3
Homestyle; Movie Theater Butter, av	35	2.5	3

Bagged Popcorn

	C	F	Cb
Average All Brands (Ready-to-Eat)			
Regular/Plain: ½ oz package	80	5	8
1 oz package	160	10	16
4 oz package	640	40	64
2 oz Box (store/airport)	320	16	32
3 oz Bag (9" high x 5" wide)	480	24	48
Caramel Popcorn, with nuts, 1 cup, 1.5 oz	230	12	39

Brands ~ Bagged Popcorn

	C	F	Cb
Boston's: Lite, 3½ cups, 1 oz	120	4	20
Homestyle, 2½ cups, 1 oz	160	9	18
Cracker Jack: Original, 1 cup, 1 oz	180	3	35
4.25 oz pkg (Hunger Grab)	510	8	98
Crunch 'N Munch:			
Buttery Toffee: ⅔ cup, 1.1 oz	150	6	22
1 cup, 1.6 oz	220	9	32
Caramel: ⅔ cup, 1.1 oz	160	8	20
1 cup, 1.6 oz	230	12	29
12 oz box	1745	87	218
Fiddle Faddle:			
Av. all varieties: 1 oz	120	2	24
1 cup, 2 oz	240	4	48
6 oz box	720	12	144
Korn Krunch, Almond Pecan (Sugar Free), 1 oz	125	6	28
PopCorners, Butter/Kettle, 1 oz	120	3.5	21
Popcorn Indiana: *Per 1 oz*			
Kettlecorn:			
Aged White Cheddar, av.	150	11	13
Other varieties, av.	130	4.5	21
Popcorn: Bacon Ranch	150	10	13
Poppycock:			
Original/Pecan Delight: ½ cup, 1 oz	155	8	20
1 cup, 2 oz	310	16	40
Original, 1 oz	160	8	20
Chocolate Lovers, ½ cup, 1.15 oz	160	7	22
Smartfood *(Fritolay),* Movie Theater Butter, 1 oz	150	9	15

Movie Theater Popcorn

	C	F	Cb
Small, (7 cups): Plain	385	21	44
With Butter (3 pumps, 0.75 oz)	570	42	44
Medium, (15 cups): Plain	825	45	94
With Butter (4 pumps, 1 oz)	1075	73	94
Large, (20 cups): Plain	1100	60	124
With Butter (6 pumps, 1.5 oz)	1485	102	124
Butter: 1 Pump, 0.25 oz	65	7	0
4 Pumps (2 Tbsp), 1 oz	250	28	0

Corn & Tortilla Chips

Average All Brands	C	F	Cb
Corn Chips:			
Average all types: 1 oz	150	8	18
8 oz bag	1200	64	144
Fritos, Original, 32 chips, 1 oz	160	10	15
Tortilla Chips: Average, 1 oz	140	7	18
(1 oz = approx. 12 chips or 13 strips)			
Doritos: Regular, 13 chips, 1 oz	140	7	18
Salsa Verde (12)	140	7	19
Baked! Nacho Cheese (15), 1 oz	120	3.5	21
Reduced-Fat, Nacho Cheese, 1 pkg	130	5	19
Kettle, Tias, av. all flavors, 1oz	145	8	17
Snyder's: White/Yellow Corn	140	4.5	23
Restaurant Style, 1 oz	130	5	20
Utz: White/Yellow Corn	140	7	18
Restaurant Style	130	6	18
Tostitos (Fritolay):			
Average all, 1 oz	145	7	19
Baked! Scoops, 1 oz	120	3	22
Restaurant Style, Blue Corn, 1 oz	140	6	19

Potato Chips/Crisps

Average All Brands	C	F	Cb
Regular:			
Plain or flavored, (2 chips)	15	1	1.5
1 oz package (20 chips)	150	10	15
4 oz quantity	600	40	60
14 oz package	2100	140	210
Brands:			
Lay's, average all, 1 oz	160	10	15
Lay's Stax, average all, 1 oz	150	9	15
Pringles:			
Original; Xtreme Varieties	150	9	15
Large, 6.38 oz can	960	58	96
Minis, 1 bag, 0.8 oz	140	9	16
Snack Stacks, av., 1 tub	140	9	12
Multi Grain, all flav., 1 oz	140	8	16
Ruffles, Reg., av., 1 oz	160	11	15
Reduced Fat:			
Lay's, Kettle, 1 oz	140	6	19
Pringles, all flavors, 16 Chips, 1 oz	130	7	17
Sun Chips: Original			
16 chips, 1 oz	140	6	19
Low-Fat/Baked:			
Lay's, Baked!: Original (15), 1 oz	120	2	23
Tostitos, Scoops, (15) 1 oz	120	3	22
Ruffles, Baked!, average all,	120	3.5	21
Fat Free: (Lay's): Light, Orig., 1 oz	75	0	17
Pringles, Fat-Free, (15), 1 oz	70	0	15

Pretzels

Average All Brands	C	F	Cb
Hard-Baked Pretzels: Each			
1 oz quantity	110	1	23
Sticks, thin, 2¼" (9/oz)	12	0	3
Twists, thin, ¼" thick, (5/oz)	25	0	5
Dutch (2¾"x 2⅝"), 0.5 oz	55	1	11
Sourdough (Snyder's), 0.75 oz	100	0	22
Soft Pretzel Twists, average: Each			
Plain: Small, 2 oz	210	2	43
Medium, 4 oz	390	3.5	80
Large, 5 oz	485	4.5	100
Big Cheese, 1.76 oz	130	3	22
New York Street Vendors, 7 oz	660	6	135
Peanut Butter filled (Tr. Joe's), 1 oz	150	8	14
Milk Choc-Coated (Snyders), 1 oz	140	6	19
White Choc. covered, 7 pieces, 1 oz	130	6	19

Brands ~ Pretzels

	C	F	Cb
Flipz: Milk Choc, 8 pcs, 1 oz	130	5	20
White Fudge, 7 pcs, 1 oz	130	5	20
Rold Gold (Frito-Lay):			
Braided Twists,			
Honey Wheat (8), 1 oz	110	1	24
Classic: Pretzel Sticks, 1 oz	100	0	23
Rods/Tiny Twists, av., 1 oz	110	1	23
Sourdough, 1 pretzel	90	1	19
Tiny Twists, Fat-Free, 1 oz	110	0	23
Snyder's of Hanover:			
100 Calorie Pack, Snaps, 0.9 oz	100	0.5	22
Gluten Free Pretzel Sticks (30)	120	1.5	25
Homestyle (15), 1 oz	120	1	25
Organic Sticks:			
Honey Whole Wheat	110	2	21
Whole Wheat & Oat	110	1.5	21
Pieces, Bacon Cheddar (28), 1 oz	140	7	17
Pretzel Chips, Original, (14)	110	0.5	24
Rods (3), 1 oz	120	1.5	24
Thins, 1 oz	110	0	23
SuperPretzel:			
Soft Pretzels (1), 2¼ oz	160	1	34
Softstix (2), 1¾ oz	130	3	22
Soft Pretzel Bites (5), 1.85 oz	150	0.5	32
Pretzelfils: Pizza (2), 1.85 oz	120	2	20
Pepperjack; Mozzarella, (2),av.	130	4.5	19
Utz: Chocolate covered, 2 pcs	110	4	17
Average other varieties , 1 oz	110	1	21

Snacks | C | F | Cb

Note: Actual weight of packaged snacks is usually 5-10% more than label Net Wt. For accuracy, weigh snack and allow extra calories, fat and carbs for any extra weight.

Item	C	F	Cb
Apple Chips (Seneca), av., 1 oz	140	7	20
Bagel Crisps (N.Y. Style), 6 crisps, 1 oz	130	6	17
Baguette Chips (Pillsbury), 21 chips	130	5	20
Banana Chips (T.Joe's), 13 chips, 1 oz	160	11	13
Beef Jerky (Jack Link's), av., 1 oz	80	1	5
Beef Sticks (Slim Jim), Orig., 0.28 oz	40	3.5	1
(Jack Links), Original, 1 oz	110	9	1
Bugles, (Tostitos), Nacho, 1 oz, 1 oz	160	9	18
Cakes ~ See Pages 62- 64			
Cheese Balls (Utz), Jug Container, 1 oz serving	130	7	16
Cheese Nips, 1.25 oz package	170	7	22
Cheese Puffs: Average, 1 oz	160	10	15
Snyder's, Multigrain, 1 oz	130	6	20
Cheese Twists, 1 oz	140	8	15
Cheerios, Snack Mix, average, ⅔ cup, 1.1 oz	130	3.5	22
Cheetos: Av. all flav., 1 oz	160	10	15
4 oz package	640	40	60
Baked!, Fantastix, av., 1 oz	130	5	19
Simply Natural, White Cheddar Puffs, 1 oz	150	9	16
Cheez-It Crackers:			
Original, 1.23 oz package	180	9	20
Baked, reduced fat, av., 1 oz	130	4.5	20
Big (13)	150	8	17
Chester's: Fries, Flamin' Hot, 1 pkt	260	14	30
Snack Mix, Crazy Cheddar, 1 oz	140	7	17
Chex Mix (General Mills),			
100 Calorie, av., 1 bag, 0.81 oz	100	3	18
Chips Ahoy!: Choc Chip Cookies:			
1.4 oz Single Serve Pack	190	9	27
Mini: 3 oz package	410	20	57
Go-Pak!, 1 pkt	550	27	77
Chicharrones ~ See Pork Skins			
Churros (Rubio's), 9", 1.6 oz	170	8	22
Combos:			
Crackers: Av., ⅓ cup, 1 oz	140	6	18
Snack size, av., 1.7 oz pkg	240	11	31
Pretzels: All varieties, ⅓ cup, 1 oz	130	4.5	19
Single snack bag, average, 1.7oz	235	9	34
Cookies ~ See Pages 81			
Cool Cuts, Carrot & Ranch, 2.3 oz	70	5	5
Corn Chips ~ See Page 149			
Corn Nuts: ⅓ cup, 1 oz	120	4.5	20
1.7 oz bag	210	8	34
Corn Puffs/Twists, (32 approx), 1 oz	160	11	15
Dunkin Stix (Dolly Madison), (3)	490	25	63

Snacks (Cont) | C | F | Cb

Item	C	F	Cb
Edamame:			
Dry Roasted (Seapointe),1 oz	130	4	10
Choc. Covered (Tr. Joe's), 1.5 oz	200	11	21
Fig Newtons:			
Regular, 2 oz pkg	200	4	39
Fat-Free, 2.1 oz pkg	180	0	44
Minis, Fig/Strawb., av., 1.34 oz pkg	130	3	27
Flipz ~ See page 149			
Fritos: Corn Chips (30), av. all, 1oz	160	10	15
Flavor Twists (23), 1 oz	150	9	16
Funyuns, 1⅛ oz pkg	220	11	27
Goldfish, average, 1 oz	140	5	20
Gold-N-Chees (Lance), 1.25 oz	190	10	19
Gripz: Cheez It; Chips Deluxe, av., 0.9 oz	120	6	17
Hot Peanuts (Lays), 1.65 oz	310	25	10
Munchies Snack Mix (Frito-Lay):			
Cheese Fix, ¾ cup	140	7	18
Flaming; Totally Ranch, ¾ c.	140	6	19
Munchos, 16 pieces, 1 oz	160	10	16
Nabisco:			
Toasted Chips: Ritz, av. all flav., 1 oz	130	5.5	20
Wheat Thins, 1 oz	125	4.5	21
Nutter Butter, Sandwich Cookies:			
Singles, 1.9 oz pkg	250	10	37
Bites: 1.25 oz pkg	170	7	24
Milk Choc-Covered, 2.54 oz pkg	350	17	48
Onion Rings (T.G.I. Friday), 1 oz	130	6	19
Oreo Cookies:			
Double Stuf, 1.5 oz pkg	210	10	30
Mini Bite Size: (9 cookies) 1.25 oz	170	7	25
Go-Pak, 4 oz cup	530	22	81
Snak-Saks, 8 oz pkg	1040	48	168
Oreo Cakesters, soft, 2 oz	250	12	36
Oriental Mix (Rice Snacks), 1 oz	125	3.5	21
Peanut Butter Nuggets, (10), 1 oz	140	6	15
Pepitas, dried or roasted, ¼ **cup,** 1 oz	155	14	3
Pirate's Booty:			
Aged White Cheddar, 4 oz bag	520	20	76
Chocolate, 4 oz bag	560	32	64
Pita Chips, average, (9) 1 oz	130	4	18
Plaintain Chips (Goya), 34 chips, 1 oz	150	8	20
PopCorners, Butter/Kettle, 1 oz	120	3.5	21
Popcorn ~ See Page 148			
Pork Cracklins, 1 oz	160	12	0
Pork Skins/Rinds: 1 oz	160	10	0
99c pkg (Baken-ets), 1.25 oz	200	13	0
Chicharrones (Mission), 3 oz pkt	480	27	0
Potato Chips ~ See Page 149			
Potato Skins (TGI Friday), (16), 1 oz	130	9	24

Snacks (Cont)

	C	F	Cb
Puffed Wheat (Sabritones), 1 oz	150	10	13
Pretzels ~ See Page 149			
Quakes, Rice Snacks, av.,1 oz	130	4	26
Rice Cakes:			
Lundberg, (1), average, 0.7 oz	75	0.5	16
Quaker, (1), average, 0.4 oz	50	1	9
Rice Chips (Lundberg), av., 1 oz	140	7	18
Sandwich Crackers:			
Austin, Cheese Crackers:			
With Cheddar, 1.38 oz	190	10	23
With Peanut Butter, 1.3 oz	190	10	23
PB & J Flavored, 1.38 oz	190	8	26
Lance:			
Nip Chee/Toasty, av.. 6 pces	185	9	21
Toast Chee, 6 pieces	220	12	23
Whole Grain: Cheese, 6 pieces	190	9	25
Peanut Butter, 6 pieces	180	9	23
Ritz Bits:			
Cheese: 1.5 oz package	220	13	24
Go-Pak: 13 crackers, 1 oz	150	9	17
3½ oz Pak	520	29	58
P'nut Butter: 1.25 oz pkg	170	10	20
Big Bag (99 cents), 3 oz	420	23	48
Sesame Sticks (SunRidge Farm), 1.1 oz	170	11	14
Smart Puffs (Pirates Booty), 1 oz	150	8	18
Snack Mix (Quaker), Kids Mix, 1 pkg	110	4	18
Soy Crisps, average,1 oz	120	3	17
Soy Nuts: Dry Roasted, ¼ cup, 1 oz	130	6	9
Choc-coated, 1 oz	140	7	13
Sun Chips (Fritolay), average (15 chips), 1 oz	140	6	19
Takis: Fajitas (12), 1 oz	140	7	17
4 oz package	560	28	68
Tings (Robert's), 2 oz bag	300	16	36
Toasted Cheese Crackers (Fritolay), 1 package	220	11	23
Tortilla Chips ~ Page 149			
Tostitos:			
Scoops, Blue; Yellow, av.	140	7	19
Multigrain, 1 oz	150	8	18
Trail Mix (Nuts/Seeds/Dried Fruit):			
Regular, 3 Tbsp, 1 oz	140	9	13
Tropical, 3 Tbsp, 1 oz	130	7	16
Turkey Jerky: Teriyaki, 1 oz	80	1	8
Original (Trader Joe's), 1 oz	60	0.5	6
Veggie Crisps (Snyder's), 1 oz	140	7	18
Wasabi Peas, ¼ cup, 1 oz	120	3	19
Yogurt Pretzels, (7), 1.5 oz	190	7	30
Yogurt Raisins (Sun-Maid), 1 oz	120	4.5	20

Fruit Snacks

	C	F	Cb
Betty Crocker: Fruit Gushers, 0.9 oz	90	1	20
Fruit by the Foot, 1 roll, 0.75 oz	80	1	17
Fruit Roll Ups, 1 roll, 0.5 oz	50	1	12
Fruit Flavored Shapes, All varities, 0.9 oz	80	0	19
Sunkist: Fruit Snacks, 1 pouch	80	0	19
Fruit Smoothie Blitz, 1.3 oz	140	1	32

Vending Machines

	C	F	Cb
Bugles, Nacho Cheese, 1.5 oz	220	12	25
Cheese Balls (Utz), 1 oz	150	9	16
Cheetos, Crunchy, 2 oz	325	20	30
Cheeze-It, Snack Mix, 1.5 oz	195	6.5	30
Chex Mix, average, 1.75 oz	220	5	42
Chester's Fries, 1.75 oz	260	14	29
Choc Chip Cookies: Chips Ahoy, 1.4 oz	190	9	27
Famous Amos, 2 oz	280	13	38
Grandma's, (2), 2⅞ oz	350	14	53
Chocolate Bars:			
Hershey's, 1.55 oz	210	13	26
Kit Kat, 1.5 oz	210	11	28
Snickers, 2.07 oz bar	280	14	35
Donut, plain cake, 1.4 oz	160	9	18
Doritos, 1.75 oz	245	12	32
Fritos Corn Chips, Orig., 1.75 oz	280	17	26
Fruit Pie (Hostess), 4.5 oz	480	20	68
Granola/Cereal Bars, av., 1 oz	140	3	26
M & M'S:			
Milk Chocolate, 1.69 oz	240	10	34
Peanuts, 1.74 oz	250	13	30
Oreo Cookies, 1.8 oz	250	10	37
Peanut Butter Cups,			
Reese's, 1.5 oz	230	13	23
Popcorn, plain, 1 oz	160	10	16
Pop Chips, 0.8 oz	100	3	16
Pork Skins, 1.5 oz	240	15	0
Potato Chips: 1 oz	150	10	15
Baked! (Ruffles), 1.12 oz	140	4	24
Potato Skins (TGI Friday's), 1.5 oz	225	12	29
Pretzels (Snyder's), Old Time, 1 oz	120	1	24
Raisins, ½ oz package	45	0	11
Rice Krispies Treat	90	2	17
Skittles, 2.17 oz	250	2.5	56
Starburst, Fruit Chews, Orig., 2.07 oz	240	4.5	48
Tortilla Chips, 1 oz	140	7	18
Soft Drinks, av.: 12 fl.oz	145	0	40
20 fl.oz bottle	245	0	62

Homemade & Restaurant

Restaurant & Take-Out:
Average All Preparations, Per 8 fl.oz

	C	F	Cb
Bean Medley	200	3	34
Beef Consomme	30	0	2
Borscht (with Sour Cream)	130	8	14
Bouillabaisse	400	15	10
Chicken & Corn	290	14	20
Chicken & Wild Rice	80	4	9
Chicken Consomme	50	0	2
Chicken Curry	180	8	18
Chicken Jambalaya	160	7	8
Chicken Noodle	80	2	12
with Chicken	160	4	12
Chicken Chowder	80	2	6
Chili with Beans	250	12	25
Clam Chowder	240	15	17
Corn & Crab	120	3	18
Corn Chowder	150	8	16
Cream of Broccoli	200	12	20
Cream of Potato	150	6.5	17
Cream of Mushroom	200	13	15
Fish Chowder	220	15	6
French Onion	420	15	15
Gazpacho	50	0	5
Lentil Soup	250	9	28
Lobster Bisque	320	15	10
Matzo Ball (with 1 large ball)	180	7	24
Minestrone	125	2.5	20
Mulligatawny	300	15	8
Pea & Ham	240	10	25
Potato & Bacon	170	7	19
Pumpkin, Creamy	210	10	26
Shark Fin Soup	100	4	8
Spicy Shrimp Soup, 1 bowl	160	7	10
Split Pea Soup	180	2.5	30
Vegetable (Fat Free)	75	0	18
Vegetable Beef	80	2	10
Vichyssoise	200	9	15
Watercress	90	4	13

Other Soups ~ See International & Fast-Foods Sections (Arby's, Au Bon Pain, Boston Market, Dunkin' Donuts, Denny's, Schlotzsky's, Sizzler, Souplantation,Sweet Tomatoes, Zoup!)
Homemade Soups: *Calculate calories, fat and carbohydrates from recipe ingredients.*

Bouillon Cubes & Powders

	C	F	Cb
Bouillon Cubes: *Average all types*			
Regular, 1 cube	5	0	1
Granulate, sodium fre	10	0	2
Powders, average, 1 tsp	10	0	1
Herb-Ox:			
Instant Broth & Seasoning,			
Beef, 1 envelope	5	0	1
Chicken; Vegetarian	5	0	1

Brands

	C	F	Cb
Amy's:			
Heat & Serve (Organic): *Per 1 Cup, Unless Indicated*			
Alphabet	80	0	16
Chunky Vegetable	60	0	13
Cream of M'shrm, ¾ cup	150	9	13
Cream of Tomato	110	2.5	19
Curried Lentil	230	8	30
Fire Roasted Southwestern Vege	140	4	21
Lentil	180	5	25
Lentil Vegetable	160	4	24
Rustic Italian Vegetable	140	6	18
Split Pea	100	0	19
Thai Coconut	140	10	10
Tuscan Bean & Rice	160	4.5	25
Vegetable Barley	70	1	13
Andersen's: *Per 1 Cup*			
Split Pea	130	0	24
Split Pea with Bacon	140	1	23
Tomato	130	3.5	22
Bertoli: *Per ½ package, 12 oz*			
Meal Soups: Chicken Minestrone	370	18	32
Roasted Chicken & Rotini Pasta	290	12	28
Tomato Florentine & Tortellini,			
with Chicken	410	19	36
Tuscan Style Beef & Vegetables	360	20	26
Campbell's:			
Chunky: *Per 8 fl.oz Cup*			
Baked Potato w/ Ched. & Bacon Bits	200	9	24
Chicken Corn Chowder	190	10	20
Classic Chicken Noodle	120	3	14
Hearty Beef Noodle	110	1	17
Hearty Style Ital. Wedding	140	2.5	21
Hearty Tomato with Pasta	140	1	30

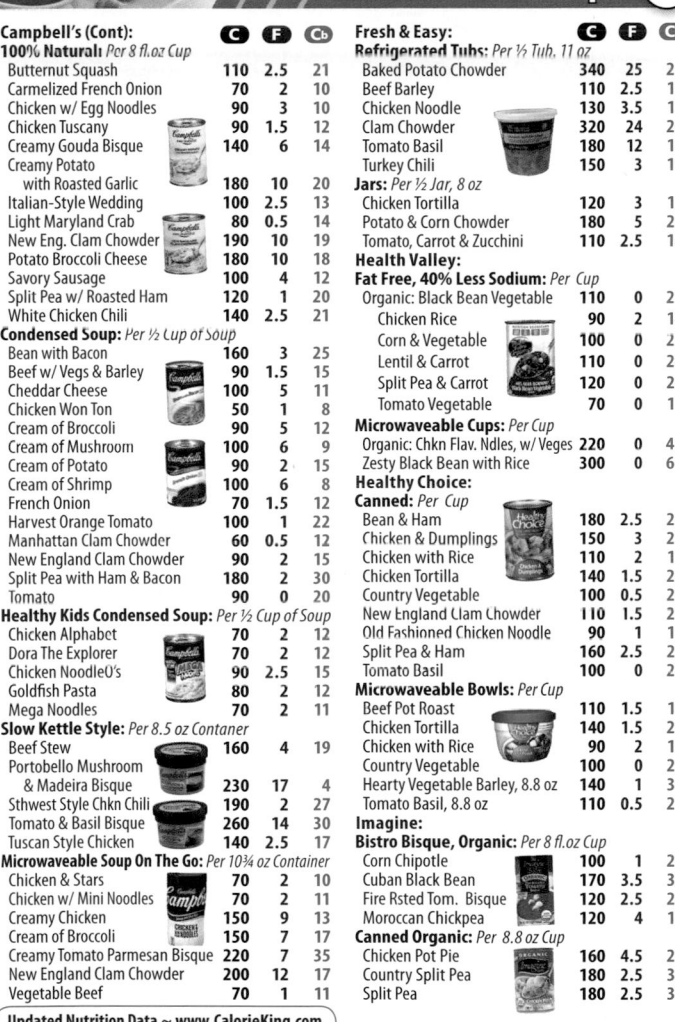

Campbell's (Cont):
100% Natural: *Per 8 fl.oz Cup*

	C	F	Cb
Butternut Squash	110	2.5	21
Carmelized French Onion	70	2	10
Chicken w/ Egg Noodles	90	3	10
Chicken Tuscany	90	1.5	12
Creamy Gouda Bisque	140	6	14
Creamy Potato with Roasted Garlic	180	10	20
Italian-Style Wedding	100	2.5	13
Light Maryland Crab	80	0.5	14
New Eng. Clam Chowder	190	10	19
Potato Broccoli Cheese	180	10	18
Savory Sausage	100	4	12
Split Pea w/ Roasted Ham	120	1	20
White Chicken Chili	140	2.5	21

Condensed Soup: *Per ½ Cup of Soup*

Bean with Bacon	160	3	25
Beef w/ Vegs & Barley	90	1.5	15
Cheddar Cheese	100	5	11
Chicken Won Ton	50	1	8
Cream of Broccoli	90	5	12
Cream of Mushroom	100	6	9
Cream of Potato	90	2	15
Cream of Shrimp	100	6	8
French Onion	70	1.5	12
Harvest Orange Tomato	100	1	22
Manhattan Clam Chowder	60	0.5	12
New England Clam Chowder	90	2	15
Split Pea with Ham & Bacon	180	2	30
Tomato	90	0	20

Healthy Kids Condensed Soup: *Per ½ Cup of Soup*

Chicken Alphabet	70	2	12
Dora The Explorer	70	2	12
Chicken NoodleO's	90	2.5	15
Goldfish Pasta	80	2	12
Mega Noodles	70	2	11

Slow Kettle Style: *Per 8.5 oz Container*

Beef Stew	160	4	14
Portobello Mushroom & Madeira Bisque	230	17	4
Sthwest Style Chkn Chili	190	2	27
Tomato & Basil Bisque	260	14	30
Tuscan Style Bisque	140	2.5	17

Microwaveable Soup On The Go: *Per 10¾ oz Container*

Chicken & Stars	70	2	10
Chicken w/ Mini Noodles	70	2	11
Creamy Chicken	150	9	13
Cream of Broccoli	150	7	17
Creamy Tomato Parmesan Bisque	220	7	35
New England Clam Chowder	200	12	17
Vegetable Beef	70	1	11

Fresh & Easy:
Refrigerated Tubs: *Per ½ Tub, 11 oz*

	C	F	Cb
Baked Potato Chowder	340	25	22
Beef Barley	110	2.5	13
Chicken Noodle	130	3.5	17
Clam Chowder	320	24	20
Tomato Basil	180	12	15
Turkey Chili	150	3	19

Jars: *Per ½ Jar, 8 oz*

Chicken Tortilla	120	3	11
Potato & Corn Chowder	180	5	27
Tomato, Carrot & Zucchini	110	2.5	18

Health Valley:
Fat Free, 40% Less Sodium: *Per Cup*

Organic: Black Bean Vegetable	110	0	25
Chicken Rice	90	2	14
Corn & Vegetable	100	0	22
Lentil & Carrot	110	0	24
Split Pea & Carrot	120	0	26
Tomato Vegetable	70	0	17

Microwaveable Cups: *Per Cup*

Organic: Chkn Flav. Ndles, w/ Veges	220	0	48
Zesty Black Bean with Rice	300	0	66

Healthy Choice:
Canned: *Per Cup*

Bean & Ham	180	2.5	28
Chicken & Dumplings	150	3	22
Chicken with Rice	110	2	17
Chicken Tortilla	140	1.5	23
Country Vegetable	100	0.5	20
New England Clam Chowder	110	1.5	20
Old Fashioned Chicken Noodle	90	1	12
Split Pea & Ham	160	2.5	27
Tomato Basil	100	0	22

Microwaveable Bowls: *Per Cup*

Beef Pot Roast	110	1.5	17
Chicken Tortilla	140	1.5	23
Chicken with Rice	90	2	13
Country Vegetable	100	0	20
Hearty Vegetable Barley, 8.8 oz	140	1	30
Tomato Basil, 8.8 oz	110	0.5	25

Imagine:
Bistro Bisque, Organic: *Per 8 fl.oz Cup*

Corn Chipotle	100	1	22
Cuban Black Bean	170	3.5	30
Fire Rsted Tom. Bisque	120	2.5	24
Moroccan Chickpea	120	4	16

Canned Organic: *Per 8.8 oz Cup*

Chicken Pot Pie	160	4.5	22
Country Split Pea	180	2.5	30
Split Pea	180	2.5	30

Imagine (Cont):

	C	F	Cb
Creamy: *Per 8 fl.oz Cup*			
Acorn Squash & Mango; Chicken	70	1.5	14
Harvest Corn	110	3	20
Portobello Mushroom	80	3	10
Potato Leek	70	1.5	12
Sweet Pea	80	1.5	14
Tomato	90	2	18

Kettle Cuisine: *Per 10 oz*

	C	F	Cb
Gluten Free:			
Angus Beef Steak Chili w/ Beans	250	9	21
Chicken: Chili w/ White Beans	320	15	23
With Rice Noodles	140	3	15
Sthwest & Corn Chdr	230	10	21
Thai Curry	330	11	44
NE Clam Chowder	310	17	26
Organic Mushroom & Potato	170	6	25
Roasted Vegetable	190	9	23
Three Bean Chili	220	3.5	36
Tomato with Garden Vegetables	110	3.5	16

Knorr:

	C	F	Cb
Cubes: *Per ½ Cube, 1 Cup, Prepared*			
Beef; Chicken, av.	15	1.5	1
Vegetable	20	1	1
Homestyle Stock: *Per 1 Tsp*			
Beef	10	1	0
Chicken	10	2	0

Lipton:

	C	F	Cb
Cup-a-Soup: *Per Envelope*			
Chicken Noodle, Original	50	1	10
Cream of Chicken	60	0.5	12
Tomato with Croutons	80	1.5	14
Recipe Secrets: *Per 1 Tbsp Dry Mix*			
Onion	20	0	4
Onion Roasted Garlic	45	0	8
Savory Herb with Garlic	25	0	6

Manischewitz:

	C	F	Cb
Cans: *Per ½ Cup Soup*			
Chicken Consume, Clear	15	0	2
Chicken Kreplach	40	1	6
Chicken Noodle	60	1.5	7
Quart Jars: *Per 6 fl.oz*			
Borscht with Beets	50	0	13
Borscht, Low Calorie	15	0	4
Ready To Serve,			
Matzo Ball Chicken, 1 cup, 8 fl.oz	120	4.5	14

Maruchan:

	C	F	Cb
Instant Lunch,			
average all flavors, 1 pkg	290	12	38
Ramen, all flavors:, 1 pkg, 3 oz	380	14	52

Nile Spice: *Per Cup*

	C	F	Cb
Black Bean; Lentil	195	1.5	35
Couscous Minestrone	180	1.5	34
Potato Leek	120	3	17
Split Pea	200	1	35

Nissin:

	C	F	Cb
Souper Meal: *Per ½ of 4.3 oz Ctn*			
Chicken	290	13	38
Picante Shrimp	270	11	36
Top Ramen: *Per ½ of 3 oz Ctn*			
Beef/ Chicken Flavor, average	190	7	27

Pacific Foods:

	C	F	Cb
Condensed Soups: *Per ½ cup, 4.65 oz*			
Cream of Celery	70	2.5	11
Cream of Mushroom	100	2.5	18
Creamy Organic: *Per ¼ of 32 fl.oz Container, 8 fl.oz*			
French Onion	30	1	5
Cashew Carrot Ginger Bisque	130	5	20
Curried Red Lentil	140	4.5	20
Thai Sweet Potato	160	6	25
Tomato	100	2	16

Progresso:

	C	F	Cb
Rich & Hearty: *Per ½ Can, 1 Cup*			
Chicken & Homestyle Noodles	110	2.5	14
Chicken Corn Chowder	200	9	23
Loaded Potato w/ Bacon	180	9	20
New Engl. Clam Chowder	180	8	22
Savory Beef Barley Veg.	130	2.5	17
Steak & HomeStyle Noodles	110	2.5	14
Traditional: *Per ½ Can, 1 Cup*			
Chicken Noodle	100	2.5	12
Homestyle Chicken w/ Veggies & Pasta	100	2	14
Italian-Style Wedding	120	4	11
Split Pea with Ham	140	1	24
Vegetable Classic: *Per ½ Can, 1 Cup*			
French Onion	50	1	9
Green Split Pea w/ Bacon	160	2	28
Garden Vegetable	90	0	20
Minestrone	100	2	20
Tomato Rotini	130	0.5	28
Light: *Per ½ Can, 1 cup*			
Beef Pot Roast	80	2	10
Chicken Pot Pie	100	3	15
Italian Style Vegetable	70	0	16
Vegetable & Noodle	60	0.5	13
World Recipes: *Per ½ Can*			
Black Bean Jalapeno	130	1	30
Chicken & Vegetable	90	1.5	14
Chicken Tortilla	110	2.5	17

Safeway (Vons):	C	F	Cb
Signature Soups: Per Cup			
Broccoli & Cheesy Cheddar	270	18	18
Chunky Chicken Noodle	160	5	14
Fiesta Chicken Tortilla	110	2	15
Italian-Style Wedding	120	4	14
Pacific Coast Clam Chowder	330	24	27
Savory Chicken & Orzo	90	0.5	13
Tuscan Tomato & Basil Bisque	330	22	27
Swanson:			
Broth: Per 8 fl.oz Cup			
Chicken, 99% Fat-Free	10	0.5	1
Vegetable	15	0	3
Organic, Chicke n,			
99% Fat-Free	15	0	1
Tabatchnick:			
Frozen Soups:			
Dairy: Per 15 oz Pouch			
Corn Chowder	130	4.5	21
Cream of Broccoli	90	4	12
New England Potato	140	4	24
Gluten Free: Per 15 oz Pouch			
Split Pea	140	0	34
Southwest Bean	220	5	35
Vegetarian Chili	180	3.5	28
Low Sodium: Per 15 oz Pouch			
Barley Mushroom	80	1	17
Split Pea	140	0	34
Vegetable	90	1.5	17
Meatl Per 15 oz Pouch			
Frenchman's Onion	60	1.5	11
Wilderness Wild Rice	80	0.5	16
Parve: Per 15 oz Pouch			
Balsamic Tom. & Rice	110	3.5	18
Black Bean	230	2.5	39
Minestrone	100	1.5	18
Shelf Stable: Per 2/3 Cup, 5.3 fl.oz			
Broth: Classic Chicken	5	0	0
Kosher Chicken	10	0	1
Soup: Creamy Tomato	70	2	14
Roasted Red Pepper & Tomato	70	2.5	13
Wisconsin Cheddar Cheese	150	11	10
Thai Kitchen:			
Rice Noodle Soup Bowls: Per Bowl			
Hot & Sour	250	4	51
Lemongrass & Chili	250	3.5	52
Spring Onion	260	4.5	50
Roasted Garlic	250	3	52
Thai Ginger	260	3	52

Trader Joe's:	C	F	Cb
28 fl. oz Cans: Per Cup			
Chunky, Low Fat:			
Lentil with Vegetables	140	3	21
Minestrone	110	2.5	19
14½ oz Cans: Per Cup			
Organic: Black Bean	130	1.5	25
Lentil Vegetable, ½ can	130	3.5	19
Split Pea	100	0	19
10¾ oz Can,			
Low Sodium, Minestrone	200	4	37
15 oz Can,			
Low Fat, Chicken Noodle, 1 cup	90	1	14
32 fl. oz Cartons: Per Cup			
Butternut Squash	90	2	16
Carrot & Ginger	80	1	17
Crmy Corn & Rstd Pepper	110	2	23
Latin Style Black Bean	70	1	12
Sweet Potato Bisque	130	1	28
Organic: Butternut Squash	70	0	17
Tom. & Rstd Red Pepper	100	2	16
Low Sodium, Crmy Tomato	90	3.5	15
Light Sodium, Tomato Bisque	130	4	21
17.6 fl. oz Cartons: Per Cup			
Beef, Barley with Veggies	100	0.5	16
Chicken Noodle with Veggies	100	1	16
Whole Foods: Per Cup			
365 Organic: Black Bean	150	1	25
Chicken Noodle	90	2	11
Cream of Mushroom	100	6	11
Minestrone	120	2	21
Tomato	90	3.5	14
Vegetable	70	1	11
Wolfgang Puck: Per Cup			
Organic:			
Butternut Squash	200	11	22
Chicken & Dumplings	140	7	14
Classic Minestrone	120	2.5	20
Corn Chowder	210	13	20
Creamy Tomato	250	16	23
Free Range Chicken with			
White & Wild Rice	110	4	15
Hearty Garden Vegetable	130	4	22
Hearty Lentil & Vegetable	150	1	24
Signature Tortilla	160	3.5	27
Tomato Basil Bisque	150	6	21

Soybean Products

	C	F	Cb
Cheeses (Soy) ~ *See Page 78*			
Miso Soy Bean Paste:			
Cold Mountain: Light Yellow, 1 tsp	10	0	1
Mellow Red, 1 tsp	15	0	3
Red, 1 tsp	10	0	1
Miso Soup (dry mix):			
1 Tbsp., dry mix	35	1	5
1 cup, prepared	35	1	5
Natto, ½ cup, 3 oz	160	7	14
Okara (Tofu fiber residue), ½ c., 2 oz	47	1	8
Tempeh: 1 piece, 3 oz	180	8	12
Fried, 3 oz	250	14	14
Seitan (Westsoy), Strips, 3 oz	120	2	4
Soybean Protein (TVP), 1 oz	95	0	8
Soy Bean Paste, 1 tsp	10	0	2
Soy Beans ~ *See Page 160*			
Soy Drinks ~ *See Page 49*			

Tofu ~ Packaged

	C	F	Cb
Azumaya Tofu:			
Extra Firm; Firm, av., 3 oz	70	4	2
Soft (Silken), 3.2 oz	40	2	1
House Foods: Per 3 oz			
Premium Tofu: Extra Firm	80	4	1
Firm	70	3.5	2
Medium Firm (Regular)	60	3	2
Soft (Silken)	50	2.5	2
Organic Tofu: Firm	60	3.5	0
Extra Firm	70	4	0
Ethnic: Tokusen Kinugoshi	90	4	3
Sukui; Soon (Extra Soft)	45	2	2
Yaki Tofu (Broiled)	90	5	2
Seasoned, Garlic & Pepper	90	4	1
Mori-Nu Tofu:			
Silken: Soft, 3 oz, 1" slice	45	2.5	2
Firm, 3 oz, 1" slice	50	2.5	2
Extra Firm, 3 oz, 1" slice	45	1.5	2
Organic, Silken 3 oz, 1" slice	50	2.5	2
Lite, Firm, 3 oz, 1" slice	30	1	1
Nasoya: Soft, 2.8 oz	60	3	1
Silken, 3.2 oz	45	2	1
Firm, ⅓ pkg., 2.8 oz	70	3	2
Extra Firm, ⅓ pkg., 2.8 oz	80	4	2
Tofuplus: Extra Firm, 3 oz	80	4	2
Firm, 3 oz	70	3	2
Sprouted, 3 oz	100	5	3

Supplements

	C	F	Cb
Aloe Vera Juice, undiluted, 2 fl.oz	5	0	1
Brewer's Yeast: Tablets, 2 tabs	4	0	0.5
Flakes, 1 heaping Tbsp, 0.3 oz	30	0.5	4
Powder, 1 heaping Tbsp, 0.5 oz	50	0.5	6
Calcium Chews: CVS, 1 chew	20	0	3
Chocolate (Trader Joe's), 1 chew	20	1	3
Cod Liver Oil, 1 Tbsp	125	13	0
2 tabs (Fiber Choice)	15	0	4
Fiber (Fibersure),			
1 heaping tsp	25	0	6
Fish Oil Capsules, av., 1	10	1	0
Flax Oil: Capsules, 2	10	1	0
3 softgels (Barlean's)	110	11	0
Garlic Tablets/Capsules, each	3	0	0
Glowelle:			
Beauty Drink, 8 fl.oz	100	0	24
Powder Stick (1)	50	0	12
Lecithin Granules, 1 Tbsp	55	4	0.5
Metamucil, Powder:			
Orange (Smooth Texture),			
1 rounded Tbsp	45	0	12
Sugar-Free, 1 rounded tsp	20	0	5
Pink Lemonade, Sugar-Free,			
1 rounded tsp	20	0	5
Fiber Wafers, (2)	120	5	17
Capsules:			
Heart & Digestive (6)	10	0	3
Strong Bones (5)	10	0	3
Protein, Powders, average, 1 oz	100	0.5	0
Seaweed: Dried, 1 oz	85	0.5	22
Soaked, drained, 1 oz	15	0.5	3
Spirulina, 1 tablet	2	0	0.5
Vitamins/Minerals: Tabs/Caps, 1	2	0	0
Vitamin E Capsules, each	5	0.5	0
Viactiv Chews, (1)	20	0.5	4

Cough & Pharmaceutical

	C	F	Cb
Antacids: Av., 1 tablet	4	0	1
Liquid, 1 Tbsp	6	0	1
Antacid Sodium Counts ~ *See Page 280*			
Cough/Cold Syrups:			
Regular: With sugar, 1 Tbsp	35	0	9
With alcohol, 1 Tbsp	46	0	9
Sugar-Free (Diabetic Tussin), 1 T.	0	0	0
Cough Drops/Lozenges ~ *See Page 75*			
Syrup (Sudafed), 1 tsp	14	0	3
Liquid (Tylenol): Child, 1 tsp	17	0	4
Extra Strength, 1 tsp	11	0	3

Sugar ◊ Syrups ◊ Topping ◊ Honey & Jam S

Sugar

	C	F	Cb
White Sugar, granulated:			
1 level teaspoon	15	0	4
1 heaping teaspoon	25	0	6
1 Tablespoon	50	0	12
1 ounce, 1 oz	110	0	28
1 cup, 7 oz	775	0	200
1 pound	1760	0	454
Single Portion Packages:			
1 stick	15	0	4
1 packet, 0.1 oz	10	0	3
1 cube, 0.08 oz	10	0	2.5
Brown Sugar: 1 Tbsp	50	0	13
1 ounce, 1 oz	110	0	28
1 cup, not packed, 5 oz	550	0	140
1 cup, packed, 7.75 oz	835	0	216
Powdered/Confectioners:			
Sifted, 1 cup, 3.5 oz	390	0	100
Unsifted, 1 cup, 4.25 oz	465	0	120
Cinnamon Sugar, 1 tsp	15	0	4
Dextrose, 1¼ tsp	15	0	4
Fructose: Dry, 1 tsp	15	0	4
Liquid, 1 oz	80	0	21
Glucose, 1 oz	110	0	27
Glucose Tablets, (1)	20	0	5
Palm Sugar, 3 Tbsp	45	0	11
Piloncillo, (Brown Sugar), 3oz	325	0	81
Turbinado Sugar, 2 Tbsp, 1 oz	110	0	27
Unrefined Cane Sugar, 1 oz	110	0	27

Sugar Substitutes

	C	F	Cb
DiabetiSweet, 1 teaspoon	9	0	4.5
(Carbohydrate as Sugar Alcohol)			
Equal: Tablet (2)	0	0	0
Granular, 1 tsp	0	0	0
Packet (1)	0	0	0
Natra Taste; Sweet One, 1 packet	0	0	0
NutraSweet, 1 tsp	0	0	0
Splenda:			
Granulated No Calorie Sweetener:			
1 tsp	0	0	0
1 cup	95	0	24
Packets, all flavors	0	0	0
Sugar Blend,Orig/Brown, ½ cup	385	0	96
Stevia, single serving	0	0	0
Sugar Twin, 1 packet	0	0	0
Sweet 'N Low, 1 packet	0	0	0
Truvia, 1 packet	0	0	0
Walgreens, Wal-Sweet, 1 packet	0	0	0
Whey Low, 1 tsp	4	0	1

Syrups, Molasses, Agave

Syrups: *Average All Brands* *(Corn/Rice/Maple/Pancake/Sundae/Waffle)* Includes Aunt Jemima, Cary's, Karo, Hershey's, Hungry Jack, IHOP, Log Cabin, Mrs Butterworth's

Regular/Dark/Light Color:	C	F	Cb
1 Tbsp, ½ fl.oz	55	0	14
¼ cup (4 Tbsp)	220	0	55
Single Portion, 1½ oz pkg	170	0	42
Lite, 1Tbsp, 1 oz	25	0	6
Sugar-Free: 2 Tbsp, 1 oz	18	0	5
2 Tbsp *(Maple Grove, Cozy Cott.)*	10	0	3
4 Tbsp *(IHOP),* 2 oz	20	0	7
Fruit Syrups, *(IHOP),* ¼ cup, 2 oz	200	0	50
Honey Cream Syrup, ¼ c., 2 oz	220	0	55
Molasses: Dark/Light: 1 T, 0.75 oz	55	0	14
1 cup, 11.5 oz	880	0	224
Blackstrap, 1 Tbsp, 0.75 oz	47	0	13
Agave Nectar, av. all flav.			
1 Tablespoon, 0.75 oz	60	0	15

Ice Cream Toppings

	C	F	Cb
Average All Types & Brands: *Per 2 Tbsp*			
(Hershey's): Caramel	110	0	27
Chocolate; Fruit Flavors, av	100	0	25
Lite	45	0	11
(Smuckers):			
Microwaveable:			
Hot, Caramel; Fudge, av.	130	3.5	25
Sugar Free Spoonables: Caramel	90	0	24
Hot Fudge	90	0.5	23
Sugar Free Sundae Syrup:			
Strawberry	110	0	26
Average other flavors	100	0	25

Honey, Jam, Preserves

Average All Brands	C	F	Cb
Honey: 1 tsp, 0.25 oz	22	0	5.5
1 Tbsp, 0.75 oz	65	0	17
1 ounce, 1 oz	85	0	23
1 cup, 12 oz	1030	0	269
Single Portion, 0.5 oz package	45	0	11
Jams/Jellies/Marmalade/Preserves:			
Regular: 1 tsp, 0.25 oz	20	0	5
1 Tbsp, 0.75 oz	55	0	14
1 ounce, 1 oz	80	0	20
Single Portion, 0.5 oz pkg	40	0	11
Apple/Fruit Butters, 1 T., 0.6 oz	20	0	6
Fruit Spreads: Regular, 1 tsp	15	0	4
Low Sugar, 1 tsp	8	0	2
Low Calorie *(Featherweight),* 1 tsp	8	0	2
Jelly: Regular, average, 1 tsp	18	0	4.5
Imitation, Low Calorie, 1 tsp	4	0	1

V Vegetables & Legumes

Vegetables

Vegetables	C	F	Cb
Alfalfa Sprouts, ½ cup, 0.5 oz	5	0	0.5
Artichokes, Globe/French:			
1 medium, 4.5 oz	60	0	13
1 large, 5.7 oz	75	0	17
Artichoke Heart, plain, 2 pces	15	0	3
Asparagus, raw/frozen:			
3 medium spears	10	0	2
Cuts & Tips (Del Monte), ½ cup, 4.3 oz	20	0	3
Bamboo Shoots, cooked, ½ c., 2 oz	7	0	1
Beans: Green/Snap/String, ½ c., 2 oz	20	0	4
10 beans (4" long), 2 oz	20	0	4
Dried, average all types:			
(Kidney, Brown, Lima, Navy, Pinto, White)			
Raw: 2 Tbsp, 1 oz	95	0.5	18
1 cup, 7 oz	665	3	126
Cooked: 1 oz	35	0	7
½ cup, 3 oz	105	0	21
Bean Sprouts, average, ½ c., 2 oz	15	0	3.5
Beets (Beetroot):			
Raw, 1 beet (2" diam), 4 oz	35	0	8
Cooked, 1 cup, slices, 3 oz	35	0	8
Canned ~ *See Page 168*			
Beet Greens, cooked, ½ cup, 2.5 oz	20	0	4
Bell Pepper ~ *See Peppers*			
Bitter Melon/Gourd, 1 cup, 1.5 oz	15	0	1.5
Blackeye Peas, cooked, ½ cup, 3 oz	100	0.5	18
Bok Choy (Chinese Chard), ckd, 3 oz	10	0	1.5
Breadfruit, ¼ small fruit, 3 oz	100	0	26
Broadbeans (Fava Beans):			
Green, raw, (in pod): 4 pods			
(3½ oz w/ shells; 1.2 oz beans)	30	0	6
1 cup beans (w/o shell), 4.5 oz	110	1	22
Mature Seeds: Raw, 1 cup, 5.3 oz	510	2.5	87
Cooked, ½ cup, 3 oz	95	0	17
Broccoflower, ⅕ head, 3.5 oz	35	0	7
Broccoli: Raw, chopped, 1 cup, 3 oz	30	0	6
3 Florets, 2.5 oz	25	0	5
1 Spear (5" long), 1.1 oz	10	0	2
1 Whole: Medium, 14 oz	135	1.5	26
Large, 21 oz	205	2	40
1 Head (no stalk), 11 oz	105	1	21
1 Stalk, small (5" long), 5.3 oz	50	0.5	10
Brocco Sprouts, ½ cup, 1 oz	15	0	2
Brussels Sprouts: Cooked, ½ c., 2.8 oz	30	0.5	6
2 Sprouts, 1.5 oz	15	0	3
Butterbeans, cooked, ½ cup, 3 oz	90	0	16
Cabbage, all types, average:			
Raw: 1 Leaf, large, 1 oz	5	0	2
Shredded, 1 cup, 2.5 oz	15	0	4
½ Large Head (7" diam), 22 oz	150	1	35
Cooked, shredded, ½ cup, 2.5 oz	15	0.5	3.5

Vegetables (Cont)

Vegetables (Cont)	C	F	Cb
Cactus Leaf (Nopales):			
1 leaf, 4½ oz	20	0	4
1 cup (slices), 3 oz	15	0	3
Carrots, regular thick variety:			
1 small, 4 oz	45	0	11
1 medium, 6 oz	70	0	16
1 large, 8 oz	95	0	22
Chopped, 1 cup, 4.5 oz	50	0	12
Grated, 1 cup, 4 oz	45	0	11
Slices, 1 cup, 4.5 oz	50	0	12
Sticks (4"), 4-5, 1.5 oz	20	0	4
Long thin variety, 1 medium, 2.2 oz	25	0	6
Baby: Snack size, 3 medium, 1 oz	10	0	2.5
Snack Pack, 3 oz	30	0	7
Cauliflower: Raw: 1 cup (pieces), 3.5 oz	25	0	5
½ medium head, 10 oz	70	0	15
Cooked, 3 florets, 2 oz	10	0	2
Celeriac, ½ cup, raw, 2.75 oz	35	0	7
Celery: 1 large stalk, 11", 2.2 oz	10	0	2
1 small stalk, 5", 0.5 oz	2	0	0.5
4 Strips, thin sticks, 0.5 oz	5	0	1
Chopped, 1 cup, 3.5 oz	15	0	3
Chard (Swiss), ½ cup, cooked, 3 oz	20	0	3.5
Chayote Squash: 1 medium, 7 oz	40	0	9
1 cup (pieces), 4.5 oz	25	0	6
Chick Peas:			
Dry, 1 cup, 7 oz	730	12	121
Cooked, 1 cup, 6 oz	270	4	45
Chicory Greens, 1 cup, 1 oz	7	0	1.5
Chili Peppers ~ *See Peppers*			
Chinese Long Bean, sl., 1 cup, 3.2 oz	45	0	8
Chives, chopped, 1 Tbsp	1	0	0
Choy Sum, 3 oz	15	0	3
Cilantro (Coriander), 1 cup	5	0	0.5
Collards, cooked, ½ cup, 3 oz	25	0	5
Corn, Yellow/White:			
Raw: Kernels, ½ cup, 3 oz	80	0.5	19
Ear (5"x 1¾"), 5.5 oz	155	1	37
Cooked: Kernels, ½ cup, 3 oz	77	0.5	18
Cob, Small, 2.25 oz	60	0.5	14
Large ear, 5.5 oz	120	1	28
Courgette ~ *See Zucchini*			
Cowpeas ~ *See Blackeye Peas*			
Cress, garden, raw, 1 cup, 1.75 oz	15	0	3
Cucumber: 1 whole, 11 oz	45	0.5	11
½ cup slices, 2 oz	10	0	2
Mini/Lebanese (1), 3 oz	15	0	3
Daikon Radish, ½ cup, slices, 2 oz	9	0	2
Dandelion Greens, raw, ½ cup, 1 oz	10	0	2.5
Edamame *(Immature green soybeans):*			
Shelled, ½ cup, 2.6 oz	110	5	8
With shells, 10 pods, 1.25 oz	30	1	3

Vegetables (Cont)	C	F	Cb
Eggplant: Raw, 4 oz	**30**	0	7
Raw, ½ cup, 1" pieces, 1.5 oz	**10**	0	2
1 slice, fried, 1 oz	**75**	4	10
Endive, Belgian/French: Raw,			
1 medium head (6"), 2.5 oz	**12**	0	3
Fennel, 1 cup, sliced, 3 oz	**25**	0	7
Gai Choy Cabbage, ckd, 1 c. 6 oz	**20**	0	3
Gai Lan, (Chinese Kale), cooked, 1 c.	**35**	0.5	7
Garlic, 1 clove	**4**	0	1
Ginger: ¼ cup slices, 1 oz	**20**	0	5
Crystallized (sugared), 7 pieces, 1.5 oz	**130**	0	35
Horseradish, raw, 1 pod, 0.5 oz	**5**	0	1
Jerusalem Artichoke, raw, ½ cup	**55**	0	13
Jicama, raw, sliced, ½ cup, 2.25 oz	**25**	0	6
Kale, 1 cup, chopped, 2.5 oz	**35**	0.5	7
Kohlrabi, ½ cup, cooked, 1.75 oz	**17**	0	5
Leek, cooked, 1 whole, 4.5 oz	**40**	0	9
Lentils, green/brown: Dry, 1 oz	**100**	0.5	17
1 cup, 6.75 oz	**675**	3	115
Cooked, ½ cup, 3.5 oz	**115**	0.5	20
Lettuce: 1 cup, chopped/shred., 2 oz	**7**	0	1
Butterhead, 2 leaves, 0.5 oz	**2**	0	0.5
Cos/Romaine, shredded, 1 c.	**10**	0	2
Iceberg: 1 outer leaf, 0.5 oz	**2**	0	0.5
1 meium head, 16 oz	**75**	1	16
Lima Beans, baby, cooked, ½ c., 3 oz	**105**	0	20
Lotus Root, 10 slices, cooked, 3 oz	**60**	0	14
Mung Bean Sprouts, ½ cup, 2 oz	**15**	0	3
Mushrooms: Raw, 1 med., 0.6 oz	**4**	0	0.5
1 large, sliced, 0.75 oz	**5**	0	1
½ cup pieces, 1.25 oz	**8**	0	1
Fried/Sauteed, 6 oz	**220**	16	11
Steamed, ½ cup pieces, 2.5 oz	**20**	0.5	4
Mustard Greens, raw, ½ cup, 1 oz	**7**	0	2
Nopales ~ *See Cactus Leaf*			
Okra: Raw, 8 pods, 4 oz	**30**	0	7
Cooked, ½ cup, 2.75 oz	**20**	0	4
Onions, Raw: 1 small, 2.5 oz	**30**	0	7
1 medium, 4 oz	**50**	0	11
1 large, 5.5 oz	**65**	0	15
1 jumbo, 16 oz	**190**	0.5	46
Chopped: ½ cup, 3 oz	**35**	0	8
1 Tbsp, 0.4 oz	**5**	0	1
Slices: 1 cup, 4 oz	**50**	0	12
1 medium slice (⅛"), 0.5 oz	**5**	0	1
1 large slice (¼"), 1.3 oz	**15**	0	4
Dehydrated flakes, ¼ cup, 0.5 oz	**50**	0	12
Rings, breaded & fried, 2 rings	**80**	5	9
Scallions, ½ cup, 2 oz	**15**	0	3
Spring, ½ cup, chopped, 2 oz	**15**	0	3
French's Fried Onions ~ *See Page 114*			
Blossom/Blooming ~ *See Fast-Foods (Chili's/Outback)*			

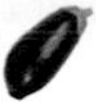
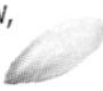

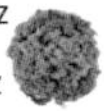
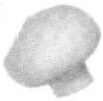
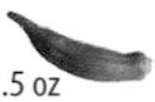
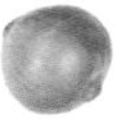

Updated Nutrition Data ~ www.CalorieKing.com
Persons with Diabetes ~ See Disclaimer (Page 22)

Vegetables (Cont)	C	F	Cb
Parsley, chopped, ½ cup, 1 oz	**10**	0	2
Parsnip: 1 medium, 4 oz	**85**	0	20
Cooked, ½ cup slices, 2.75 oz	**55**	0	13
Peas: Green, raw, ¼ cup, 1.5oz	**30**	0	5
With pods, 0.5 lb	**70**	0	13
Snow Peas, 10 pods, 1.2 oz	**15**	0	3
Split: Dry, hulled, 1 oz	**100**	0.5	17
Cooked, 1 cup, 7 oz	**230**	1	42
Peppers: Sweet, 1 medium, 4.2 oz	**30**	0	7
Bell: 1 medium, 4.2 oz	**30**	0	7
½ cup, chopped, raw, 2.5 oz	**20**	0	5
2 rings (5" diam. x ¼" thick)	**3**	0	1
Chili: Green/Red, 1.5 oz	**20**	0	5
Habanero, 1 only, 0.3 oz	**10**	0	2
Pigeon Peas, cooked, ½ cup, 3 oz	**95**	1	17
Pimientos, 3 medium, 3.5 oz	**25**	0	5
Poi, ½ cup, 4.2 oz	**135**	0	33
Potatoes:			
Raw (with skin):			
1 Baby, 2 oz	**45**	0	10
1 Small, 6 oz	**135**	0	30
1 Medium, 8 oz	**180**	0	40
1 Large, 12 oz	**270**	0	60
1 Extra large, 16 oz	**360**	0	80
Baked, (no added fat), large, 10 oz (raw wt):			
Plain: With skin, 7 oz (ckd wt)	**185**	0	42
Without skin, 5.5 oz (ckd wt)	**145**	0	34
With Skin/Toppings:			
+ 2 tsp fat	**270**	8	58
+ Sour Cream & Chives, 2 T.	**320**	6	60
+ Plain Yogurt, 2 Tbsp	**260**	1	60
+ Grated Cheese, 1 oz	**370**	9	58
Mashed:			
With milk plus fat, ½ cup, 4 oz	**120**	4.5	18
KFC Style without gravy, 4 oz	**90**	3	15
Loaded (fat/cream/cheese/bacon):			
Side serving, 6 oz	**180**	9	22
Large serving, 12 oz	**360**	18	44
Potato Skins, (Baked with cheese topping),			
½ whole, 4 oz	**240**	13	22
French Fries: Small serving, 2.6 oz	**250**	13	30
Medium serving, 4 oz	**380**	20	47
Frozen, uncooked, 18 fries, 4 oz	**165**	5.5	28
Oven-heated, 18 fries, 4 oz	**165**	5.5	28
Take-Out, 1 cup, 5 oz	**440**	25	60
Fried, 18 pieces, 4 oz	**165**	5.5	28
Au Gratin, ½ c., 4.3 oz	**160**	9	14
Pancakes, 2 small, 2 oz	**120**	6.5	12
Puffs, fried, 4 puffs, 1 oz	**55**	2.5	8
Scalloped, 1 cup, 8.5 oz	**220**	9	26

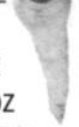
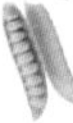

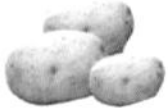
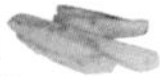

Vegetables (Cont) | C | F | Cb

	C	F	Cb
Pumpkin:			
Raw, 1" cubes, 1 cup, 4 oz 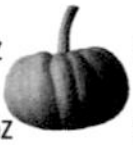	30	0	7
Cooked:			
Baked, without fat, 4 oz	90	7	9
Mashed: 1 scoop, 2 oz	10	0	2
½ cup, 4⅓ oz	25	0	6
Pumpkin Flowers, 1 cup, 1.2 oz	5	0	1
Purslane: Cooked, ½ cup, 2 oz	10	0	2
Raw, 1" cubes, 1 cup, 1.5 oz	5	0	1.5
Radicchio: 2 leaves, 0.5 oz	5	0	1
Shredded, 1 cup, 1.5 oz 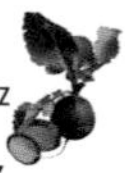	20	0	4
Radishes: 1 small	0	0	0
10 medium/5 large, 1.6 oz	5	0	1
½ cup (slices), 2 oz	10	0	2
Rhubarb: raw, ½ cup, 2 oz	15	0	3
Rutabaga: ckd, ½ c., (cubes), 3 oz	30	0	7
Salsify: ckd, ½ cup, (slices), 2.5 oz	50	0	11
Sauerkraut, ½ cup, 2.5 oz 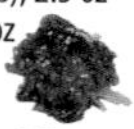	15	0	3
Seaweed: Dried, 1 oz	5	0	2
Soaked, drained, 1 oz	15	0	4
Nori/Laver, dried, 6 sheets, 0.5 oz	35	0	5
Shallots, 1 Tbsp, (chopped) ,0.5 oz 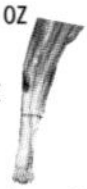	5	0	1
Sorrel, raw, ½ cup, 4 oz	20	0	4
Soybeans: Dry, ½ cup, 3.3 oz	390	18	28
Mature, dry, 1 oz	120	5.5	9
Cooked, ½ cup, 3 oz	150	7.5	8
Soy Products/Tofu/Tempeh ~ *See Page 156*			
Spinach: Cooked, ½ cup, 3 oz	20	0	4
Creamed, ½ cup, 4.5 oz	190	15	8
Raw: 3 leaves,1 cup, 1 oz 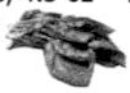	7	0	1
1 Bunch, 12 oz	80	1.5	12
Squash: 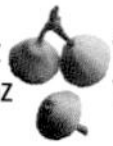			
Summer, Raw: ½ cup, 2.5 oz	10	0	2
Cooked, ½ cup slices, 3 oz	15	0	3
Winter, Cooked:			
Acorn: ½ cup cubes, 3.5² oz	35	0	9
½ medium (10 oz raw weight)	115	0	30
Butternut: ½ cup, (cubes), 3.5 oz	40	0	10
¼ medium (9 oz raw weight)	115	0	30
Spaghetti, ½ cup, 1.75 oz	15	0	3
Succotash, cooked, ½ cup,3.3 oz	110	1	23
Sweetcorn ~ *See Corn* 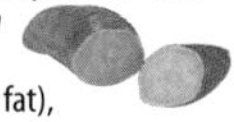			
Sweet Potatoes:			
Cooked with skin (w/o fat), 1 medium, 4 oz	105	0	24
Without skin, mashed, ½ c., 5.5 oz	125	0	29
Fries (Alexia, Julienne syle), approximately 12 pieces, 3 oz	140	5	24

Vegetables (Cont) | C | F | Cb

	C	F	Cb
Swiss Chard, cooked, chopped, 1 c., 6 oz	35	0	7
Taro, cooked, ½ cup, 2.3 oz	95	0	23
Tomatoes: 1 small (2¼" diam.), 3 oz	15	0	3
1 medium (2¾" diameter), 5 oz	25	0	5
1 large (3½" diameter), 8 oz	40	0.5	9
1 extra lge (4" diam.), 12 oz	60	0.5	14
Chopped, 1 cup, 6.5 oz	35	0.5	7
Tomatillo: 1 medium, 1.2 oz 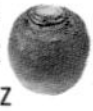	10	0	2
Turnip: Cooked, ½ cup, 2.75 oz	15	0	4
Greens, cooked, ½ cup, 2.5 oz	15	0	3
Water Chestnuts: 5-6 nuts, 1 oz	56	0.5	13
½ cup, (slices), 2.25 oz, raw	60	0	15
Canned, 1 oz	15	0	3
Watercress, 10 sprigs, 1 oz	3	0	0.5
Yams: Cooked, ½ cup, 2.5 oz	80	0	19
Baked: 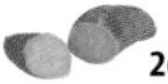			
1 medium (6") 8 oz	265	0.5	63
1 large (9") 12 oz	400	0.5	94
Yardlong Bean, 1 pod, 0.5 oz 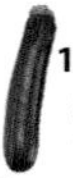	5	0	1
Yucca Root, ½ cup, 3.5 oz	165	0	39
Zucchini: 1 medium, 7 oz, raw	30	0.5	7
Cooked, ½ cup, (slices), 3 oz	15	0	4

Frozen Vegetables | C | F | Cb

	C	F	Cb
Birds Eye: 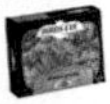			
Pure & Simple:			
Baby: Broccoli Florets, 1 cup, 3 oz	35	0.5	5
Gold & White Corn, ⅔ c., 3.2 oz	105	1	22
Sweet Peas, ⅔ cup, 3 oz	80	0	14
Blends: Asparagus Stir-Fry, 1¾ cup, 5.3 oz	60	0.5	11
Pepper Stir-Fry, 1 cup, 3 oz	30	0.5	6
Sauced & Seasoned:			
Broccoli & Cheese Sauce			
Steamfresh:			
Chef's Favorites, Lightly Sauced:			
Broccoli, Caulif. & Carrots, ¾ cup	50	2	7
Rotini 7 Broccoli, 2 cups, 6.4 oz	115	2	20
Pure & Simple Blends:			
Baby Broccoli Blend, 1 cup	65	1.5	8
Baby Potato Blend, 3/4 cup	50	0.5	10
Brocc. & Cauliflower, 1 c., 3.35 oz	30	0.5	4.5
With Carrots, ¾ cup, 3 oz	35	0.5	5.5

Frozen Vegetables (Cont)	C	F	Cb
Green Giant:			
Create A Meal Stir Fry: *Per 1 Cup Prepared*			
Lo Mein	260	7	27
Sweet & Sour	280	0	34
Szechuan	220	10	14
Teriyaki	190	0	14
Just for One,			
Broccoli & Cheese Sauce, 4.25 oz	40	1	7
Caulifl. & Cheese Sauce, 4.25 oz	40	1	8
Sauced/Seasoned:			
Baby Sweet Peas & Butter Sauce, ¾ cup, 4 oz	80	1.5	14
Brocc. & Cheese Sauce, ⅔ cup, 3.9 oz	60	2.5	7
Simply Steam: *Prepared*			
Asparagus Cuts, ⅓ cup	20	0	4
Green Beans & Almonds, ⅓ cup	40	2	4
Sweet Peas & Pearl Onions, ½ cup	60	0	11
Valley Fresh Steamers: *Prepared*			
Broccoli & Cheese Sauce, ⅔ cup	90	3	14
Buttery Rice & Vegetables, 1 cup	180	2	37
Cheesy Rice & Broccoli, ½ cup 3.5 oz	100	3.5	18
Garden Vegetable Medley, ½ cup	60	0.5	12
Ore-Ida:			
Fries: *Per 3 oz Unless Indicated*			
Classic: Golden Crinkles	120	4.5	19
Golden; Shoestring, av.	135	4	22
Steak	110	3	19
Extra Crispy Easy, Crinkles; Golden	180	8	25
Extra Crispy: Fast Food Fries	150	6	24
Golden Crinkles	160	7	22
Seasoned Crinkles	150	6	22
Tater Tots	170	9	21
Premium: Country	150	5	25
Crispers	230	14	23
Golden Twirls	150	6	23
Texas Crispers	150	7	20
Hash Browns: Golden Patties (1)	140	8	15
Potatoes O'Brien, ¾ cup	60	0	13
Shredded Hash Browns Patties	70	0	16
Southern Style, ⅔ cup	70	0	16
Onion: Chopped, 2.85 oz	20	0	5
Gourmet Rings, 2.7 oz	185	9	24
Onion Rings, 2.85 oz	180	10	21
Steam n' Mash: Cut Russet, 3.35 oz	70	0	16
Cut Sweet Potatoes, 4.3 oz	70	0	16
Garlic Seasoned Potatoes, 3.35 oz	90	1.5	17
Tater Tots: Regular, 3 oz	160	8	20
Crispy Crowns	170	9	21
Extra Crispy, 3 oz	170	9	20

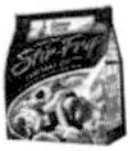

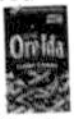

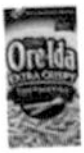

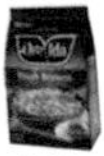

Canned/Bottled	C	F	Cb
Solids & Liquid			
Artichoke Hearts *(Fanci Foods):*			
Plain, 1 oz (1)	8	0	1
Marinated, ¼ bottle, 1 oz	25	1.5	2
Asparagus: Drained, 3 spears	10	0	1.5
Pieces, ½ cup, 4.3 oz	25	0.5	3
Bamboo Shoots, 1 cup, 4.5 oz	25	0	4
Bean Salad, ½ cup, 4.35 oz	90	0	20
Beans: Baked, ½ cup, 4.5 oz	120	0.5	27
Butter, ½ cup, 4.5 oz	90	0	16
Green, ½ cup, 2.5 oz	15	0	3
Italian, ½ cup, 2.5 oz	30	0	6
Kidney, ½ cup 3.5 oz	105	0.5	19
Lima, ½ cup, 4.5 oz	80	0	15
Pinto, ½ cup, 4.5 oz	105	1	18
Beets: Sliced, ½ cup, 3 oz	25	0	6
Crinkle/Pickled *(Del Monte)* ½ c.	80	0	20
Carrots: Sliced, ½ cup, 2.5 oz	20	0	4
Honey Glazed *(Del Monte)* ½ cup	75	0	18
Corn: Kernels, ½ cup, 4.5 oz	80	0.5	18
Creamed style, ½ cup, 4.5 oz	90	0.5	23
Garbanzo/Chick Peas, ½ c., 4.2 oz	145	1.5	27
Hearts of Palm, (1), 1.2 oz	7	0	1
Mushrooms: ½ cup, 2.5 oz	20	0	4
In Butter Sauce, 2 oz	20	1	2
Onions: Cocktail (1)	0	0	0
Pickled, 1 medium, 0.5 oz	0	0	2
French's Fried Onions ~ *See Page 112*			
Peas, ½ cup, 3 oz	60	0.5	10
Peppers: Hot Chili, Jalapeno, (1), 1 oz	5	0	1
Red/Green, 1 oz	5	0	1
Sweet, undrained, 2.5 oz	13	0	3
Jalapeno, with liquid, ½ cup chopped	20	0.5	3
Fried, drained, 2 Tbsp, 1 oz	60	5	3
Salsa, average all types, 2 Tbsp	10	0	2
Sauerkraut, drained, 1 cup, 5 oz	25	0	6
Spinach, ½ cup, 3.5 oz	25	0	3.5
Succotash: Cream Style, ½ cup	100	0.5	23
W/ whole kernels, undrained, ½ c.	80	0.5	18
Sweetcorn ~ *See Corn*			
Sweet Potato, ½ cup, 3.5 oz	90	0	24
Tomatoes, Sundried: Nat., 5-6 pces	20	0	5
In Oil, drained, 6 pieces, 0.5 oz	40	2.5	4
Tomato Products ~ *See Page 144*			
Vegetables, mixed, ½ cup, 4 oz	45	0	8
Yams: In Light Syrup, ½ cup, 4 oz	105	0	25
Candied, ½ cup, 4 oz	170	0	46
Zucchini, in Tomato Sauce, ½ c., 4 oz	30	0	8

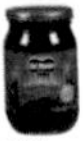

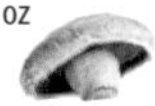

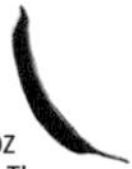

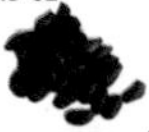

Quick Guide   C   F   Cb

Yogurt: *Average All Brands: Per 8 oz Container*

	C	F	Cb
Plain Yogurt: Whole	140	8	10
Low-Fat	145	3.5	16
Fat-Free	125	0.5	17
Fruit Flavored: Whole	225	8	32
Low-Fat	230	3	43
Fat-Free, regular	215	0.5	43
Fat-Free, no sugar added	80	0	15

Yogurt Parfait/Deli Cups:

	C	F	Cb
With Fruit Pieces: (⅔ Yogurt + ⅓ Fruit)			
Small, 8 oz cup	140	3	20
Large, 12 oz cup	210	4.5	30
With Fruit + Granola:			
Small, 8 oz cup (+ ¾ oz Granola)	235	7	30
Large, 12 oz cup (+ 1½ oz Granola)	400	13	58

Yogurt ~ Brands   C   F   Cb

	C	F	Cb
Alta Dena: *Per 8 oz*			
Low-Fat: Plain	170	4.5	20
All Natural, all flavors, av.	215	2	41
Non-Fat: Plain	110	0	16
Fruit, all flavors, av.	185	0	38
Vanilla	160	0	30
Amande *(Non Dairy/Soy):*			
24 oz Containers: Plain, 8 oz	170	9	19
Vanilla, 8 oz	220	8	25
Fruit Flavors, 6 oz cont.	150	6	23
Axelrod:			
Fat free: Plain, 8 oz	130	0	19
Fruit flavors, av. all, 6 oz	90	0	17
Low Fat: Plain, 8 oz	140	2.5	18
Fruit flavors, 6 oz	180	1.5	36
Brown Cow: *Per 6 oz Container*			
Cream Top:			
Fruit On The Bottom:			
Apricot Mango	170	6	23
Cherry-Vanilla	180	6	28
Low Fat, Peach	150	2	26
Smooth & Creamy: Plain	130	7	9
Coffee; Vanilla; Maple, av	165	7	20
Cabot: *Per 8 oz Serving*			
32 oz Containers:			
Greek Style: Plain	290	23	12
Lowfat (2%): Plain	150	5	11
Strawberry	220	4	33
Non-Fat, Plain	110	0	18
Cascade Fresh:			
6 oz Containers:			
Low-Fat, all flavors, 6 oz	140	2	21
Fat-Free, all flavors, 6 oz	110	0	20
32 oz Cont., Whole Milk, Plain, 8 oz	170	8	12

	C	F	Cb
Chobani Greek Yogurt:			
Champions: *Per 3.5 oz Container*			
Vanilla Chocolate Chunk	120	3	14
Other flavors, average	100	1.5	13
Low-Fat (2%):			
Plain, 6 oz	130	3.5	7
Fruit flavors, av., 6 oz	160	3	21
16 /32 oz Ctn, Plain, 8 oz	170	5	9
Non-Fat: *Per 6 oz Container*			
Plain	100	0	7
Fruit flavors, average	140	0	21
Honey	150	0	20
16 oz/32 oz Ctn:			
Plain, 8 oz	140	0	9
Strawberry, 8 oz	190	0	27
Vanilla, 8 oz	170	0	18
Dannon:			
Activia Yogurt: *Per 4 oz Container Unless Indicated*			
Fiber, average	110	2	19
Fruit Flavors, average	120	2	23
Light, average	70	0	13
Parfait, average, 6 oz container	220	3	42
All Natural: *Per 6 oz Container*			
All flavors	160	2.5	26
Low-Fat, all flavors	100	2.5	12
Non-Fat, Plain	80	0	12
Danimals: Crush Cups, all flav., 4 oz	110	1.5	19
Smoothies, 3.1 fl.oz	70	0.5	15
Fruit On The Bottom,			
average, 6 oz	150	1.5	29
Light & Fit: All flavors, 4 oz Cont.	60	0	10
All flav., 6 oz Container	80	0	16
Quarts, all flavors, 8 oz serving	110	0	21
Carb & Sugar Control,			
average all flavors, 4 oz cup	50	1.5	3
Oikos: *Per Single, 5.3 oz Container, Unless Indicated*			
Traditional, Fruit Flavors	160	4.5	18
Nonfat: Plain	80	0	6
Fruit flavors, average	125	0	20
Quarts, Vanilla, 8 oz	190	0	29
Emmi: *Per 6 oz Container*			
Swiss: Plain, lowfat	170	2.5	10
Average other flavors	170	3	27
Fage: *Per 5.3 oz Container Unless Indicated*			
Total Classic: Plain, Single Serve, 7 oz	190	10	8
Fruit flavors, all	170	6	17
Honey	210	6	29
Total 2%:			
Plain, Single Serve, 7 oz	150	4	8
Fruit Flavors, all	140	2.5	17
Honey	190	2.5	29
Total 0%:			
Plain, Single Serve, 6 oz	100	0	7
Fruit flavors, average	120	0	18
Honey	170	0	30

Brands (Cont)

	C	F	Cb
Fresh & Easy: *Per 6 oz Container*			
Greek, Vanilla	230	14	20
Lowfat, average all flavors	170	1.5	32
Nonfat, average all flavors	100	0	19
Jewel: *6 oz Carton*			
Blended Low Fat: Av. all flavors	150	1.5	30
Light, average all flavors	110	0	20
Fruit On The Bottom, av.	180	2	33
Fat-Free, Plain	90	0	14
32 oz Tubs: *Per 8 oz*			
Lowfat, average fruit flav.	205	2	39
Plain, Non-Fat	120	0	18
Kemps,			
'Light' 80 Cals, av., 6 oz	80	0	16
Kirkland,			
Low-Fat, Blueb.; Peach; Strawb, 6 oz	180	1.5	36
Kroger: *Per 6 oz carton*			
Blended, all flavors	190	2	35
Carb Master, av. all flav.	80	1.5	4
Fruit On The Bottom,			
average all flavors	170	2	30
Lite, average all flavors	80	0	13
La Yogurt *(Probiotic): Per 6 oz Carton*			
Low Fat: Original, all flav., av.	150	1.5	27
Rich & Crmy, all flav., av.	180	1.5	35
Non Fat, all flavors, av.	90	0	16
Sabor Latino,			
Low Fat, all flav., av.,	185	1.5	37
LALA,			
Blended, Fruit Flavors, av., 6 oz	150	3	27
Liberte: Plain, 5.3 oz Ctn	90	0	7
Lemon, 5.3 oz container	140	0	23
Other var., av., 5.3 oz ctn	130	0	22
Lucerne: *Per 6 oz Container*			
Low-Fat, all flav., av.	170	2	32
Fat-Free: Plain	80	0	13
Light Fat-Free, fruit, 6 oz	90	0	17
Mountain High: *Per 8 oz*			
32 oz Containers:			
Original Style: Plain	180	8	17
Strawb./Vanilla, average	210	7	28
Low-Fat: Plain	140	2.5	18
Rasp./Strawb./Vanilla, average	175	2.5	29
Fat-Free: Plain	120	0	18
Strawberry; Vanilla, average	160	0	29
Nancy's: *Per 8 oz Container*			
Natural:			
Whole Milk: With Honey	170	8	17
With Fruit on Top, average	230	5	41
Organic Low Fat: Plain; Lemon	150	3	16
Average other flavors	175	3	27
Organic Nonfat:			
Fruit On The Top: Cherry; Peach, av.	145	0.5	26
Raspberry; Strawberry, av.	165	0	31

	C	F	Cb
Oikos ~ *see Dannon & Stonyfield*			
O Organics, Low-Fat, av., 6 oz	140	2.5	23
Publix: Fat-Free, Plain, 8 oz	140	0	23
Swiss Style, Low-Fat, 8 oz	240	2.5	41
Ralphs ~ *Same as Kroger*			
Roberts: *Per 6 oz Ctn*			
Low-Fat, average all flavors	165	1.5	32
Fat-Free, all flavors	90	0	15
Silk Live! (Soy):			
32 oz Ctn, Plain, 8 oz serving	150	4	22
6 oz Cups, Fruit Flavors	150	3	30
So Delicious, (Dairy/Soy Free)			
Cultured Coconut Milk: Plain, 4 oz	80	4.5	12
Chocolate, 6 oz	170	7	27
Pina Colada; Raspb., av., 6 oz	150	6	25
Vanilla, 6 oz	140	6	22
Greek. Plain, 6 oz	130	5	22
Stater Bros: *Per 6 oz Container Unless Indicated*			
Plain	105	1.5	14
Fruit on the Bottom, av all flavors	170	1.5	34
Blended Low-Fat, av. all flavors	155	1.5	29
32 oz Tubs: Non-Fat, Plain, 8 oz	120	0	18
Low Fat, 8 oz	140	2	19
Stonyfield Organic:			
Fruit On Bottom: *Per 6 oz Container*			
Whole Milk: Choc. U'ground	220	5	37
Strawb. & Cream	150	6	20
Low Fat, average all flavors	125	2	21
Fat Free: Choc Underground	150	0	30
Average other flavors	115	0	22
Oikos: *Per 5.3 oz Container Unless Indicated*			
Smooth & Creamy, 0% Fat, average	110	0	13
Fruit On The Bottom, 0% Fat,			
average all flavors	125	0	17
Organic Activia, 4-Pack,			
Strawberry; Vanilla, av, 4 oz	90	1	16
Smooth & Creamy: *Per 6 oz Container Unless Indicated*			
Whole Milk: 32oz Ctn, Plain, 8 oz	170	9	12
Average all flavors 6 oz ctn	170	6	23
Low Fat: Plain,	90	2	11
Average all flavors	130	2	22
Fat Free: Plain	80	0	11
Average all flavors	100	0	18
Stop & Shop:			
Blended, Light, Non Fat,			
average all flavors, 6 oz	90	0	16
Fruit On The Bottom,			
Low Fat, average all flavors, 6 oz	170	1.5	31
Trader Joes:			
French Village: Non-Fat, all flav., 6 oz	130	0	24
32 oz Containers:			
Plain, 8 oz	120	0	17
Vanilla, 8 oz	180	0	34
Cream Line, Plain, 8 oz	170	10	12

Brands (Cont) — C | F | Cb

	C	F	Cb
Trader Joes (Cont):			
Greek Style: Plain, 8 oz	260	18	14
Apricot Mango; Honey, av. 8 oz	300	15	28
Non-Fat: Plain; Peach, av 8 oz	120	0	7
Blueb.; Honey 5.3 oz	120	0	16
Vanilla, 5.3 oz	130	0	20
With Fiber: Plain, 5.3 oz	80	0	8
Peach	110	0	8
Low-Fat, Pre-Stirred, Fruit, 8 oz	220	3	40
Low-Fat: With Almonds/Granola:			
Pomegranate, 4.6 oz	140	2.5	27
Vanilla, 4.6 oz	160	7	20
Rich & Creamy, average, 4 oz	140	6	19
Squishers, Org., low fat, 1 tube, 2 oz	60	1	10
Voskos, Greek, Nonfat,			
Vanilla Bean, 5.3 oz	130	0	20
Wallaby Organic, Blended,			
Low-Fat, average all flavors, 6 oz	150	2.5	26
Wegmans: Per 6 oz Container			
Blended, Light, all flavors	100	0	18
Fruit On The Bottom, Lowfat:			
Strawberry; Mixed Berry, average	180	2	35
Average other fruit flavors	160	2	29
Greek, Non-Fat: Plain	90	0	7
Fruit flavors; Vanilla, avereage	135	0	20
Vanilla	130	0	18
Whole Foods (365):			
Non-Fat, Plain, 6 oz	90	0	13
Fruit flavors, average 6 oz	145	0	30
Vanilla, 6 oz	130	0	23
Whole Soy: Plain, 6 oz	150	4.5	19
Other flavors, average, 6 oz	170	3.5	33
YoCrunch: Per 6 oz Container Unless Indicated			
Cookies & Candy Crunch:			
Strawberry: W/ Nestle Crunch pcs	200	4.5	36
With Oreo Cookie pieces	180	3	34
Vanilla, with pieces, av. all varieties	195	4	34
Fruit Parfaits: W/ Granola, all flav.	170	1.5	35
Nonfat Greek, w/Granola, all flavors	175	1.5	33
100 Calorie, av. all flav., 3¾ oz	100	1.5	20
Yoplait: Per 6 oz Container Unless Indicated			
Original: 99% Fat-Free, all flavors	170	1.5	33
Thick & Creamy, all flavors	180	2.5	31
Light: Fat-Free, Fruit Flavors	100	0	19
Thick & Creamy, all flavors	100	0	21
With Fiber, 4oz container	50	0	13
Large 2lb Ctn: All Nat., ff., Plain, 8 oz	130	0	19
99% Fat-Free, average, 8 oz	210	1.5	42
Delights, all flavors, 4 oz ctn	100	1.5	17
Fiber One, average, 4 oz container	50	0	13
Fruplait, average, 4 oz container	115	1	22

Brands (Cont) — C | F | Cb

	C	F	Cb
Yoplait (Cont):			
Go-Gurt!, all flavors, 2.25 oz tube	70	0.5	13
Greek, 0% Fat: 100 Cal., fruit flav., 6 oz	100	0	14
Plain, 6 oz	120	0	12
Fruit Flavors, av., 6 oz	160	0	25
Honey Vanilla, 6 oz	150	0	22
Simplait, all flavors, 6 oz	200	7	28
Splitz, av. all flavors, 3.25 oz ctn	90	1	17
Trix, Fruit Flavors, av. all, 4 oz cup	100	0.5	20
Whips!: Chocolate flavors,			
4 oz cup	160	4	25
Fruit flavors, 4 oz cup	140	2.5	25
Yo-Plus, all flav., 4 oz	110	1.5	22
Yoplait Kids, all flav., 3 oz cup	70	1	13

Yogurt Drinks & Probiotics — C | F | Cb

	C	F	Cb
BioKult, Cultured,			
all flavors, 2.1 oz bottle	35	0	8
Cacique, Yonique,			
av. all flav, 7 fl.oz	200	1.5	35
Dannon: Activia, all flavors, 7 fl oz	160	3	27
Danimals, Smoothies,			
all flavors, 3.1 fl.oz	70	0.5	15
DanActive,			
average all flav., 3.1 fl.oz	80	1.5	15
Dan-o-nino, all flavors, 3.1 fl.oz	70	0.5	15
Danone (Canada),			
Danacol, all flavors, 80 ml	35	1	4
Glen Oaks, 32 fl.oz Containers,			
average all flavors, 8 6l.oz	150	2.5	28
Good Belly: Per 2.7 fl.oz Bottle			
Probiotics: BigShot, all flavors	60	1	11
Plus, average all flavors	50	0	12
Kemps, Yo-J Drink, 16 fl.oz ctn,			
all flavors, 8 fl. oz	120	0	27
LaLa:			
Yogurt Smoothies,			
av. all flavors, 7 fl.oz	150	2.5	26
Lifeway, Kefir Smoothie (Probiotic):			
32 fl. oz Container: Plain, 8 fl.oz	150	8	12
Lowfat: Choc. Truffle, 8 fl.oz	160	2	34
Other flavors, 8 fl.oz	140	2	20
Ralphs,			
Smoothies, av., 7 fl.oz	200	2.5	37
Stonyfield Organic:			
Oikos, 4-pack, av. all flavors, 6 oz	155	2	26
Super Smoothies: Av. all flav, 10 oz	230	3	40
4-pack, average all flavors, 6 oz	140	2	22
Trader Joe's,			
Lowfat Smoothies, fruit flav., 6 fl.oz	140	2	23
Yakult, 2.7 fl.oz bottle	50	0	12
Yoplait:			
Frozen Smoothies,			
all flav., ½ pouch, 8 fl.oz prep'd	110	1.5	14

Cafeteria-Style Foods   C   F   Cb

Average All Preparations:

	C	F	Cb
Beef Stroganoff, 5 oz	195	13	7
Beef Stroganoff with 4 oz noodles	350	14	36
Chicken Lasagna, 1 piece	300	11	32
Chicken Chop Suey with 4 oz rice	245	4	37
Deep Dish Burrito, 7 oz	265	13	20
Grnd Beef Casserole, 2 scps, 6 oz	245	13	17
Italian Meat Sce for Spaghetti, 5 oz	150	9	9
with 5 oz Spaghetti	350	10	49
Lasagna, 1 piece	275	11	25
Meatloaf, 3 oz	205	13	4
Ranch Beans, 2 scoops, 6 oz	350	11	45
Red Beans & Rice, 7 oz	280	9	37
Scalloped Potato/Ham, 2 scps, 6 oz	160	6	20
Stuffed Shells in Sauce (1)	105	3	17
Swedish Meatballs (3)	205	12	9
Sweet & Sour Pork/Rice, 9 oz	240	3	40
Swiss Steak w/ Mushr. Gravy, 6 oz	280	11	4
Tator Tot Casserole, 2 scoops, 6 oz	260	15	20
Tenderloin Tips/Mushr. Gravy, 5 oz	210	13	3
with 5 oz noodles	395	15	38
Tuna Noodle Casserole, 2 scps, 6 oz	180	6	17
Turkey Tetrazzini, 2 scoops, 6 oz	195	7	17
Vegetable Lasagna, 1 piece	250	13	21

Croissants

	C	F	Cb
Unfilled, medium 1.5 oz	180	10	21
Filled: With Ham (2 oz), garnish	280	14	24
With Ham (2 oz), Cheese (2 oz)	470	30	20
With Chick (2 oz) Cheese (2 oz)	470	30	20
With Turkey/Ham/Cheese (2 oz ea.)	580	36	20
Au Bon Pain: Ham & Cheese	390	21	35
Spinach & Cheese	290	17	28

7-Eleven ~ See Page 236

Bagels

	C	F	Cb
Plain: Large, 4 oz (without filling)	320	2	65
With 2 oz Cream Cheese	500	27	54
With 2 oz Lox (Smoked Salmon)	400	4	65

Also see Bagels Section ~ *Page 54*
Fast-Foods Restaurants ~ *Page 175*
Au Bon Pain ~ *Page 179*
Brueggers ~ *Page 185*
Einstein Bros Bagels ~ *Page 199*

Sandwiches   C   F   Cb

No Spreads Unless Indicated:
(Includes 2 Slices Bread ~ 3 oz)

	C	F	Cb
BLT (5 strips Bacon, 2 Tbsp Mayo)	600	40	46
Breaded Chicken & Garnish	540	28	46
Chicken Salad with Mayo., 5 oz	580	30	49
Chopped Liver, Egg, Mayonnaise	630	25	44
Corned Beef with Mustard, 5 oz	560	28	44
Egg Salad with Mayonnaise	570	29	49
Egg Salad Club w/ Bacon & Mayo.	780	53	49
Grilled Cheese (3 oz)	540	30	44
Ham (4 oz); Cheese (4 oz), & Mayo.	910	56	44
Lobster Salad (4 oz) w/ Mayonnaise	530	25	45
Overstuffed Tuna Salad (7 oz)	870	39	75
Philadelphia Cheese Steak Sandwich	550	23	42
Reuben (6 oz Beef/Pastrami,			
2 oz Cheese, 2 Tbsp Dressing)	920	60	28
Roast Beef (4 oz) with Mustard	460	12	45
Roast Pork (4 oz) with Apple Sauce	500	16	55
Shrimp Salad Club w/ Bacon & Mayo	800	57	46
Sloppy Joe with Sauce (7 oz)	600	30	45
Steak Sandwich (5 oz cooked)	680	32	41
Triple Cheese Melt (4 oz)	720	45	46
Tuna Salad (5 oz) with Mayonnaise	610	30	49
Turkey Breast (5 oz) w/ Mayonnaise	460	18	44
Turkey Breast (5 oz) w/ Mustard	360	7	44
Turkey Club with Bacon, Mayonnaise	830	38	31
Vegetarian with Avocado & Cheese	820	49	72

7-Eleven ~ *Page 236*
Schlotzsky's ~ *Page 237*
Subway ~ *Page 245*

Wraps & Roll-Ups   C   F   Cb

Average All Types
Meat/Chicken/Fish/Veggie:

	C	F	Cb
Small, approximately 9 oz	500	25	48
Regular, approximately 15 oz	830	40	80
Large, approximately 22 oz	1400	70	134

Fast-Foods Restaurants ~ *Page 175*
Au Bon Pain ~ *Page 179*
Sonic Drive-In ~ *Page 241*
Subway ~ *Page 245*
WAWA ~ *Page 254*

Updated Nutrition Data ~ www.CalorieKing.com
Persons with Diabetes ~ See Disclaimer (Page 22)

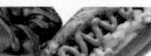

Fair & Carnival Foods

Barbeque Chicken/Meats:	C	F	Cb
Chicken, ½ chicken, 15 oz	740	24	34
Grilled Chicken Pita, with dressing	680	19	82
Teriyaki Chicken on stick, w/ dressing	250	6	4
Pork Ribs, 18 oz	1360	68	21
Turkey Leg: Regular, 19 oz	1135	54	0
Caveman (2lb Turkey Leg with 1lb Bacon)	2360	177	3
Bacon: Fried, on-a-stick, w/ syrup	230	16	5
Choc-covered Bacon, 4.5 oz dish	640	43	30
Beef Stew over Rice, 2 cups	440	14	61
Butter Balls, deep fried, 4 Balls	460	38	24
Cheese Curds, Breaded & fried, (Culver's), 6.7 oz	670	38	54
Corn Dogs: Regular, 4 oz	250	14	23
Jumbo, 6 oz	375	21	36
Pretzel-Wrapped Dog	300	16	30
Papa Pup, on-a-stick	400	24	32
Pronto Pup, on-a-stick	170	9	16
Corn On The Cob, 8"(1), 16 oz	200	1	42
Finger Foods:			
Artichoke, fried, 9 pieces	250	14	24
Chicken Nuggets (6)	340	17	26
Chicken Strips (4), 4.5 oz	445	21	33
Onion Rings, 3 rings	310	13	40
Onion Flower	1320	72	140
Shrimp, Fried, 10-12 pieces, 5 oz	555	30	36
Spam, deep-fried in batter, 2 pcs	330	24	18
Gator:			
Big Gator, Nuggets/Hushpuppies	550	31	54
Stick Gator, 1 sausage	250	20	4
Greek:			
Baklava, 2" square	245	13	32
Falafel, 11.6 oz	660	27	85
Greek Salad, 14 oz	520	48	17
Gyro, 7.5", 12 oz	680	40	55
Spanakopita, 8 oz	200	7.5	23
Hamburgers:			
⅓ Pound Burger, 7.5 oz	670	41	26
Cheeseburger, 6 oz	550	36	25
Hot Dogs: *With Bun*			
Regular: No extras	215	14	28
With Chili, 6 oz	450	32	32
With Chili & Cheese, 7.3 oz	500	36	31
⅓ Pound Hot Dog	550	41	31
Foot Long Hot Dog	470	26	41
Jumbo, Bratwurst/Kielbasa, av.	800	60	28

Fair & Carnival Foods (Cont)

Mexican:	C	F	Cb
Burrito with Bean/Beef, 17 oz	1100	41	104
Carne Asada, 14.5 oz	820	44	58
Cheese Quesadilla, 1.75 oz	480	27	40
Chicken Taco, 3.3 oz	210	12	16
Fish Taco, 5 oz	270	13	31
Jalapeno Pepper, choc-covered (3)	270	15	31
Nachos with Cheese, 9" plate	860	59	70
Tamale (1), 3.5 oz	180	8	21
Taquito, 5 oz	370	17	43
Pizza:			
Pizza Bread, Pepperoni, ½ loaf, 12 oz	1115	32	151
Pizza on-a-stick, 1 piece	535	28	55
Personal Pizza:			
Cheese, 7"	670	24	80
Pepperoni, 7"	795	35	80
Ham & Pineapple, 7"	800	31	87
Potatoes & Fries:			
Australian Battered Potatoes	1290	66	155
Baked Potato, 14 oz	435	0.5	100
Fries: French, 7 oz	560	24	
Cheese Fries, 10 oz	645	38	62
Chili Fries, 10 oz	700	36	83
Curly Fries, 7 oz	620	30	78
Jamaican Jerk Fries, 7 oz	640	34	77
Sweet Potato, baked, 14 oz	405	0.5	97
Tornado, on-a-stick	210	15	18
Salads/Sides:			
Chili, 1 cup	280	11	24
Cole Slaw, 5 oz	350	21	37
Pickle, whole (6")	30	0	8
Potato Salad, 5 oz	290	15	35
Sandwiches: 7½" Roll			
Ham, 11 oz	645	39	47
Hot Pastrami, 9 oz	760	17	62
Roast Beef, 11 oz	620	36	46
Philadelphia Cheese Steak, 13 oz	680	36	49
Turkey, 11 oz	665	24	65
Drinks, Slushies:			
Horchata, 16 fl.oz	280	8	54
Lemonade, 18 fl.oz	210	0	52
Orange Julius, 20 fl.oz	490	10	96
Strawberry Julius, 20 fl.oz	430	0	98
Icee, 16 fl.oz	235	0	65
Shakes, average, 16 fl.oz	690	33	85
Slushies, 16 fl.oz	260	0	65
Soft Frozen Lemonade, 12 fl.oz	300	0	78
Smoothies, Berry Flavors, 16 fl.oz	350	1	80

Fair & Carnival Foods (Cont)

Cakes, Pastries:	C	F	Cb
Funnel Cake, Plain (1)	760	44	80
Toppings:			
Apple Cinn., 2 oz	85	3	36
Cinn. & Sugar, 2 tsp	40	0	10
Strawberry & Cream, 2 oz	70	0	16
Cheesecake on-a-stick, 6 oz	655	47	56
Churro (1), 9", 1.6 oz	170	8	22
Cream Puff, 4.3 oz	500	43	22
Fried Twinkie, 1	420	34	45
Puff-on-a-Stick (4), 8.6 oz	995	86	44
Strawberry Crepe, 4.3 oz	280	14	36
Twinkie Dog (Sundae)	500	14	89
Candied Apple, 7 oz	330	0	80

Cookies:			
Sweet Martha (1), ¾ oz	90	4	14
Deep Fried: Oreos, tray (5)	890	48	108
Cookie Dough on stick, 3 pieces	670	32	89

Cotton Candy:			
Small, 1 oz	110	0	27
Large, 2.25 oz	250	0	62
Family Size, 5.5 oz	610	0	151
Dirt Dessert, 1 cup, 9.3 oz	405	12	69
Donuts, Jumbo Twist, (1), 7.5 oz	905	49	109

Fried Dough/FryBread:			
Plain: 7", 3.7 oz	390	19	47
9", 4¾ oz	510	25	61
Toppings: Cinnamon Sugar, 2 tsp	40	0	10
Butterscotch; Caramel, 2 Tbsp	115	0	29
Hot Fudge, average, 2 Tbsp	110	4	22
Cheese Powder, 2 tsp	70	3	2
Honey, 1 Tbsp, ¾ oz	65	0	17
Fudge, 1.5 oz	200	11	25

Ice Cream & Frozen Treats:			
Deep-fried Klondike Bar w/ syrup	430	16	18
Dippin' Dots Ice Cream, 6 oz cup	380	20	46
Frozen Banana, chocolate coated, 5 oz	240	4	53
Frozen Yogurt in sugar cone, 14 oz	475	2	94
Ice Cream: Small, sugar cone, 10 oz	775	42	83
Large, sugar cone, 14 oz	935	54	96
Sherbet, 8 oz	270	4	59
Snow Cone (includes 3 oz syrup)	270	0	68
Strawberry, Choc. Dipped, 1 piece	125	7	15

Popcorn:			
Plain: Small, 3 oz	450	24	48
Large, 6 oz	900	48	96
Kettle Corn: Small, 5 oz	600	15	110
Large, 10 oz	1200	30	220
Pretzels, Soft, 4.5 oz	340	2	70
S'more, on stick	275	16	27

Stadium Foods

Burgers:	C	F	Cb
Bacon Burger, 8.3 oz	470	25	34
Cheeseburger, 8.3 oz	450	23	33
Hamburger, 7.8 oz	400	19	33
French Fries, 6.4 oz	470	34	39
Fruit Cup, 6 oz	80	0	20

Hot Dogs:			
Chili Dog, 7.7 oz	520	29	45
Hot Dog, 6.4 oz	465	21	50
Jumbo Dog, 6 oz	440	25	38
Kraut Dog with Sauerkraut , 7.8 oz	490	27	41

Individual Pan Pizza (6"): *Per Pizza*			
BBQ Chicken	630	24	71
Cheese	630	27	71
Pepperoni	660	30	70
Nachos, 40 chips w/ 4 oz cheese	1100	59	132

Sandwiches:			
Chicken: With Bacon, 8.3 oz	530	31	41
With Cheese, 8.3 oz	510	29	40
Without Cheese, 7.7 oz	460	25	40
Polish Sausage S'wich, 7 oz	565	33	46

Snacks:			
Brownie, 2.5" x 4.5"	360	18	44
Cheese Sauce, 1.25 oz	100	8	4
Cheetos, 2.75 oz package	440	28	42
Chocolate Chip Cookie, 2.3 oz	280	12	40
Churro (1), 10", 2.1 oz	210	10	26
Doritos, Nacho, 2.75 oz package	390	20	48

King Size Candy:			
Butterfinger, 3.75 oz	480	18	75
Nestle Crunch, 2.75 oz	390	21	85
Lay's Chips, 2.75 oz package	440	28	42
Peanuts in shell, 8 oz	930	80	24

Popcorn: Small (9 cup size)	575	35	56
Large (15 cup size)	950	58	93
Pretzel, Reg., 5.5 oz	490	3.5	101
Red Vines, 5 oz box	500	0	117
Snow Cone: With 3 oz syrup	270	0	68
With 6 oz syrup	540	0	136

Beverages: Orange Juice, 12 fl.oz	180	0	2
Beer: Heineken, 16 fl.oz	200	0	16
Miller: Draft, 16 fl.oz	195	0	17
Lite, 16 fl.oz	125	16	4
Jack Daniels, Punch, 12 fl.oz	235	0	34
Wine, White, 9 fl.oz	190	0	6
Soda, (with ½ ice), average: 20 fl.oz	160	0	40
32 fl.oz	260	0	65
Starbuck's, coffee frappuccino, 9.5 fl.oz bottle	200	3	37

Chinese & Asian Dishes

	C	F	Cb
Appetizers:			
Crab Cake, 2¼ oz	125	10	1
Dumplings: Pork, steamed, (1)	80	4.5	5
Pork, fried, (1)	90	6	5
Vegetable, steamed (1)	35	1	5
Egg Rolls, mini, 3 rolls	100	3	11
Spring Roll:			
Small, 1.5 oz	85	4	9
Medium, 3 oz	170	8	17
Large, 5 oz	290	15	29
Wonton, 1 only	75	4	5
Soup: Egg Flower, bowl 12 oz	90	2	16
Hot & Sour Soup, bowl 12 oz	110	3.5	14
Rice: Plain, 1 cup (½ Pint), 6.5 oz	320	2	66
2 cups (1 Pint), 13 oz	640	4	132
Fried: 1 cup, 5 oz	365	11	55
Large dish, 16 oz	950	28	67
Noodles, Chinese Egg, ckd, 1 cup	200	4	37
Entrees & Mains: *Per Serving*			
Almond Chicken, 6 oz	270	10	21
BBQ Pork, 5.5oz	440	23	15
Beef in Black Bean Sauce, 8.5 oz	390	17	17
Broccoli Beef, 6 oz	370	21	13
Chicken & Broccoli, 5.5 oz	160	8	10
Chicken Skewers, 3 oz	210	9	18
Chop Suey:			
Chicken, 5 oz	140	9	2
Pork, 5 oz	170	12	3
Chow Mein, Beef/Chicken, 8 oz	390	12	59
Crab Puff/Rangoon, 1 dumpling	190	11	13
Crispy Fried Chicken, 8 oz	485	33	12
Egg Drop Soup: With Noodles, 1 cup	110	3	16
Without Noodles, 1 cup	60	3	4
Egg Foo Yung with Sauce, 1 cup	270	15	16
Kung Pao Chicken, 5.5 oz	240	15	12
Lemon Chicken, 5 oz	525	21	57
Lo Mein (stir-fried), 8 oz	705	42	49
Omelet, Chicken/Shrimp, 16 oz	990	82	10
Orange Chicken, 5.5 oz	500	27	42
Steamed Whole Fish,			
½ Sockeye Salmon	646	36	23
Sweet & Sour:			
Fish, 20 oz	1160	58	106
Pork, 5.5 oz	400	23	35
Vegetable Combination, w/ oil, 6 oz	367	5	66
Vegetables, Steamed, w/o oil, 6 oz	137	1	29
Sauces: Mandarin Sauce 1.5 oz	70	0	17
Potsticker Sauce 1.5 oz	35	0	8
Bubble Tea, average, 12 fl oz	280	0.5	68
Fortune Cookie, each	32	0.5	7

Cajun & Creole

	C	F	Cb
Alligator, cooked, 4 oz	160	2	0
Baked Herb Chicken, 1 serving	850	53	2
Bouillabaisse	400	15	10
Cajun Fried Turkey, 1 serving	630	25	0
Cocktail Sauce, 2 Tbsp	30	0	6
Couche-couche, ½ cup	80	0	17
Crawfish Bisque, 1 serving	500	10	10
Crawfish, cooked, 2 oz	45	0.5	0
Creole Jambalaya,			
1 serving	550	30	15
Frog Legs, steamed (2)	45	0	0
Guinea Fowl, flesh, 4 oz, cooked	160	4	0
Hogshead Cheese, ¼ cup	80	5.5	0
Jambalaya, Shrimp & Crabmeat	520	14	12
Red Beans & Rice, 1 serving	400	17	52
Roasted Quail, w/ Bacon on Toast	550	25	15
Remoulade Sauce, 2 Tbsp, 1 oz	110	11	2
Shrimp Creole, 1 serving	450	20	10
Stuffed Smothered Steak,			
with 1 cup Rice	890	50	50
Turtle, cooked, 3 oz	120	3	0

Cuban

	C	F	Cb
Bl. Beans w/ Rice (Moros con Cristianos)	510	22	76
Black-Eyed Pea Fritters (Bollitos de Carita)	80	5	6
Casserole Corn Tamale	445	20	55
Chicken w/ Yellow Rice (Arroz con Pollo)	925	49	87
Cuban Bread (Pan Cubano)	80	1.5	15
Donuts in Syrup (Bunuelos),	170	5	10
with Melado	100	5	10
Grilled Plantains	145	0	40
Gypsy's Arm Cake (Brazo Gitano)	260	18	42
Roast Pork S'wich (Pan con Lechon)	640	30	62
Seasoned Beef with Olives & Raisins			
(Picadillo)	435	36	10
Shredded Beef (Ropa Vieja)	550	35	10
Taro Root Mash (Pure de Malanga)	315	3	69
Yuca with Citrus Garlic Dressing			
(Yuca con Mojo)	190	9	25

French Foods

	C	F	Cb
Blanquette d'Agneau (Lamb Stew)	800	30	17
Brioche, 1 cake	280	14	34
Bouillabaisse	400	15	10
Coq au Vin	800	30	16
Coquilles St. Jacques	320	13	36
Crème Brulée, 1 serving	460	40	21

French Foods (Cont)

	C	F	Cb
Baguette, 3 slices, 2.2 oz	150	1	35
Creme Caramel (Caramel Custard)	260	10	38
Crepe Suzette, 1x6" crepe with sauce	220	10	13
Duck a l'Orange	780	35	47
Escargot (Snails), in garlic butter (6)	200	10	4
Frog Legs, fried, 4 medium pairs	400	20	10
Lamb Noisettes, fried, 2 chops	500	40	1
Potage Creme Crecy (Carrot Soup)	360	18	14
Salade Nicoise (Tuna/Olives/Vegs)	450	13	14
Veal Cordon Bleu (Veal/Ham)	650	25	18
Vichyssoise (Potato /Leek Soup), 1 c.	200	9	15

Baguette & French Stick ~ *See Page 54*
Croissants ~ *Pages 135, 165*

German

	C	F	Cb
Beef: Goulash with Veggies	520	20	46
Weiner Schnitzel, 1 medium	750	35	38
Chicken: Fried, Viennese-style	530	20	28
Livers with Apple/Onion, 6 oz	460	28	10
Herring, Pickled: Rollmops, 4 oz	260	16	3
With Sour Cream, 4 oz	310	20	3
Pork, Sauerbraten (Pot Roast)	650	35	15
Sausage: Bratwurst, grilled, 6 oz	450	37	2
Hot Sausage Curry	300	7	6
Cakes: Black Forest, 1 slice	380	16	30
Bavarian Bread Dumpling, 3 small	330	10	28
Kugelhupf Cake, 1 large slice, 4 oz	400	23	40
Torte: Linzer (Almond/Raspb. Jam)	430	18	58
Sacher (Chocolate/Apricot Jam)	260	12	23

Greek

	C	F	Cb
Baklava Pastry: Small	240	13	32
Large, 3¾ oz	400	21	45
Calamari, deep fried, 1 cup	300	13	17
Chicken Kebob Plate	345	13	8
Dolmades (Stuffed Grape Leaves), 2 rolls, 6 oz	200	5	13
Galactobureko, 1 only (Filo, Custard, Pastry in Syrup)	360	15	48
Greek Chicken Salad	400	18	9
Gyros: 6" Pita, 8 oz	475	32	35
7½" Pita, 12 oz	680	40	55
Hummus & Pita, 4 oz	260	12	30
Kataifi, (Filo, Nut, Pastry in Syrup)	350	11	56
Moussaka: Small serving, 8 oz	350	22	22
Large serving, 16 oz	700	44	44
Soup, Avgolemono (Egg Lem. Soup with Chicken & Rice), 1 cup	85	6	5
Souvlaki (Lamb), each, 2 oz	120	6	1

Greek (Cont)

	C	F	Cb
Stuffed Tomatoes, 2	250	12	17
Taramosalata, 1 T., 0.5 oz	40	3	2
Tyropita (Filo/Egg/Cheese Pastry)	350	26	31

Daphne's Greek Cafe ~ *See Fast-Foods Section*

Hawaiian

	C	F	Cb
Ahi Tuna, grilled w/o fat, (6 oz fillet)	220	2	0
Chicken Long Rice, 1 cup, 7 oz	240	14	12
Gyoza, 1 only	55	2	6
Haupia (Coconut Pudd.), 1 pce (4"x 2½")	120	6	17
Hawaiian Sweet Bread, ½" sl., 2 oz	180	4.5	29
Kalua: Chicken, 4 oz	280	16	0
Pork, 4 oz	350	24	0
Kim Chee (pickled cabbage), ½ c., 4 oz	20	0	5
Kulolo (Taro Pudding), 1 slice	125	5	19
Lau Lau: Chicken (1) 7 oz	280	21	3
Pork (1) 7 oz	320	26	5
Loco Moco (rice/burger/egg/gravy)	650	27	63
Lomi Salmon, ¼ cup, 4 oz	20	1	2
Malasadas (Donut), 2 oz	240	13	26
Manapua (Char Siu Pork Bun), 2.3 oz	180	8	25
Poi (mashed cooked taro), 1 c., 8.5 oz	270	0.5	65
Poke, average all types, 3 oz	90	1	0
Portuguese Sausage, 2 oz	180	15	2
Potato Salad, ½ cup, 5 oz	170	10	17
Shave Ice (Matsumoto), all flavors:			
With Ice Cream, 1 large	300	4	64
With Beans, 1 large	290	0	72
Spam Musubi: With Regular Spam	265	11	34
(4 oz rice+1.3 oz Spam/7-Eleven Hawaii)			
Homemade: w/ Lite Spam (50% less fat)	220	5	34
Taro Pancake Mix, ⅓ cup (makes 2)	140	2	26
Plate Lunches:			
Chicken Katsu, (9 oz): With Rice	1110	48	108
+ Macaroni Salad, ¾ cup	1360	68	123
or Tossed Salad + Fr. Dress. (2 T.)	1240	61	111
Hamburger, (5 oz): With Rice	710	24	81
Gravy + Macaroni Salad	1135	49	112
Mahi Mahi, (7 oz): With Rice	650	12	90
+ Macaroni Salad + Tartar Sce	1150	58	109
or Macaroni Salad, w/o Tartar ce	935	34	108
or Tossed Salad + Fr. Dress. (3 T.)	815	27	96
or Tossed Salad, without dressing	670	12	93
Teri Beef, (5 oz): With 2 scps Rice	790	23	94
+ Macaroni Salad, ¾ cup	1095	47	113
or Tossed Salad, without dressing	800	23	95

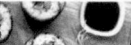
Indian & Pakistani **C** **F** **Cb**

Per Serving, Meat dishes allow 4 oz meat/serving

	C	F	Cb
Aloo Samosa, each	155	12	12
Alu Gosht Kari (Meat/Potato Curry)	600	40	23
Chicken Korma	500	35	6
Chicken Pilaf	700	53	50
Chicken Tikka	260	16	2
Chicken Vindaloo	400	20	8
Chapati/Roti, 7" diameter, 1 piece	60	0.5	11
Dahl (Lentil Puree): 1 cup, without oil	230	1	37
1 Tbsp Tadka (oil topping)	120	13	0
Dhakla (Lentil Dish), 1" square, 1 oz	105	5	13
Dhansak, ½ cup	105	3.5	11
Gosht Kari	460	25	17
Lamb Pilaf	520	35	40
Lassi (Sweet or Mango), 1 cup, 8 oz	160	4	24
Masala Gosht (Beef/Tomato/Gravy)	400	25	8
Mulligatawney Soup	300	15	8
Murgh Tikka, 1 cup	300	4	7
Naan Flatbread, ½, 2 oz	160	3.5	29
Pappadum, 1 large/2 small	50	3	5
Pesrattu (Lentil Crepe), 9", 2.6 oz	130	5	15
Pork Vindaloo Curry, without Rice	620	47	3
Rajmah, 1 cup	225	5	35
Rogan Josh, without Rice/Potatoes	500	30	3
Shahi Korma (Braised Lamb)	430	28	3
Tandoori Chicken: Breast	260	13	5
Leg/Thigh portion	300	17	6

Italian Dishes **C** **F** **Cb**

Entrees:

	C	F	Cb
Baked Ziti: Small	370	27	32
Regular	575	42	49
Breadstick (1), 2 oz	120	2.5	25
Broccoli Fettucine Alfredo, regular	815	23	125
Bruschetta, 2 slices	380	17	53
Calzones, average, all types	840	34	101
Cannelloni, 1 tube, 4 oz	280	15	18
Cheese Breadstick (1), 2.4 oz	180	8	20
Cheese Ravioli with Sauce	495	17	65
Chicken Alfredo	775	29	82
Chicken Parmigiana, 11 oz	520	22	16
Chicken Scallopine, dinner	1110	71	68
Eggplant Parmigiana	900	39	78
Fettucine Alfredo: Lunch, 9 oz	885	65	63
Dinner, 15 oz	1475	108	104
Linguine & Seafood, dinner	1130	71	79
Manicotti Formaggio	800	38	57
Meat Lasagne: Small, 10 oz	440	23	39
Large, 16 oz	700	36	60
Meat Ravioli	725	22	102
Minestrone Soup, 1 bowl	110	2	18
Penne Rustica: Lunch	1300	71	76
Dinner	1540	80	101
Ravioli, over-stuffed, av.	990	67	57

Spaghetti & Meatballs:

	C	F	Cb
With Tomato Sauce: Kids	500	20	58
Medium/Lunch	1080	63	89
Large/Dinner	1430	81	119
With Meat Sauce: Kids	550	25	56
Medium/Lunch	1300	79	84
Large/Dinner	1700	103	110
Veal Marsala, dinner	1320	66	132
Veal Parmigiana, dinner	1270	65	116
Vegetable Primavera	610	8	116

Panini Sandwich:

	C	F	Cb
Chicken, 16 oz	900	38	81
Meats, average, 18 oz	940	39	81
Vegetarian, 15 oz	750	31	83

Pizza: Ready-To-Eat ~ *Page 135*
Gourmet Deep Dish (Gino's East) ~ *Page 202*

Salad,

	C	F	Cb
Caprese, 11 oz	445	34	10

Desserts:

	C	F	Cb
Gelato: Vanilla (Milk Base), ½ c.	200	15	18
Choc. Hazelnut (Milk), ½ cup	370	29	26
Water Base, ½ cup	100	0	25
Lemon Ice	180	0	45
Tiramisu, 1 piece, 5 oz	400	29	30

Further listings ~ *See Fast-Foods Section*

Japanese

	C	F	Cb
Sashimi: (Sl. Raw Seafood/Beef)			
Ika (Squid), 4 oz	105	2	0
Hamachi (Yellowtail), 4 oz	165	6	0
Maguro (Yellowfin Tuna), 4 oz	120	1	0
Niku (Beef), 5 oz	200	10	0
Saba (Mackerel), 4 oz	160	7	0
Suzuki (Sea Bass), 4 oz	110	0.5	0
Tako (Octopus), 4 oz	95	1	0
Sushi Rice: Cooked, 1 Tbsp	25	0	5
1 cup, 5.25 oz	380	3	82
Sushi (Maki) Rolls: *Per Piece*			
Average all types (California Rolls; Cream Cheese with Crab; Eel; Salmon; Shrimp; Tuna; Yellowtail; Vegetable)			
Small (1⅛" diam. x 1⅛" high), 0.8 oz	25	0.5	3.5
Med. (1¾" diam. x 1¾" high), 1.6 oz	50	1	7
Large (2¼" diam. x ⅞" high), 2 oz	60	1.5	9
Sushi Packs: *Per Pack*			
Average all types: 6 large pieces	370	5	55
9 medium pieces	360	6	60
12 small pieces	265	3	45
Futomaki (thick roll), 6 pieces	380	5	72
Hand Roll (Cone), 4 oz	120	2	18
Inari (rice filled soybean pocket), 4 pces	420	9	73
Sushi-Nigiri, (fish on rice), average all types, 1 piece	70	0.5	12
Sushi Plate: Assorted: 6 pieces	420	3	36
Combination (Sushi & Sushi Rolls) 2 Sushi + 6 small & 3 med. rolls	400	7	72
Dipping Sauces: Average, 2 Tbsp	30	0	7
Ginger Vinegar Dressing, 2 Tbsp	20	0	5
Edamame, (young green soybeans):			
Boiled beans (no pods), 4 oz	160	7	12
Steamed (in pods), 4 oz	60	3	5
Katsu-don, Pork with Rice	1100	39	141
Miso Soup, with Tofu pieces, 1 cup	85	3	11
Sake Wine, (16% alcohol), 3 fl.oz	115	0	5
Seaweed Salad, 1.5 oz	20	2	4
Sukiyaki, (Beef/Tofu/Veg.), 8 oz	400	24	32
Tempura:			
3 large shrimp & veggies	320	18	25
1 shrimp only	60	4	3
Teppan Yaki, (Steak, Seafood & Veggies), 10 oz serving	470	30	15
Teriyaki: Beef, 4 oz	350	25	4
Chicken, 4 oz	260	9	7
Salmon, medium, 6 oz	270	8	3
Yakatori, 1 skewer, 2.5 oz	140	5	1

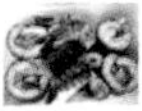

Kosher/Deli Foods

	C	F	Cb
Bagel/Bialy, 1 small, 2 oz	160	2	32
Beiglach, (Cheese Knish)	350	17	35
Blintzes, Average, 1 only	120	1	25
With Sour Cream & Preserves	370	10	30
Borscht, (Without Sour Cream): 1 cup	85	3	14
Diet/Reduced Calorie, 1 cup	30	1	7
Cabbage Roll, (meat/rice), 5 oz	170	6	21
Chicken Broth: 1 cup	80	8	0
With vegetables	100	8	5
With noodles	150	9	16
Lowfat, plain, 1 cup	25	1	0
Cholent, 1 medium serving, 1 cup	350	16	48
Chopped Liver, 1 serving, 3 oz	110	6	5
With Egg Salad, ¼ cup	100	7	3
Farfel, dry, ½ cup	90	0.5	21
Gefilte Fish Balls: Regular, med., 2 oz	55	2	4
With Jelled Broth	80	2	6
Cocktail size, 1 oz	30	1	2
Sweet, medium, 2 oz	65	2	4
With Jelled Broth	95	2	9
Hallah, (Yeast Bread), 1 slice, 1 oz	85	2	14
Herring: Smoked, 2 oz	120	8	0
In Sour Cream, 2 oz	150	10	0
Kasha, cooked, ½ cup	100	0.5	20
Kipfel, (Vanilla/Almond Cookie), 1 pce	60	2	7
Knaidlach ~ *See Matzo Balls*			
Knish: Kasha/Potato, 1 only	130	4	22
Cheese, 1 only	350	17	35
Kreplach, beef, 1 piece	40	1	6
Kugel, potato/noodle, 1 serving	300	20	25
Latkes, (Potato Pancake): 2 oz	200	11	22
3 Latkes with Sour Cran Apple Sce	750	25	95
Lochshen: Plain, 1 cup	130	2	26
Pudding, 1 cup	380	13	48
Lox (Smoked Salmon), 2 oz	65	2	0
Mandelbrot, (Almond Bread), 1 slice, ¼" thick	45	2	5
Matzo, 1 oz board	110	0.5	21
Matzo Balls: 2 small, or 1 large, 2"	90	3	12
Extra large ball, 3"	180	6	24
Matzo Ball Soup:			
Cup with 2 small or 1 large ball	150	5	27
Bowl with Chicken & Noodles	325	13	34
Jerry's Deli, large bowl	560	17	56
New York Cheesecake, 4 oz	350	24	26
Pierogi, potato/cheese, 1 piece	90	4	11
Reuben S'wich, w/ ½ lb Corned Beef	920	60	28
Schmaltz, (Rend'd Chicken Fat), 1 T.	90	10	0

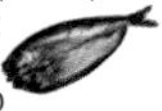

Korean Food

	C	F	Cb
Bibimbab (Veg. & Beef on Rice), 1 cup	**565**	**15**	89
Bulgogi (Barbeque Beef), 3.5 oz	**325**	**12**	15
Galbi (Short Ribs), 16 oz	**975**	**61**	16
Gujeolpan (Pancake with Meat & Vegetables), 1 cup w/ 1 pancake	**340**	**11**	39
Japchae (Noodle w/ Veggies & Meat), 1¼ cup	**365**	**19**	34
Sides:			
Kimchee (Cabbage Relish), ½ cup	**30**	**0**	6
Namool (Assorted Veg.), 1 cup	**125**	**6.5**	9
Soups: *Per Serving*			
Muguk (Radish & Chive Soup), 6 oz	**105**	**7**	6
Samgyetang (Ginseng Chkn Soup):			
Without Chicken Skin, 1 cup	**520**	**11**	60
With Chicken Skin, 1 cup	**725**	**35**	60
Yuk Gae Jang (Spicy Beef Soup), 1¼ cup	**180**	**13**	5

Lebanese/Middle East

	C	F	Cb
Baba Ghannouj, 2 Tbsp, 1 oz	**70**	**6**	2
Baklava (Pastry, Nuts, Syrup), 1 pastry, 1¾ oz	**245**	**18**	18
Cabbage Rolls (Cabb. Leaf, Meat, Rice), 1 roll, 3 oz	**100**	**3**	12
Cous Cous (Semolina, Milk, Fruit, Nuts), 1 serving	**400**	**21**	43
Felafel (Chick Pea Fritter), Fried, 1 medium, 1 oz	**60**	**4**	4
Hummus, ¼ cup, 2.2 oz	**105**	**3**	5
Fried Kibbi (Wheat, Meat Pinenuts), 1 piece, 3 oz	**180**	**8**	15
Kafta (Ground Lamb, Ssge on Skewer), 1 skewer, 1½ oz	**85**	**5**	2
Kibbeh Naye (raw Lamb, Bulgur & Spice) 1 cup, 9 oz	**450**	**18**	28
Lebanese Omelet, 1 serving, 4 oz (Egg, Spinach, Pinenuts, Onion)	**200**	**12**	13
Pilaf (Rice, Onion, Raisins, Apr., Spice) 1 cup	**400**	**11**	60
Shawourma (Spit-Roast Beef), 4 oz serving	**280**	**15**	2
Shish Kabob, 1 stick, 2½ oz	**130**	**7**	2
Spinach Pie, 1 piece, 3½ oz	**290**	**21**	20
Sweet Almond Sanbusak, (Pastry, Almonds, Spices), 1 pce	**200**	**15**	11
Tabouli, 1 serving, 4 oz	**125**	**7**	13
Tahini Sauce, average, 1 Tbsp	**90**	**8**	2

Mexican

	C	F	Cb
Burritos *(Taco Bell):* Bean	**370**	**10**	56
Supreme Beef	**420**	**16**	53
Chili, plain, ¼ cup	**90**	**6**	8
Chili con Carne: With Beans, 1 cup	**310**	**17**	15
Without Beans, 1 cup	**370**	**28**	10
Chimichangas, Beef, 5 oz	**400**	**19**	43
Chorizo Sausage, 2 oz	**265**	**23**	0
Churros, 1½ oz	**150**	**8**	18
Corn Chips, ½ cup, 1 oz	**160**	**10**	17
Costillas Ribs, 6 oz	**675**	**52**	0
Enchilada, average	**330**	**10**	49
Fajitas, Chicken	**200**	**7**	20
Guacamole, average, 2 Tbsp, 1 oz	**45**	**4**	2
Horchata: *(Don Jose)*, 1 c. 8 fl. oz	**140**	**4**	25
Cacique, 1 pint bottle, 16 fl. oz	**320**	**7**	62
Margarita, with 1½ oz Tequila	**160**	**0**	6
Masa (Pre-mixed for Tamales), 1 oz	**80**	**5**	9
Menudo, ½ cup	**55**	**1.5**	10
Nachos: *(Del Taco)*, Regular, 4 oz	**370**	**22**	28
Macho Nachos, 17 oz	**1000**	**56**	94
Taco Bell: BellGrande®, 10.75 oz	**770**	**42**	79
Supreme®, 6.75 oz	**440**	**25**	42
Nachos: With cheese, peppers, 1 portion, 6-8 nachos, 7 oz	**600**	**33**	60
W/ cheese, beans, beef, peppers, 1 portion, 6-8 nachos, 9 oz	**570**	**31**	56
Nopal Cactus Salad, 1 serving	**130**	**9**	11
Papas Fritas, (1), 6 oz	**325**	**18**	40
Piloncillo: (Brown Sugar)			
1 T., 0.46 oz	**50**	**0**	13
Cone, small, 3", 3 oz	**325**	**0**	81
Quesadilla, Cheese	**490**	**28**	39
Queso Fresco, ¼ cup	**80**	**4.5**	8
Refried Beans, ¾ cup, 6 oz	**160**	**3**	26
Rice Pudding *(Arroz Con Leche)*, 4 oz	**140**	**3**	24
Soup, Black Bean, 1 bowl	**200**	**3**	34
Tacos *(Taco Bell):*			
Crunchy: Regular	**170**	**10**	12
Supreme	**200**	**12**	15
Soft: Crispy Potato	**270**	**13**	31
Grilled Steak	**250**	**14**	19
Taco Salad with Salsa	**840**	**52**	85
Taco Sauce, average, ¼ cup	**15**	**0**	3
Taco Shell, regular	**50**	**2**	8
Tamales, Beef/Chicken, av. 4½ oz	**250**	**11**	27
Taquitos, Beef & Cheese, 4½ oz	**330**	**15**	36
Tostada (Taco Bell)	**250**	**10**	29
Tortilla, Corn, 6" diameter	**70**	**1**	14
Tortilla Chips, 1 oz	**150**	**8**	18
Soup, Black Bean, 1 bowl	**200**	**3**	34

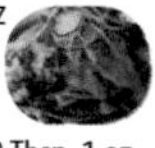

Extra Listings of Mexican Dishes ~ Fast-Foods Section (Taco Bell, Del Taco)

Canned Bean/Chili Products ~*See Page 111*

Mexican (Cont)

	C	F	Cb
Breads: Bolillos, 1 roll, 3½ oz	240	4	42
Telera, 2 oz	150	1.5	19
Mexican Cornbread, 4" square	210	11	19
Cakes, Cookies, Pastries:			
Banderilla (Pastry Puff), 1 shell	140	10	8
Bigotes, 7"	570	22	44
Calvos, 2½ oz	320	18	38
Capirotada (Bread Pudding), 10 oz	810	38	107
Cinnamon Cookies, 2	125	8	13
Cocadas, 1 oz	120	6	15
Cortadillo, 1 cookie, 1.9 oz	300	11	48
Concha (All Colors):			
Small (3" diameter), 2½ oz	250	8	38
Medium (4" diameter), 3½ oz	350	11	53
Large (5" diameter), 5½ oz	550	18	84
Cream Puff with Custard, 4¼ oz	255	14	25
Cuerno, 2 oz	200	4.5	34
Cuerno Fine, 2¾ oz	330	17	40
Donut, large, 4", 3½ oz	440	21	58
Elotes, 3½ oz	450	24	51
Empanadas (Average all types):			
Small, 2 oz	230	10	28
Regular, 3 oz	300	14	42
Fiesta Cookie (1), 2¼ oz	280	8	47
Galletas Mixtas (1), 1 oz	100	2.5	16
Guayaba, 3¼ oz	360	14	53
Jelly Roll (1), 3¼ oz	240	4	46
Mantecadites, 4½ oz	670	42	64
Mini Pound Cake, 1 slice, 3 oz	260	12	33
Mini Cupcake (1), 1¾ oz	180	8	25
Muffins/Nino Enbuelto, large, 6 oz	465	11	48
Nuez, 3¼ oz	380	17	52
Ojo De Buey, 4 oz	360	15	55
Oreja (Elephant Ear), 3 oz	310	15	38
Pan Dulce, 1 bun	330	10	45
Panquecitos, 2½ oz	260	11	36
Piedras, 2 oz	470	15	76
Polvorones (1), 3 oz	370	18	48
Puerquitos, 5 oz	600	24	88
Rebanadas, 3½ oz	390	18	51
Roles De Canela (Cinn. Roll), 4½ oz	490	15	81
Roscas, 2¾ oz	360	18	44
Semitas, 3 oz	300	10	46
Sopapillas (flaky pastry puffs): 1 piece	100	7	14
With Honey & Cream	200	14	18
Strawberry Crema Roll (⅙), 2½ oz	240	5	45
Extra Food Listings ~ See CalorieKing.com			

Polish

	C	F	Cb
Cabbage Rolls with Sour Cream, 2 sm.	220	10	30
Chicken Casserole w/ Mushrooms, 1 c.	520	27	5
Kielbasa (Sausages, Onions, fried), 2 large	350	28	2
Meatballs in Sour Cream, 3 x 1½" balls	300	16	11
Pierogi, Fruit/Vegetables, 3" ball	80	2	15
Pork Goulash (Pork/Vegetable Stew)	550	21	38
Pot Roast with Vegetables	630	21	28

Soul Foods

	C	F	Cb
Breakfast Sausage, fried, 2 patties	250	17	0
Brunswick Stew, 1 cup, 8.5 oz	320	14	19
Cornbread, homemade, 3 oz	200	7.5	28
Fatback, raw, 0.25 oz	60	6.5	0
Ham Hock	90	6.5	2
Hog Maw	45	2.5	0
Hominy, cooked, ¾ cup	110	0.5	25
Hush Puppies, 5 pieces	260	12	35
Kale, cooked, ½ cup	20	0.5	4
Oxtail	70	3.5	0
Pig's Ear, ¼ ear	50	3	0
Pig's Foot, ½ foot	70	4.5	0
Pig's Tail, ⅓ tail	115	10	0
Poke Salad, cooked, ½ cup	16	0.5	3
Pork Brains	40	2.5	0
Pork Chitterlings, simmered, 3 oz	260	25	0
Pork Cracklings, 0.5 oz	80	6	0
Pork Neck Bones	65	4	0
Pork Skin, 1 cup	70	4.5	0
Pork Tongue, ⅓ tongue	75	5.5	0
Possum	65	3	0
Sousemeat	60	4.5	0
Succotash, ½ cup	80	1	17
Sweet Potato Pie, ⅛ of 9" pie	250	12	34
Tripe, 2 oz	55	2	0
Vienna Sausage, 2 small	90	8	1
1 small	45	4	0.5

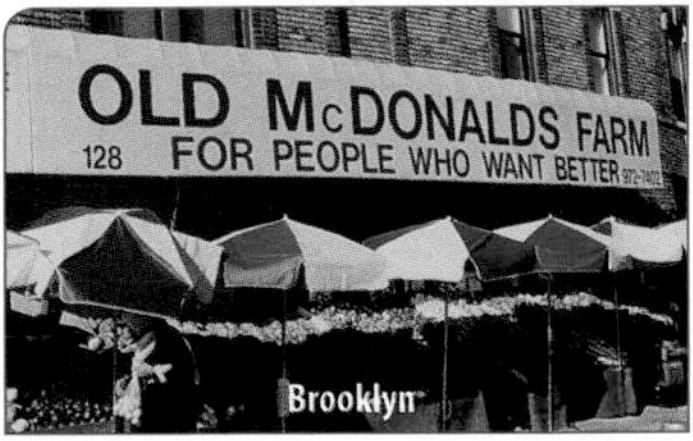

OLD McDONALDS FARM
128 FOR PEOPLE WHO WANT BETTER

Brooklyn

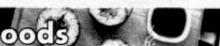

Spanish

	C	F	Cb
Arroz Abanda (Fish with Rice)	340	8	31
Arroz Con Pollo (Rice/Chicken Salad)	500	23	50
Clams Marinara, 8 clams	330	16	22
Cochifrito (Lamb with Lemon/Garlic)	650	25	5
Cochinillo Asado, 2 sl. (Rst Suckling Pig)	300	15	3
Cocido Madrileno			
(Madrid-Style Boiled Dinner)	450	27	18
Flan de Leche (Caramel Custard)	325	9	52
Fritadera de Ternera (Sauteed Veal)	450	27	2
Gazpacho, 1 bowl	60	0	15
Mole Poblano, ½ cup	205	14	16
Paella a la Valenciana			
(Chicken & Shellfish Rice)	900	42	70
Pollo a la Espanola (Chicken)	475	30	4
Ternera al Jerez (Veal with Sherry)	660	29	6
Zarzuela (Fish & Shellfish Medley)	530	27	40

Thai Foods

	C	F	Cb
Appetizers: Satay Pork, 1 oz	100	4	2
Spring Roll, 1¼ oz	110	6	13
Soups Tom Yam (Hot & Sour):			
Spicy Shrimp/Seafood: 1 cup	100	4	6
1 bowl	160	7	10
Vegetarian, 1 cup	50	0	11
Curries: Chicken with Ginger, 1 c.	390	34	4
Thick Red Curry withBeef, 1 cup	600	50	7
Thai Chicken Curry, 1 cup	340	23	4
Massaman Curry, 1 cup	680	57	8
Green Curry with Pork, 1 cup	480	44	5
Pad Thai, large serving, 18 oz	990	38	125
Fish: Steamed with Spicy Thai Sce	450	8	46
Crispy Fried, 5 oz	290	15	9
Spicy Chicken, stir-fry	450	22	14
Spicy Garlic Tofu, stir-fry	340	18	18
Sticky Thai Rice: Plain 1 cup, 6 oz	170	0.5	36
With Coconut & Sesame Seeds, 1 c.	880	28	120
Stir-fried Rice Noodles, 1 c. 5.5 oz	270	9	40
Stir-fried Vegetables, 1 cup	100	3	18
Salads: Green Papaya Salad	160	0	40
Spicy Prawn, 9 shrimp	170	3	15
Thai Chicken, 1 serving	330	9	17
Thai Beef Salad, 1 serving	260	9	15
Thai Noodle, 1 serving	410	13	45
Satay Chicken & Peanut Sauce,			
1 satay stick	390	24	20
Sauce, Peanut Satay, ½ c., 4 oz	160	10	13

Vietnamese

	C	F	Cb
Banh Cuon (Steam Rice w/ Pork), 1 roll	105	7	8
Bo Nuong (Beef Satay), 2 sticks	265	9	4
Bo Xao Dau Phong			
(Ginger Beef with Onion, Fish Sce)	750	30	10
Ca Chien Gung (Whole Snapper/Ginger)	600	16	6
Canh Chay (Vegetable/Tofu Soup)	80	3	13
Cari Chicken, 1 cup	475	29	16
Cari Chicken w/ Rice Noodle,			
cup curry & cup cooked noodles	660	29	60
Cari Chicken, w/ Steamed Rice,			
cup curry & cup rice	650	29	55
Cuu Xao Lan (Curried Lamb,			
Veggies in Coconut)	900	40	80
Ga Chien (Crisp Chick + Plum Sauce)	900	40	105
Ga Nuong (Chicken Satay + Sauce)	240	10	4
Ga Xao Rau (Marinated Chicken			
Braised with Vegetables)	800	26	100
Gio Lua (Lean Pork Pie), ⅛ of pie	245	12	0
Goi Cuon (Cold Spring Rolls), 1 roll	60	1	7
Rau Cai Xao Chay (Stir Fried Veges)	400	15	65
Thit Bo Vien (Beef Balls), 6 balls	225	14	2
Thit Heo Goi Baup Cai			
(Spicy Cabb. Rolls with Pork), 1roll	200	7	11
Soup: Per Bowl, ½ Cup			
Bun Bo Hue (Hot & Spicy Soup):			
Without Pork Feet	340	9	35
With Pork Feet	830	45	35
Chicken & Rice Noodle Soup	400	3	55
Pho Bo (Beef Noodle Soup)	410	7	59
Pho Ga (Chicken Noodle Soup)	460	6	58
Pho Tai (Rare Beef & Noodle Soup)	440	7	73
Salad, Goi Du Du,			
(Green Papaya), ½ cup	155	3	29
Sauce, Nuoc Cham (Hot Sauce)	5	0	1

Gourmet & Miscellaneous

	C	F	Cb
Ants Eggs/Larvae, 1 Tbsp	20	0	0
Ants, chocolate coated, 3 Tbsp	140	7	2
Bee Maggots, canned, 3 Tbsp	65	2	0
Caviar, black/red, 1 Tbsp	40	3	0
Caterpillars, canned, 2 oz	60	2	0
Frog Legs, fried, 1 pair (large)	125	7	0
Haggis, boiled, 4 oz	350	24	22
Locusts, roasted, 1 oz	35	1	0
Silkworms, raw, 1 oz	60	2	0
Snails in garlic butter, 6 large	200	10	4
Snake, roasted, 4 oz	160	6	0

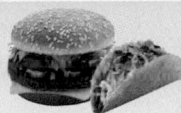

©2012
Allan Borushek

**For More Restaurants &
Full Nutritional Data
~ See CalorieKing.com**

A&W® (Oct '12)

Burgers:	C	F	Cb
Hamburger	380	19	33
Cheeseburger	420	21	37
Double Cheeseburger	680	38	44
Bacon Cheeseburger	530	30	39
Bacon Dble Cheeseburger	760	45	45
Papa Burger	690	39	44
Papa Single Burger	470	25	38
Sandwiches:			
Crispy Chicken	550	25	52
Grilled Chicken	400	15	31
Chicken Strips, 3 pces	500	29	32
Hot Dogs: Plain	310	19	23
Coney Chili Dog	340	20	26
Coney Chili Cheese Dog	380	23	28
Fries/Sides:			
French Fries: Small/Kids, 2.5 oz	200	8	28
Regular, 4 oz	310	12	45
Large, 5.5 oz	430	17	61
Cheese Fries: 6 oz	390	18	50
Chili Cheese Fries, 7 oz	410	17	52
Cheese Curds, Regular, 5 oz	570	40	27
Corn Dog Nuggets: 5 pieces	180	8	20
8 pieces	280	13	32
Onion Rings: Reg., Breaded, 4 oz	350	16	45
Large, 5.5 oz	480	27	62
Dipping Sauces: BBQ, 1 oz	40	0	10
Honey Mustard, 1 oz	100	6	12
Ranch, 1 oz	160	17	2
Sweets & Treats:			
Polar Swirl: M&M; Oreo	700	25	107
Reese's	740	31	97
Sundaes: Chocolate	320	8	53
Caramel; Hot Fudge, av.	345	10	56
Soft Serve Cone, Vanilla, 5.5 oz	260	7	41
Floats:			
A&W Root Beer: Medium, 20 oz	350	5	77
Large, 32 oz	640	10	136
Diet, 20 oz	170	5	30
Freeze, A&W Root Beer, 16 oz	370	8	68
Milkshakes: Strawb., Small, 16 oz	670	29	90
Chocolate; Vanilla, average:			
Small, 16 fl.oz	710	30	100
Medium, 20 oz	890	38	123
Smoothies: Pineapple Banana, 16 oz	400	6	85
Strawberry, 16 oz	360	6	70
Strawberry Banana, 16 oz	390	6	78
Sodas:			
A&W Root Beer: Reg., 20 oz	270	0	72
Diet, 20 oz	0	0	0
Pepsi: Small, 16 oz	200	0	56
Regular, 20 oz	250	0	70

Applebee's® (Oct '12)

Appetizers: As Served	C	F	Cb
Classic Wings: Classic Buffalo	710	49	8
Honey BBQ	790	35	59
Hot Buffalo	720	49	9
Boneless Wings: Classic Buffalo	1170	69	66
Honey BBQ	1250	55	116
Hot Buffalo	1170	70	67
Dips: Bleu Cheese	240	26	0.5
Ranch	200	21	1
Chili Cheese Nachos	1620	102	131
Crunchy Onion Rings	1290	56	181
Mozzarella Sticks (9)	930	48	84
Chicken: Includes Standard Sides			
Chicken Fried Chicken	1160	57	104
Chicken Parmesan Stack	1690	95	130
Chicken Tenders: Basket	1070	61	93
Platter	1390	79	118
Crispy Orange Chicken	1510	53	208
Pasta: As Served			
Blackened Steak Penne	1430	76	116
Chicken Broccoli Alfredo	1350	71	111
Three-Cheese Chicken Penne	1460	74	128
FreshBurgers: Without Fries			
Bacon Cheddar Cheeseburger	970	59	52
Cheeseburger	940	58	51
Cowboy Burger	1180	70	77
Fire Pit Bacon Burger	1130	75	53
Hamburger	790	46	50
Ribs: Includes Standard Sides			
Applebees Riblets: Basket	1180	55	109
Platter	1820	87	162
Sandwiches: Without Sides			
Applebees Reuben	880	53	50
Bacon Cheese Chicken Grill	750	33	51
Philly Cheese Steak	980	60	67
Zesty Ranch Chicken	1150	74	77
Seafood: As Served			
Blackened Tilapia	410	15	37
Double Crunch Shrimp	1280	69	133
Garlic Herb Salmon	680	29	62
Hand-Battered Fish & Chips	1570	106	108
New England Fish & Chips	1930	138	121
Sizzling Entrees: Includes Sides			
Bourbon Street Chicken & Shrimp	760	45	31
Bourbon Street Steak	740	44	31

Continued Next Page...

176

Applebees® cont... (Oct '12)

Sizzling Entrees Cont: Includes Sides C F Cb

Skillet Fajitas

		C	F	Cb
Chicken		1320	47	147
Combo		1460	66	151
Shrimp		1390	64	150
Steak		1400	54	151

Steaks & Toppers: *Without Sides*

	C	F	Cb
House Sirloin, 9 oz	310	13	0
New York Strip, 12 oz	480	24	0.5
Ribeye, 12 oz	670	47	3
Shrimp 'N Parmesan Sirloin	670	42	5
Steak Combos: With Fried Shrimp	650	34	37
With Grilled Shrimp	540	36	2
With Honey BBQ Chicken	600	15	37
Toppers: Baked Potato	330	18	41
Garlic Mashed Potatoes	250	15	26
Sauteed Garlic Mushrooms	130	12	4

Under 550 Calories: *Includes Sides*

	C	F	Cb
Cabernet Mushroom Sirloin	460	15	39
Creamy Parmesan Chicken	470	13	35
Grilled Dijon Chicken & Portobellos	470	16	30
Roasted Garlic Sirloin	450	18	33
Signature Sirloin w/ Garlic Shrimp	500	20	31

Salads: *Regular, Without Dressing*

	C	F	Cb
Bruschetta Chicken	790	36	56
Grilled Shrimp 'N' Spinach	630	46	20
Grilled Steak Caesar	470	21	22
Oriental Chicken	730	41	57

Sides: *As Served*

	C	F	Cb
Chili Bowl	410	27	14
Chili Cheese Fries	590	32	59
Cole Slaw	140	9	15
Crunchy Onion Rings	530	28	63
Fries	390	18	53
Garlic Mashed Potatoes	250	15	26
Loaded Baked Potato	400	23	41

Soups: *Per Bowl*

	C	F	Cb
Clam Chowder	370	26	22
French Onion	260	15	15
Tomato Basil	260	16	27

Desserts: *As Served*

	C	F	Cb
Maple Butter Pecan Blondie	1020	55	120
Shooters: Chocolate Mousse	460	32	42
Hot Fudge Sundae	350	18	43
Triple Choc. Meltdown	830	48	97

Arby's® (Oct '12)

Sandwiches: C F Cb

	C	F	Cb
Beef 'n Cheddar: Classic	440	10	47
Mid	530	23	48
Max	650	29	52
Roast Beef: Classic	350	12	39
Mid	440	17	40
Max	580	22	49
Ultimate Angus:			
Philly	590	29	48
Three Cheese & Bacon	640	33	45
Chicken:			
Chicken Bacon & Swiss: Crispy	610	30	51
Roast	480	20	43
Cravin Chicken: Crispy	510	22	51
Roast	380	12	42
Roast Chicken Club	460	19	42

Market Fresh Sandwiches:

	C	F	Cb
Reuben	640	30	62
Roast Turkey & Swiss	700	27	77
Roast Turkey, Ranch & Bacon	800	36	78

Wraps:

	C	F	Cb
Roast Turkey & Swiss	490	25	39
Roast Turkey, Ranch & Bacon	590	33	39

Chicken:

Prime Cuts: Chicken Tenders (3) 350 17 25
Chicken Tenders (5) 590 28 42

Optional/Regional Items:

Chicken Cordon Bleu Sandwich:

	C	F	Cb
Crispy	620	32	48
Roast	500	22	40
Homestyle Fries: Small	360	17	49
Medium	480	22	66
Large	610	28	82

Loaded Potato Bites:

	C	F	Cb
5 Bites	330	19	31
8 Bites	530	30	50
Melts: Arby's	330	11	40
Ham & Swiss	300	9	37

Regular Combos: *Includes Small Curly Fries and Small Pepsi*

	C	F	Cb
Beef 'n Cheddar, mid	1110	45	144
Chicken, Bacon & Swiss, Crispy	1190	52	147
Reuben Sandwich	1220	52	158
Roast Chicken Club Sandwich	1040	41	138
Roast Turkey & Swiss Sandwich	1280	49	173

Sides & Snacks:

	C	F	Cb
Curly Fries: Small, 4.5 oz	400	22	47
Medium, 6 oz	540	29	62
Large, 7 oz	630	35	74
Mozzarella Sticks, regular, 4 sticks	420	21	35
Potato Cakes: 3 Cakes	340	20	37
4 Cakes	460	27	50

Continued Next Page...

Arby's® cont... (Oct '12)

	C	F	Cb
Market Fresh Chopped Salads: *Without Dressing*			
Chopped Farmhouse Chicken:			
Crispy	430	24	26
Roasted	250	14	11
Dressings: *Per 1.5 oz packet*			
Balsamic Vinaigrette	130	12	5
Buttermilk Ranch	210	22	2
Dijon Honey Mustard	180	16	8
Kids Meals:			
Curly Fries, 2.75 oz	240	13	28
Jr Rst Beef Sandwich	210	6	25
Jr Turkey & Cheese Sandwich	210	5	24
Macaroni & Cheese	170	5	25
Prime Cut Chicken Tenders (2), 3 oz	230	11	17
Sliced Apples, 2.2 oz	35	0	9
Breakfast: *Per Serving*			
Biscuits: Bacon, Egg & Cheese	450	26	34
Ham, Egg & Cheese	420	21	34
Sausage, Egg & Cheese	600	42	35
Croissants: Bacon, Egg & Cheese	380	24	24
Ham, Egg & Cheese	350	20	24
Sausage, Egg & Cheese	540	40	26
Sourdoughs:			
Bacon, Egg & Cheese	460	21	44
Ham, Egg & Cheese	430	16	44
Sausage, Egg & Cheese	610	37	46
Wraps:			
Bacon, Egg & Cheese	490	26	43
Ham, Egg & Cheese	420	20	42
Sausage, Egg & Cheese	620	40	44
Sauces:			
Arby's, ½ oz	15	0	3
Bronco Berry, 1 oz	60	0	15
Cheddar Cheese, 1.5 oz	50	3.5	4
Marinara, 1 oz	25	0.5	3
Spicy Three Pepper, ½ oz	25	1	3
Dipping Sauces:			
Buffalo, 1 oz	10	1	1
Ranch, 1 oz	100	11	1
Desserts:			
Turnovers: Apple with Icing	430	18	64
Cherry Turnover with Icing	390	13	64
Shakes: *Per 17 fl. oz*			
Chocolate	570	15	99
Vanilla	470	15	75
Drinks: *Per Small, 16 fl.oz Cup*			
Mountain Dew	200	0	54
Pepsi	180	0	49

Atlanta Bread Co® (Oct '12)

Sandwiches:	C	F	Cb
Chicken Salad on Sourdough	440	19	42
Honey Maple Ham on Honey Wheat	410	5	64
Tuna Salad on French	630	33	57
Turkey on Nine Grain	370	6	50
Veggie on Nine Grain	500	25	52
Signature Sandwiches: *On Focaccia Unless Indicated*			
ABC Special on French Baguette	750	38	57
Bella Chicken	610	38	34
California Avocado	930	50	98
NY Hot Pastrami on Rye	660	29	59
Turkey Bacon Rustica	960	56	62
Paninis: Chicken Pesto	710	26	80
Chicken Cordon Bleu	670	19	80
Cubano	650	19	80
Italian Vegetarian	570	16	84
Turkey Club	710	24	81
Salads: *Without Dressing*			
Balsamic Bleu Salad	330	18	35
Chopstix Chicken Salad	240	10	22
Greek Salad	240	16	15
House Salad	90	2	13
Salsa Fresca Salmon Salad	560	29	40
Soups: *Per 1¼ Cups*			
Baja Chicken Enchilada	330	19	23
Broccoli Cheese	250	17	14
Chicken & Sausage Gumbo	190	6	24
Chili, Beef/Frontier, average	290	10	30
Homestyle Chicken & Dumpling	400	34	17
Tomato Fennel & Dill	290	23	18
Wisconsin Cheese	290	15	24

For Complete Menu & Data ~ see CalorieKing.com

Au Bon Pain® (Oct '12)

Bagels: *Per Bagel*	C	F	Cb
Asiago Cheese	370	8	56
Cinnamon Crisp	410	7	77
Everything	300	2	58
Jalapeno Double Cheddar	320	8	52
Honey 9 Grain	310	2	63
Cream Cheese Spreads: *Per 2 oz*			
Lite Cream Cheese	120	9	5
Honey Pecan, 2.5 oz	200	16	10
Vegetable	170	16	3

Continued Next Page... ...

Au Bon Pain® cont... (Oct '12)

Breakfast Sandwiches:	C	F	Cb
Egg on a Bagel:	440	17	58
With Bacon	510	18	58
With Cheese	480	16	58
Egg Whites & Cheddar, on Skinny Wheat Bagel	230	9	22
Smkd. Salmon & Wasabi/On. Dill	410	10	62

Cafe Sandwiches: *Per Whole Sandwich*			
Black Angus Roast Beef & Cheddar	480	17	47
Black Forest Ham & Cheddar	640	17	92
Classic Chicken Salad	450	11	61
Grilled Chicken	450	12	47
Tuna Salad	430	12	54
Turkey & Swiss	740	30	79

Signature Sandwiches: *Per Whole Sandwich*			
Black Angus Roast Beef & Herb Cheese	520	14	71
Caprese	550	27	52
Chipotle Turkey & Avocado	660	31	58
Lobster Salad BLT on Brioche	650	33	54
The Veggie	650	26	78
Turkey Club	600	24	53

Wraps: Chicken Caesar	620	29	54
Mediterranean	550	24	65
Southwest Tuna	710	38	59
Thai Peanut Chicken	550	15	75

Harvest Rice Bowls:			
Angus Steak Teriyaki	730	20	107
Mayan Chicken	630	16	92

Soups: *Per Medium 12 oz Bowl*			
Baked Stuffed Potato	380	22	32
Carrot Ginger	140	5	24
Chicken Gumbo	190	9	22
Corn & Green Chili Bisque	290	17	29
Cream of Chicken & Wild Rice	250	15	24
Italian Wedding	190	10	16
Southern Black-Eyed Pea	190	2	31
Tomato Florentine	140	3	20
Vegetarian Chili	240	3	43
Wild Mushroom Bisque	190	9	22

Specialty Soups: *Per 12 fl.oz Bowl*			
BBQ Chkn & Beef Stew	300	10	36
Beef & Vegetable	330	17	27
Chicken Pot Pie	370	22	26
Lobster Bisque	410	30	25
Macaroni & Cheese	560	35	37
Turkey Chili	380	14	43

Au Bon Pain® cont... (Oct '12)

Salads: *Without Dressing*	C	F	Cb
Chef's, 9 oz	260	15	8
Chicken Cobb, with Avocado	410	25	12
Greek	230	15	16
Mediterranean Chicken, 10.25 oz	290	16	12
Thai Peanut Chicken, 10.5 oz	200	5	18
Tuna Garden, 12 oz	270	13	19
Turkey, Apple, Brie & Spinach	430	25	30

Dressings: Balsamic Vinaig., 2 oz	120	9	8
Bleu Cheese, 2 oz	310	33	2
Caesar, 2 oz	270	28	4
Sesame Ginger, 2 oz	230	20	12
Thai Peanut, 2 oz	160	8	20

Bakery: *Per Item*			
Brownie, Choc Chip, 4 oz	440	21	62
Cakes: Red Velvet Cupcake, 3.1 oz	400	22	46
Pound Cakes: Lemon, 4.3 oz	490	25	63
Marble, 4.1 oz	420	23	50
Cookies: Chocolate Chip, 2 oz	280	13	40
Shortbread, 2.25 oz	340	20	37
Croissants, Filled: Almond	540	33	50
Apple	280	11	44
Chocolate	440	22	58
Raspberry Cheese	370	17	46
Sweet Cheese	400	19	49
Muffins: Blueberry	490	17	74
Carrot/Cranberry Walnut, av.	550	26	69
Raisin Bran	480	11	85
Triple Berry, low-fat	300	3	65
Beverages: Caffe Latte, 16 fl.oz	250	14	21
Hot Chocolate, 16 fl.oz	460	15	74
Peach Iced Tea, 24 fl.oz	270	0	67
Strawberry Smoothie, 16 fl.oz	310	1	66

For Complete Nutritional Data ~ see CalorieKing.com

Aunty Anne's® (Oct '12)

Pretzels: *With Butter*	C	F	Cb
Almond	390	6	74
Cinnamon Sugar	470	12	84
Garlic	350	5	65
Jalapeno	330	5	63
Original	340	5	65
Original Stix, 6 sticks	340	5	65
Sesame	400	10	67
Sour Cream & Onion	360	5	68

Continued Next Page ...

Aunty Anne's® cont... (Oct '12)

Dipping Sauces:

	C	F	Cb
Caramel Dip, 1.5 oz	130	3	23
Cheese Dip; Hot Salsa Cheese, av., 1.1 oz	95	7.5	3
Light Cream Cheese, 1.25 oz	80	6	1
Marinara Sauce, 2 oz	45	1	7
Sweet Glaze, 1.5 oz	130	0	32
Sweet Mustard, 1.25 oz	60	2	10

Beverages: Per Serving
Dutch Ice: Per 20 fl.oz

Blue Raspberry	240	0	62
Pina Colada	300	0	73
Strawberry	230	0	58
Wild Cherry	280	0	69

Dutch Smoothie: Per 20 fl.oz

Blue Raspberry	440	15	72
Mocha	540	22	79
Pina Colada	470	15	79
Strawberry	430	15	69

Back Yard Burgers® (Oct '12)

Burgers:

	C	F	Cb
American Cheeseburger, ⅓ lb	730	44	47
Back Yard Burger, ⅓ lb	680	39	47
Black Jack	780	49	48
Bleu Cheeseburger: ⅓ lb	780	47	47
⅔ lb	1270	86	47
Cheddar Cheeseburger: ⅓ lb	790	48	47
⅔ lb	1290	88	47
Jr Burger	530	27	47
Mushroom Swiss	790	49	45
Pepper Jack, ⅓ lb	740	45	47
Swiss Cheeseburger: ⅓ lb	790	48	47
⅔ lb	1290	88	47

Chicken Sandwiches:

Blackened Chicken	540	24	53
Crispy Chicken	590	26	65
Grilled Chicken	350	4.5	47
Hawaiian Chicken	450	11	59

Specialities:

Big Dog	500	33	32
Bak-Pak: Chicken Tender Meal	1110	71	91
Dog	320	18	29
Chicken Tender Meal	1260	79	102
Chili Cheese Big Dog	630	44	34
Garden Veggie Burger	400	8	57

Back Yard Burgers® cont... (Oct '12)

Sides: Per Serving

	C	F	Cb
Chili	150	9	8
Seasoned Fries: Regular, 6 oz	640	45	58
Large, 9 oz	960	68	87

Salads: Without Dressing

Chicken: Blackened	330	15	25
Fried	410	19	41
Grilled	220	4	23
Garden Fresh	100	2	20
Side Salad	30	0	6

Dressings: Per Serving

Balsamic Vinaigrette	170	17	3
Bleu Cheese	220	24	1
Honey Mustard	240	23	7
Ranch	150	15	2

Desserts: Per Serving

Cobblers: Apple	360	14	59
Blackberry	290	8	51
Cherry	350	12	59
Peach	330	11	56

Shakes: Per 12 fl.oz

Chocolate; Strawberry, average	630	29	83
Vanilla	620	28	83

Baja Fresh® (Oct '12)

Burritos: With Standard Menu Board Components

	C	F	Cb
Baja: With Carnitas	830	45	67
With Chicken	790	38	65
With Steak	850	46	67
Bean & Cheese: With Carnitas	1010	42	98
With Chicken	970	35	96
With Steak	1030	43	97
Vegetarian, without Meat	840	33	96
Mexicano: With Carnitas	830	20	119
With Chicken	790	13	117
With Steak	860	21	118
Ultimo: With Chicken	880	36	84
With Steak	950	44	85
Vegetarian, Grilled Veggie	800	33	94

Fajitas: As Served, Without Tortilla Chips

Chicken, with Corn Tortillas	860	24	105
Chicken, with Flour Tortillas	1140	33	147

Nachos: As Served

Grande: With Cheese	1890	108	163
With Chicken	2020	110	164
With Steak	2120	118	163

Continued Next Page...

Updated Nutrition Data ~ www.CalorieKing.com
Persons with Diabetes ~ See Disclaimer (Page 22)

Baja Fresh® cont... (Oct '12)

Quesadillas: With Grilled Flour Tortilla and Standard Menu Board Components

	C	F	Ch
With Cheese	1200	78	84
With Chicken	1330	80	84
With Steak	1430	87	84
Vegetarian	1260	78	96

Tacos: With 2 Grilled Corn Tortillas & Standard Menu Board Components

Original Baja:

With Chicken	210	5	28
With Shrimp	200	5	28

Salads: With Standard Menu Board Components, Without Dressing

Baja Ensalada:

With Carnitas	370	18	20
With Chicken	310	7	18
With Shrimp	230	6	18
With Steak	450	18	18

Tostada:

With Carnitas	1180	62	100
With Shrimp	1120	55	99
With Steak	1230	63	98

For Complete Nutritional Data ~ see CalorieKing.com

Baskin Robbins® (Oct '12)

Ice Creams: Per 4 oz Scoop

	C	F	Cb
Classic Flavors: Cherries Jubilee	240	12	30
Chocolate	260	14	33
Jamoca Almond Fudge	260	15	29
Made With Snickers	290	14	36
Mint Chocolate Chip	260	16	28
Old Fashioned Butter Pecan	280	18	25
Oreo Cookies 'n Cream	280	15	32
Peanut Butter 'n Chocolate	320	20	30
Pistachio Almond	280	19	22
Pralines 'n Cream	280	14	35
Rainbow Sherbet	160	2	34
Reese's P'nut Butter Cup	300	17	32
Vanilla	260	16	27
Very Berry Strawberry	220	11	27
World Class Chocolate	280	16	31
Seasonal Flavors: Cotton Candy	260	12	32
Baseball Nut	270	14	30
Egg Nog	250	13	30
Fudge Brownie	310	18	35
German Chocolate	300	17	34
Lemon Custard Cream	260	13	30
Rum Raisin	240	11	30
Strawberry Shortcake	280	14	34

Baskin Robbins® cont... (Oct '12)

Classic Sundaes:

	C	F	Cb
Banana Royale	620	20	07
Banana Split	1010	34	173
Brownie	920	47	119
Choc. Chip Cookie Dough	990	43	138
Made With Snickers	1000	46	138
Two Scoop	530	29	61

Soft Serve:

Parfaits: Per Regular 15 oz Size

Oreo	740	27	114
Reese's	990	63	86
Strawberry 'n Almonds	600	27	76

'31 Below' Mix-In: Per 16 oz Medium Cup

Butterfinger	840	32	127
Choc. Chip Cookie Dough	860	30	132
Heath	940	43	121
Oreo	750	28	110
Reese's P'nut Butter Cup	880	40	115
Cups: Vanilla: Kid's, 3 oz	130	4.5	18
Regular, 6 oz	250	9	37
Large, 9 oz	380	14	55
Cake Bites: Chocolate Mint, 3 oz	330	20	33
Double Chocolate, 3 oz	310	18	35
Oreo Cookie, 2.7 oz	290	17	31
Praline Caramel, 3 oz	360	22	39

Beverages:

Freezes, with Or. Sherbet:

Small, 16.3 oz	370	4	82
Medium, 23 oz	510	5	112

Fruit Blast: Per Med., 24 fl.oz

Peach Passion Fruit	370	0.5	94
Strawberry Citrus	350	0	87
Wild Mango	500	1.5	123

Milk Shakes: Per Medium, 24 fl.oz

Choc. with Choc. Ice Cream	930	40	129
Mint Chocolate Chip	890	44	109
Strawb. w/ Strawb. Ice Cream	780	31	109

Smoothie: Per Medium, 24 fl.oz

Mango Banana	630	2	150
Strawberry Banana	520	1	126
Tropical Banana	550	1.5	132
Cones: Cake	25	0	5
Sugar	45	0.5	9
Waffle	160	4	28

Big Apple Bagels® (Oct '12)

Bagels:

	C	F	Cb
Regular flavors, average all, 5 oz	340	2	70

Choice Bagels: Per Bagel

	C	F	Cb
Blueberry Cobbler	390	8	70
Cheddar Nacho	350	6	60
Cinnamon Apple Pie	385	8	68
Cinnamon Bun	400	8	70
Cinnamon Danish	395	8	72
French Toast	370	4	74
Quiche Lorraine	355	8	54
Strawberry White Chocolate	365	4	72
Swiss Melt	370	8	58
White Chocolate Swirl	395	8	70

Cream Cheese: Per 2 Tbsp, 1 oz

	C	F	Cb
Plain	90	9	2
Plain, Lite	60	4.5	3
Other varieties, average	90	8	2
Whipped: Classic Plain	70	7	1
Brown Sugar Cinnamon	70	5	5
Reduced-Fat Spring Veggie	60	5	2

Overstuffed Sandwich,

	C	F	Cb
Manhattan Club	1122	40	120

Specialty Sandwiches:

	C	F	Cb
Big Apple Club	795	37	75
Chicken Caesar	610	19	78
Grilled Chicken	570	17	77
Turkey Club	780	34	75

Toasted Sandwiches:

	C	F	Cb
Cafe Chicken Melt	815	32	80
Roast Beef Parmesan Grinder	585	15	76
Tuna Melt	640	23	75
Breakfast, Morning Classic	485	11	73

For Complete Nutritional Data ~ see CalorieKing.com

Biggby Coffee® (Oct '12)

Hot Drinks:

Per Tall, 16 fl.oz, w/o Cream & Sugar Unless Indicated

	C	F	Cb
Caffe Latte: With 2% Milk	175	7	16
With Non-Fat Milk	115	0	16
With Soy	160	5	19
Cappuccino: With 2% Milk	105	4	10
With Non-Fat Milk	70	0	10
With Soy	95	3	11
Chai Latte: With 2% Milk	315	7.5	51
With Non-Fat Milk	255	0	51
Cocoa Carmella: *With Sugar*			
With 2% Milk	325	9	51
Add Whipped Cream	405	15	55
Mocha Mocha: *With Sugar*			
With 2% Milk	295	8	48
Add Whipped Cream	375	14	52

Biggby Coffee® cont... (Oct '12)

Cold Drinks: *Per Tall, 16 fl.oz*

	C	F	Cb

Frozen Hot Chocolate: With 2% Milk & Whipped Cream

	C	F	Cb
Regular	565	18	93
Mint	560	18	93
Raspberry	565	18	94

Frozen Lattes, Almond Blizzard

	C	F	Cb
with Whipped Cream & Sugar	475	15	80

For Complete Menu & Data ~ see CalorieKing.com

Blimpie® (Oct '12)

Cold Deli Subs:

Per 6" White Sub, with Standard Menu Board Toppings

	C	F	Cb
Blimpie Best	450	18	47
BLT	430	22	43
Club	410	13	49
Ham & Swiss	410	14	47
Roast Beef & Provolone	430	15	44
Tuna without Cheese	460	21	41
Turkey & Provolone	410	14	47

Wraps: *Includes Dressing*

	C	F	Cb
Caesar	590	26	56
Southwestern	500	19	60

Hot Deli Subs: *Per 6" White Sub with Standard Menu Board Toppings*

	C	F	Cb
Meatball	560	29	47
Pastrami	430	16	42
VegiMax	520	21	55

Salads: *Regular, Without Dressing*

	C	F	Cb
Buffalo Chicken	220	9	10
Garden	30	0	6
Tuna Salad	270	19	6
Ultimate Club	270	14	11

Dressings & Sauces: *Per 1.5oz*

	C	F	Cb
Creamy Caesar	210	21	2
Creamy Italian	180	18	4

Soups: *Per 8.5 oz Serving*

	C	F	Cb
Chicken Noodle	130	4	18
Cream of Broccoli with Cheese	250	19	13
Harvest Vegetable	100	1	19
New England Clam Chowder	170	3	28
Vegetable Beef	80	2	13

Desserts:

	C	F	Cb
Brownie	230	10	28
Cookies: Oatmeal Raisin	160	8	23
Sugar	320	15	42

For Complete Nutritional Data ~ see CalorieKing.com

Bob Evans® (Oct '12)

Starters:

	C	F	Cb
Breaded Garlic Mushrooms, 11 oz	460	18	63
Country Fair Cheese Bites	950	66	49
Crispy Buttermilk Shrimp, 5 pieces	345	24	18

Sandwiches & Burgers:

	C	F	Cb
Big Farm Burgers: Regular	725	42	50
Bacon Cheeseburger	900	58	51
Favorite Burger	830	51	48
Smokehouse Burger	1170	78	65

Sandwiches

	C	F	Cb
Farm Favorites: Chicken, Fried	660	26	61
Chicken, Grilled	520	17	48
Farm-Grill: Chicken Club, Fried	670	27	61
Chicken Club, Grilled	535	18	48
Knife & Fork Turkey	775	42	62
Pot Roast	650	36	49
Turkey Bacon Melt, full size	570	27	49

Dinners: Without Sides Unless Indicated

	C	F	Cb
Beef: Country Fried Steak w/ Gravy	605	41	42
Meatloaf, 1 slice	345	23	15
Pot Roast Stroganoff, 24 oz	825	48	61
Spaghetti with Meat Sce, 21.5 oz	785	35	87
Chicken: Chicken & Brocc. Alfredo	845	45	61
Chicken-N-Noodles: Deep-Dish	665	30	72
Slow Roasted, 13.5 oz	225	4	31
Chicken Parmesan, w/ sauce, 27 oz	1145	53	100
Chicken Pot Pie, slow roasted	860	56	63
Garlic Butter Grilled Chkn Breast	160	4	1
Fish: Garlic Butter Salmon, 8 oz	255	9	1
Potato-Crusted Flounder, 5 oz	175	7	9
Wildfire Salmon, 8.5 oz	310	9	15
Turkey: Slow-Roasted, 3.5 oz	115	4	3
Turkey & Dressing, 16.5 oz	645	31	53
Side Dishes: Coleslaw, 3.5 oz	210	14	19
Baked Potato, Plain, 10 oz	195	0	50
Bread & Celery Dressing, 6 oz	295	16	29
French Fries, 7 oz	495	21	71
Hash Browns, 4.5 oz	315	9	53
Home Fries, 5 oz	180	6	28
Loaded Baked Potato, 12 oz	395	16	53
Loaded Home Fries, 5.1 oz	270	16	22
Macaroni & Cheese, 7 oz	305	15	29
Mashed Potatoes, 5 oz	190	9	24
Gravy: Beef, 2.25 oz	20	1	2
Chicken Roasted, 2 oz	50	4	3
Country, 3 oz	55	2	8

Bob Evans® cont... (Oct '12)

Sauces:

	C	F	Cb
Hollandaise, 1 oz	25	1	3
Wildfire BBQ, 1 oz	60	0	15

Soups: Per Bowl

	C	F	Cb
Beef Vegetable	165	3	25
Cheddar Baked Potato	330	19	26
Farm Festival Bean	200	3	28

Salads: Large, Without Dressing

	C	F	Cb
Cobb, 14.5 oz	515	31	10
Cranberry Pecan Chicken, 14 oz	620	36	34
Heritage Chef, 12.5 oz	400	25	11
Wildfire Grilled Chicken, 13.5 oz	390	13	37

Dressings: Per 3 oz

	C	F	Cb
Blue Cheese	410	44	5
Buttermilk Ranch	290	29	3
Sweet Italian	255	23	12

Breakfast:

	C	F	Cb
Biscuit Bowls: Sausage, 19 oz	975	59	76
Spinach, Bacon & Tomato, 18.5 oz	1015	60	79
Hotcakes: Without Topping			
Buttermilk (1)	330	8	58
Cranberry Multigrain (1)	330	4	68
Loaded Hash Browns, 6.5 oz	520	25	57
Omelets: Border Scramble	630	45	15
With Egg Lites	415	23	14
Farmer's Market	535	38	13
Western	495	35	7
Pot Roast Hash, 14.5 oz	760	53	29
Sunshine Skillet, 11.5 oz	435	24	38

Fit From The Farm:
Breakfast:

	C	F	Cb
Be Fit Breakfast	350	3	68
Veggie Omelet w/ Fruit/Toast/Jelly	310	6	43
Salad: Apple Cranberry Spinach, with Reduced Fat Raspb. Drssng	370	14	48
Kid's Menu: French Fries, 4.5 oz	320	13	46
Fried Chicken Strips (1), 1.5 oz	135	8	10
Mac & Cheese, 7 oz	300	9	45
Mini Cheeseburger (1)	275	15	21
Plenty-O-Pancakes, Plain, w/o Topping, 11.5 oz	710	18	130
Smiley Face Potatoes, 3 oz	270	16	29
Sundae, Fudge Blast, 4 oz	215	9	31
Dessert: Coconut Cream Pie, 7 oz sl.	515	29	59
French Silk Pie, 5.5 oz slice	660	44	60
Peanut Butter Brownie Bites (8)	1025	49	134

Bojangles® (Oct '12)

Sandwiches:

	C	F	Cb
Cajun Filet: Regular	495	27	43
Club	640	39	44
Grilled Chicken: Regular	375	15	33
Club	520	27	34

Biscuit: Plain

	C	F	Cb
	280	14	33
Bacon, Egg & Cheese	550	37	35
Cajun Filet	515	28	45
Country Ham	355	18	33
Egg & Cheese	515	34	35
Gravy Biscuits	390	20	43
Sausage	420	27	33
Steak	555	35	44

Fixins': Per Individual Serve Unless Indicated

	C	F	Cb
Bo-Tato Rounds, medium	350	22	35
Cole Slaw	255	20	18
Dirty Rice	165	6	24
Macaroni & Cheese	240	7	33
Mashed Potatoes 'N Gravy	150	6	21
Picnic Grits	230	2	47
Seasoned Fries: Individual	215	14	20
Medium size	300	20	27
Picnic size	530	35	49

Salads: Chicken Supreme

	C	F	Cb
	460	18	33
Garden	190	9	9
Grilled Chicken	305	11	11

Sweet Biscuits: Bo Berry (1)

	C	F	Cb
	375	15	55
Cinnamon Twist (1)	270	12	36

For Complete Nutritional Data ~ see CalorieKing.com

Boston Market® (Oct '12)

Sandwiches: With Menu Board Set Toppings

	C	F	Cb
All White Rotisserie Chicken Salad	950	60	74
Brisket Dip Carver, whole	840	45	62
Roasted Turkey Carver:			
Whole	850	43	65
Half	430	21	32
Rotisserie Chicken Carver: Whole	770	35	66
Half	360	17	31

Individual Meals: Without Sides

	C	F	Cb
Beef Brisket, regular, 4 oz	230	13	0
Meatloaf, regular, 7.5 oz	480	30	25
Rotisserie Chicken, half, 12 oz	640	33	2

Boston Market® cont... (Oct '12)

Salads: Includes Dressing

	C	F	Cb
Chicken Caesar: Whole, 13.5 oz	670	43	32
Half, 7 oz	340	21	16
Mediterranean: Whole, 15 oz	640	44	27
Half, 7.5 oz	340	21	16
Southwest Santa Fe: Whole, 17.8 oz	760	46	50
Half, 8.9 oz	380	23	25

Sides:

	C	F	Cb
Creamed Spinach, 6.3 oz	260	21	11
Fresh Steamed Vegetables, 4.8 oz	80	5	8
Fresh Vegetable Stuffing, 5.5 oz	220	10	28
Garlic Dill New Potatoes, 4.5 oz	100	2	20
Garlic Lemon Spinach, 6 oz	120	9	8
Gravy: Beef, 1 oz	10	0	2
Poultry, 1 oz	10	0	2
Green Beans, 4.25 oz	90	6	9
Macaroni & Cheese, 7.4 oz	280	11	33
Mashed Potatoes: Reg., 7.oz	240	10	32
Loaded, 7 oz	310	16	31
Rice Pilaf, 6.6 oz	190	3	37
Sweet Potato Casserole, 7.4 oz	480	14	87

Soups:

	C	F	Cb
Chicken Noodle, 14 oz	230	8	22
Chicken Tortilla: W/ Toppings, 12.8 oz	430	25	36
Without Toppings, 10.8 oz	270	14	22

Desserts:

	C	F	Cb
Apple Pie, 1 Slice, 5.75 oz	430	21	59
Chocolate Brownie (1), 4.7 oz	470	19	64
Chocolate Cake, 1 Slice, 5 oz	580	32	67

For Complete Nutritional Data ~ see CalorieKing.com

Boston's Gourmet Pizza® (Oct '12)

Starters: Per Order

	C	F	Cb
Oven Roasted Wings, Cajun, 15 oz	800	57	21
Spinach & Artichoke Dip, with Garlic Parmesan Bread	1260	60	124

Burgers & Sandwiches:

	C	F	Cb
Burgers: Bacon Cheeseburger	1240	92	45
Boston Cheeseburger	1170	86	48

Sandwiches:

	C	F	Cb
Beef Dip with Fries, Horseradish & Au Jus	1410	58	189
Boston's Cheesesteak, with Fries & Au Jus	1630	75	193
Double Decker Club	780	33	57
Gr. Chipotle Chicken w/o Bacon	530	24	40
Pulled Pork Slider, with Fries	1140	46	124

Continued Next Page...

Boston's Pizza® cont... (Oct '12)

Pizzas: Per Whole Medium Pizza

	C	F	Cb
Basic Cheese	1810	49	243
Double Meat & Peppers	2480	103	257
Florentine	2050	43	324
Hawaiian	1880	43	324
Pepperoni	2040	74	241
Tropical Chicken	2980	140	262
Tuscan	2600	103	295

Pastas: Full Order, Without Garlic Bread

Chicken Milano	1700	54	236
Fettuccini with Alfredo Sauce	1750	74	226

Salads: Includes Dressing

Santa Fe, with Gr. Chicken, 16.3 oz	840	44	66
Spinach & Cranberry, 9.1 oz	810	66	44

Desserts: With Ice Cream & Sauce

Apple Crisp, 12 oz	960	42	140
Choc. Brownie Addiction, 14 oz	1450	70	188

For Complete Nutritional Data ~ see CalorieKing.com

Braum's® ~ see CalorieKing.com

Bruegger's® (Oct '12)

Bagels:

	C	F	Cb
Chocolate Chip, 4.1 oz	330	3.5	65
Jalapeno Cheddar, 5.5 oz	450	9	75
Plain, 4.1 oz	300	2	60
Sesame, 4.1 oz	310	3	30
Whole Wheat, 4.1 oz	310	3.5	60

Breakfast Bagel S'wiches: Plain Bagel, with Menu Board Components Unless Indicated

Better Bacon Cheddar	650	29	66
Smoked Salmon	360	9	47
Spinach & Cheddar Omelet	500	16	63
Western Egg	670	34	66
Egg White: Sundried Tomato	480	13	65
Skinny Zesty	410	14	45

Deli Sandwiches: Includes Menu Board Components

BLT on Hearty White Bread	720	42	62
Chicken Breast on Plain Bagel	550	6	81
Garden Veggie on Plain Bagel	360	2	72
Ham On Honey Wheat Bread	510	13	61

Hot Paninis: Includes Menu Board Components

Four Cheese & Tom. on Hearty White	630	29	56
Ham & Cheddar on Honey Wheat	600	17	72
Tuna & Chedd. Melt on Honey Wheat	800	44	60

Signature & Classic Sandwiches: Includes Menu Board Components

Herby Turkey on Sesame Bagel	570	15	75
Leonardo da Veggie on Plain Softwich	560	15	76
Thai Peanut Chicken on Plain Bagel	580	11	91
Turkey Chipotle Club on Honey Wheat	530	18	60

Bruegger's® cont... (Oct '12)

Cafe Salads: With Dressing

	C	F	Cb
Chicken Caesar, with Caesar Dress.	260	14	13
Harvest Chicken w/ Strawb. Vinaig.	260	9	30
Mandarin Medley w/ Bals. Vinaig.	260	14	12
Cookies, average, 3 oz	385	18	51

Dessert Bars: Seven Layer, 4.7 oz

Seven Layer, 4.7 oz	650	43	58
Chocolate Chunk Brownie, 2.5 oz	310	18	38
Marshmallow Chews, 2.4 oz	280	6	55
Toffee Almond, 3.1 oz	400	19	53

For Complete Menu & Data ~ see CalorieKing.com

Buco di Beppo®

Antipasti: Bruschetta, 5.6 oz

	C	F	Cb
Bruschetta, 5.6 oz	385	38	12
Fried Calamari, 7 oz	170	7	15
Mozzarella Caprese, 3 oz	330	35	1

Insalate: Includes Dressing

Antipasto, 7 oz	340	31	8
Apple Gorgonzola, 6.9 oz	450	38	25

Entrees:

Chianti Braised Short Ribs, 11.3 oz	565	44	5
Chicken Limone, 7 oz	735	62	23
Chicken Saltimbocca, 9.3 oz	450	32	10
Prosciutto Stuffed Chicken, 11.3 oz	965	70	43
Tuscan Pork Chops, 12.6 oz	1075	83	19
Veal Parmesan, 7 oz	285	11	25

Specialty Pasta:

Baked Ravioli, 6.3 oz	320	13	36
Buscatini Ala Enzo, 8.3 oz	765	42	65
Linguini Frutti di Mare, 14.6 oz	855	38	80
Penne Ala Vodka, 17.8 oz	1640	55	187
Shrimp Fra Diavolo, 10.2 oz	870	54	68

Desserts:

Tiramisu, 9.4 oz	685	50	129
Celebration Cake, wedge size, 15.2 oz	1100	46	139

Burgerville® (Oct '12)

Burgers:

	C	F	Cb
Original Hamburger	330	17	30
Cheeseburger	370	21	31
Double Beef Cheeseburger	470	29	31
Half Pound Colossal Cheeseburger	750	45	43
Pepper Bacon Cheeseburger	710	45	40
Tillamook Cheeseburger	600	36	42

Sandwiches: Crispy Chicken

Crispy Chicken	490	24	50
Deluxe Crispy Chicken	720	42	52
Turkey Club	650	42	34

French Fries: Small, 2.75 oz

Small, 2.75 oz	200	8	28
Regular, 5 oz	360	15	52
Large, 6.5 oz	470	19	67

For Complete Menu & Data ~ see CalorieKing.com

Burger King® (Oct '12)

	C	F	Cb
Flame Broiled Whoppers: Includes Mayo			
Whopper	630	35	57
With Cheese	710	42	59
Double Whopper	830	50	57
With Cheese	990	65	53
Texas Double Whopper, w/o chse	1000	66	55
Triple Whopper, w/o cheese	1020	65	57
Whopper JR.	340	19	28
With Cheese	380	23	39
Flame Broiled Burgers: With Standard Toppings			
BK Stackers: Single	370	21	32
Double	490	30	32
Triple	630	41	32
Cheeseburger	280	12	32
Double Cheeseburger	370	18	32
Hamburger	240	8	31
Chicken & Fish Sandwiches: With Standard Toppings			
Prem. Alaskan Fish, w/ Tartar Sce	590	31	57
Orig. Chicken, w/ Mayo	630	39	46
Spicy Chick'N Crisp	460	29	38
Homestyle Chicken Strips:			
2 pieces	240	13	23
3 pieces	360	19	34
5 pieces	610	32	57
Dipping Sauces: Per 1 oz			
BBQ; Sweet & Sour, average	45	0	11
Buffalo	80	8	2
Honey Mustard	90	6	8
Ranch; Zesty Onion Ring, average	145	15	2
Sides:			
French Fries: Salted			
Small, 4.25 oz	340	15	49
Medium, 5.75 oz	410	18	58
Large, 7 oz	500	22	72
Fresh Apple Slices, 2 oz	30	0	7
Onion Rings: Small (15)	320	16	41
Medium (20)	410	21	53
Large (24)	500	25	64
Salads: With Dressing			
Garden Fresh:			
Caesar: With TenderCrisp Chkn	670	43	40
With TenderGrill Chicken	490	28	22
Chicken BLT:			
With TenderCrisp Chkn	690	48	31
With TenderGrill Chicken	510	33	13

Burger King® cont... (Oct '12)

Dressings: Per 1.75 oz Packet

	C	F	Cb
Ken's: Apple Cider Vinaigrette	210	18	10
Honey Mustard	220	18	13
Ranch	170	18	2
Breakfast:			
Biscuits: Bacon, Egg & Cheese	420	25	32
Ham, Egg & Cheese	390	19	33
Sausage, Egg & Cheese	520	34	33
Burritos:			
Sausage	290	17	21
Southwestern	620	37	47
Croissan'wich: Bacon Egg & Chse	320	18	25
Egg & Cheese	280	15	25
Ham Egg & Cheese	310	15	26
Double Croissan'wich:			
Bacon, Egg & Cheese	390	24	25
Ham, Egg & Cheese	390	19	27
Sausage, Bacon, Egg & Cheese	530	36	26
Sausage, Egg & Cheese	660	48	27
French Toast Sticks:			
3 pieces	230	11	29
5 pieces	380	18	49
Hash Browns: Small, 2.95 oz	250	16	24
Medium, 5.95 oz	500	33	48
Large, 7.9 oz	670	44	65
Hot Oatmeal: Original	140	3.5	23
Maple & Brown Sugar	270	4	55
Muffins: Bacon, Egg & Cheese	250	11	22
Ham, Egg & Cheese	250	9	23
Sausage, Egg & Cheese	390	23	23
Pancakes, (3),			
with 1 oz Breakfast Syrup	500	19	77
Platters:			
Pancake, with Sausage & Syrup	670	34	78
Ultimate Breakfast, 18 oz	1450	84	134
Desserts/Pies: Dutch Apple Pie	340	14	51
Hershey's Sundae Pie	310	19	32
Shakes:			
Chocolate: Small, 12 fl.oz	580	17	97
Medium, 16 fl.oz	760	21	131
Large, 20 fl.oz oz	980	24	174
Vanilla: Small, 12 fl.oz	550	16	91
Medium, 16 fl.oz	730	20	124
Large, 20 fl.oz	930	23	163
Beverages:			
Coca Cola Classic: Small, 20 fl.oz	190	0	51
Medium, 30 fl.oz	290	0	77
For Complete Nutritional Data ~ see CalorieKing.com			

Updated Nutrition Data ~ www.CalorieKing.com
Persons with Diabetes ~ See Disclaimer (Page 22)

Fast - Foods & Restaurants

California Pizza Kitchen
~ See CalorieKing.com

Captain D's Seafood® (Oct '12)

Starters:	C	F	Cb
Cheesesticks, 4 pieces	220	12	16
Jalapeno Poppers, 5 pieces	155	7	20

Dinners/Platters: Includes Cole Slaw, French Fries & Hush Puppies

	C	F	Cb
Bite Size Shrimp Dinner	1140	61	120
Catfish Feast	995	57	88
Clam Platter, ½ lb	1450	87	133
Country Style Fish Dinner	1070	59	97
Deluxe Seafood Platter, with Cracklins	1610	94	138
Fried Flounder	1530	93	115
Ultimate Premium Shrimp Platter	1290	65	141

Salads: Without Dressing

	C	F	Cb
Fried Chicken Salad	235	12	21
Side Salad	20	0	3
Wild Alaskan Salmon Salad	175	1	8

Sides:

	C	F	Cb
Baked Potato, plain	240	0	54
Breadsticks, 3 oz	300	11	42
Broccoli, 3.5 oz	40	1	5
Macaroni & Cheese, 4 oz	160	7	17
Dessert, Cheesecake w/ Strawb.	430	26	45

Caribou Coffee® (Oct '12)

Without Whipped Cream Unless Indicated

Classic Hot Coffees: Per Medium	C	F	Cb
Coffee Of The Day, with 2% Milk	15	0.5	1
Espresso, 3 shots	0	0	0
Cappuccino, with 2% Milk	70	3	6
Latte, with 2% Milk	200	8	19
Macchiato, with 2% Milk	25	5	1

Hot Chocolate: Per Medium, With Whipped Cream

	C	F	Cb
Berry Mocha, Milk Choc., 2% Milk	570	31	67
Mint Cond., Milk Choc., 2% Milk	580	31	68

Cold Beverages: Per Medium

	C	F	Cb
Iced Americano	10	0	0
Iced Latte, with 2% Milk	90	3.5	8
Iced Mocha, Milk Choc., 2% Milk	320	10	47

Coolers: Per Medium, With Whipped Cream

	C	F	Cb
Caramel	500	16	88
Coffee	420	17	67
Espresso	370	16	57

Smoothies: Per Medium

	C	F	Cb
Mango Orange Key Lime	450	0	113
Strawberry Banana	370	0	87
White Peach Berry	330	0	80

Snowdrift: Per Medium, With Milk Chocolate

	C	F	Cb
Cookies & Cream, with 2% Milk	630	18	103
Mint, with 2% Milk	510	13	84

Carl's Jr.® (Oct '12)

Charbroiled Burgers:	C	F	Cb
Big Hamburger	490	18	59
Famous Star with Cheese	680	39	57
Kid's Hamburger	280	10	34
Super Star with Cheese	940	59	59
The Big Carl	930	58	55
Western Bacon Cheeseburger	740	34	74
The Six Dollar Burger: Original	910	54	63
Guacamole Bacon	1030	69	56
Low-Carb	570	43	9
Portobello Mushroom	880	53	56
Western Bacon	1030	55	81

Chicken Sandwiches:	C	F	Cb
Charbroiled: BBQ Chicken	390	7	50
Chicken Club	580	29	45
Santa Fe Chicken	570	28	46
Spicy Chicken Sandwich	460	26	47

Chicken Tenders, hand breaded, 5 pieces, without Sauce	440	21	21
Chicken Stars, 6 pieces, w/o Sce	260	16	18
Fish: With Chips	710	38	69
Carl's Catch Fish Sandwich	700	37	73
Turkey Burgers: Teriyaki	470	14	55
Regular; Santa Fe, average	490	23	44
Breakfast: Bacon & Egg Burrito	560	32	37
Breakfast Burrito	810	42	69
French Toast Dips, 5 pcs, w/o Syrup	460	21	60
Hash Brown Nuggets, 4 oz	350	23	32
Loaded Breakfast Burrito	780	47	51
Sourdough Breakfast Sandwich	450	21	38
Steak & Egg Burrito	640	35	42
Sunrise Croissant Sandwich	590	44	28
Fries: Chili Cheese, 11.3 oz	820	46	81
CrissCut Fries, 5 oz	450	29	42
Natural Cut: Small, 4.25 oz	310	15	40
Medium, 6 oz	430	21	56
Large, 6.5oz	470	23	61
Onion Rings, 4.5 oz	530	28	61

Salads: Without Dressing or Croutons	C	F	Cb
Cranb. Apple Walnut Gr. Chicken	330	15	31
Original Grilled Chicken	280	13	23

Dressings: Per 2 oz Package	C	F	Cb
Blue Cheese	320	34	1
House	220	22	3
Low-Fat Balsamic	35	1.5	5

Shakes: Vanilla; Choc.; Strawb. av.	695	34	85
Oreo	720	38	79
Malts: Oreo	790	39	94
Other flavors, average	765	35	99

187

Fast - Foods & *Restaurants*

Carvel® (Oct '12)

Carvelanche: Per Medium, 16 oz

	C	F	Cb
Butterfinger	850	45	104
M&M's; Reese's, average	880	48	99

Classic Sundaes: Per Small, 12 oz

Caramel	700	36	84
Hot Fudge	540	30	60
Strawberry	610	34	67

Sundae Dashers: Per Small, 12 oz

Banana's Foster	660	23	105
Fudge Brownie	850	45	102
Mint Chocolate Chip	770	42	95
Peanut Butter Cup	1060	60	95
Strawberry Shortcake	580	29	74

Take Home Treats: Brown Bonnet

Brown Bonnet	390	23	43
Flying Saucers: Chocolate	230	10	33
Deluxe, with Sprinkles	350	16	49

Thick Shakes: Chocolate

Chocolate	650	27	93
Strawberry	600	31	70
Vanilla	660	31	86

Thick ShakeFloats: Chocolate

Chocolate	790	34	109
Strawberry	750	39	85
Vanilla	810	39	102

Checkers®

Same Menu & Data as Rally's ~ See Page 231

Cheesecake Factory® (Oct '12)

10" Cheesecake: Per Slice

	C	F	Cb
Chocolate Raspberry Truffle	1080	n/a	103
Original, with Strawberries	750	n/a	72
Low Carb	540	n/a	41
Reese's P.B. Chocolate Cake	1560	n/a	170

Small Plates & Snacks: Per Dish, As Served

Crispy Crab Bites	360	n/a	11
Sausage & Ricotta Flatbread	460	n/a	35
Vietnamese Tacos	950	n/a	155

GlamBurgers & Sandwiches: Without Sides

Chicken Almond Salad	1530	n/a	83
Factory Burger	780	n/a	64
Turkey Burger	1250	n/a	60

Specialties: Per Dish, As Served

Crispy Chicken Costoletta	2560	n/a	105
Famous Factory Meatloaf	1800	n/a	119
White Chicken Chili	590	n/a	59

Salads: As Served, Includes Dressing

Herb-Crusted Salmon	770	n/a	21
Santa Fe Salad	1700	n/a	97
Skinnylicious Spicy Chicken	440	n/a	42

Charley's Grilled Subs® (Oct '12)

Subs: Regular 7½" Includes Standard Toppings, Without Sauce or Dressings Unless Indicated

	C	F	Cb
BBQ Cheddar, with Sauce	580	20	68
Bacon 3 Cheese Steak	635	32	54
Buffalo Chicken, with Sauce	525	16	60
Chicken Bacon Club	570	25	53
Chicken Cordon Blue	570	18	54
Chicken Teriyaki, with Sauce	520	16	58
Italian Deli	585	25	53
Mushroom Swiss Steak	520	19	57
Philly Cheesesteak	520	19	56
Philly Chicken	515	16	58
Philly Ham & Swiss	515	15	60
Philly Steak Deluxe	525	19	58
Sicilian Steak	640	31	54
Turkey Cheddar Melt	470	12	53
Ultimate Club	560	23	54

Salads: Cheese/Dressings not included

Chicken, Teriyaki; Buffalo, average	210	7	13
Fresh Garden	60	2	9
Grilled Steak	210	10	10
Dressings, Italian/Ranch, av., 1 oz	150	16	1
Mayo, 1 Tbsp, ½ oz	100	11	0
Original Lemonade, 8fl.oz	85	0	20

For Complete Menu & Data ~ see CalorieKing.com

Chevys Fresh Mex® (Oct '12)

Burritos: As Served

	C	F	Cb
Fajita Carnitas	1260	51	144
Fajita Chicken	1240	46	142
Fajita Steak	1300	54	142

Fresh Mex Combos: As Served

Chevys Super Cinco	1920	100	171
Mar Y Tierra Combo	1230	54	108
Taste of Chevys	1480	68	155

Made From Scratch Enchiladas: As Served

Chicken	1070	65	93
Farmers Market	1130	72	101
Shrimp & Crab	1250	80	94

Tacos: As Served

Chicken	980	28	123
Fish	920	27	123
Steak	1050	38	123

Grande Salads: Without Dressing Unless Indicated

Grilled Fajita Chicken w/ dressing	1220	90	51
Santa Fe Chopped	660	39	26
Tostada Steak	1560	100	91
Soup, Tortilla, 1 bowl	420	18	38
Tortilla, El Machino (1), 6"	140	4	22
Tortilla Chips	430	20	56

188

Updated Nutrition Data ~ www.CalorieKing.com
Persons with Diabetes ~ See Disclaimer (Page 22)

Chick-fil-A® (Oct '12)

Chick-fil-A Sandwiches: W/o Sauce	C	F	Cb
Chargrilled Chicken	290	4	36
Chargrilled Chicken Club	400	12	36
Chicken Salad	510	19	55
Cool Wraps: Without Dressing			
Chargrilled Chicken	410	10	50
Chicken Caesar	470	13	47
Spicy Chicken	420	10	49
Chicken:			
Chick-n-Strips, breaded, 4 count	470	22	22
Nuggets: Breaded, 8 count	260	12	11
12 count	400	18	17
Breakfast:			
Biscuits: Chicken	440	20	48
Bacon, Egg & Cheese	440	22	45
Sausage, Egg & Cheese	670	45	45
Burritos: Chicken	430	19	42
Sausage	500	28	40
Chicken, Egg & Cheese Bagel	480	20	48
Chick-n-Minis, 1 box, 3 pieces	280	10	30
Cinnamon Cluster	430	17	63
Hash Browns, 2.7 oz	240	14	26
Oatmeal: Multigrain w/ toppings	290	11	50
Without toppings	140	2.5	28
Salads: Chicken-n-Strips	450	22	27
Chargrilled Chicken & Fruit	230	6	23
Southwest Chargrilled Chicken	250	9	19
Condiments:			
Garlic & Butter Croutons, ½ oz	60	2	9
Harvest Nut Granola, salad portion	60	3	8
Honey Rstd Sunfl. Knls, salad portion	90	7	4
Tortilla Strips, ½ oz	80	4	8
Dressings: Blue Cheese, 2.5 oz	290	29	3
Buttermilk Ranch. 1.5 oz	280	30	2
Light Italian, 1.5 oz	25	1	3
Thousand Island, .5 oz	270	26	9
Sauces: BBQ; Honey Mustard, 1 oz	45	0	11
Buffalo, ¾ oz	10	1	1
Buttermilk Ranch, ¾ oz	110	12	1
Chick-fil-A, 1 oz	140	13	6
Honey Roasted BBQ, ½ oz	60	5	2
Sides: Carrot & Raisin Salad, med.	260	12	40
Chicken Salad Cup, 6 oz	350	22	9
Cole Slaw, medium	360	31	19
Waffle Potato Fries: Small	300	16	37
Medium	390	20	48
Large	520	27	63
Desserts, Fudge Brownie, 3 oz	390	18	53
Milkshakes: Chocolate, large	730	27	110
Peach, large	850	21	153

Chili's® (Oct '12)

Appetizers: As Served	C	F	Cb
Bottomless Tostada Chips w/ Salsa	910	45	112
Crispy Onion Str. & Jalap. Stack/Ranch	1060	84	67
Classic Nachos: Beef (12)	1420	91	61
Chicken (12)	1440	91	58
Skillet Queso with Tostada Chips	1580	96	135
Sthwestern Eggrolls w/ Avoc. Ranch	770	40	81
Triple Dipper: Big Mouth Bites w/ Ranch	780	53	47
Chicken Crispers w/out Dressing	340	15	21
Hot Spin. & Artichoke Dip w/ Chips	590	39	48
Burgers: As Served, On white Bun with Fries			
Big Mouth Bites with Ranch	1770	109	137
Classic Bacon Burger	1410	85	108
Jalapeno Smokehouse with Ranch	1770	115	120
Chicken, Seafood & Pasta: As Served			
Cajun Pasta:			
With Grilled Chicken	1300	61	116
With Grilled Shrimp	1240	62	114
Chicken:			
Chkn Crispers w/ Hon. Mustard	1400	63	145
Margarita Grilled Chicken	590	16	68
Monterey Chicken	890	44	58
Southwest Grill:			
Fajitas: Without Tortillas & Condiments			
Beef	540	33	25
Chicken	400	13	26
Trio	600	28	31
Condiments only (1)	180	16	7
Flour Tortillas only (3)	260	7	42
Quesadillas: As Served			
Bacon Ranch Chicken	1450	100	69
Bacon Ranch Steak	1440	99	71
Steaks: As Served			
Classic Ribeye	1160	68	59
Classic Sirloin, 6 oz	790	41	59
Country-Fried Steak	1240	64	126
In-House Slow Smoked Ribs: Full Rack, As Served			
Original	2180	122	139
Memphis Dry Rub	1980	110	134
Shiner Bock BBQ	2330	123	161
Salads: Large, Includes Dressing			
Boneless Buffalo Chicken	920	63	52
Caribbean with Grilled Shrimp	620	28	74
Quesadilla Explosion	1360	88	87
Stupendously Sweet Endings: Per Slice			
Cheesecake	750	47	69
Chocolate Chip Paradise Pie	1190	60	150
Molten Chocolate Cake	1110	59	136

For Complete Menu & Data ~ see CalorieKing.com

Chipotle® (Oct '12)

Breads:	C	F	Cb
Crispy Taco Shells (3)	180	6	27
Flour Tortillas (Burrito), (1)	290	9	44
Soft Corn Tortillas (Taco), (3)	180	1.5	39
Meal Components:			
Barbacoa, 4 oz	170	7	2
Black Beans, 4 oz	120	1	22
Brown Rice, 4 oz	160	4	31
Carnitas, 4 oz	190	8	1
Cheese, 1 oz	100	9	0
Chicken, 4 oz	190	6.5	1
Guacamole, 3.5 oz	150	13	8
Lettuce, 1 oz	5	0	0
Pinto Beans, 4 oz	120	1	22
Steak, 4 oz	190	6.5	2
Condiments:			
Salsa: Chili Corn, 3.5 oz	80	1.5	15
Green Tomatillo, 2 oz	15	0	3
Red Tomatillo, 2 oz	40	1	8
Tomato, 3.5 oz	20	0	4
Sour Cream, 2 oz	120	10	2
Extras, Chips, serving, 4 oz	570	27	73

Chuck E. Cheese® (Oct '12)

Appetizers: Includes Condiments	C	F	Cb
Buffalo Wings (12)	900	60	48
Italian Bread Stick (1)	175	9	18
Mozzarella Stick (1)	95	6	6
Oven Baked Sandwiches:			
Ham & Cheese	685	27	79
Italian Sub	790	39	78
Roasted Chicken Ciabatta	715	28	80
Pizzas: Per Medium Slice			
BBQ Chicken	185	6	24
Cheese	155	5	21
Super Combo	185	8	22
Veggie Combo	160	6	22
Platters: Sampler, ½ Platter	330	19	25
Veggie, ⅛ Platter	130	11	7
French Fries,			
with Ketchup & Ranch: 4 oz	420	20	55
Desserts: Apple Dessert Pizza, 1 sl.	190	5	33
Chocolate Cake (8"), 1 slice	290	13	41
Cinnamon Stick, w/ Toppings (1)	70	2	11

Church's Chicken® (Oct '12)

Chicken: Per Serving	C	F	Cb
Original: Breast, 1 piece	200	11	3
Leg, 1 piece	110	6	3
Thigh, 1 piece	330	23	8
Wing, 1 piece	300	18	7
Spicy: Breast, 1 piece	320	20	12
Leg, 1 piece	180	11	8
Thigh, 1 piece	480	35	20
Wing, 1 piece	430	27	17
Tender Strips:, average, 1 piece	130	7	7
Sides: Per Small Serving			
Cajun Rice, 6 oz	130	7	16
Cole Slaw, 4.15 oz	150	10	15
Corn on the Cob (1)	140	3	24
French Fries, 1.6 oz	140	6	19
Honey Butter Biscuits (1), 2.1 oz	240	12	28
Macaroni & Cheese, 6 oz	190	7	24
Mashed Potatoes & Gravy, 6 oz	110	2	21
Okra, 1.95 oz	170	11	17
Sauces: Per Packet			
BBQ; Sweet & Sour	25	0	6
Creamy Jalapeno; Honey Mstrd, av	85	9	2
Ketchup	15	0	4
Ranch	100	10	1

Cici's Pizza® (Oct '12)

Buffet: Per ⅒ of 12" Pizza	C	F	Cb
Alfredo	120	3.5	19
BBQ	140	2.5	25
Beef; Cheese, average	150	4	20
Ham & Pineapple	150	3.5	21
Pepperoni & Jalapeno	150	4.5	20
Sausage	170	6	19
Spin. Alfredo; Zesty Ham & Chedd.	120	3.5	19
To-Go: Per ⅒ of 15" Pizza			
Alfredo	170	6	23
BBQ	240	6	36
Beef; Pepperoni & Jalapeno	210	7	24
Sausage	230	10	24
Spinach Alfredo	170	6	23
Zesty: Ham & Cheddar; Pepperoni	180	6	23

Cinnabon® (Oct '12)

Baked Goods: Cinnabon Bites (6)	C	F	Cb
	620	24	88
Caramel Pecanbon (1)	1080	50	147
Bites (6)	800	39	100
Classic Cinnabon (1)	880	36	127
Stix (5)	390	21	46
Sweet Roll Icing, Frosting Cup, 1.4 oz	180	11	20

Updated Nutrition Data ~ www.CalorieKing.com
Persons with Diabetes ~ See Disclaimer (Page 22)

Claim Jumper® (Oct '12)

Appetizers: As Served

	C	F	Cb
Southwest Eggrolls	1190	53	114
Three Cheese Potatocakes (3)	1075	71	80

Burgers & Sandwiches: Without Sides

	C	F	Cb
Grilled Cobb Sandwich	1210	78	78
Widow Maker Burger	1370	87	84

Meals:

Favorites: With Menu Set Sides & Toppings

	C	F	Cb
Country Fried Steak	2030	107	189
Giant Stuffed Chicken Baker	990	34	118
Meatloaf & Mashed Potatoes	1300	75	117

Pasta/Pizza:

	C	F	Cb
California Works, Classic Crust	1295	64	127
Grilled Chicken Pasta	1400	94	93

Specialties: With Roasted Vegetables

	C	F	Cb
BBQ Baby Back Pork Ribs, Full Rack	1745	111	111
Roasted Tri-Tip	800	47	19

Seafood: With Menu Set Sides & Sauces

	C	F	Cb
Fish & Chips	1195	74	82
Lobster Tail Dinner	715	46	42

Entree Salads: Without Dressing Or Bread

	C	F	Cb
Californian Citrus Chkn, Charbroiled	865	53	58
Seared Ahi Spinach	515	24	31

Soups: Per Bowl

	C	F	Cb
Potato Cheddar	710	61	31
New England Clam Chowder	525	45	23

Sweets:

	C	F	Cb
Choc. Motherlode Cake	2770	144	340
Italian Lemon Cake	1240	62	158

Coldstone Creamery® (Oct '12)

Ice Creams:

	C	F	Cb
Amaretto: Like it	330	20	33
Love it	530	31	53
Gotta have it	790	47	80

Sorbet:

	C	F	Cb
Strawberry Mango: Like it	220	0	55
Love it	350	0	87
Gotta have it	520	0	131

Cosi® (Oct '12)

Flatbread Pizza: Individual

	C	F	Cb
Original Crust: Margherita	705	22	91
Pepperoni	815	32	90
Traditional Cheese	675	20	90

Melts: With Rustic Bread

	C	F	Cb
Chicken TBM	695	31	49
Pesto Chicken	640	27	48
Steakhouse Gorgonzola	780	44	65
Tuna Melt	775	41	50

Cosi® cont... (Oct '12)

Sandwiches: With Rustic Bread

	C	F	Cb
Buffalo Bleu	565	25	47
Fire Roasted Veggie	350	11	51
Italiano	810	47	49
TBM	595	35	47

Soup: Per 5 oz Bowl, w/o Flatbread

	C	F	Cb
Pollo e Pasta	65	2	7
Tomato Basil	215	20	9

Salads: Includes Dressing

	C	F	Cb
Cosi Cobb, 14 oz	720	55	18
Greek, 14 oz	515	47	19
Signature, 12.8 oz	645	45	51
Steakhouse, 14 oz	650	52	16

Costco Food Court® (Oct '12)

Pizza: Per Slice

	C	F	Cb
Combo, 11 oz	680	29	72
Cheese, 10 oz	700	28	70
Pepperoni , 9 oz	620	24	68
Dogs, Hot Dog, Polish Ssg., 7 oz	550	33	39

Salads:

	C	F	Cb
Chicken Caesar, w/ dress., 20.5 oz	670	40	35
Quinoa, ½ cup	110	6	12

Meals:

	C	F	Cb
Cheese Burger Fry Combo	860	45	72
Chicken Bake 12.75 oz	770	25	78
Ital. Sausage Sandwich, 12.5 oz	700	42	46
Turkey Wrap, 14.5 oz	810	38	65

Beverages:

	C	F	Cb
Hot Latte, 9.5 fl oz	190	5	24
Hot Mocha, 11.25 fl oz	310	9	45
Latte Freeze, 15.5 fl.oz	240	7	32
Mocha Freeze, 16.25 fl .oz	320	7	49

Desserts:

	C	F	Cb
Ice cream Bar, 8 oz	870	65	60
Berry Sundae, 12.25 oz	410	0	87
Chocolate Gelato, 8.5 oz	410	9	82
Pistachio Gelato, 7.75 oz	480	13	82
Yogurt, 12 oz	390	0	82

Cousins Subs® (Oct '12)

Subs: Per 7½" With Italian Bread

	C	F	Cb
BLT, with Mayo	590	38	47
Cheese Steak	680	32	50
Chicken Cheddar Deluxe, w/ Mayo	670	39	51
Club, with Mayo	720	39	55
Double Cheese Steak	1090	63	50
Garden Provolone	880	54	65
Italian Special, with Dressing	980	65	52
Philly Cheese Steak, with Sauce	710	37	52

Continued Next Page...

Fast - Foods & Restaurants

Cousins Subs® cont... (Oct '12)

7½" Subs (cont):

	C	F	Cb
Roast Beef & Cheddar	710	35	52
Tuna with Mayo Blend	670	40	49
Turkey Breast with Mayo	530	29	53

Better Bunch: 7½ Subs, W/o Mayo & Cheese

Club	380	4.5	54
Garden	330	2	64
Ham; Turkey Breast, average	33	3.5	51

French Fries: Small, 2.75 oz

	250	13	30
Medium, 4 oz	365	19	43
Large, 5.25 oz	485	25	57

Salads: Without Dressing

Almond Berry Chicken	440	20	37
Gourmet Garden with Chicken	340	15	21
Turkey Bacon Delight	370	21	23

For Complete Nutritional Data ~ see CalorieKing.com

Culver's® (Oct '12)

Butter Burgers:

	C	F	Cb
Original: Single; Kids	330	15	31
Double	460	23	31
Triple	590	31	32
Cheddar with Bacon, Single	540	33	31
Cheese: Single	400	21	32
Double	600	35	33
Culver's Bacon Deluxe: Single	595	39	35
Double	790	53	35
Culver's Deluxe: Single	515	32	35
Double	710	46	35
Mushroom & Swiss, Single	430	23	33
Sourdough Melt, Single	415	20	35
Corn Dog, Kids	260	14	26

Chicken Tenders, 4 pieces

	560	28	40

Sandwiches: Beef Pot Roast

	365	16	33
Crispy Chicken	450	17	57
Grilled Reuben Melt	590	31	42
North Atlantic Cod Filet	665	40	47
Pork Tenderloin, Breaded	600	29	63
Shaved Prime Rib	505	28	35

Sides:

Crinkle Cut Fries: Small

	170	6	26
Regular	235	8	37
Large	300	11	47
Chili Cheddar Fries	480	22	53
Mashed Potatoes, w/ Gravy, reg.	140	2	26
Wisconsin Cheese Curds, 6.5 oz	670	38	54

Dinners: As Served

Beef Pot Roast	745	36	73
Butterfly Jumbo Shrimp, 6 pieces	1170	58	136
Chopped Steak	850	49	63
Fried Chicken, 2 pieces	1640	90	125
North Atlantic Cod, Fried, 2 pieces	1715	112	120

Culver's® cont... (Oct '12)

Salads: Without Dressing

	C	F	Cb
Chicken Cashew w/ Grilled Chkn	460	23	16
Cranberry Bacon Bleu, with Grilled Chicken	360	12	19
Garden Fresco w/ Grilled Chicken	335	11	15
Side Salad	60	2	6

Dressings:

Chunky Bleu Cheese, 1.75 oz	310	33	2
French Dressing, 1.75 oz	190	13	19
Ranch, 1.75 oz	230	24	3
Thousand Island, 2 oz	220	18	14

Desserts:

Concrete Mixers: Per Medium

Brownie Batter	1100	59	123
Cherry Cheesecake	965	52	109
Chocolate	995	49	122
Turtle	1155	71	114

Sundaes: Per 2 Scoops With Whipped Topping

Banana Split	1090	63	115
Caramel Cashew	960	52	104
Fudge Pecan	980	62	94

Beverages: Per Medium

Choc. Malt, medium	970	45	122
Chocolate Shake, medium	910	44	114
Root Beer Float, medium	550	18	90

D'Angelo's® (Oct '12)

Sandwiches: Based on White Sub Roll with Standard Toppings

Subs: Per Medium Size

	C	F	Cb
Cheeseburger	870	40	67
Chicken Stir Fry	740	19	78
Classic Veggie	700	27	81
Roast Beef	490	8	67
Turkey	500	5	65

Pokkets: Per Plain Pokket With Standard Toppings

Cheeseburger	530	24	39
Caesar Salad	650	39	57
Lobster	510	25	38
Steak & Cheese	530	24	37

Wraps: Per Small White Wrap with Standard Toppings

Buffalo Chicken Salad	830	45	66
Caesar Salad	790	48	72
Chicken Caesar Salad	930	51	74
Chicken Cobb	910	53	71
Greek	790	54	60
Turkey Club	500	16	52

Salads: Entree Size, Without Pokket Bread

Caesar, with dressing	630	53	28
Chicken Caesar, with dressing	770	55	30

Soups: Per Small Serve

Baked Potato	260	18	20
Chicken Noodle	110	2	14
New England Clam Chowder	320	18	31

For Complete Menu & Data ~ see CalorieKing.com

Dairy Queen® (Oct '12)

Burgers & Sandwiches:

	C	F	Cb
Grillburgers:			
Bacon Cheese, ¼ lb	630	37	44
½ lb Burger	710	44	43
½ lb Flame Thrower	1000	74	40
Bacon Double Cheeseburger	720	41	34
Cheeseburger	400	18	34
Hamburger: Regular	350	14	33
Double	540	26	33
Sandwiches: Crispy Chicken	600	30	59
Grilled Chicken	360	15	32
Baskets:			
Chkn Strips: 4 piece w/ Country Gravy	1030	53	105
6 piece, with Country Gravy	1260	66	121
Iron Grilled Chicken Quesadilla	1160	60	110
Hot Dogs: Beef	290	17	22
With Chili & Cheese	380	24	23
Salads: Without Dressing			
Crispy Chicken	470	26	29
Grilled Chicken	330	15	13
Sides:			
DQ French Fries, regular, 4 oz	310	13	43
DQ Onion Rings, 4 oz	360	16	47
Desserts: Per Medium			
Blizzard Treats: Banana Cream Pie	770	28	117
Butterfinger	740	26	114
Cappuccino Heath	870	39	122
Cookie Dough	1020	40	148
Oreo Cookies	680	25	100
Reese's Peanut Butter Cups	740	31	101
Strawberry CheeseQuake	690	28	92
DQ Blizzard Cakes (10"): Per ⅒ Cake			
Oreo	760	33	104
Reese's Peanut Butter Cup	720	33	94
Strawberry Cheese Quake	610	27	79
DQ Dipped Cones: Per Medium Cone			
Butterscotch	470	21	62
Chocolate	470	22	61
DQ Sundaes: Per Medium, 8.25 oz			
Caramel	430	11	74
Hot Fudge	440	15	67
Strawberry	350	10	56
Malts: Per Medium, With Whipped Topping			
Caramel	830	25	134
Chocolate	790	26	130
Strawberry	700	22	107
Moo Latte: Per Medium, With Whipped Topping			
Cappuccino	580	19	91
French Vanilla	630	19	101
Mocha	670	25	104

For Complete Nutritional Data ~ see CalorieKing.com

Daphne's Greek Cafe® (Oct '12)

Starters:

	C	F	Cb
Original Hummus & Pita	300	15	37
Fire Feta & Original Pita	310	17	31
Pita Sandwiches: Without Fries, Rice or Salad			
Crispy Shrimp	390	19	40
Fire Roasted Vegetables	350	18	39
Fresh Carved Gyros	660	47	40
Grilled Chicken	370	15	33
Plates: Without Sides, Pita Bread or Tzatziki			
Mix & Match:			
Crispy Shrimp	120	6	7
Falafel	180	11	16
Fresh-Carved Gyros	320	27	7
Grilled Chicken Kabob	150	4	4
Grilled Steak Kabob	170	9	4
Grilled Salmon	330	22	0
Classic Greek Salads: Without Dressing			
Crispy Shrimp	350	19	28
Falafel	540	31	49
Grilled Chicken	330	15	21
Dressings: Classic Greek	110	12	2
Lite Greek	60	6	2
Sides: Fire Roasted Vegetables	50	3	5
Fries	310	16	39
Multigrain Pita Chips	170	5	27
Original Pita Bread	180	6	28
Seasoned Rice Pilaf	250	6	47
Tabouli Salad	80	1	17

Davanni's® (Oct '12)

Half Hoagies: Includes 6" White Bun and Standard Toppings

	C	F	Cb
Assorted	490	30	39
BLT	645	44	40
Chicken & Bacon w/ Honey Mstrd	505	22	46
Chicken Parmigiana	445	16	40
Club	495	27	40
Italian Sausage	620	38	46
Southwestern Chicken	535	26	43
Three Cheese	525	33	39
Tuna Melt	645	44	42
Turkey	455	24	39
Turkey Bacon Chipotle	565	33	39
Veggie	445	24	43
Calzones: Sausage, Peppers & On.	925	50	83
Pepperoni Sausage	960	56	80
Pizzas: Per Slice			
Five Meat: Thin Crust	520	33	20
Traditional Crust	565	33	30
Solo, Thin Crust	1115	69	47
Veggie: Thin Crust	220	10	19
Traditional Crust	265	10	29
Works: Thin Crust	265	14	19
Traditional Crust	310	15	29

Del Taco® (Oct '12)

	C	F	Cb
Breakfast:			
Biscuit Sandwiches:			
Bacon, Egg & Cheese	475	29	35
Sausage	485	31	34
Sausage, Egg & Cheese	560	38	35
Burritos: Breakfast	280	13	28
½ lb Sausage & Egg	510	33	23
½ lb Steak & Egg	395	23	22
Egg & Cheese	315	17	22
Hash Brown Sticks: 5 pieces	205	15	18
8 pieces	330	24	29
Quesadilla, Bacon & Egg	410	20	37
Burgers: Cheeseburger	430	22	40
Double Del Cheeseburger	715	48	40
Burritos:			
Classic Grilled Chicken	445	31	23
Macho Beef	970	44	82
Macho Chicken	910	32	109
Macho Combo	965	36	110
Nachos: 4 oz	330	22	28
Macho, 17 oz	1010	56	94
Quesadillas:			
Cheddar; Spicy Jack	465	25	37
Chicken Cheddar; Spicy Jack Chicken	560	30	40
Tacos: Big Fat Chicken	325	14	34
Big Fat Steak	355	18	33
Chicken Al Carbon	150	4	19
Classic	200	12	10
Classic Soft	220	11	16
Crispy Fish	300	17	29
Macho	295	17	16
Steak Al Carbon	180	8	18
Salad, Deluxe Taco Salad	835	47	69
Sides:			
Fries: Small, 5 oz	260	15	28
Macho, 10 oz	520	30	56
Chili Cheddar, 10.5 oz	520	32	42
Deluxe Chili Cheese, 12 oz	560	35	44
Desserts: Cinnamon Churro	175	9	21
Caramel Cheesecake: 2 Bites	460	30	42
4 Bites	915	59	84
Chocolate Chip Cookie, 1.5 oz	205	10	27
Premium Shakes: Per 16 oz			
Chocolate	580	11	105
Strawberry; Vanilla, average	530	11	95

Denny's® (Oct '12)

	C	F	Cb
Breakfast:			
Favorites:			
Banana Pecan Pancake, 17 oz	780	15	130
Country Fried Steak & Eggs, without sides, 11 oz	660	43	29
Loaded Chorizo Burrito without sides , 17 oz	1230	75	89
Omelettes: Fit Fare, with sides	390	18	25
Meat Lovers, w/ Hash Browns	1060	75	39
Ultimate, w/o sides	620	48	8
Veggie-Cheese, w/o sides	460	33	9
Slams:			
All American, w/o sides	800	68	5
French Toast, 15 oz	790	58	35
Lumberjack, without sides, 15 oz	960	50	80
The Grand Slamwich, with Hash Browns, 21 oz	1520	101	97
Sides: Buttermilk Biscuit, (1)	190	9	24
English Muffin, w/o Margarine, (1)	130	1	25
Hash Browns, 5 oz	210	12	26
Pancakes: Without Margarine, Syrup or Toppings			
Buttermilk, 2 cakes	330	4	67
Hearty Wheat, 2 cakes	310	1.5	64
Lunch: Without sides Unless Indicated			
Burgers:			
Bacon Cheddar, 15 oz	880	49	45
Bacon Slamburger, 15 oz	1010	58	56
Classic Cheeseburger, 15 oz	820	44	47
Mushroom Swiss, 18 oz	860	48	51
Veggie Burger w/ Veges & dress.	540	13	76
Sandwiches: Bacon Lovers BLT, 10 oz	810	47	66
Chicken Avoc. w/ Veges	520	16	48
Club, 11 oz	630	33	55
Hickory Grilled Chkn w/ dress.	900	47	67
Melts: Prime Rib Philly, 13 oz	670	36	52
Spicy Buffalo Chicken, 15 oz	860	48	76
The Super Bird, 11 oz	610	29	54
Dinners:			
American Classics: With Bread, Without Sides			
Chicken Strips, 10 oz	760	29	84
Gr. Lemon Pepper Tilapia	800	35	59
Spagh. & Meatballs, w/ Parm Chse, & Garlic Toast, 23 oz	1220	61	108
T-Bone Steak: 12 oz	820	35	24
With Breaded Shrimp, 15 oz	1000	59	47
With Shrimp Skewer, 14 oz	900	54	27

Continued Next Page...

Denny's® cont... (Oct '12)

Dinners (Cont):

	r	F	Ch
Sizzlin' Skillets: *As Served*			
Banana Caramel French Toast,			
without meat 14 oz	840	13	164
Santa Fe, 14 oz	710	52	30
Ultimate, 15 oz	740	56	34

Dinner Sides:

Broccoli, 3 oz	25	0	4
French Fries, salted, 5 oz	430	23	50
Garlic Dinner Bread, 2 pieces	170	9	21
Green Beans, 4 oz	45	1	7
Vegetable Rice Pilaf, 5 oz	190	3	35

Soups: Per Bowl, Without Bread

Broccoli & Cheddar	370	16	48
Chicken Noodle	160	4	17
Vegetable Beef	170	4	23

Salads: Without Dressing or Bread Unless Indicated

Chicken Strip Deluxe, 18 oz	590	29	43
Cranberry Apple Chicken,			
with Balsamic Vinaigrette, 13 oz	370	12	32
Grilled Chicken Deluxe,	340	13	13

Dressings: Per 1 oz

Bleu Cheese	110	11	1
Caesar	100	10	0
French	75	5	8
Honey Mustard	160	15	5
Ranch	130	14	0

Desserts:

Apple Pie, 7 oz	480	22	67
Banana Split, 15 oz	810	31	125
Caramel Apple Crisp, 13 oz	740	21	134
Hot Fudge Brownie a` la Mode, 9 oz	830	37	122
NY Style Cheesecake, 5 oz	510	34	43
Turtle Cheesecake, 8 oz	780	42	90
Toppings: Caramel, 1.5 oz	190	1	44
Fudge, 1.5 oz	150	6	23

Beverages:

Pacific Chiller, 15 oz	210	0	54
Strawberry Lemonade, 15 oz	200	0	50

For Complete Nutritional Data ~ see CalorieKing.com

Dippin' Dots® (Oct '12)

	C	F	Cb
Flavored Ices: *Per ½ Cup, 3 oz*			
Sour Blue Razz	60	0	13
Other varieties	100	0	26
Frozen Yogurt,			
Strawberry Cheesecake, ½ cup	100	0	21
Ice Cream: *Per ½ Cup*			
Banana Split	160	8	20
Chocolate Chip Cookie dough	190	9	24
Peanut Butter Chip	170	8	21
Strawberry	160	8	18
Frappes: *Per ½ Cup, 3 oz*			
Caramel	210	9	23
Mocha	220	9	25

Donato's Pizza® (Oct '12)

	C	F	Cb
Thin Crust Pizza: *¼ Large Pizza*			
Chicken Vegy Medley	495	20	51
Classic Trio	675	37	52
Founder's Favorite	700	38	52
Hawaiian	590	27	56
Thicker Crust Pizza: *¼ Large Pizza*			
Founder's Favorite	770	36	70
Mariachi Beef	710	30	73
Mariachi Chicken	700	28	74
Pepperoni	710	32	69
Serious Cheese	700	30	69
The Works	760	35	74
Vegy	620	22	75
No Dough Pizza: *Individual*			
Chicken Vegy Medley	495	29	20
Classic Trio	530	37	18
Founder's Favorite	560	38	18
Hawaiian	435	26	22
Mariachi Beef	530	34	23
Mariachi Chicken	495	30	21
Pepperoni	500	35	17
Pepperoni Zinger	585	42	17
Serious Cheese	455	31	17
Serious Meat	655	46	19
The Works	545	37	21
Stromboli: *3 Meat*	690	31	67
Cheese	695	31	66
Deluxe	615	25	68
Pepperoni	715	34	67
Vegy	605	24	69

Desserts:

Apple Timpano, 2 slices	405	9	72
Cinnamon Timpano, 2 slices	525	22	73

For Complete Nutritional Data ~ see CalorieKing.com

Fast - Foods & Restaurants

Domino's® (Oct '12)

	C	F	Cb
12" Hand-Tossed: Per Slice, ⅛ Pizza, Includes Base Sauce and Cheese			
Bacon, Beef & Sausage	325	18	30
Beef, Green Peppers & Mushrooms	260	13	28
Fetta, Black Olives, Onions, Tomatoes, Pineapple, Green Peppers	255	12	29
Ham & Cheddar	275	13	28
Ham & Pineapple	250	11	29
Pepperoni	265	13	28
Pepperoni & Sausage	290	15	29
Sausage	280	14	29
Sliced Ital. Ssg, Beef, & Pepperoni	315	18	28
14" Thin Crust: Per Slice, ⅛ Pizza, Includes Base Sauce and Cheese			
Bacon, Sausage & American Cheese	390	20	36
Beef, Green Pepp., On. & Mushroom	280	11	34
Ham & Cheddar	305	13	34
Ham & Pineapple	280	10	36
Pepperoni	300	13	34
Pepperoni & Sausage	335	16	35
Sausage	320	14	36
12" Deep Dish: Per Slice, ⅛ Pizza, Includes Base Sauce and Cheese			
Beef, Green Pepp., On. & Mushroom	265	13	28
Ham & Cheddar	290	14	28
Ham & Pineapple	265	12	29
Pepperoni	280	14	28
Pepperoni & Sausage	305	16	29
Sausage	295	15	29
12" Feast Hand-Tossed: Per Slice, ⅛ Pizza			
America's Favorite	250	12	27
Bacon Cheeseburger	270	13	26
Deluxe	230	10	27
ExtravaganZZa	290	14	28
MeatZZa	280	14	27
Ultimate Pepperoni	260	13	25
14" Feast Hand Tossed: Per Slice, ⅛ Pizza			
America's Favorite	350	17	36
Bacon Cheeseburger	380	19	36
Deluxe	320	14	36
ExtravaganZZa	390	19	37
MeatZZa Feast	380	19	36
Ultimate Pepperoni	360	18	34
12" Legends Thin Crust: Per ¼ Party Pizza			
Buffalo Chicken	380	22	26
Cali Chicken Bacon Ranch	490	33	28
Fiery Hawaiian	390	22	32
Memphis BBQ Chicken	370	19	33
Philly Cheese Steak	360	21	26

Domino's® cont... (Oct '12)

	C	F	Cb
Oven Baked Sandwiches: Per Sandwich			
Buffalo Chicken with Blue Cheese	830	41	74
Chicken Bacon Ranch	870	45	72
Chicken Parmesan	750	30	73
Italian	820	41	70
Italian Sausage & Peppers	860	45	74
Mediterranean Veggie	680	29	72
Philly Cheese Steak	690	28	70
Sweet & Spicy Chicken Habanero	800	32	83
BreadBowl Pasta: Per ½ Bowl			
Chicken Alfredo, 10.75 oz	700	26	93
Chicken Carbonara, 11.75 oz	740	28	94
Italian Sausage Marinara, 12 oz	730	27	97
Pasta Primavera, 11 oz	670	24	94
Salads: Per Serving Without Dressing			
Garden Fresh	70	3.5	5
Grilled Chicken Caesar	90	3.5	5
Salad Dressings & Condiments: Per 1.5 oz Package			
Blue Cheese	230	24	2
Buttermilk Ranch	230	24	2
Creamy Caesar	210	21	2
Golden Italian	210	22	2
Light Italian	20	1	3
Bread Side Items:			
Breadsticks: 1 stick, without sauce	110	6	11
8 sticks, without sauce	880	48	88
Cheesy Bread:			
1 stick, without sauce	120	6	11
8 sticks, without sauce	960	48	88
Bread Dipping Sauces: Per Container			
Garlic	250	28	0
Marinara	25	0	5
Cinna Stix:			
1 stick, without icing	120	6	14
8 sticks, without icing	960	48	112
Sweet Icing, Dipper Cup	250	2.5	57
Chicken Wings: Without Dipping Sauce			
Barbeque, 4 wings	250	13	14
Hot, 4 wings	200	13	5
Chicken Dipping Cups: Per 1.5 oz Container			
Blue Cheese	240	25	2
Kicker Hot	50	4.5	3
Ranch	200	21	2
Dessert, Chocolate Lava Crunch Cake	350	17	47

Fast - Foods & Restaurants

Don Pablos® (Oct '12)

	C	F	Cb
Appetizers: Per Entire Plate, w/o Dress.			
Don's Boneless Wings: Buffalo	750	48	49
Chipotle Honey BBQ	1010	59	94
Flautas	505	29	40
Taquitos	560	39	28
The Don's Sampler	1870	104	140
Nachos: Cantina: With Chicken	1085	48	110
With Beef	1185	55	109
Quesadillas, Mesquite Grilled:			
Cheese, small	950	66	50
Steak, small	860	53	54
Dips: Per Entire Plate, Without Chips			
Bowls: Queso Blanco	1080	88	14
Prairie Fire Bean	715	43	53
Entrees: Per Meal, Without Sides			
Burritos: Chicken	1070	56	84
Fajita Steak	1025	50	79
Carnitas: Pork	790	31	82
Cold Set, Side	160	11	18
Chimichangas: Chicken	990	59	69
Spicy Beef De Oro	1360	79	89
Classic Fajitas: *With Onions, Peppers & 3x7" Fajitas*			
Combo - Steak & Chicken	625	31	47
Mesquite-Grilled: Chicken	570	27	58
Steak	680	36	36
Fajita Fixin's: 7" Flour Tortilla (3)	375	11	60
Combo Cheese Toppings, 1 oz	110	9	1
Corn Tortillas (4)	60	1	12
Guacamole, #30 scoop	70	6	4
Sour Cream, #30 scoop	80	8	2
Enchiladas: Cadillac: Chicken	945	47	80
Steak	1015	53	65
Primo Tacos: Buffalo Chicken Trio	1035	57	94
Chipotle Pork Trio	810	39	69
Crispy Chicken Trio	1005	54	93
Fried: Fish Trio	1170	40	123
Shrimp Trio	935	36	123
Grilled: Chicken Trio	995	43	106
Fish Trio	915	40	70
Shrimp Trio	680	35	70
Fresh Salads: Without Dressing			
Caesar: With Chicken	875	32	114
With Steak	945	38	99
Southwest: *Without Extra Dressing*			
With Buffalo Sauce	950	57	73
With Chipotle-Honey BBQ Sauce	1215	67	118
Sides:			
Mexican Rice, 3 oz	120	2	23
Refritos, 5 oz	215	7	27
Seasoned Vegetables, 6 oz	110	5	16

Dunkin' Donuts® (Oct '12)

	C	F	Cb
Bagels: Plain; Salt	310	1	64
Cinnamon Raisin	320	1	66
Everything	340	3	67
Multigrain	330	6	58
Onion	310	1	64
Sesame	350	4.5	65
Sour Cream & Onion	330	1.5	67
Danish: Apple Cheese	330	16	41
Cheese	330	17	39
Strawberry Cheese	320	16	40
Donuts: Apple 'n Spice	270	14	32
Bavarian Kreme	270	15	31
Boston Kreme	310	16	39
Bow Tie Donut	310	15	39
Chocolate Frosted Cocoa	270	13	33
Chocolate Kreme Filled	370	21	42
French Cruller	250	20	18
Jelly Filled	290	14	36
Old Fashioned Cake	320	22	33
Powdered Cake	340	22	38
Strawberry Frosted	280	15	32
Sugar Raised	230	14	22
Vanilla Kreme Filled	380	23	42
Muffins: Blueberry: Regular	460	15	76
Reduced Fat	410	10	75
Chocolate Chip	550	20	83
Corn	460	16	72
Honey Bran Raisin	440	13	74
Munchkins: Plain Cake (4)	240	14	24
Cinnamon Cake (4)	240	14	24
Glazed, average all varieties (4)	280	16	28
Jelly Filled (5)	400	20	45
Powdered Cake (4)	240	14	28
Sugared (5)	300	18	30
Sandwiches: On French Roll Unless Indicated			
Ham & Cheese	440	14	54
Roast Beef	460	16	54
Tuna Melt on a Croissant	650	41	44
Tuna Salad: On a Bagel	560	23	69
On English Muffin	380	19	37
Turkey Cheddar Bacon	470	14	55
Wake Up Wraps:			
Egg White: Turkey Sausage	150	5	14
Veggie	150	6	14

Continued Next Page... ...

Dunkin Donuts® cont... (Oct '12)

Breakfast:	C	F	Cb
AM Snacks:			
Hash Browns, 9 pieces	200	11	22
Oatmeal:			
Original, with Dried Fruit Topping	270	4	54
Brown Sugar Flavored Oatmeal, with Dried Fruit Topping	300	4	61
Bagels: Egg & Cheese	470	14	67
Bacon, Egg & Cheese	520	17	67
Ham, Egg & Cheese	500	15	68
Sausage, Egg & Cheese	680	33	68
Big N Toasted	530	28	43
Biscuits: Bacon, Egg & Cheese	490	30	35
Chicken	500	25	48
Sausage, Egg & Cheese	650	46	36
Croissant: Bacon, Egg & Cheese	550	34	41
Ham, Egg & Cheese	530	31	41
Sausage, Egg & Cheese	710	49	41
Egg White Flatbreads: Veggie	280	10	32
Turkey Sausage	280	8	32
English Muffin:			
Bacon, Egg & Cheese	370	18	34
Ham, Egg & Cheese	350	16	34
Sausage, Egg & Cheese	530	34	34
Sandwiches, Angus Steak & Egg	630	26	67
Coffee: Per Medium, 14 fl.oz			
Black Cocoa Creme: With Cream	250	9	40
Without Cream	170	0.5	38
Caramel Mocha: With Cream	260	9	41
Without Cream	170	0	39
Frozen Hot: Per 24 fl.oz			
Caramel:			
With Milk	550	11	110
With Skim Milk	510	5	110
Coolattas: Per Medium, 24 fl.oz			
Blue Raspberry; Cherry	360	0	92
Fruit Punch	350	0	92
Orange	310	0	81
CoolattaA's: Per Medium, 24 fl.oz			
OreoA: Coffee: With Cream	730	39	95
With Milk	490	10	97
With Skim Milk	440	4	98
Vanilla Bean	640	13	131
Strawberry Fruit	350	0	86
Other Hot Beverages: Per Medium Size, 14 fl.oz			
Chocolate: Regular; Turbo	320	11	58
Caramel; Coconut	330	11	59
Mint	310	10	52
Vanilla Chai	330	8	53

Eat 'N Park® (Oct '12)

Breakfast:	C	F	Cb
Fruit Cup	60	0.5	15
Hash Browns	200	8	28
Home Fries	210	12	24
Oatmeal with Milk	200	4	33
Omelette: Ham & Cheese	535	35	4
Meat Lover's	725	55	3.5
Pancakes, Buttermilk: Plain (1)	75	1	15
Blueberry (1)	85	1	16
Waffles: Belgian (1)	280	12	35
Strawberry (1)	375	18	48
Appetizers:			
Buffalo Chicken Tenders, 5 pieces	535	26	29
Fried Cheese Sticks	535	36	26
Grilled Chicken Quesadillas	905	55	51
Onion Rings Basket	365	24	34
Burgers:			
Black Angus: American Grill	610	37	31
BBQ Bacon Cheddar	865	53	53
Mushroom & Onion	710	41	45
Superburger	1085	73	28
Classic: Black Angus	420	21	22
Bacon Cheeseburger	535	31	22
Cheeseburger	465	25	22
Garden Burger	290	5	44
Original, Superburger	565	38	27
Sandwiches: With Menu Board Standard Add-Ins			
BLT	490	15	66
Buffalo Chicken Wrap	835	48	61
Chargrilled Chicken	320	6	32
Grilled Cheese	725	39	65
Hot Turkey	500	9	71
Santa Fe Turkey & Bacon	880	60	45
Shredded Pot Roast	530	31	28
Turkey Club	835	50	52
Whale of a Cod Fish	880	41	76
Dinners: Without Sides			
Baked Lemon Sole, 2 fillets	385	20	11
Chargrilled Chicken, 2 pieces	350	9	0
Chicken Fillets, 5 pieces	530	26	28
Chicken Parmigiana:			
W/ Marinara Sauce & Parm. Cheese	960	37	100
W/ Meat Sauce & Mozz. Cheese	985	40	95
Chicken Stir-Fry	390	8	47
Cod Floridian, 2 fillets	240	3	8
Spaghetti Marinara	695	9	129
Spaghetti with Meat Sauce	830	16	145
T Bone Steak	575	39	1

Continued Next Page....

Updated Nutrition Data ~ www.CalorieKing.com
Persons with Diabetes ~ See Disclaimer (Page 22)

Eat 'N Park® cont... (Oct '12)

Salads: Without Dressing

	C	F	Cb
Buffalo Chicken Salad	610	35	42
Chicken Fajita	745	34	64
Garden Salad	95	3	15
Grilled Chicken	445	19	30
Grilled Chicken Portobella	320	11	23

Dressings: Per 2 oz

Bleu Cheese	245	25	3
French, Fat Free	75	0	18
Italian, Fat Free	20	0	5
House Ranch	215	21	4
Thousand Island	190	19	4

Desserts:

Grilled Stickies a la Mode	725	39	81
Ice Cream, 2 scoops	230	12	27

Pies: Per Slice

Apple	525	27	67
Cherry	520	28	63
Strawberry	290	12	45

Edo Japan® (Oct '12)

Bento Box: Without Teriyaki Sauce

	C	F	Cb
Beef Yakisoba, 20.25 oz	840	29	102
Chicken Yakisoba, 20.5 oz	790	24	102
Sizzling Shrimp, 22 oz	790	15	122
Sukiyaki Beef, 20.25 oz	880	27	120

Teriyaki Dishes: Without Teriyaki Sauce

Chicken & Shrimp	640	14	82
Hawaiian Chicken, 15.5 oz	580	11	85
Sukiyaki Beef, 14.75 oz	580	15	80
Teriyaki Chicken, 15 oz	570	11	80

Soup: Per 33 oz Bowl

Beef Udon	750	16	117
Chicken Udon	700	12	117

Maki Sushi: Per 6 Pieces

California Roll, 7.6 oz	430	17	61
Spicy Tuna Roll, 6.5 oz	300	2.5	54

Nigiri Sushi: Per 1 Piece

Ebi (Steamed Prawn), 1.65 oz	70	0.5	12
Salmon Sashimi, 0.7 oz	30	1.5	1

Einstein Bros® (Oct '12)

Breakfast:

	C	F	Cb
Egg Paninis: Spinach & Bacon	770	38	72
Green Chili & Turkey Sausage	650	22	71
Egg Wraps: Santa Fe	660	33	60
Spicy Elmo	630	34	56

Bagels:

Bagel Thin Singles:

Everything	160	2	29
Other varieties, average	140	1.5	29
Classics, Plain; Honey Whole Wheat	255	1	56

Gourmet Bagels: Dutch Apple

	350	6	69
Green Chile	350	8	58
Power Bagel	310	5	61
Six-Cheese	330	6	56
Spinach Florentine	320	6	56

Pizza Bagels: Cheese

	400	11	59
Pepperoni	450	15	59

Signature Bagels: Asiago Cheese

	310	5	56
Blueberry	300	1	65
Chocolate Chip	290	2.5	58
Cinnamon Sugar	290	2.5	63
Cranberry; Onion, average	270	1	60
Garlic; Good Grains, average	270	2.5	57
Poppy; Sesame	280	3	56
Potato	270	4	52

Bagel Dogs: With Cheddar Cheese

Original	540	27	56
Asiago	550	28	56

Bagel Thin Melts:

Cheesy Chicken Asparagus	340	13	32
Cheesy Turkey	330	11	32

Lunch Paninis:

Italian Chicken	850	37	72
Turkey Club	800	37	74

Open Face Deli Melts: Ham & Swiss

	490	15	60
Chicken & Mozzarella	530	15	61
Turkey & Cheddar	490	15	58

Sandwiches:

Egg: With Bacon & Cheddar	510	19	58
With Ham & Swiss	490	16	59
With Turkey Sausage & Cheddar	540	20	59
With Spinach, Mushroom & Swiss	500	19	60
Wraps: California Chicken	700	35	64
Chipotle Turkey	630	29	69

Cream Cheese: Per 1.25 oz Schmear

Reduced Fat:

Garlic Herb/Garden Veggie	110	9	5
Honey Almond; Strawberry, av.	120	9	10
Plain; Sun Dried Tomato & Basil	110	9	4
Onion and Chive	120	11	5

El Pollo Loco® (Oct'12)

	C	F	Cb
Burritos:			
BRC, 7.6 oz	430	12	64
Califresco, 17.8 oz	850	34	87
El Tradicional, 14.7 oz	780	31	86
Grilled Chicken Tortilla Roll, 6 oz	400	15	38
Poblano, 18.6 oz	910	39	93
Chicken Meal, Skinless Breast,			
without Torilla Strips or Dressing	265	8	11
Flame-Grilled Chicken: Skin On			
Breast	220	9	0
Leg	90	4	0
Thigh	220	15	0
Wing	90	5	0
Bowl: Original Pollo	610	10	87
Ultimate: 24.4oz	960	34	92
Loco Value Menu:			
Crunchy Chicken Taco	300	17	21
Flan, 5.1 oz	260	12	34
Taco al Carbon	160	6	18
Soup:			
Chicken Tortilla with Tortilla Strips:			
Small, 10.8 oz	210	9	19
Large, 23.6 oz	450	19	40
Salads: W/o Dressing			
Chicken Tostada, 17.3 oz	860	42	77
Grilled Chicken, 10.3 oz	230	7	18
Dressings: Per Container			
Creamy Cilantro: 1.3 oz	190	20	1
Light, 1.5 oz	70	5	6
Ranch, 1.5 oz	210	22	2
Condiments:			
Guacamole	70	6	3
Salsa: Avocado, 1.5 oz	35	3.5	2
House/Roja, average, 1.5 oz	10	0	2
Sour Cream, 1.3 oz	80	7	1
Sides:			
BBQ Black Beans, 6 oz	200	3	36
Cole Slaw, 4 oz	130	10	9
Corn Cobbette, 2 pcs, 6.2 oz	160	5	25
Flame Gr. Corn, 4 oz	130	5	21
French Fries, 3.8 oz	330	17	40
Mashed Pot. w/ Gravy, 6 oz	130	1.5	28
Pinto Beans, 6 oz	200	4	29
Spanish Rice, 4.5 oz	170	2.5	33
Sweet Corn Cake, 3.7 oz	250	10	36
Sweet Potato Fries, 3.6 oz	330	20	34
Tortilla Chips & Guacamole, 7.5 oz	740	46	77
Dessert, Churros (2), 2.4 oz	300	18	32

For Complete Nutritional Data ~ see CalorieKing.com

Fatburger® (Oct'12)

	C	F	Cb
Burgers: Without Extras			
Burgers: Small	400	21	37
Medium	590	31	46
Large	850	41	69
Turkeyburger	480	21	50
Veggieburger	510	20	60
Hot Dogs: Without Extas			
Chili Cheese	480	27	35
Regular Hot Dog	320	15	32
Sandwiches: Without Extras			
Chicken: Crispy	560	27	53
Grilled	430	14	42
Fish	560	31	55
Fries: Fat Fries; Skinny Fries, av.	385	17	53
With Chili, average	485	23	57
With Chili & Cheese, average	595	32	58
Add-Ons: American Cheese, 1 slice	70	5	1
Cheddar Cheese, 1 slice	110	9	1
Mayonnaise, 1 serving	90	10	1
Relish, 1 serving	20	0	5
Sides: Chili Cup	200	11	10
With Cheese & Onions	320	20	12
Onion Rings	540	29	64
Shakes: Chocolate	910	45	115
Cookies & Ice Cream	1180	59	163
Maui Banana	940	44	126
Peanut Butter	950	53	114
Strawberry; Vanilla, average	885	44	112

For Complete Nutritional Data ~ see CalorieKing.com

Fazoli's® (Oct'12)

	C	F	Cb
Fresh Made Pasta: Per Serving			
Classic Sampler Platter, 21.6 oz	890	25	122
Fettuccine with Alfredo, 17.8 oz	800	26	108
Ravioli w/ Meat Sauce	570	24	58
Toasted Ravioli (12)	690	16	108
Ultimate Sampler Platter	1130	34	153
Oven-Baked Pasta: Per Serving			
Baked Spaghetti, 15.5 oz	640	22	80
With Meatballs, 18.8 oz	890	39	86
Cheesy Baked Ziti, 15 oz	670	27	71
Chicken Broccoli Penne, 21.3 oz	920	42	77
Chicken Carbonara, 17.8 oz	800	27	88
Chicken Parmigiano, 21.6 oz	1000	39	108
Penne Romano, 19.3 oz	880	44	76
Penne w/ Creamy Basil Chkn, 18.7 oz	970	51	73
Twice-Baked Lasagna, 18.4 oz	700	39	47

Continued Next Page....

200

Fazoli's® cont... (Oct '12)

400 Calories or Less Pasta:

	C	F	Cb
Chicken Mshrm Alfredo Bake, 9.5 oz	400	17	37
Three Cheese Baked Ravioli, 6.5 oz	340	19	26
Chicken Penne & Peppers, 10.1 oz	340	12	37

Pizzas: Per Slice

	C	F	Cb
Triple Cheese, 4 oz	290	12	32
Pepperoni Classico, 4.2 oz	300	13	32

Flatbread Pizzas: Per Pizza

	C	F	Cb
Chicken Broccoli Florentine, 9.4 oz	500	19	53
Tuscan Chicken, 10.6 oz	480	17	55

Oven Baked Submarinos:

	C	F	Cb
Club Italiano, 13 oz	780	36	68
Fazoli's Original, 12.8 oz	880	49	70
Smoked Turkey Basil, 12.8 oz	750	37	68
Ultimate M'ball Smasher, 13.7 oz	1070	65	76

Salads: With Dressing Unless Indicated

	C	F	Cb
Cherry Almond Chicken, 12.2 oz	480	25	38
Country Caesar, 16 oz	780	51	48
Fazoli's Italian House	600	45	16
Pasta Ranch Italia, 18.3 oz	770	50	44
Side, Chopped, w/o dressing, 5 oz	60	3.5	5

For Complete Nutritional Data ~ see CalorieKing.com

Firehouse Subs® (Oct '12)

	C	F	Cb

Subs: *Per Medium White Sub, With Standard Toppings and Dressings*

	C	F	Cb
Chicken Salad	820	48	60
Engine Company; Engineer, av.	695	36	59
Ham	730	36	70
Hero	770	37	64
Hook & Ladder	700	36	64
Italian	910	57	64
Meatball	820	50	60
Roast Beef	710	36	54
Tuna	1000	68	67
Turkey	670	34	58
Veggie	720	45	60
Chili, Bowl	340	17	25

Salads: Without Dressing

	C	F	Cb
Chief's Salad: With Chicken	370	18	17
With Chicken Salad	490	29	20
With Ham	410	17	31
With Tuna	670	48	27
With Turkey	350	15	19

Five Guys® (Oct '12)

Burgers:

	C	F	Cb
Bacon Burger	780	50	39
Bacon Cheeseburger	920	62	40
Cheeseburger	840	55	40
Hamburger	700	43	39

Five Guys® cont... (Oct '12)

Burgers: (Cont):

	C	F	Cb
Little: Bacon Burger	560	33	39
Bacon Cheeseburger	630	39	40
Cheeseburger	550	32	40
Hamburger	480	26	39

Dogs: Bacon Dog; Cheese Dog

	C	F	Cb
Bacon Dog; Cheese Dog	620	40	41
Bacon Cheese Dog	695	48	41
Hot Dog	545	35	40

Fries: Regular, 8.5 oz

	C	F	Cb
Fries: Regular, 8.5 oz	620	30	78
Half order, 4.25 oz	310	15	39

Flame Broiler® (Oct '12)

Bowls: Per Bowl

	C	F	Cb
Chicken; Beef; Half & Half, average	610	17	69
Beef/Chicken Vege, average	540	16	53
The Works	630	15	78

Mini Bowls:

	C	F	Cb
Chicken; Beef; Half & Half, av.	380	7	48

Plates: Per Plate

	C	F	Cb
Beef; Chicken; Chicken & Beef, av.	855	27	91
Rib	730	23	92
Works	820	24	96

Freshens® (Oct '12)

Smoothies: 100% Juice (20 fl.oz)

	C	F	Cb

Blended Fruit Classics:

	C	F	Cb
Caribbean Craze; Maui Mango	260	0	65
Citrus Mango	390	7	83
Jamaican Jammer	290	0	63
Orange Sunrise	260	3	57
Strawberry Kiwi	290	0	73
Strawberry Squeeze	250	0	54
Tropical Pineapple	380	4	88
High Protein: Peanut Butter	460	12	69
Strawberries 'n Cream	370	1	61

Rainforest Energy:

	C	F	Cb
Acai; Brazillian, average	285	3	65
Mangosteen	320	0	80

Fro-Yo Blasts: Per 12 fl.oz

	C	F	Cb
Cookie Dough	490	6	103
Oreo Overload	370	4	78

Indulgent Shakes: Per 16 fl.oz w/o Whipped Cream

	C	F	Cb
Chocolate	440	2.5	95
Oreo Cream	530	6	110
Strawberry	400	2	87

Breakfast Crepes:

	C	F	Cb
Denver; Steak & Eggs, av.	470	25	26
Wake Up	420	22	23

Savory Golden Crepes: Fajita Chkn

	C	F	Cb
Savory Golden Crepes: Fajita Chkn	500	13	58
Fajita Steak	530	19	59
Honey Mustard Chicken	470	14	52

Dessert Crepes:

	C	F	Cb
Cheesecake Supreme	510	20	69
The Guilty Pleasure	540	13	91

201

Godfather's Pizza® (Oct '12)

Golden Crust Pizza: Per Slice	C	F	Cb
Cheese: Medium, 1/8 pizza	220	8	25
Large, 1/10 pizza	250	9	28
Combo: Medium, 1/8	290	13	27
Large, 1/10 pizza	330	15	30
Super Combo: Medium, 1/8 pizza	320	15	28
Large, 1/10 pizza	370	18	31
Original Crust Pizza:			
Cheese: Mini, 1/4 pizza	150	4	20
Medium, 1/8 pizza	260	7	34
Jumbo, 1/12 pizza	350	10	44
Combo: Mini, 1/4 pizza	200	8	21
Medium, 1/8 pizza	350	14	36
Jumbo, 1/12 pizza	480	20	47
Super Combo: Mini, 1/4 pizza	220	9	22
Medium, 1/8 pizza	350	14	36
Jumbo, 1/12 pizza	520	23	48
Thin Crust Pizza:			
Cheese: Medium, 1/8 pizza	170	8	15
Large, 1/10 pizza	210	10	17
Combo: Medium, 1/8 pizza	240	13	17
Large, 1/10 pizza	280	16	20
Super Combo: Medium, 1/8 pizza	290	16	19
Large, 1/10 pizza	330	19	20
Calzones: Per Medium Calzone			
Cheese	1660	51	200
Combo	1450	40	199
Pepperoni	1410	39	195
Sides:			
Breadstick (1)	110	2	20
Cheesestick, medium, 1/8	200	7	24
Garlic Toast: 1 piece	150	9	15
With Cheese, 1 piece	210	12	16
Hot Chicken Wings (4), breaded	180	12	4
Potato Wedges, 4 oz	175	8	24

Gold Star Chili® (Oct '12)

Meals:	C	F	Cb
Burrito, Gold Star Chili	970	33	126
Burrito Bowl, Grilled Chicken	905	29	111
Chili By The Bowl:			
Gold Star	205	10	10
Low Carb Coney	740	59	9
Tex Mex	225	9	18
Coneys: Regular	225	12	21
Cheese	310	19	21
Regular: 2-Way	395	10	54
3-Way	680	34	55
4-Way, Bean	825	34	81
5-Way	795	34	77
Super, 5-Way	1180	48	122

Gold Star Chili® cont... (Oct '12)

Sandwich,	C	F	Cb
Chili Cheese	265	14	22
Salads: Without Dressing			
Cafe	305	13	34
With Crispy Chicken	495	25	43
With Grilled Chicken	410	16	36
Caesar Salad	190	5	25
With Crispy Chicken	375	16	35
With Grilled Chicken	290	7	27
South of the Border Chili	685	36	62
Sides: Fries	400	16	58
Chili Cheese	680	36	63
Garlic Bread	205	9	26
With Cheese	320	18	26

Golden Corral® (Oct '12)

Breakfast:	C	F	Cb
Bacon & Cheese Quiche, 1 slice	290	21	15
Corned Beef Hash, Grilled, 1 cup	440	28	26
Creamed Chipped Beef, 1 cup	320	18	20
French Toast, Plain, 1 slice	200	6	29
Hash Brown Casserole, 1 cup	260	10	28
Sausage Links (1)	120	11	1
Sausage Patties (1)	100	9	0
Meals: Without Sides			
Hot Buffet:			
Awesome Pot Roast, 3 oz	100	4.5	5
Baked Fish w/ Shrimp & Sce, 3 oz	160	10	2
Baked Florentine Fish, 1 piece	180	12	2
BBQ: Chicken Leg Quarter, 1 pce	490	22	21
Pork, 3 oz	170	8	5
Bone-In Catfish, 3 oz	210	14	7
Bourbon Street Chicken, 3 oz	170	9	4
Breaded Bay Scallops (10)	140	6	13
Coconut Shrimp (5)	200	12	16
Crab Cakes (1)	180	15	8
Hickory Bourbon Chkn Tenders (1)	140	2	17
Meatloaf, 1 slice	220	11	11
Sirloin Steak, 4.5 oz	230	9	1
Salad Buffet: Per 1/2 Cup Unless Indicated			
Coleslaw	110	9	6
Salads: Caesar, w/out dress., 1 cup	110	8	8
Cajun Potato	230	17	15
Chicken	240	20	3
Seafood	140	10	9
Spinach Bacon, 1 cup	120	9	4
Tuna	190	13	5
Dressings: Balsamic Vinaig., 2 T.	200	0	5
Caesar, 2 Tbsp	150	15	2
Ranch, 2 Tbsp	110	12	2

(The) Great American Bagel Co® (Oct '12)

	C	F	Cb
Bagels:			
Asiago Cheese	520	16	72
Cheddar Herb	390	8	66
Cinnamon Raisin	380	3.5	76
Jalapeno Cheddar	370	7	63
Plain	360	4	71
Spinach Tomazzo	640	20	86
Tomazzo	520	13	77
Paninis: On Regular Baguette			
Chicken Pesto	770	35	70
Ham & Swiss	600	26	58
Philly Beef	920	40	92
Turkey Club	680	29	67
Sandwiches: Asiago Omelet	720	29	80
Blt	550	17	72
Chicken Parmigiana	740	22	81
Ham	460	9	71
Roast Beef	465	9	71
Turkey	435	5	72
Cream Cheese Filling: Per 1 oz			
Plain	100	10	1
Strawberry; Vegetable, average	90	8	4
Pastries:			
Cookies: Chocolate Chunk, 4 oz	110	3.5	19
Oatmeal Raisin, 4 oz	120	5	18
Muffins: Blueberry, 4.25 oz	430	16	64
Banana Nut, 4.25 oz	430	18	61

Green Burrito® (Oct '12)

	C	F	Cb
Burritos:			
Bean & Cheese	470	19	54
Beef, Bean & Cheese	500	22	51
California: Chicken	470	21	45
Steak	480	21	44
Chicken Especial	580	26	58
Mexican: Chicken	550	23	56
Steak	560	23	55
Specialties:			
Super Nachos:			
Chicken	950	51	93
Ground Beef	1000	57	93
Taco Salad: Chicken	830	48	68
Ground Beef	880	53	67
Steak	840	47	67
Tacos: Crispy Taco	210	12	15
Ground Beef, hard shell	210	12	15
Southwest Chicken, soft	310	21	19
Street Tacos: Chicken	120	4	15
Steak	130	4	14
Sides: Beans, 9.7 oz	420	19	45
Chips, 2 oz	300	17	35
Guacamole, 1.4 oz	60	5	3

(The) Great Steak & Potato Company® (Oct '12)

	C	F	Cb
Breakfast Sandwiches:			
Bacon, Egg & Cheese, 7.6 oz	600	36	39
Egg & Cheese, 7 oz	500	29	39
Ham & Cheese, 5.5 oz	430	22	41
Ham, Egg & Cheese, 9 oz	570	32	42
Sausage, Egg & Cheese, 9 oz	700	47	39
Steak, Egg & Cheese, 10 oz	600	34	40
Breakfast Potatoes,			
Deluxe/Fresh Cut, average	385	23	43
Sandwiches: 7"			
Bacon Cheddar Cheesesteak, 12.2 oz	720	32	62
Buffalo Chicken Philly, 13.8 oz	660	24	65
Chicagoland Cheesesteak, 13.3 oz	680	29	63
Chicken Bacon Ranch, 15.2 oz	990	56	66
Chicken Cordon Bleu, 13.4 oz	580	16	78
Great Steak Cheesesteak, 13.6 oz	740	37	62
Ham Delight/Explosion, av., 14 oz	710	34	71
Pastrami, 13.3 oz	790	41	65
Pepper Steak, 15.17 oz	880	50	67
Philly Cheesesteak, 11.8 oz	650	26	62
Reuben, 11.9 oz	690	33	61
Super Steak Cheesesteak, 15 oz	750	37	64
Veggie Delight, 11.7 oz	510	19	64
Baked Potatoes:			
The Great Potato: Chicken, 12.5 oz	500	22	37
Ham, 12.3 oz	420	16	43
Steak, 13 oz	520	26	37
The King, 8.4 oz	490	29	31
Turkey, 12.3 oz	390	13	39
Fries:			
Great Fry: Kids, 6.25 oz	270	13	36
Regular, 10.25 oz	440	20	60
Large, 12.5 oz	540	25	72
Coney Island Fry, Regular, 12.7 oz	570	30	61
King Fry, regular, 11.4 oz	630	39	52
Nacho Fry, regular, 11.8 oz	510	27	53
Salads: Without Dressing			
Chef Salad, 16 oz	260	11	15
Great Salad: Grilled Chicken, 19 oz	380	18	18
Grilled Steak, 19.4 oz	400	23	18
Wedge: Grilled Chicken, 14.8 oz	270	11	11
Grilled Steak, 15.3 oz	290	16	11
Salad Dressings: Ranch, 1 oz	170	18	1
Thousand Island, 1 oz	130	12	4

Haagen-Dazs® (Oct '12)

Ice Cream: Per ½ Cup	C	F	Cb
Banana Split	280	16	31
Butter Pecan	310	23	21
Caramel Cone	320	19	32
Cherry Vanilla	240	15	23
Chocolate	260	17	22
Chocolate Chip Cookie Dough	310	20	29
Chocolate Peanut Butter	360	24	27
Coffee	270	18	21
Cookies & Cream	270	17	23
Creme Brulee	280	19	23
Dark Chocolate	260	17	21
Dulce de Leche	290	17	28
Mango	250	14	28
Pineapple Coconut	230	13	25
Pistachio	290	20	22
Rum Raisin	270	17	22
Vanilla Bean	290	18	26
Single Serve Cups: Per 1 Cup			
Caramel Cone	260	16	24
Chocolate	230	15	20
Dulce de leche; Strawb.	240	14	24
Five: Lemon	240	11	29
Other flavors, average	220	12	22
Frozen Yogurt: Per ½ Cup			
Coffee	200	4.5	31
Vanilla	170	2.5	29
Vanilla Raspberry Swirl	170	2.5	32
Sorbet: Per ½ Cup			
Blackberry Cabernet	100	0	26
Raspberry; Zesty Lemon	120	0	30
Strawberry	130	0	31

Ice Cream Bars/Cones ~ See Page 109

Hardee's® (Oct '12)

Burgers:	C	F	Cb
Cheeseburgers: Small	350	19	32
Double, 7 oz	480	29	34
Hamburger, Small	310	15	31
Turkey Burger	460	17	47
Thickburgers: Original, ⅓ lb	860	58	52
Amazing Grilled Cheese Bacon:			
10.33 oz	1000	73	44
¼ lb, 8.55 oz	850	59	44
⅓ lb, 10 oz	990	69	45
Bacon Cheese, ⅓ lb	840	56	49
Frisco, ⅓ lb	930	64	44

Hardee's® cont... (Oct '12)

Burgers (Cont):	C	F	Cb
Thickburgers (Cont):			
Little Thickburger	570	39	34
Little Thick Cheeseburger, 6 oz	430	23	34
Low-Carb, ⅓ lb	470	36	9
Memphis: BBQ Six Dollar	1000	58	83
⅓ lb	960	52	83
Little, 8.8 oz	710	39	61
Monster, ⅔ lb	1290	92	47
Mushroom 'N' Swiss, ⅓ lb	650	36	47
Six Dollar	930	63	59
Breaded Chicken Tenders: W/o Sauce			
3 pieces, 4.5 oz	260	13	13
5 pieces, 7.5 oz	440	21	21
Sandwiches:			
Big Hot Ham 'N' Cheese	450	18	46
Chicken: Charbroiled BBQ Chicken	380	6	58
Charbroiled Chicken Club	610	30	55
Hand Breaded Chicken Fillet	680	37	55
Fish, Supreme	630	38	52
Sides:			
Beer Battered Onion Rings, 4.5 oz	410	24	45
Natural Cut Fries: Small, 4.5 oz	320	14	45
Medium, 5.75 oz	430	19	60
Large, 6.25 oz	470	21	65
Kids Meals: Includes Kid's Fries & Small Drink			
Breaded Chicken Tenders, 2 pieces,			
without Sauce	380	18	36
Cheeseburger	560	29	59
Hamburger	510	25	58
Breakfast:			
Biscuits: Bacon Bacon	450	27	39
Bacon, Egg & Cheese	400	25	38
Biscuit 'N' Gravy	410	23	50
Chicken Fillet	500	26	50
Cinnamon 'N Raisin	300	15	40
Country Fried Steak	470	29	46
Loaded Omelet	610	42	36
Monster	640	44	40
Sausage and Egg	470	32	38
Smoked Sausage	510	36	39
Big Country Platter, with Bacon	810	40	74
Bowl, Low Carb	650	54	2

Continued Next Page...

Updated Nutrition Data ~ www.CalorieKing.com
Persons with Diabetes ~ See Disclaimer (Page 22)

Fast - Foods & Restaurants

Hardee's® cont... (Oct '12)

Breakfast (Cont):	C	F	Cb
Burrito, Loaded	770	49	39
Sandwiches, Frisco	430	19	41
Sunrise Croissants: With Bacon	450	29	28
With Ham	430	27	27
With Sausage	550	38	29
Breakfast Sides:			
Grits	110	5	16
Hash Rounds: Small, 2.92 oz	250	16	25
Medium, 4.23 oz	390	26	36
Large, 5.75 oz	530	35	49
Desserts:			
Apple Turnover w/o Cinn. Sugar	270	13	35
Chocolate Chip Cookie: (1), 2.4 oz	290	11	44
Fresh Baked (1), 2 oz	290	15	35
Hand Scooped Ice Cream: Malt	780	35	98
Shake, 14 oz	705	33	86
Peach Cobbler, small, 6.35 oz	285	7	56
Single Scoop Ice Cream:			
Bowl, 4 oz	235	13	27
Cone, 4.4 oz	285	13	37
Drinks:			
Hot Chocolate	150	3	18
Ice Cream Malts: Per 14.6 oz Cup			
Chocolate	780	35	98
Strawberry	780	35	98
Vanilla	780	35	98
Ice Cream Shakes: Per 14 oz Cup			
Chocolate; Strawberry, average	700	34	86
Vanilla	705	33	86

For Complete Nutritional Data ~ see CalorieKing.com

Hissho Sushi® (Oct '12)

Starters: Per Serving	C	F	Cb
Baby Octopus Salad, 3.5 oz	150	2	18
Spring Rolls: Regular (2), 4.9 oz	135	2	18
Garden (2), 4.9 oz	130	3	23
Grilled Chicken (2), 4.9 oz	140	4	19
Ocean Salmon (2), 4.9 oz	150	5	16
Ocean Tuna (2), 4.9 oz	155	4	16

Hissho Sushi® cont... (Oct '12)

Maki Sushi: Per 6 Pieces Unless Indicated	C	F	Cb
Rolls: Blazing California	265	2	53
Boston	265	2	53
California	275	3	56
Crab Salad	270	3	53
Crunchy	285	3	53
Rolls:			
Dynamite: Salmon	295	5	51
Shrimp	285	3	52
Tuna	290	4	49
Yellowtail	295	4	51
Inari	285	4	54
Nippon Favorite: Salmon, 16 pcs	330	2	65
Tuna, 16 pieces	330	2	64
Philadelphia	345	10	56
Snow Crab	280	3	56
Sushicado: Salmon, 12 pieces	510	7	92
Shrimp, 6 pieces	300	3	56
Specialty Items: Per 4 Pieces			
Rolls:			
Caterpillar	330	5	60
Grande Finale	280	5	48
Living Color	250	3	43
Mango Tango	250	5	37
Salmon Lover	305	8	42
Sriracha Party	450	8	77
Tempura Shrimp	255	1	54
TNT: Salmon	290	4	52
Shrimp	280	2	52
Tuna	290	3	50
Wasabi Crunch	335	7	53

Hot Dog on a Stick® (Oct '12)

Menu Items:	C	F	Cb
American Cheese on a Stick	260	16	21
Beef Hot Dog on a Bun	470	29	36
Turkey Hot Dog on a Stick	250	14	22
Veggie Dog on a Stick	220	8	24
Pepperjack Cheese on a Stick	240	14	19
Sides, French Fries, 4.5 oz	400	21	49
Dessert, Funnel Cake Sticks, (10)	210	8	31
Beverages: Per 16 fl.oz			
Lemonade: Original	150	0	38
Sugar Free	15	0	3
Lime	230	0	57

Fast - Foods & Restaurants

Hungry Howie's Pizza® (Oct '12)

Counts may vary in Florida.

	C	F	Cb
Pizzas: *Per Slice*			
Cheese: Small, ⅙ pizza	170	4	23
Medium, ⅛ pizza	180	4.5	24
Large, ⅒ pizza	200	5	25
X-Large, ¹⁄₁₂ pizza	240	6	33
Oven Baked Subs: *Per ½ Sub*			
Deluxe Italian	505	18	61
Ham & Cheese	475	15	61
Steak & Cheese	490	15	64
Turkey Club	555	15	63
Vegetarian	530	21	64
Sides: Boneless Wings, 3 pieces	145	5	12
Howie Wings, 5 wings	180	13	0
Salads: *Serves 2, Small Size, Without Dressing*			
Antipasto	230	15	6
Chef	230	13	8
Garden	40	0.5	7
Greek	250	15	16
Dressings: *Per 1 oz*			
Creamy Italian	120	12	2
Greek	110	11	2
Ranch	180	19	1
Thousand Island	140	14	4

In-N-Out Burger® (Oct '12)

	C	F	Cb
Burgers:			
Hamburger: With Onion	390	19	39
With Mustard/Ketchup, w/o Spread	310	10	41
Protein Style w/ Lettuce Wrap, w/o Bun	240	17	11
Cheeseburger: With Onion	480	27	39
With Mustard/Ketchup, w/o Spread	400	18	41
Protein Style w/ Lettuce Wrap, w/o Bun	330	25	11
Double Double: With Onion	670	41	39
With Mustard/Ketchup, w/o Spread	590	32	41
Protein Style w/ Lettuce Wrap, w/o Bun	520	39	11
French Fries, 4.5 oz	395	18	54
Drinks: Milk, 10 fl.oz	180	6	18
Coca-Cola, 16 fl.oz	200	0	52
Dr Pepper; 7-Up, 16 fl.oz	200	0	52
Lemonade, 16 fl.oz	180	0	40
Root Beer, 16 fl.oz	220	0	60
Shakes: Choc., 15 fl.oz	590	29	72
Strawberry, 15 fl.oz	590	27	81
Vanilla, 15 fl.oz	580	31	67

IHOP® (Oct '12)

	C	F	Cb
Pancakes:			
Buttermilk: *With Menu Toppings*			
Full Stack (5)	750	22	115
Short Stack (3)	470	15	69
Chocolate Choc. Chip, Buttermilk Style (4)	710	23	110
Double Blueberry (4)	680	17	115
Strawberry Banana (4)	760	17	137
Condiments:			
Syrup: Blueberry, 1 fl.oz	110	0	26
Boysenberry; Strawberry, 1 fl.oz	100	0	26
Maple, Regular, 1 fl.oz oz	110	0	27
Sugar-Free Syrup, 1 fl.oz	15	0	5
Whipped Butter/Margarine, 1 Tbsp	80	9	0
French Toast & Waffles: *W/ Toppings Unless Indicated*			
French Toast: Original	900	47	88
Cinnn-A-Stack	1120	54	126
Strawberry Banana	1060	45	135
Waffle, Belgian, Plain (1)	360	15	47
With Butter	400	20	47
Fruit Toppings: *With Whipped Topping*			
Blueberry Compote; Strawb., av.	165	2.5	37
Cinnamon Apple Compote	140	2.5	32
International Crepe Passport: *As Served*			
Fresh Fruit	870	50	71
German	930	70	40
Strawb. Banana Danish	1000	67	68
Savory Crepes: Chicken Florentine	880	53	48
Garden Stuffed	1050	75	51
Hearty Omelettes: *Without Pancakes or Sides*			
Big Steak	1210	81	52
Garden	830	65	17
Hearty Ham & Cheese	910	64	18
Spinach & Mushroom	910	70	24
Sandwiches & Burgers: *Without Sides*			
Bacon Cheddar Chicken Sandwich	930	61	47
Chicken Clubhouse Super Stacker	1180	83	56
Patty Melt	900	65	38
Philly Cheese Steak Stacker	930	56	56
Turkey & Bacon Club Sandwich	740	41	51
Breakfast Combinations: *As Served, w/o Syrup*			
Biscuits & Gravy Combo w/ Country Gravy	1380	93	96
Breakfast Sampler	1160	70	83
Country Fried Steak & Eggs with Country Gravy	1540	84	139
Split Decision	1120	68	80
T-Bone Steak & Eggs, 12 oz	1220	65	74
Hearty Dinner Favorites: *As Served*			
Chicken Fried Chkn, w/ Gravy	690	33	74
Crunchy Battered Shrimp	600	21	76
Simple & Fit Grilled Tilapia	500	23	27
Sirloin Steak Tips	800	40	69
T-Bone Steak, 12 oz	760	41	44

Jack in the Box® (Oct '12)

Sandwiches & Burgers:	C	F	Cb
Bacon Ultimate Cheeseburger	910	56	44
Hamburger: Original	280	11	32
With Cheese	320	14	32
Deluxe	320	15	33
With Cheese	410	22	34
Jumbo Jack: Original	490	23	44
With Cheese	570	30	45
Junior Bacon Cheeseburger	390	21	32
Sirloin Cheeseburger, with Bacon	1030	71	52
Sourdough Jack	660	41	40
Sourdough Steak Melt	650	38	38
Ultimate Cheeseburger	820	49	44

Chicken & Fish:	C	F	Cb
Chicken Sandwich	410	21	47
With Bacon	470	25	42
Chicken Strips: Crispy, 4 pieces	560	24	53
Grilled, 4 pieces	250	7	5
Fish & Chips, small fries, 8.5 oz	710	37	74
Jack's Spicy Chkn S'wich	530	20	61
With Cheese	600	25	62
Sourdough Gr. Chicken Club	540	26	38

Breakfast:	C	F	Cb
Biscuit: Bacon, Egg & Cheese	430	25	35
Sausage, Egg & Cheese	570	38	36
Breakfast Jack: Regular	280	11	30
With Bacon	310	14	30
Croissants: Sausage	570	40	32
Supreme	450	27	32
Sandwiches: Extreme Sausage	660	47	32
Sourdough	410	21	35
Ultimate	520	25	42
Hash Brown Sticks, 5 pieces	280	19	26
Meaty Burrito, without salsa	610	37	38

Snacks & Sides:	C	F	Cb
Bacon Cheddar Pot. Wedges, 9.25 oz	680	42	58
Beef Taco, regular	190	11	17
Chiquita Apple Bites, med.	70	0	17
Egg Rolls (3), w/o sauce	440	22	46
Mozzarella Cheese Sticks:			
3 Pieces	280	16	22
6 Pieces	560	33	43
Stuffed Jalapenos:			
3 Pieces	220	12	21
7 Pieces	510	29	49
Onion Rings (8), 4.25 oz	450	28	45
Seasoned Curly Fries, med., 4.5 oz	430	25	46

Jack in the Box® cont... (Oct '12)

Healthy Dining	C	F	Cb
Chicken Fajita, without Salsa	320	11	33
Chicken Teriyaki Bowl	690	6	133
Grilled Chicken Strips, w/ Teriyaki Dipping Sce	310	8	16
Hamburger Deluxe	320	15	33

Salads: No Dressing or Condiments	C	F	Cb
Chicken Club with Grilled Chicken	360	20	12
Side Salad	20	0	4
Southwest Chicken, with Grilled Chicken Strips	350	15	28

Sauces & Dressings:	C	F	Cb
Dipping Sauce: Barbecue, 1 oz	40	0	10
Buttermilk House, 1 oz	130	13	3
Frank's Red Hot Buffalo, 1 oz	10	0	2
Sweet & Sour, 1 oz	45	0	11
Tartar, 0.5 oz	150	16	2
Sauce: Mayo-Onion, ½ oz	90	10	0
Soy, ¼ oz	5	0	1
Taco, ¼ oz	0	0	0

Shakes & Desserts:	C	F	Cb
Chocolate Overload Cake	300	7	57
Churros, Mini (5)	350	18	42
New York Style Cheesecake	310	17	32
Shakes: 16 oz, with Whipped Topping			
Chocolate	800	38	101
Oreo Cookie	810	43	92
Strawberry	780	38	95
Vanilla	700	38	76

For Complete Nutritional Data ~ see CalorieKing.com

Jack's® (Oct '12)

Sandwiches:	C	F	Cb
Big Bacon Burger	610	41	31
Big Jack Burger	530	33	35
Cheeseburger	380	21	31
Chicken Fillet Sandwich	490	24	40
Double Big Jack Cheese Burger	850	59	35
Double Cheeseburger	540	33	31
Grilled Chicken Sandwich	380	16	32
Hamburger	340	18	31
Chicken, Chicken Fingers, 3 pieces	300	14	14
Fries, regular	310	13	42
Breakfast: Egg & Cheese Biscuit	360	21	31
Sausage, Egg & Cheese Biscuit	520	35	32
Steak Biscuit	480	28	43

For Complete Menu & Data ~ see CalorieKing.com

Fast - Foods & *Restaurants*

Jamba Juice® (Oct '12)

	C	F	Cb
All Fruit: *Original Size, 22 fl.oz*			
Mega Mango	340	0.5	85
Peach Perfection; Strawberry Whirl	300	0.5	75
Pomegranate Paradise	340	0.5	85
Classics: *Per 16 fl.oz*			
Banana Berry	290	1	68
Mango-a-go-go	28	1	65
Peach Pleasure; Pomeg. Pick-Me-Up	260	1	61
Strawberry Surf Rider	300	1	72
Creamy Treats: *Per 16 fl oz*			
Chocolate Moo'd	430	4	86
Orange Dream Machine	350	1	76
Peanut Butter Moo'd	480	10	83
Fruit & Veggie Smoothies: *Per 16 fl.oz*			
Apple & Greens; Berry upBEET, av.	225	1	50
Orange Carrot Karma	180	0.5	43
Jamba Light: *Per 16 fl oz*			
Berry Fulfilling	140	0.5	29
Mango Mantra; Strawb. Nirvana, av.	155	0	33
Pre Boosted Smoothies: *Per 16 fl.oz*			
Acai Super-Antioxidant	260	4	54
Protein Berry Workout	290	0	54
The Coldbuster	250	1	59
Probiotic Fruit & Yogurt Blends,			
average all flavors, 16 fl.oz	240	0	49
Fresh Squeezed Juices: *Per 12 fl.oz*			
Carrot	100	0.5	22
Orange	170	0.5	39
Shots: *Single*			
Matcha Energy Shot-Soymilk, 4 fl.oz	70	0	15
Wheatgrass Detox, 1 fl oz	5	0	1
Breakfast:			
Hot Oatmeal: *With Fruit & Brown Sugar*			
Berry Cherry with Pecan	500	15	87
Fruit flavors, average	385	4.5	81
Plain, brown sugar only	260	4.5	52
California Flat Bread: *Per Flatbread*			
Four Cheesy, 5.75 oz	420	16	46
MediterraneaYum, 6 oz	320	8	49
Smokehouse Chicken, 6 oz	390	10	53
Baked Goods: *Per Item*			
Apple Cinnamon Pretzel, 5 oz	380	4	76
Berry Agave Bar, 3 oz	220	12	26
Blueberry Streusel Muffin	400	19	45
Cheddar Onion Bread, 3 oz	240	8	34
Sourdough Parmesan Pretzel, 5 oz	410	10	67
Parfaits: *Per 16 oz*			
Acai/Mango Peach Toppers, average	480	9	94
Chunky Strawberry	570	17	93

Jersey Mike's Subs® (Oct '12)

	C	F	Cb
Cold Subs: *Per Regular, on Wheat,*			
w/out Vinegar, Oil or Mayo Unless Indicated			
#1 BLT	570	26	64
#2 Jersey Shore Favorite	560	18	67
#3 American Classic	560	18	65
#5 Super Sub	580	19	67
#6 Roast Beef & Provolone	720	25	64
#7 Turkey Breast & Provolone	540	16	65
#8 Club Sub with Mayonnaise	890	52	67
#9 Club Supreme w/ Mayonnaise	940	52	66
#10 Albacore Tuna	910	59	66
#13 Original Italian	680	27	66
#14 Veggie	720	33	65
Hot Subs/Cheese Steaks: *Per Regular on Wheat Roll*			
#15 Meatball & Cheese	890	52	72
#17: Chicken Philly	630	25	65
Steak Philly	620	24	64
#43: Chipotle Chicken	910	56	68
Chipotle Steak	900	55	66
#18 Chicken Parmesan	650	22	77
#19 BBQ Beef	710	16	83
#20 Pastrami & Swiss	580	18	60
#56: Big Kahuna Steak	670	28	65
Big Kahuna Chicken	680	29	66
Cold Wraps: *With Flour Tortilla, w/o Vin./Oil or Mayo*			
#1 BLT	590	29	60
#2 Jersey Shore Favorite	580	22	64
#3 American Classic	580	22	63
#5 Super Sub	600	22	65
Salads: *Without Dressing*			
Chef, 16 oz	240	10	12
Grilled Chicken Caesar, 12.5 oz	510	35	11
Tossed, 12 oz	50	0.5	11
Tuna, 18 oz	690	60	15
Dressings: *Per 2 Tbsp, 1 oz*			
Caesar	150	15	2
Chipotle Mayo	180	20	0
Golden Italian	110	11	3
Ranch	120	12	2
Russian	160	16	4
Desserts: Cookie, Choc Chip, 1.5 oz	200	11	24
Chocolate Brownie, 1.5 oz	170	7	23
Drinks: Mountain Dew, 22 oz	310	0	84
Mug Root Beer, 22 oz	290	0	79
Tropicana Twister Orange, 22 oz	360	0	96

Updated Nutrition Data ~ www.CalorieKing.com
Persons with Diabetes ~ See Disclaimer (Page 22)

Fast - Foods & Restaurants

Jimmy John's® (Oct '12)

Subs: (8")

Figures Based on French Bread w/ Standard Toppings & Mayo, Unless Indicated

	C	F	Cb
#1 Pepe	615	31	50
#2 Big John	535	24	49
#3 Totally Tuna without dressing	690	31	55
#4 Turkey Tom	515	22	50
#5 Vito with Italian Vinaigrette	600	28	52
#6 Vegetarian	580	30	53
JJBLT	635	35	49

Giant Club Sandwiches: *Figures Based on French Bread w/ Standard Toppings & Mayo, Unless Indicated*

	C	F	Cb
#7 Gourmet Smoked Ham	775	32	69
#8 Billy Club	795	34	68
#9 Italian Night w/ Mayo & Vinaig.	950	51	70
#10 Hunter's Club	805	35	67
#11 Country Club	765	31	69
#12 Beach Club	730	31	71
#13 Gourmet Veggie	775	38	71
#14 Bootlegger	685	25	67
#15 Club Tuna without dressing	885	39	73
#16 Club Lulu	755	33	67
#17 Ultimate Porker, with 9-grain wheat bread	735	39	62

Plain Slims: *Figures Based on French Bread without Toppings, Dressing or Mayo*

	C	F	Cb
Slim 1 Ham & Cheese	505	10	66
Slim 2 Roast Beef	425	3	64
Slim 3 Tuna Salad	765	31	69
Slim 4 Turkey Breast	400	0.5	65
Slim 5 Salami Capicola & Cheese	600	20	66
Slim 6 Double Provolone	545	16	65

Low Carb Options: *With Standard Toppings & Mayo, without Bread*

	C	F	Cb
Hunter's Club Unwich	470	35	4
The JJ Gargantuan Unwich	740	54	7

Low-Fat Options: *With French Bread Only*

	C	F	Cb
#4 Turkey Tom	305	0.5	48
Slim 4, Turkey Breast	400	0.5	65

Sides:

	C	F	Cb
Jimmy Chips: BBQ, 1 oz	160	9	17
Jalapeno, 1 oz	150	7	18
Regular, 1 oz	160	8	18
Sea Salt & Vinegar, 1 oz	140	8	16
Thinny, 1 oz	130	5	19
Pickle: Spear	5	0	1
Whole	20	0	4

Johnny Rockets® (Oct '12)

Original Hamburgers:

	C	F	Cb
Hamburger #12	960	62	60
Original Burger	870	55	57
Rocket: Single	940	61	56
Double	1410	98	57
Route 66	990	68	51
Smoke House: Single	1140	71	70
Double	1700	115	70
Streamliner	430	11	59
Chicken Tenders, without Sauce	880	56	42

Hot Dogs: *Without Sides or Condiments*

	C	F	Cb
Regular	410	2	34
Chili Cheese Dog	770	50	42

Rocket Melts: *Without Sides*

	C	F	Cb
Patty Melt	870	53	52
Tuna Melt, on Sourdough	790	48	43

Sandwiches: Chicken Club

	C	F	Cb
Chicken Club	750	28	71
Grilled Chicken	590	26	53
Philly Cheese Steak, w/ Swiss Chse	820	42	56
Tuna Salad, on Wheat Bread	770	49	50

Extras: Bacon, 2 slices

	C	F	Cb
Bacon, 2 slices	90	7	0
Chili, 2 oz	120	10	4
Cheese: American, 0.67 oz	70	6	1
Cheddar; Pepperjack, 0.7 oz	90	7	0
Swiss, 1 oz	110	8	2
Grilled Mushrooms, 2.5 oz	70	6	2
Grilled Onions, 1 oz	20	0.5	3

Starters:

	C	F	Cb
Chili Bowl, 9 oz	610	48	16
Fries: American Fries, 7 oz	480	19	69
Cheese Fries, 12 oz	740	38	82
Chili Cheese Fries, 14 oz	1000	57	93
Onion Rings, 9 oz	880	40	90
Rocket Wings, Traditional, 9 oz	660	49	19

Desserts: Apple Pie

	C	F	Cb
Apple Pie	610	73	33
Super Sundae w/ Hot Fudge, 11 oz	670	37	79

Beverages:

	C	F	Cb
Coke, 21 oz	240	0	67
Fanta Orange, 21 oz	270	0	80
Iced Tea, 21 oz	0	0	0
Minute Made Lemonade, 23 oz	240	0	65

Deluxe Shakes:

	C	F	Cb
Chocolate Vanilla Twist	910	50	102
Oreo Cookies & Cream	1040	61	110
Strawberry Banana	890	50	100

209

KFC® (Oct '12)

Chicken Pieces:	C	F	Cb
Original Recipe:			
Breast, 1 piece, 5.75 oz	360	21	11
Drumstick, 1 piece, 1.75 oz	120	7	3
Thigh, 1 piece, 3.4 oz	250	17	7
Whole Wing, 1 piece, 2 oz	120	7	3
Grilled:			
Breast, 4.25 oz	220	7	0
Drumstick, 1.5 oz	90	4	0
Thigh, 2.5 oz	170	10	0
Whole Wing, 1.25 oz	80	4.5	1
Spicy Crispy:			
Breast, 1 piece, 6.25 oz	420	25	12
Drumstick, 1 piece, 2 oz	160	10	5
Thigh, 1 piece, 4 oz	360	27	13
Whole Wing, 1 piece, 1.75 oz	170	12	6
Popcorn Chicken: Kids, 2.85 oz	260	17	12
Individual, 4.3 oz	400	26	18
Large, 6.15 oz	560	37	26
Strips & Filets:			
Crispy: 2 Strips, 4 oz	260	14	11
3 Strips, 6 oz	390	21	17
Original Filet 3.5 oz	200	9	8
Wings: Without Dipping Sauce			
Fiery Buffalo, Hot	70	4	5
Honey BBQ, Hot	80	4	8
Hot	70	4	4
Dipping Sauces: Per 0.9 oz Container			
Bacon/Creamy Ranch	140	15	1
Creamy Buffalo	70	7	2
Honey BBQ	40	0	9
Honey Mustard	120	10	6
KFC Signature Sauce	70	5	5
Orange Ginger	50	0	11
Spicy Chipotle	70	3.5	8
Sweet & Sour	45	0	12
KFC Famous Bowls & Pot Pie:			
Bowls: Snack Size, 6.5 oz	260	13	26
Mashed Potato, with Gravy, 18.5 oz	680	31	74
Chicken Pot Pie, 14 oz	790	45	66

KFC® cont... (Oct '12)

Sandwiches: With Sauce	C	F	Cb
Chicken Littles	320	19	24
Crispy Twister	610	33	52
Double Down, Original Filet	610	37	18
Doublicious, Original Filet	520	25	40
Honey BBQ	320	3.5	47
Value Boxes:			
Drumsticks: Original	400	22	37
Extra Crispy	440	25	39
Grilled	380	19	34
Popcorn Chicken	680	41	53
Thighs: Original	540	32	42
Extra Crispy	630	39	45
Grilled	460	25	34
Wings: Fiery Buffalo	510	28	51
BBQ	540	28	58
Hot	490	27	45
Salads: Without Dressing or Croutons			
Caesar, Side	40	2	2
Crispy Chicken BLT	360	19	18
Crispy Chicken Caesar	340	18	16
House Side Salad	15	0	3
Dressings & Add-Ins:			
Creamy Parmesan Caesar, 2 oz	260	26	4
Light Italian, 1 oz	15	0.5	2
Original Ranch Fat Free, 1.5 oz	35	0	8
Croutons, Parm. Garlic, 1 pouch	70	3	8
Sides: Per Single Portion			
BBQ Baked Beans, 4.5oz	210	1.5	41
Biscuit, 2 oz	180	8	23
Cole Slaw, 4.2 oz	180	10	20
Corn on the Cob (3"), 2.5 oz	70	0.5	16
Cornbread Muffin, 2 oz	210	9	28
Macaroni & Cheese, 4.75 oz	160	7	19
Mashed Potatoes, with Gravy, 5 oz	120	4	19
Potato Wedges, 3.8 oz	290	15	35
Desserts:			
Lil' Buckets Parfait Cups:			
Chocolate Creme, 4 oz	280	13	37
Lemon Creme, 4.5 oz	400	13	65

Updated Nutrition Data ~ www.CalorieKing.com
Persons with Diabetes ~ See Disclaimer (Page 22)

Krispy Kreme® (Oct '12)

Doughnuts:	C	F	Cb
Apple Fritter	710	14	18
Caramel Kreme Crunch	390	20	50
Chocolate Iced Glazed Cruller	260	12	38
Chocolate Iced Cake	280	15	34
Chocolate Iced Custard Filled	310	17	36
Chocolate Iced Glazed	240	11	33
Chocolate Iced, Kreme Filled	360	21	40
Chocolate Iced Glazed w/ Sprinkles	270	11	41
Cinnamon Apple Filled	290	16	33
Cinnamon Bun	260	16	28
Cinnamon Twist	240	15	23
Dulce de Leche	300	18	31
Glazed: Chocolate Cake	300	15	41
Cinnamon	200	11	25
Cruller	220	12	27
Kreme Filled	340	20	38
Lemon Filled	290	16	35
Maple Iced	230	11	32
Original	190	11	21
Raspberry Filled	290	16	36
Sour Cream	310	14	43
Powdered: Cake	220	11	27
Strawberry Filled	290	16	33
Sugar	190	11	20
Traditional Cake	190	12	19
Doughnut Holes: Orig. Glazed (4)	200	11	26
Glazed Cake, Regular/Choc. (4)	200	10	26

Kool Kreme:

Doughnut Shakes: Per 12 oz			
Original Glazed	600	26	80
Chocolate Cake	650	30	86
Raspberry Filled	630	26	87
Doughnut Sundaes:			
Orig. Glazed	460	17	69
Chocolate Cake	560	21	89
Strawberry Cake	560	20	90

Chiller Beverages: Without Whipped Cream Topping
Orange You Glad; Very Berry, average:

12 fl.oz	175	0	43
20 fl.oz	295	0	71

Kremey Chillers: Includes Whipped Cream Topping

Orange & Kreme: 12 fl.oz	630	28	92
20 fl.oz	970	40	150
Choc./Mocha: 12 fl.oz	670	29	105
20 fl.oz	1050	41	171

For Complete Menu & Data ~ see CalorieKing.com

Krystal® (Oct '12)

Burgers:	C	F	Cb
Big Angus: Original	550	35	48
Dble, w/ Bacon & Cheese	850	59	48
Krystal:			
Original:			
Double	290	13	33
Bacon Cheese	200	11	20
Chik	300	16	27
Double Cheese	350	17	34
Pups: Chili Cheese	230	14	16
Corn	240	14	22
Plain	150	8	15
Fries:			
Chili Cheese, 8.25 oz	570	29	62
French, medium, 4.25 oz	310	13	46
Sides:			
Chik'n Bites, small, 3 oz	200	7	20
Salad, Crispy Chicken, 11 oz	370	21	20
Breakfast Items:			
Biscuits:			
Bacon, Egg & Cheese	440	24	34
Chik	400	18	43
Gravy	350	18	41
Plain	260	13	32
Sausage	420	28	32
Sandwich, Krystal Sunriser	200	11	16
Scramblers:			
Original: With Bacon	330	16	27
With Sausage	420	26	27
4-Carb Scrambler,			
With Sausage	620	52	3
Desserts:			
Apple Turnover, fried	220	8	34
Lemon Icebox Pie	320	9	56
Drinks: Per 16 fl.oz, with ¼ ice			
Coca-Cola,			
Classic	120	0	32
Diet Coke	0	0	0

For Complete Menu & Data ~ see CalorieKing.com

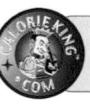

For Menu Updates,
Check Author's Website
www.CalorieKing.com

LaRosa's Pizzeria® (Oct '12)

Pizzas:

Focaccia Style: *Per Slice, 1/10 of Medium Pizza*

	C	F	Cb
Florentine	240	13	24
Roma	300	18	23

Hand Tossed: *Per Slice, 1/8 of Medium Pizza*

Cheese	230	8	29
Double Pepperoni	300	14	29
Big 4 Meat	325	15	29
Big 4 Pick 4	280	11	30
Big 4 Veggie	240	7	30

Multigrain Wheat: *Per 1/12 of 12" Pizza*

Pepperoni-Sausage	190	11	14
Other varieties, average	125	5	15

Pan Crust: *Per Slice, 1/8 of Medium Pizza*

Cheese	300	16	30
Double Pepperoni	370	22	30
Big 4 Meat	325	15	29
Big 4 Pick 4	275	11	30
Big 4 Veggie	235	7	30

Traditional Crust: *Per Slice, 1/8 of Medium Pizza*

Cheese	200	10	19
Double Pepperoni	280	16	20
Big 4 Meat	285	16	20
Big 4 Pick 4	240	12	20
Big 4 Veggie	200	8	21

Calzones: *Per Calzone, No Dipping Sauce*

3 Meat & 3 Cheese	1080	55	102
3 Veggie & 3 Cheese	860	34	105
Cheese & Pepperoni	960	45	101
Cheese	840	34	101
Philly Cheesesteak	870	39	90
Sausage Pelucci	1040	52	92

Pasta Dinner: *Without Bread, Soup or Salad*

Cheese Ravioli	660	26	80
Lasagna, with Meat Sauce	735	38	61
Spaghetti: With Alfredo Sauce	975	50	104
With Meatballs	870	28	119
With Meat Sauce	700	18	104
With Traditional Sauce	640	12	113
Ziti Chicken Alfredo	980	42	102
Ziti Sausage Pelucci	765	20	115

Appetizers: *Per Serve, Without Dipping Sauce*

Boneless Wings: BBQ, 1 piece, 1 oz	60	2.5	6
Hot, 1 piece, 1 oz	60	3.5	4
Chicken Tenders, 7.6 oz	480	22	40
Four Taste Sampler, 6.63 oz	475	26	48
Fries: French, 10 oz	440	13	71
Garlic, 11 oz	630	34	74
Onion Twists, regular, 10 oz	910	57	91

For Complete Nutritional Data ~ see CalorieKing.com

La Salsa Fresh Mexican® (Oct '12)

Appetizers:

	C	F	Cb
Salsa & Chips: Regular, 14.5 oz	700	32	87
With Guacamole, 14.5 oz	970	55	103
Chips (15), 1.4 oz	200	10	25

Nachos:

Black Beans: With Carnitas	1570	83	141
With Chicken	1600	83	148
With Steak	1580	84	142
Pinto Beans: With Carnitas	1560	83	139
With Chicken	1590	83	146
With Steak	1565	84	139

Burritos:

Black Beans: With Cheese	1100	48	132
With Carnitas	1205	51	132
With Chicken	1240	52	139
With California Steak	815	35	89
Pinto Beans: With Cheese	1070	48	115
With Chicken	1200	52	122
With Steak	1175	54	115
Baja Fish Burrito	875	53	58

Overstuffed Grilled Burrito:

With Carnitas	1200	59	108
With Chicken	1260	59	110
With Steak	1290	66	109

Grande, Black Beans:

With Carnitas	810	34	91
With Chicken	810	33	93
With Steak	820	35	91

Tacos: Baja Fish

Baja Fish	395	22	29
Baja Shrimp	320	19	30
Guadalajara Carnitas	320	15	30
Mexico City, Chicken	190	3	27

Quesadillas: *Without Chips*

Classic: Carnitas

Carnitas	960	58	57
Chicken	955	57	58
Steak	965	59	57
Grande, Pinto Beans: W/ Carnitas	1135	61	89
With Chicken	1130	61	91
With Steak	1130	62	90
Chips	200	10	25

Favorites: *Without Chips*

Stuffed Fajita Quesadilla:

With Carnitas	855	51	53
With Chicken	865	52	56
With Shrimp	800	49	54
With Steak	885	55	53

Fire Roasted Bowls:

Black Beans: W/ Chicken	730	32	74
With Steak	735	34	73
Without Meat	630	29	71
Pinto Beans: W/ Chicken	730	32	73
With Steak	720	34	70
Without Meat	620	29	69

Little Caesars® (Oct '12)

14" Pizza: Per Slice, ⅛ Pizza

	C	F	Cb
Original Crust. 3 Meat Treat	340	17	32
Hula Hawaiian: W/ Ham	280	9	35
W/ Canadian Bacon	280	9	35
Ultimate Supreme	310	13	33
Veggie	270	10	32
Deep Dish: Just Cheese	320	13	38
Pepperoni	360	16	38
Hot-N-Ready:			
Just Cheese	250	9	32
Pepperoni	280	11	32
Baby Pan! Pan!:			
Cheese & Pepperoni, 1 pan	360	18	33
Caesar Wings: Per Wing			
BBQ: Regular	80	5	3
Spicy	70	5	1
Buffalo, Mild or Hot	70	5	0
Garlic Parmesan	90	7	1
Lemon Pepper	90	8	0
Oven Roasted	70	5	0
Caesar Dips: Per 1 oz Container Unless Indicated			
BBQ; Buffalo Ranch	160	17	2
Buffalo	100	10	2
Buttery Garlic, ½ oz	130	14	0
Cheezy Jalapeno	140	15	2
Ranch	170	18	2
Bread: Per Piece			
Crazy Bread, 1 stick	100	3	15
Crazy Sauce, 4 oz	45	0	10
Italian Cheese Bread	130	6	13
Pepperoni Cheese Bread	150	8	13

Lone Star Steakhouse® (Oct '12)

Appetizers: Per Serving

	C	F	Cb
Chicken Tenders: Original, 3.5 oz	320	19	27
Buffalo Style, 3.5 oz	300	19	23
Lone Star Wings, mild, 3.5 oz	305	20	5
Spin. & Artichoke Dip, 3.5 oz	160	13	4.5
Texas Rose, 3.5 oz	285	19	25

Meals: Without Sides, Toppings & Sauce

Mesquite Grilled Steaks:

Chopped Steak, 9.6 oz	710	52	0
Five Star Filet, 6 oz	335	18	2
NY Strip, 9.6 oz	525	28	0
Texas Ribeye, 12.5 oz	710	40	5.5

Lone Star® cont... (Oct '12)

Meals (Cont): Without Sides, Toppings & Sauce

Ribs Combo:	F	F	Cb
Baby Back Ribs:			
With Chicken, 10.45 oz	740	30	46
With Sirloin, 10.2 oz	655	33	7.5
Grilled Pork Chops: 3.5 oz	190	10	0
5.9 oz	315	16	0
Seafood:			
Fried Shrimp Entree, 11.65 oz	865	40	97
Grilled Shrimp: 3.5 oz	60	2	5.5
11 oz	190	7	17
Lobster Tail, 3.5 oz	150	1	14
Lobster & Lobster, 3.95 oz	165	1	15
Sweet Bourbon Salmon: 6oz	240	11	0
9 oz	360	16	0
Burgers:			
Bubba, 15.65 oz	1085	57	67
Bacon Bleu, 13.45 oz	820	37	51
Cheeseburger, 14 oz	895	45	50
Lonestar, 12.15 oz	640	27	48
Swiss & Mushroom, 15.2 oz	845	38	53
Chili, 10 oz bowl	345	18	14
Salads: Per Serving, Includes Dressing			
Dinner, Caesar, 6.25 oz	145	11	8
Grilled Chicken Caesar	480	24	19
Lettuce Wedge	395	34	10
Steakhouse	710	53	2
Sides: Per Serving			
Garlic Mashed Potatoes, ½ cup	130	5	19
Macaroni & Cheese: 3.5 oz	80	4	8
8 oz	185	9	18
Steak Fries, 8 oz	610	26	86
Texas Rice, 8 oz	100	3.5	14

Long John Silver's® (Oct '12)

	C	F	Cb
Sandwiches: Includes Toppings and Condiments			
Alaskan Pollock: Regular, 6.25 oz	470	23	49
Ultimate, 7 oz	530	27	50
Seafood:			
Battered Fish, 1 piece, 3.25 oz	260	16	17
Battered Shrimp, 3 pieces, 1.5 oz	130	9	8
Breaded Clam Strips, 3 oz	320	19	29
Buttered Lobster Bites, snack box, 3.25 oz	230	9	24

Continued Next Page....

213

Long John's® cont... (Oct '12)

Seafood (Cont):

	C	F	Cb
Langostino Lobster, Stuffed Crab Cake, 2.25 oz	170	9	16
Popcorn Shrimp, 1 snack box, 3 oz	270	16	23
Shrimp Scampi, 8 pieces	200	13	3
Chicken, Chicken Strip, 1 piece	140	8	9

Freshside Grille: Per Entree Plate, w/ Rice & Veggies

Salmon, 2 filets	280	7	27
Shrimp Scampi	330	15	29
Tilapia, 1 filet	250	4.5	27

Sauces & Condiments:

Dipping Sauces: *Per 1 oz*

Cocktail	25	0	6
Tartar	100	9	4
Louisiana Hot Sauce, 1 tsp	0	0	0
Ketchup, 1 packet, ¼ oz	10	0	2
Malt Vinegar, ½ oz	0	0	0

Sides:

Breaded Mozzarella Sticks (3)	150	9	13
Broccoli Cheese Soup, 1 bowl, 7.5 oz	220	18	8
Cole Slaw, 4 oz	200	15	15
Corn Cobbette w. Butter Oil, 3.5 oz	150	10	14
Crumblies, 1 oz	170	12	14
Fries: Platter Portion, 3 oz	230	10	34
Combo Portion, 4 oz	310	14	45
Hushpuppy, 1 pup, 0.8 oz	60	2.5	9
Jalapeno Cheddar Bites (5)	240	14	23
Rice, 5 oz	180	1	37
Vegetable Medley, 4 oz	50	2	8

For Complete Menu & Data ~ see CalorieKing.com

Macaroni Grill® (Oct '12)

	C	F	Cb

Tapas & Antipasti: Per Whole Appetizer as Served

Calamari Fritti	850	51	58
Goat Chse Peppadew Peppers	360	18	42
Lobster Stuffed Clams	260	20	7
Mac & Chse Bites w/ Dip	990	78	45
Parmesan Fries	790	57	61

Meals: Per Whole Entree, as Served

Classics: Carmela's Chkn	930	31	111
Eggplant Parmesan	950	56	76
Fettuccine Alfredo, Chicken	1470	88	94
Lasagna Bolognese	720	38	46
Mama's Trio	1510	98	96
Mom's: Ricotta Meatballs & Spaghetti Bolognese	1190	70	95
M'balls & Spag. Pomodoro	960	55	91
Penne Rustica	1160	49	110

Macaroni Grill® cont... (Oct '12)

Meals (Cont): Per Whole Entree

	C	F	Cb

Fresh Pasta: Carbonara

Carbonara	1260	68	101
Eggplant Quadratini	910	33	115
Lobster Ravioli	710	41	39
Pasta Di Mare	1310	57	100
Whole Wheat Fettuccine	1060	46	105

Principale: Per Whole Entree, as Served

Chianti BBQ Steak	1920	121	81
Chicken: Marsala	810	35	61
Scallopine	1180	81	55
Under a Brick	1440	115	24
Grilled King Salmon	1110	68	71
Pan-Roasted Pork Chops	1370	91	58
Parmesan-Crusted Sole	1550	104	99
Pollo Caprese	560	22	31
Spiedini: Grilled Chicken	410	11	38
Grilled Shrimp	380	9	41
Ravioli: Lobster	710	41	39
Mushroom	900	62	52

Pizzas & Flatbreads: Per Whole Meal, as Served

Flatbread:

Mushr. & Goat Cheese	910	46	83
Roasted Chicken & Arugula	1060	50	83

Pizza:

Italian Sausage	1100	52	100
Margherita	840	31	101
Primo Pepperoni	980	41	97

Salads: Includes Dressing

Bibb & Blue	680	56	23
Caprese	480	40	10
Market Chop	1010	71	33
Salad Sampler	1030	80	36
Warm Spinach	340	25	17

Soups: Per 8 oz Bowl

Pomodorina	190	12	16

Dolce: Per Serving

Gelato: Dark Chocolate	260	12	36
Double Vanilla	290	12	40
Homemade Chocolate Cake	990	56	114
Lemon Passion	580	33	65
New York Style Cheesecake	760	52	61
Sorbet White Peach	160	0	39
Tiramisu	690	48	54
Warm Berry Torta	640	34	77

For Complete Nutritional Data ~ see CalorieKing.com

Updated Nutrition Data ~ www.CalorieKing.com
Persons with Diabetes ~ See Disclaimer (Page 22)

Manhattan Bagel® (Oct '12)
Ragels: Per Ragel

	C	F	Cb
Blueberry, 3.75 oz	300	1	65
Chocolate Chip, 3.75 oz	290	2.5	58
Cinnamon Raisin, 4 oz	330	1	70
Egg; Jalapeno Cheddar, av., 4 oz	320	2	67
Everything, 4.25 oz	350	3	68
Poppy, 4.25 oz	360	5	69
Pumpernickel, 3.5 oz	240	1.5	53
Salt, 4.25 oz	320	1	68
Sesame Seed, 4.5 oz	360	5	68
Cream Cheese: Plain, 1.25 oz	120	11	3
Plain, Reduced-Fat, 1.25 oz	110	9	4

For Complete Nutritional Data ~ see CalorieKing.com

Marie Callender's® (Oct '12)
Appetizers: Per Complete Dish as Served

	C	F	Cb
Crispy Chicken Tenders	940	59	64
Crispy Green Beans	810	52	75
Mozzarella Sticks	690	42	53
Burgers and Sandwiches: With Fries			
Original Burger	1200	77	84
Albacore Tuna Melt	1430	92	99
Grilled Ham Stack	1260	81	96
Roasted Turkey Croissant Club	1450	97	95
Main Meals: Per Complete Meal as Served			
Comfort Classics:			
Artichoke & Mushroom Chicken	1070	74	38
Callender's Fish & Chips	1280	92	85
From The Grill: Gr. Rosemary Chkn	900	49	43
Gr. Atlantic Salmon, Cajun style	630	39	25
St. Louis BBQ Ribs, Full Rack	1260	82	58
Pasta Perfecto: Includes Garlic Bread			
Chicken & Broccoli Fettuccini	1540	87	119
Double Shrimp Pasta	1500	96	97
Pies, Chicken Pot Pie, w/out sides	1140	79	68
Fresh Crisp Salads: Includes Dressing			
Chinese Chicken	910	33	107
Gorgonzola, Pecan & Field Greens	990	54	79
Traditional Caesar	490	35	28
Sides: Cornbread, 1 serving, 3 oz	340	21	33
French Fries, 4 oz	380	20	45
Honey Butter, 1 oz	170	16	8
Loaded Mashed Potatoes, 6.15 oz	340	23	23
Macaroni & Cheese, 6.35 oz	230	9	26
Soups: Per Bowl			
Chicken Noodle	130	0.5	22
Clam Chowder	270	13	22
Hearty Vegetable	90	3	13
Split Pea & Ham	220	13	17

Marie Callender's® cont... (Oct '12)
Breakfast: As Served

	C	F	Cb
Griddle Greats:			
Belgian Waffles	600	19	99
Buttermilk Pancake Stack	720	30	99
Old Fashioned French Toast	830	31	123
Hashers: Country	1320	82	90
Tex-Mex	1180	71	99
Homestyle Classics:			
Country Fried Steak & Eggs	1680	74	186
Grilled Ham & Eggs	1170	47	146
Marie's Magnificent Six:			
With Bacon	750	36	80
With Sausage	910	52	81
Omelettes: BTA	1610	84	160
Denver	1380	65	149
Spanish	1550	78	165
Quiche: Bacon, 1 slice	990	79	45
Ham, 1 slice	1030	83	39
Desserts: Per Slice Unless Indicated			
Pies: Apple	570	31	70
Banana Cream, with Meringue	510	24	66
Chocolate Cream, with Meringue	570	26	77
Pumpkin, with Whipped Cream	530	23	70
Razzleberry	660	39	71

Breakfast & Other Menu Items ~ see CalorieKing.com

Max & Erma's® (Oct '12)
Appetizers:

	C	F	Cb
Black Bean Roll-Ups w/out drssng	560	13	92
Wing: Buffalo (6)	1340	128	9
Sweet Chili (6)	650	32	72
Specialties: As Served			
Crispy Chicken Tender Dinner	1410	81	126
Ribs: Half Rack	1320	76	88
Full Rack	2200	124	132
Salads: Entrée Size, w/ Dressing, w/out Breadstick			
Apple Pecan, with Chicken	1060	59	87
Caesar: Without Chicken	670	57	24
With Chicken	880	67	28
Sides: Onion rings	280	17	28
Herb Rice	250	1.5	51
Sweet And Treats:			
Banana Cream Pie	990	61	107
Triple Choc. Cake, with Ice Cream	1270	65	157

Fast - Foods & *Restaurants*

McAlister's Deli® (Oct '12)

Sandwiches: Per Whole Sandwich

	C	F	Cb
Classic: Grilled Chicken	680	37	46
Harvest Chicken Salad	760	53	51
Italian Submarine	750	34	58
Tuna Salad	540	27	45
Veggie Pita	620	41	48
Club: Black Angus	810	40	68
Grilled Chicken	790	34	73
McAlister	770	34	72
Grilled Sandwiches:			
Four Cheese Griller	850	48	63
Smoky Pepper Jack Turkey	670	34	53
Spicy Southwest Chicken	930	47	75
Sweet Chipotle Chicken	640	19	75
Hot Sandwiches:			
California Turkey Reuben	760	39	69
French Dip	600	22	54
Ham Melt	610	25	52
Reuben	780	41	62
Roast Beef Melt	590	24	49
The Big Nasty	790	24	82
The New Yorker	550	21	49
Spuds: *Per Whole Spud*			
Bacon Angus Roast Beef	910	26	124
Cheese	710	18	118
Grilled Chicken	760	12	119
Max	940	33	120
Soups: *Per Bowl*			
Asiago Cheese Bisque	440	30	32
Cheddar Potato	400	26	32
Chicken Noodle	200	6	26
Clam Chowder	380	22	37
Traditional Chili	540	36	48

McDonald's® (Oct '12)

Burgers/Sandwiches:

	C	F	Cb
Angus: Bacon & Cheese	790	39	63
Deluxe	750	39	61
Mushroom & Swiss	770	40	59
Big Mac	550	29	46
Cheeseburger	300	12	33
Double Cheeseburger	440	23	34
Hamburger	250	9	31
McDouble	390	19	33
Quarter Pounder: With Cheese	520	26	42
Double with Cheese	750	42	42
Filet-O-Fish	380	18	39
McChicken	360	16	40
McRib	500	26	44
Southern Style Crispy Chicken	420	19	43

McDonald's® cont... (Oct '12)

Premium Chicken Sandwiches:

	C	F	Cb
Classic: Crispy Chicken	510	22	56
Grilled Chicken	350	9	42
Club: Crispy Chicken	620	29	57
Grilled Chicken	460	16	43
Snack Wraps:			
Angus: Bacon & Cheese	390	21	28
Deluxe	410	25	27
Mushroom & Swiss	430	26	27
Crispy: Chipotle BBQ	330	15	34
Honey Mustard	330	15	33
Ranch	350	19	31
Grilled: Chipotle BBQ	250	8	27
Honey Mustard	250	8	27
Ranch	270	12	25
Mac	330	19	26
Chicken:			
McBites: Snack Size	270	17	18
Regular	410	25	27
Shareable	910	55	61
McNuggets: 4 pieces	190	12	12
6 pieces	280	18	18
10 pieces	470	30	30
Strips: 3 pieces	380	23	21
5 pieces	640	38	36
French Fries:			
Kids, 1.1 oz	100	5	13
Small, 2.5 oz	230	11	29
Medium, 4 oz	380	19	48
Large, 5.5 oz	500	25	63
Sauces:			
BBQ/Mustard/Sweet 'N Sour, 1 oz	50	0	12
Chipotle BBQ, 1 oz	50	0	11
Creamy Ranch, 0.8 oz	110	12	1
Honey, 1 pkt, 1/2 oz	50	0	12
Ketchup, 1 pkt, 0.35 oz	15	0	3
Spicy Buffalo, 0.8 oz	35	3	1
Tangy BBQ, 1 pkt, 1 oz	50	0	12
Breakfast:			
Big Breakfast: With Regular Biscuit	740	48	51
With Hotcakes	1090	56	111
Biscuits:			
Bacon Egg & Cheese: Regular	420	23	37
With Large Biscuit	480	27	43
Sausage with Egg: Regular	510	33	36
With Large Biscuit	570	37	43
Southern Style Chicken:			
Regular	410	20	41
W/ Large Biscuit	470	24	46

Continued Next Page...

McDonald's® cont... (Oct '12)

Breakfast (Cont):

	C	F	Cb
Cinnamon Melts, 4 oz	460	19	66
Fruit & Maple Oatmeal: Regular	290	4.5	57
Without Sugar	260	4.5	48
Hash Brown, (1), 2 oz	150	9	15
Hotcakes: Plain (3)	350	9	60
W/ Margarine (2 pats),w/o Syrup	430	18	60
W/ Margarine (2 pats), w/ Syrup (1)	610	18	105
McGriddles: Bacon, Egg & Cheese	420	18	44
Sausage	420	22	44
Sausage, Egg & Cheese	560	32	48
McMuffins: Egg	300	12	30
Sausage	370	22	29
Sausage with Egg	450	27	30
Sausage Burrito, 4 oz	300	16	26

Happy Meals:

	C	F	Cb
4 Chicken McNuggets:			
+ Fries + Apple Juice	390	17	48
+ Fries + 1% Low Fat Milk	390	20	37
+Apple Slices + Fat-Free Choc Milk	335	12	39
Hamburger:			
+Fries + Apple Juice	450	14	67
+Fries + 1% Low Fat Milk	450	17	56
+ Apple Slices + 1% Low-Fat Milk	365	12	47
Cheeseburger:			
+Fries + Apple Juice	500	17	69
+Fries + 1% Low-Fat Milk	500	20	58
+ Apple Slices & Fat-Free Choc Milk	445	12	60

Mighty Kids Meals:

	C	F	Cb
With 6 Chicken McNuggets:			
+Fries, 1.1 oz + Apple Juice	480	23	54
+ Apple Slices+ Fat-Free Choc Milk	425	18	45
With Double Cheeseburger:			
+Fries, 1.1 oz + Apple Juice	640	28	70
+ Apple Slices + 1% Low-Fat Milk	555	26	50

Premium Salads: Without Dressing

	C	F	Cb
Bacon Ranch: Without Chicken	140	7	10
With Crispy Chicken	390	22	24
With Grilled Chicken	230	9	10
Caesar: Without Chicken	90	4	9
With Crispy Chicken	350	18	24
With Grilled Chicken	190	5	10
Southwest: With Crispy Chicken	450	21	42
With Grilled Chicken	290	8	28

McDonald's® cont... (Oct '12)

Salad Dressings: Per Package

	C	F	Cb
Newman's Own: Crmy Caesar, 2 fl.oz	190	18	4
Ranch, 2 fl.oz	170	15	9
Low-Fat: Balsamic Vinaig., 1.5 fl.oz	35	2.5	3
Family Recipe Italian, 1.5 fl.oz	50	2.5	7

Desserts & Cookies:

	C	F	Cb
Baked Apple Pie, 2.7 oz	250	13	32
Cookies: Choc. Chip Cookie (1)	160	8	21
Oatmeal Raisin (1), 1 oz	150	6	22
Sugar Cookie (1), 1 oz	160	7	21
Ice Cream, Vanilla Reduced Fat,			
Cone, 3.7 oz	170	4.5	27
McFlurry: M&M Candies, 12 fl.oz	650	23	96
Oreo Cookies, 12 fl.oz cup	510	17	80
Sundaes:			
Hot Caramel, 6.4 oz	340	8	60
Hot Fudge, 6.3 oz	330	9	53
Strawberry, 6.3 oz	280	6	49

McCafe:

	C	F	Cb
Shakes: Chocolate; Strawberry, average:			
12 fl.oz cup	565	17	86
16 fl.oz cup	705	21	114
22 fl.oz cup	860	25	140
Vanilla: 12 fl.oz	530	17	84
16 fl.oz	670	20	107
22 fl.oz	820	24	133
Hot Coffees:			
Cappuccino:			
Whole Milk: Small, 12 fl oz	120	7	9
Medium, 16 fl oz	140	8	11
Large, 20 fl oz	180	10	13
Nonfat Milk: Small, 12 fl oz	60	0	9
Medium, 16 fl oz	80	0	11
Latte:			
Whole Milk: Small, 12 fl oz	150	8	11
Medium, 16 fl oz	180	10	13
Nonfat Milk: Small, 12 fl oz	90	0	13
Medium, 16 fl oz	110	0	15
Mocha:			
Whole Milk: Small, 12 fl oz	280	11	40
Medium, 16 fl oz	330	12	48
Nonfat Milk: Small, 12 fl oz	240	5	41
Medium, 16 fl oz	280	6	50
Iced Coffee: Regular or Flavors			
Premium Roast:			
Small, 16 fl.oz	140	5	22
Medium, 21 fl.oz	200	8	30
Large, 32 fl.oz	280	11	45
Caramel Mocha: With Whole Milk & Cream			
Small, 12 fl.oz	250	11	33
Medium, 16 fl.oz	290	12	39

Continued Next Page...

McDonald's® cont... (Oct '12)

	C	F	Cb
Iced Tea, Sweetened, 21 fl.oz	180	0	45
Milk: 1% Low-Fat, 8 fl.oz	100	2.5	12
Fat-Free Chocolate	130	0	23
Juice: Apple Juice, 6.8 fl.oz box	100	0	23
Orange Juice: Small, 12 fl.oz	150	0	30
Medium, 16 fl.oz	190	0	39
Large, 22 fl.oz	280	0	58
Sodas: Without Ice			
Coca-Cola or Sprite:			
Child, 12 fl.oz cup	110	0	29
Small, 16 fl.oz cup	150	0	40
Medium, 21 fl.oz cup	210	0	58
Large, 32 fl.oz cup	310	0	86
Diet Coke	0	0	0
Hi-C Orange Lavaburst:			
Child, 12 fl.oz cup	120	0	32
Small, 16 fl.oz cup	160	0	44
Medium, 21 fl.oz cup	240	0	64
Large, 32 fl.oz cup	350	0	94
Powerade, Mountain Berry Blast:			
Child, 12 fl.oz	70	0	20
Small, 16 fl.oz	100	0	27
Medium, 21 fl.oz	150	0	39
Large, 32 fl.oz cup	220	0	58

For Complete Menu & Data ~ see CalorieKing.com

Mimi's Cafe® (Oct '12)

	C	F	Cb
Breakfast: Without Sides			
Gourmet: Eggs Benedict	820	56	35
Eggs Florentine Benedict	710	51	36
Quiche Lorraine	895	60	58
Three Egg Omelettes: Mardi Gras	490	34	5
Five Alarm Santa Fe	385	27	8
Hot off The Griddle:			
Cinnamon Brioche French Toast	880	35	126
Mimi's Original Pain Perdu	480	20	63
Lunch: Without Sides			
Burgers: Classic	820	50	56
Monterey Chicken	1005	59	59
Cafe Classics: Chicken Pot Pie	1300	66	122
Oven Fresh Pot Roast	835	51	44
Sandwiches: Turkey Pesto Ciabatta	1100	59	90
West Coast Reuben	1390	90	102
Dinner: Without Sides			
Pasta: Crispy Parm. Crusted Chkn	1560	43	187
Mediterranean Fettuccine	1275	99	84
Steaks & Chops:			
Flat Iron Steak	715	50	11
Honey Dijon Pork Chops	585	17	32

Mr. Goodcents® (Oct '12)

	C	F	Cb
Cold Subs: Per ½ Wheat Bread Sub With Standard Ingredients			
Centsable	440	17	57
Italian Sub	640	37	55
Mr. Goodcents Original	510	25	56
Oven Roasted Chicken Breast	350	6	55
Penny Club	350	6	57
Pepperoni	700	43	55
Roast Beef	350	6	55
Tuna Salad	490	21	63
Veggie Sub	290	4	57
Toasted Sub: Per ½ Wheat Bread Sub With Standard Ingredients			
Chicken Bacon Ranch, w/ Cheddar	660	27	61
Chipotle Cheesesteak, w/ Provolone	670	29	66
Meatball w/ Mozzarella	680	33	67
Pasta: On Mostaccioli			
Alfredo Sauce	1290	80	106
Chicken Alfredo	1370	79	112
Chicken Parmesan	660	10	100
Red Sauce	520	4	100

Mr. Hero® (Oct '12)

	C	F	Cb
7" Hot Subs & Burgers:			
Burgers: Cheeseburger	775	55	47
Romanburger	860	62	48
Meatball Sub	725	47	47
Steak Subs: Tuscan	625	31	42
Hot Buttered Cheesesteak	670	42	45
Zesty Bacon & Swiss	615	32	42
7" Deli Subs: Original Italian	640	39	47
Tuna & Cheese	725	54	44
Turkey	470	20	46
Ultimate Italian	675	40	46
4½" Taste Buddies: Per Sandwich			
Bacon Cheeseburger	430	30	33
Crispy Chicken Wrap	385	23	31
Grilled Chicken Wrap	235	9	25
Grilled Italiano	440	32	32
Tuna 'n Cheese	485	38	31
Zesty Chicken	495	25	48
Pasta, Spag./Rigatoni w/ Meatballs in Marinara Sce w/ Breadstick	1115	36	153
Sides:			
Breadsticks, w/ Marinara Sauce (2)	445	17	64
Jalapeno Poppers. 4.5 oz	430	28	37
Mozzarella Sticks, w/ Marinara Sce	565	43	12
Onion Petals, w/ Tangy Sce, 5.75 oz	595	37	58
Fries, Potato Waffer, 5.75 oz	430	30	38
Desserts: Oreo Cookie Cheesecake	260	17	24
Snickers Cheesecake	270	18	23
Strawb. Swirl Cheesecake	280	19	22

Fast - Foods & Restaurants

Mrs Fields Cookies® (Oct '12)

	C	F	Cb
Brownies: *Per 2.15 oz Brownie*			
Butterscotch Blondie	260	10	38
Double Fudge; Pecan Fudge, av.	265	14	33
Special Walnut Fudge & Blondie	260	13	33
Toffee Fudge; Walnut Fudge, av.	265	14	33
Brownie Bites:			
Double Fudge (3)	200	10	27
Toffee Fudge (3)	200	11	26
Coffee Cake,			
Choc. Chip, small, 2.35 oz	240	11	30
Cookies:			
Bite Size Nibblers: Cinn. Sugar (3)	180	8	25
Oatmeal Raisin & Walnuts	200	9	27
Semi-Sweet Chocolate (3)	170	8	23
Triple Chocolate (3)	160	8	22
White Chunk Macadamia (3)	180	9	22
Butter (1)	200	8	29
Cut Out (1)	280	11	44
Debra's Special (1)	200	9	27
Peanut Butter (1)	200	12	24
Semi-Sweet: Chocolate (1)	210	10	29
With Walnuts (1)	220	11	28
Triple Chocolate (1)	210	10	28
White Chunk Macadamia (1)	230	12	28
Muffins: *Per 2 oz*			
Blueberry	190	9	24
Chocolate Chip	200	10	26

For Complete Nutritional Data ~ see CalorieKing.com

My Favorite Muffin® (Oct '12)

	C	F	Cb
Jumbo Muffins: *Per 5¾ oz*			
Regular: Blueberry	505	24	66
Choc. Chip; Cinn Swirl Cheesecake	635	33	81
Deep Dish Apple Pie	530	24	75
Pumpkin Spice	545	24	78
Fat Free: Blueberry	325	0	78
Chocolate Marble	375	0	87
Cinnamon Bun	505	0	126

Nathan's Famous® (Oct '12)

	C	F	Cb
Burgers:			
Bacon Cheeseburger, 5 oz	900	61	43
Double Beefburger, 10 oz	1030	73	41
Hamburger, 5 oz	620	38	41
Super Cheeseburger, 5 oz	960	67	48
Nathan's Famous Hot Dogs: *With Natural Casings*			
Original, 3.5 oz	290	17	24
Cheese Dog, 5.5 oz	390	25	30
Chili Dog, 5.5 oz	420	28	30
Chili Cheese, 6.5 oz	460	31	33
Corn Dog, on a stick, 3.2 oz	380	21	39

Nathan's Famous® cont... (Oct '12)

	C	F	Cb
Chicken:			
Chkn Tenders, Krispy, 3 pcs, 6.3 oz	520	31	32
Grilled Chicken Platter, 19 oz	1000	59	87
Fries:			
French: Regular, 7.5 oz	510	34	42
Large, 11.5 oz	780	52	64
Family, 15.5 oz	1050	70	86
Cheese: Regular, 9 oz	570	38	46
Large, 13.5 oz	860	58	70
Philly Cheesesteak, 14.4 oz	680	33	52
Wrap, Grilled Chicken Caesar, 9.2 oz	580	22	57

New York Fries
~ See CalorieKing.com

Ninety Nine (Oct '12)

	C	F	Cb
Standout Starters: *As Served*			
Baked Stuffed Clams	800	52	52
Boneless Wings & Skins Sampler	1660	111	72
Buffalo Chicken Flatbread	1090	77	58
Fried Mozzarella	780	48	57
Outrageous Potato Skins	1130	84	45
Burgers: *Without Sides*			
All Star	1310	96	57
Brewhouse BBQ Steak Burger	1160	69	73
Steakburger: Steakburger	860	54	46
With Cheese	940	61	48
Sandwiches: *Without Sides*			
Honey BBQ Chicken Wrap	930	40	94
Triple-Decker Turkey Club	970	37	106
Meals: *Served With Menu Set Sides Unless Indicated*			
Chicken & Sausage Al Forno	1900	89	179
Chkn Caesar Crowd Pleaser	2700	210	67
Fish & Chips	1830	124	120
Macadamia Crusted Chkn	1130	69	80
New England Shoreline Combo	2180	145	159
NY Strip Sirloin, without sides	680	28	1
Panko Crusted Cod	1410	63	143
Prime Rib: 12 oz, without sides	920	72	2
18 oz, without sides	1370	107	2
Smothered Sirloin Tips, w/o sides	1010	56	12
Steak & Kickin Shrimp Combo	680	31	33
Salads: *As Served*			
Chicken Caesar	830	54	50
Fire Grilled SW Cobb	890	58	30
Tropical Chicken	760	39	60
Sides:			
Double Bleu Iceberg Wedge	460	42	9
Honey Butter Bisc., w/ Honey Butter	220	9	29
Loaded Baked Potato	580	34	52
Dessert:			
Little Midnight Fudge Hero	420	22	52

219

Noodles & Company® (Oct '12)

Meals: Per Regular Bowl

	C	F	Cb
American: Buttered Noodles	930	39	114
Mushroom Stroganoff	790	31	102
Spaghetti	660	16	105
Spaghetti w/ Meatballs	970	39	111
Steak Stroganoff	1030	46	104
Wisconsin Mac & Cheese	1030	43	122
Asian: Bangkok Curry	480	14	80
Chinese Chop Salad	370	22	39
Indonesian Peanut Saute	830	18	148
Japanese Pan Noodles	620	15	110
Pad Thai	830	18	151
Mediterranean: Pasta Fresca	780	25	114
Penne Rosa	790	35	97
Pesto Cavatappi	800	31	102
The Med Salad	320	13	44
Whole Grain Tuscan Linguine	680	32	77
Proteins: Chicken Breast	110	3	0
Meatballs	300	23	6
Organic Tofu	180	11	6
Parmesan-Crusted Chicken Breast	200	10	8

Salads: Per Side Serving

	C	F	Cb
Cucumber Tomato	110	0	24
Tossed Green, with Balsamic	60	6	4
Sides: Potstickers (6), w/out Sauce	340	10	45
Ciabatta Roll (1)	120	1	24

Sandwiches:

	C	F	Cb
Mmmeatball	670	32	59
The Med	330	10	41
Spicy Chicken Caesar w/o dressing	330	9	40
Wisconsin Cheesesteak on Ciabatta	570	22	54
Cookies: Chocolate Chunk	370	9	65
Smoodledoodle	350	8	64

Nothing But Noodles® (Oct '12)

Noodle Bowls:

	C	F	Cb
American: Beef Stroganoff	510	31	33
Buttery Noodles	650	44	46
Santa Fe Pasta	705	54	40
Southwest Chipotle	715	58	41
Spicy Cajun Pasta	660	50	44
Asian: Pad Thai Noodles	600	10	118
Sesame Lo Mein	410	11	64
Spicy Japanese Noodles	420	8	74
Thai Peanut	570	20	89
Italian: Basil Pesto	575	42	36
Cappellini Primavera	500	28	56
Fettuccini Alfredo	725	56	36
Margherita Pasta	475	31	36
Marinara Pasta	485	11	77
Three-Cheese Macaroni	445	21	45

For Complete Menu & Data ~ see CalorieKing.com

O'Charley's® (Oct '12)

Appetizers: As Served

	C	F	Cb
Chicken Tenders, w/ Chipotle BBQ Sce	1040	37	119
Over-Loaded Potato Skins	1260	98	44
Spicy Jack Cheese Wedges (7)	880	60	55
Top Shelf Combo Platter	1890	131	106

Meals:

Chicken & Ribs: *Without Sides*

	C	F	Cb
Chicken Italia	1330	75	93
Chicken Tenders w/ Honey Mstd Sce	1090	61	82
O'Charley's Baby Back Ribs:			
Full Rack	1480	96	76
Half Rack	740	48	38
Teriyaki Sesame Chicken			
on Rice Pilaf	1030	25	151
Pasta: New Orleans Chicken	1600	102	90
Prime Rib	1530	101	90
Shrimp Scampi Pasta	840	33	93

Seafood: *Without Sides Unless Indicated*

	C	F	Cb
Bayou Tilapia, w/ Rice, Veges & Sce	880	54	44
Cedar Planked Salmon	530	32	2
Gr. Atl. Salmon w/ Chipotle, 9 oz	610	33	17
Hand Battered Fish & Chips	1190	85	43
Panko Crusted Fried Shrimp,			
on Rice Pilaf	570	26	53

Steak & Combos: *Per Serving, Without Sides*

	C	F	Cb
Louisiana Sirloin	680	40	3
Panko Crusted Shrimp &			
Battered Cod	810	44	39
Steak & Grilled Atlantic Salmon	800	50	3
Steak & Shrimp Scampi	770	55	11
Sides: Broccoli	140	10	11
French Fries, 1 serve	520	33	53
Potato: Loaded, baked	590	40	52

Salads: *Without Dressing Unless Indicated*

	C	F	Cb
Black & Bleu Caesar w/ Dressing	1115	82	35
California Chicken	685	36	47
Pecan Chicken Tender	1005	59	79

Soup: *Per Cup*

	C	F	Cb
Chicken Harvest	160	8	12
Chicken Tortilla	150	9	12
Overloaded Potato	170	9	16
Desserts: Apple Caramel Cobbler	750	29	113
Ooey Gooey Caramel Pie, 1 slice	440	21	57

For Complete Menu & Data ~ see CalorieKing.com

Updated Nutrition Data ~ www.CalorieKing.com
Persons with Diabetes ~ See Disclaimer (Page 22)

Olive Garden® (Oct '12)

	C	F	Cb
Appetizers:			
Bruschetta	950	13	173
Muscles di Napoli	180	8	13
Sicilian Scampi	500	22	43
Stuffed Mushrooms	280	19	15
Entrees:			
Lunch: Capellini Pomodora, 13 oz	480	11	78
Eggplant Parmigiana	620	26	70
Fettuccine Alfredo	800	48	69
Five Cheese Ziti al Forno	770	32	89
Lasagna Classico	580	32	35
Linguine alla Marinara	310	4	55
Venetian Apricot Chicken	290	4.5	34
Dinner: Capellini Pomodoro	840	17	141
Fettucini Alfredo	1220	75	99
Linguine alla Marinara, 17 oz	430	6	76
Ravioli di Portobello	670	30	74
Shrimp Primavera, 28 oz	730	12	110
Venetian Apricot Chicken	400	7	34
Desserts: Black Tie Mousse Cake	760	48	73
Strawb. & White Choc. Cream Cake	210	11	27
Tiramisu	510	32	48

Old Spaghetti Factory® (Oct '12)

	C	F	Cb
Appetizers: As Served			
Shrimp, Spinach & Artichoke Dip	590	40	39
Sicilian Garlic Cheese Bread	1320	77	111
Entrees, Lunch/Dinner:			
Classics:			
Spaghetti: With Clam Sauce, 15 oz	810	31	107
With Marina Sauce, 15 oz	560	5	108
With Meat Sauce, 15 oz	650	11	108
With Sicilian Meatballs, 21 oz	1040	36	115
Factory Favorites:			
Chicken Parmigiana, 18 oz	750	29	70
Spinach & Cheese Ravioli, 11 oz	470	16	63
Spinach Tortellini w/ Alfredo Sce	940	56	86
Managers Favorites:			
Marinara: Clam, 15 oz	690	18	107
Meat, 15 oz	600	8	108
Mushroom, 16.5 oz	610	10	109
Signature Selection:			
Chicken Penne, 18.8 oz	870	38	102
Baked Chicken, 16.55 oz	970	60	61
Crab Ravioli, 11 oz	810	45	73

On the Border® (Oct '12)

	C	F	Cb
Appetizers: As Served			
Border Sampler	2060	142	101
Fajita Quesadillas: Chicken	1180	82	55
Steak	1210	88	54
Burritos: Includes Rice, Without Beans & Sauce			
Classic Chicken	920	36	103
Classic Shredded Beef	1020	41	102
Chimichangas: Includes Rice, Without Beans & Sauce			
Chicken	1300	79	103
Ground Beef	1420	90	105
Dinner: Includes Rice, Without Beans			
Enchiladas: Gr. Pepper Jack Chkn	1050	48	106
Ranchiladas	1260	66	96
Suiza	1000	45	106
Fajitas, Signature: Without Rice, Beans, Tortillas or Condiments			
Monterey Chicken Ranch	650	43	12
The Ultimate	1160	96	26
Fresh Grill: Served As Listed			
Carne Asada	970	38	105
Chicken Salsa Fresca	520	9	60
Queso Chicken	1030	41	110
Tomatillo Chicken	850	24	109
Salads: Without Dressing			
House, side size	200	12	20
Grande Taco Salad: With Chicken	1180	75	79
With Ground Beef	1280	85	80
Sides: Per Serving			
Chile con Carne for Buritos/Chimmis	100	5	8
Mexican Rice	280	5	55
Pico de Gallo	10	1	1
Sour Cream for Burritos/Chimmis	80	6	5
Dressings: Per Serving			
Ranch Dressing	230	24	2
Smoked Jalapeno Vinaigrette	250	24	8

For Complete Nutritional Data ~ see CalorieKing.com

Orange Julius® (Oct '12)

	C	F	Cb
Fruit Drinks: Per Small, 16 fl.oz			
Bananarilla	350	6	75
Blackberry	380	6	85
Mango	250	0	67
Raspberry	300	0	79
Strawberry Banana	380	6	83
Premium Fruit Smoothies: Per Medium, 20 fl.oz			
Blackberry Storm	620	6	139
Orange Swirl	460	7	95
Raspberry Creme	530	6	114
Fat Free: Berry Banana Squeeze	320	0	82
Strawberry Sensation	420	0	99
Nutrition Boosts: Banana, 4.45 oz	110	0	29
Protein, ¾ oz	100	4	9

Fast - Foods & *Restaurants*

Outback Steakhouse® (Oct '12)

Aussie-Tizers: Per Whole Dish, With Sauce/Dressing — **C** **F** **Cb**

Alice Springs Chicken Quesadilla:

	C	F	Cb
Small, serves 2	940	65	48
Regular, serves 4	1565	97	87
Aussie Cheese Fries:			
Small, serves 3	1280	93	80
Regular, serves 6	1965	134	139
Bloomin' Onion, serves 6	1960	161	117
Coconut Shrimp, serves 2	415	22	40
Seared Ahi Tuna: Small, serves 2	365	24	24
Regular, serves 4	500	28	35

Burgers & Sandwiches:

	C	F	Cb
Aged Cheddar Bacon Burger	1005	72	36
With Fries	1385	90	84
Grilled Chicken & Swiss Sandwich	685	37	41
With Fries	1070	56	90
The Bloomin Burger	1030	71	50
With Fries	1415	89	99
The Outbacker Burger	685	40	38
With Fries	1070	59	87

Steaks: Without Sides

	C	F	Cb
New York Strip, 14 oz	765	49	0
Outback Special: 6 oz Sirloin	255	13	0
9 oz Sirloin	380	19	0
12 oz Sirloin	510	25	0
Prime Rib: 8 oz	420	14	0
16 oz	830	28	1
Ribeye, 14 oz	760	49	0
Teriyaki Filet Medallions	680	30	32
Porterhouse, 20 oz	1010	71	4
Victoria's Filet, 6 oz	220	9	0

Outback Favorites: With Set Sides as Per Menu

	C	F	Cb
Alice Springs Chicken	1145	66	62
Baby Back Ribs, full rack	1540	96	71
Grilled Chicken on the Barbie	400	7	21
New Zealand Rack of Lamb	1005	59	45
No Rules Parmesan Pasta	880	51	73
With Grilled Chicken	1320	70	79
With Grilled Chicken & Scallops	1330	71	83
With Grilled Chicken & Shrimp	1315	70	93
With Grilled Scallops	1305	71	86
With Grilled Shrimp	1205	69	97
Sweet Glazed Rstd Pork Tenderloin	665	28	53

Fish & Seafood: Without Sides

	C	F	Cb
Lobster Tails	450	27	2
Tilapia, with Lump Crab Meat	515	28	9

Outback Steakhouse® cont... (Oct '12)

Perfect Combinations: W/O Sides — **C** **F** **Cb**

	C	F	Cb
Filet & Grilled Shrimp On The Barbie	560	38	17
Filet, 6 oz & Lobster Tail, 4 oz	630	43	3
Sirloin:			
6 oz: With Coconut Shrimp	495	24	29
With Grilled Shrimp	500	29	17
9 oz: With Coconut Shrimp	590	30	20
With Grilled Shrimp	625	36	17

Salads: Without Dressing Unless Indicated

	C	F	Cb
Aussie Chicken Cobb: Crispy	840	54	45
Grilled	545	29	19
California Chicken	690	39	52
Chicken Caesar, with dressing	705	41	19
Classic Roasted Filet Wedge, with dressing	735	59	16

Soups: Per Bowl

	C	F	Cb
Creamy Onion	485	36	25
Potato	485	33	38

Add Ons:

	C	F	Cb
Blue Cheese Crumb Crust	225	21	4
Grilled Scallops	210	10	8
Horseradish Crumb Crust	220	21	7
Lobster Tail	325	24	2
Sauteed Mushrooms	200	10	15

Sides:

	C	F	Cb
Aussie Fries	385	19	49
Baked Potato: Plain	230	1	49
With Bacon & Sour Cream	285	5	51
With Butter	360	15	49
With Butter, Cheese & Bacon	400	19	49
With Chse, Chives & Sour Cream	290	5	51
Fresh Seasonal Mixed Veggies	95	3	11
Garlic Mashed Potatoes	305	17	32
Sweet Potato: With Honey Butter	420	16	66
Without Honey Butter	320	5	63

Desserts: Per Single Serving

	C	F	Cb
Classic Cheesecake, plain, ½ slice	165	12	11
Chocolate Thunder, ¼ of dish	390	26	33
Sydney's Sinful Sundae, ½ of dish	480	31	46

For Complete Menu & Data ~ see CalorieKing.com

Panda Express® (Oct '12)

Appetizers:

	C	F	Cb
Chkn Egg Roll (1), 3 oz	200	12	16
Chicken Potsticker (3), 3.3 oz	220	11	23
Cream Cheese Rangoon (3), 2.4 oz	190	8	24
Veggie Spring Rolls (2), 3.4 oz	160	7	22

Continued Next Page...

Updated Nutrition Data ~ www.CalorieKing.com
Persons with Diabetes ~ See Disclaimer (Page 22)

Panda Express® cont... (Oct '12)

Entrees:

	C	F	Cb
Beef: Beijing Beef, 5.6 oz	690	40	57
Broccoli Beef, 5.4 oz	120	4	13
Shanghai Angus Beef, 5.4 oz	720	7	19
Chicken. Kung Pao Chicken, 5.8 oz	240	14	13
Mandarin Chicken, 5.8 oz	310	16	8
Orange Chicken, 5.7 oz	420	21	43
Potato Chicken, 5.2 oz	190	9	19
SweetFire Chicken Breast, 5.8 oz	440	18	53
Pork: BBQ Pork, 4.6 oz	360	19	13
Sweet & Sour Pork, 6.2 oz	390	21	44
Shrimp: Crispy Shrimp (6), 3.5 oz	260	13	26
Golden Treasure Shrimp, 5 oz	390	19	39
Honey Walnut Shrimp, 3.7 oz	370	23	27

Rice & Noodles: Per Serving

	C	F	Cb
Chow Mein, 9.4 oz	490	22	65
Fried Rice, 9.3 oz	530	16	82
Steamed Rice, 8.1 oz	380	0	86

Panera Bread® (Oct '12)

Bagels: Asiago Cheese

	C	F	Cb
Bagels: Asiago Cheese	330	6	55
Cinnamon Crunch	420	7	80

Breakfast Sandwiches:

	C	F	Cb
Bagels: Asiago Cheese, w/ Sausage	650	32	55
French Toast, with Sausage	670	30	69
Whole Grain, Power	340	15	31
Bacon, Egg & Cheese on Ciabatta	510	25	43

Cafe & Signature Sandwiches: Per Full Sandwich:

	C	F	Cb
Asiago Roast Beef, on Asiago Cheese	700	27	64
Bacon Turkey Bravo on Tom. Basil	800	29	83
Chicken Caesar on Three Cheese	750	33	73
Italian Combo on Ciabatta	980	41	95
Smoked Ham & Swiss on Rye	590	17	64
Smoked Turkey Breast on Country	420	3	66
Tuna Salad on Honey Wheat	510	16	63
Hot Paninis: Cuban Chicken	860	36	87
Rstd Turkey Artichoke on Focc.	780	33	78
Steak & White Cheddar on Baguette	970	33	111
Tomato & Mozzarella on Ciabatta	760	29	95

Salads: Full Size, With Dressing, Without Bread

	C	F	Cb
Asian Sesame Chicken	450	24	33
Caesar	410	28	28
Greek	370	34	14
Roasted Turkey Fuji Apple	590	40	32

Signature Mac & Cheese,

	C	F	Cb
Large, 15.5 oz	980	61	75

Panera Bread® cont... (Oct '12)

Soups: Without Bread

	C	F	Cb
Broccoli Cheddar, 12 oz	300	19	21
Cream of Chkn & Wild Rice, 13.25 oz	310	17	24
Creamy Tomato w/ Croutons, 13 oz	410	29	30
French On. w/ Croutons, 14.75 oz	230	11	27
Low Fat: Chicken Noodle, 13.5 oz	120	1.5	22
Vegetable with Pesto, 14.75 oz	150	5	26
Vegetarian Black Bean, 13.25 oz	240	2.5	50
New England Clam Chowder, 12 oz	630	54	27

Pastries & Sweets:

	C	F	Cb
Bear Claw, 4.5 oz	550	28	68
Cheese Pastry, 3.75 oz	400	22	44
Chocolate Pastry, 3.5 oz	410	23	47
Cobblestone, 7 oz	640	13	122
Oatmeal Raisin Cookie, 3.25 oz	390	14	62
Pecan Braid, 3.75 oz	470	26	53
Pecan Roll, 5.5 oz	740	40	89
Muffins: Apple Crunch, 5 oz	450	12	80
Pumpkin, 5 oz	590	22	91
Wild Blueberry, 4.5 oz	440	17	66

Papa Gino's® (Oct '12)

Appetizers: Small, Per 2 Servings

	C	F	Cb
BBQ Chicken Tenders, 8.25 oz	520	18	60
Buffalo Chicken Tenders, 9.65 oz	660	42	38
Cheese Breadsticks, 20 oz	1240	44	158
Chicken Tender, 6.6 oz	420	18	36
Burgers: Cheeseburger, 6.75 oz	570	32	37
Classic Double, 12.85 oz	1040	67	43
Hamburger, 6.25 oz	520	28	36
French Fries, 4 oz	170	7	25

Pastas: Entree Size, Without Breadstick

	C	F	Cb
Papa Platter, Penne, 22 oz	1020	34	145
Ravioli, 12.4 oz	560	21	67
Spaghetti & Meatballs, 19.8 oz	780	28	109

Pizzas:

Thin Crust: *Per Slice of Large Pizza*

	C	F	Cb
Buffalo Chicken	270	8	32
Cheese	230	7	32
Chicken and Roasted Garlic	260	7	34
Meat Combo	330	16	32
Papa Roni	340	16	32
Pepperoni	280	11	32
Super Veggie	250	8	35
Works	330	14	34

Subs: Per Small Sub

	C	F	Cb
BLT	690	35	67
Italian	590	24	64
Meatball Parmesan	790	38	79
Steak & Cheese	710	33	63
Super Steak	750	33	72
Tuna	730	39	64
Turkey Club	600	22	67

Papa John's® *(Oct '12)*

Pizzas: | C | F | Cb
Original Crust (14"): *Per ⅛ Pizza*

	C	F	Cb
Buffalo Chicken, 5.25oz	370	17	39
Spicy Italian, 5.25 oz	380	18	38
Spinach Alfredo, 4 oz	280	10	36
The Meats, 3.75 oz	370	17	38
The Works, 5.5 oz	330	14	39

Thin Crust (14"): *Per ⅛ Pizza*

	C	F	Cb
BBQ Chicken & Bacon, 4 oz	290	13	29
Spicy Italian, 4 oz	320	20	22
Spinach Alfredo, 2.75 oz	220	12	21
The Meats, 3.75 oz	310	19	22
The Works, 4.25 oz	270	15	23

Wings: *Without Sauce*

	C	F	Cb
BBQ, 2 wings, 2.5 oz	190	12	6
Spicy Buffalo, 2 wings, 2.5 oz	170	13	3

Dipping Sauces: *Per 1 oz Container*

	C	F	Cb
Barbeque	45	0	11
Blue Cheese	160	16	1
Buffalo	15	0.5	2
Ranch	100	10	1

Sides: *Without Dipping Sauce*

	C	F	Cb
Breadsticks (2)	290	4.5	54
Cheesesticks (4), 4.75 oz	370	16	41
Chicken Strips (2), 2.5 oz	130	4.5	10

Papa Murphy's® *(Oct '12)*

Pizzas: | C | F | Cb
Original Crust : *Per ½ Family Size Pizza*

	C	F	Cb
BBQ Chicken	330	12	36
Cheese	270	10	29
Cowboy	335	16	30
Gourmet: Chicken Garlic	320	13	30
Classic Italian	350	18	31
Vegetarian	300	13	31
Hawaiian	295	11	33
Murphy's Combo	350	17	31
Papa's Favorite	350	17	31
Pepperoni	320	15	31
Rancher	325	15	30
Specialty of the House	310	14	30
Veggie Combo	280	12	32

Stuffed Pizza: *Per 1/16 Family Size Pizza*

	C	F	Cb
5 Meat	370	16	38
Big Murphy	370	15	39
Chicago Style	365	15	39
Chicken and Bacon	370	12	38

Papa Murphy's® *cont... (Oct '12)*

Pizzas: | C | F | Cb
Thin Crust deLITEs: *Per 1/10 Large Pizza*

	C	F	Cb
Cheese	145	7	13
Hawaiian	160	7	15
Pepperoni	170	9	13

Salads: *Per Whole Salad, 2 Servings, Without Dressing or Croutons*

	C	F	Cb
Club ,13 oz	280	16	12
Garden, 14.5 oz	190	11	15
Italian, 13 oz	265	19	13

Pei Wei Asian Diner *(Oct '12)*

Small Plates: *Per Serving, Without Sce*

	C	F	Cb
Crab Wontons (2)	340	20	26
Crispy Potstickers (2)	300	16	24
Minced Chicken w/ Lettuce Wraps (2)	620	22	72
Vegetable Spring Rolls (1)	110	3.5	17

Noodle & Rice Bowls: *Per Whole Meal, 2 Servings*

	C	F	Cb
Dan Dan Noodle, Chicken	780	20	106
Fried Rice: Chicken	1000	24	132
Steak	1040	32	136
Lo Mein Noodles: Chicken	1120	40	134
Steak	1080	40	134
Pad Thai Noodles: Chicken	1440	40	210
Steak	1580	52	218

Teriyaki Bowl: *Includes Per Whole Meal, 2 Servings, With White Rice*

	C	F	Cb
Beef	1020	18	180
Chicken	1060	18	178
Shrimp	980	14	178

Signature Entrees: *Per Whole Meal, 2 Servings, W/o Rice*

	C	F	Cb
Honey Seared: Chicken	860	30	98
Shrimp	900	36	98
Pei Wei Spicy: Beef	1220	52	148
Chicken	920	32	110
Sweet & Sour: Chicken	720	20	96
Shrimp	740	26	94

Soup:

	C	F	Cb
Hot & Sour, 1 Cup, 6 fl.oz	190	8	12
Thai Wanton, 1 Cup, 6 fl.oz	110	6	5

Salads: *Per Whole Meal, Serves 2, Without Dressing*

	C	F	Cb
Asian Chopped Chicken	380	12	26
Pei Wei Spicy Chicken	1040	44	116

Dressings: *Per 2 oz Serving*

	C	F	Cb
Lime Vinaigrette	220	20	14
Sesame Ginger	220	21	6
Sauces: Lettuce Wrap	50	3	3
Potsticker	30	1	3
Sweet Chile	130	0	32
Thai Peanut	160	10	16

Pepe's Mexican® *~ see CalorieKing.com*

Updated Nutrition Data ~ www.CalorieKing.com
Persons with Diabetes ~ See Disclaimer (Page 22)

Perkins® (Oct '12)

Breakfast:

	C	F	Cb
Benedicts: *With Muffin, Hashbrowns & Fruit Cup*			
Classic, 11.2 oz	1160	51	138
Country Cookin', 23.3 oz	1560	91	141
Classics: *W/- B'milk Pancakes, Butter, Syrup & Hashbrowns*			
Country Fried Steak & Eggs	1870	79	227
Tremendous Twelve	1620	68	201
Griddle Greats: *With Butter, Syrup & Powdered Sugar, Unless Indicated*			
Belgian Waffle: 9.2 oz	700	33	92
Blueberry, w/o Butter, 14.8 oz	780	18	147
Strawb., w/o Butter, 14.8 oz	720	18	132
Berry Blueberry Pancakes, w/ Non Dairy Tppng, w/o Butter	1140	29	200
Oo-la-la French Toast	1000	42	121
Potato Pancakes w/ Bacon and Applesauce, 15 oz	1670	74	216
Omelettes:			
Everything, with Hashbrowns, B'milk P'cakes, Syrup & Butter	1640	73	192
Farmer's, with Hashbrowns, White Toast & Butter	1460	81	127
Granny's Country, with H'browns B'milk P'cakes, Butter & Syrup	2060	81	276
Sides:			
Potatoes, 5 oz	250	12	32
English Muffin, 2.7 oz	230	11	28
Fruit Cup, 4 oz	50	0	12
Hash Browns, 4 oz	490	13	67
Oatmeal, w/ 2% Milk & Br. Sugar	330	6	60
Sausage Links (4)	460	44	2
Burgers: *Without Sides*			
BBQ Bacon Supreme	950	57	56
Hamburger	670	37	44
Melts: *With French Fries*			
Chicken Strip	1710	111	119
Reuben Melt, on Rye	1340	82	87
Sandwiches: *With Fries Unless Indicated*			
French Dip, with Au Jus, 17.3 oz	930	51	77
Kickin' Chicken, w/out Fries, 17.7 oz	980	47	89
Triple Decker Club, 18.5 oz	1210	75	85
Wraps: *With French Fries*			
Ham & Turkey BLT w/ Ranch Drssng	1080	69	89
The Buffalo Wrap, with Blue Cheese Dressing	1460	98	105

Perkins® cont... (Oct '12)

Dinners: With Menu Set Sides

	C	F	Cb
Butterball Turkey	1000	49	91
Chicken Pot Pie	1470	106	80
Chicken Strips	1820	120	132
Country Fried Steak	1080	61	92
Grilled Pork Chops	1020	51	72
Homestyle Pot Roast	820	46	63
Top Sirloin	690	27	64
Seafood: *With Menu Set Sides*			
Captain's Catch, 34.3 oz	2400	146	217
Grilled Salmon, 16.2 oz	890	50	62
Jumbo Shrimp Dinner, 20.7 oz	1020	52	112
Tilapia Grille, 21.15 oz	890	45	71
Sides:			
Baked Potato, with Sour Cream, & Whipped Butter, 8.64 oz	390	22	42
Broccoli, butter steamed, 4.25 oz	140	12	6
Cheddar Mashed Potatoes, 6 oz	260	14	24
French Fries, 7 oz	570	36	56
Macaroni & Cheese, 5 oz	200	8	24
Mashed Potatoes & Gravy, 7.12 oz	230	13	26
Side Salad with Croutons, and Ranch Dressing, 6.5 oz	300	25	15
Super Soups: *Per Bowl*			
Broccoli & Cheddar Cheese	280	18	20
Homestyle Chicken Noodle	150	5	16
Loaded Baked Potato	280	18	25
New England Clam Chowder	260	14	19
Southwest Style Chicken Tortilla	180	6	19
Vegetable Beef	150	5	19
Salads:			
Chef Deluxe, with Ranch Dressing	880	58	30
Chicken & Spinach, w/out Dressing	960	65	37
Dessert: *Per Slice*			
Pies: Caramel Apple, 7.15 oz	500	22	68
Chocolate French Silk, 6 oz	760	54	66
Peanut Butter Silk, 7.2 oz	960	68	73
Southern Pecan, 5.5 oz	670	33	86
Wildberry, no sugar added, 7 oz	360	15	50
Beverages:			
Cherry Coke, 12.35 oz	160	0	42
Raspberry Iced Tea, 11.64 oz	130	0	34

Peter Piper Pizza® (Oct '12)

Appetizers: Per Serving **C** **F** **Cb**

Boneless Wings: Per Regular Size

	C	F	Cb
Buffalo	395	19	22
Plain	305	11	19
Garlic Cheese Bread, 3.25 oz	310	14	37

Signature Pizzas: Per Slice

Original Crust: Per 1/8 of Large 14" Pizza

	C	F	Cb
5 Meat Supreme	350	13	58
California Veggie	200	6	23
Chicago Classic	300	10	38
New York 3 Cheese w/ Pepperoni	380	16	38
Pepperoni & Sausage	310	11	37
The Werx	320	11	38

Original Crust: Per 1/12 of Extra Large 16" Pizza

	C	F	Cb
5 Meat Supreme	320	13	33
California Veggie	240	6	33
Chicago Classic	270	9	33
New York 3 Cheese w/ Pepperoni	340	14	32
The Werx	290	10	33

Hand-Tossed: Per 1/8 of Large 14" Pizza

	C	F	Cb
5 Meat Supreme	350	13	38
California Veggie	270	7	39
Chicago Classic	300	10	39
New York 3 Cheese w/ Pepperoni	380	16	39
Pepperoni & Sausage	310	11	38
The Werx	310	11	39

Hand-Tossed Crust: Per 1/12 of Extra Large 16" Pizza

	C	F	Cb
5 Meat Supreme	320	13	34
California Veggie	240	6	34
Chicago Classic	270	9	34
New York 3 Cheese w/ Pepperoni	340	14	34
The Werx	280	10	34

Pan Crust: Per 1/8 of Large 14" Pizza

	C	F	Cb
5 Meat Supreme	380	13	46
California Veggie	300	7	47
Chicago Classic	340	10	46
New York 3 Cheese w/ Pepperoni	410	16	46
Pepperoni & Sausage	340	11	45
The Werx	350	11	46

Pan Crust: Per 1/12 of Extra Large 16" Pizza

	C	F	Cb
5 Meat Supreme	340	13	39
California Veggie	260	6	39
Chicago Classic	290	9	39
New York 3 Cheese w/ Pepperoni	360	15	39
The Werx	310	10	39

Peter Piper® ...cont (Oct '12)

Signature Pizzas: (Cont): **C** **F** **Cb**

Thin Crust: Per 1/8 of Large 14" Pizza

	C	F	Cb
5 Meat Supreme	180	8	14
California Veggie	130	4.5	15
Chicago Classic	150	6	15
New York 3 Cheese w/ Pepperoni	200	10	14
Pepperoni & Sausage	150	7	14
The Werx	160	7	14

Thin Crust: Per 1/16 of Extra Large 16" Pizza

	C	F	Cb
5 Meat Supreme	190	9	14
California Veggie	130	4	14
Chicago Classic	150	6	14
New York 3 Cheese w/ Pepperoni	200	10	14
The Werx	160	7	14

P.F. Chang's® (Oct '12)

Starters: Per Whole Dish **C** **F** **Cb**

	C	F	Cb
Crab Wontons (6), without sauce	475	29	40
Egg Rolls (4), without sauce	560	20	75
Lettuce Wraps: Chicken (4)	530	24	47
Vegetarian (4)	610	36	39

Pork Dumplings: Without Sauce

	C	F	Cb
Pan-Fried (6)	360	15	33
Steamed (6)	330	12	33

Shrimp Dumplings: Without Sauce

	C	F	Cb
Pan-Fried (6)	230	6	28
Steamed (6)	220	1.5	31
Spare Ribs: Northern Style (6)	1120	63	41
Changs BBQ (6)	1180	81	33
Spring Rolls, without Sauce, (4)	230	10	25

Main Menu:

Beef: Per Whole Meal, Without Rice

	C	F	Cb
A La Sichuan	680	32	54
Mongolian	720	39	31
Orange Peel	720	36	55

Chicken: Per Whole Dish, Without Rice

	C	F	Cb
Chang's Spicy	830	35	74
Kung Pao Chicken	1100	66	56
Orange Peel Chicken	860	41	66
Sesame Chicken	790	36	50
Sweet & Sour Chicken	840	44	71
Duck, Chinese 5 Spice Duo, w/o rice	1310	66	85

Continued Next Page...

Updated Nutrition Data ~ www.CalorieKing.com
Persons with Diabetes ~ See Disclaimer (Page 22)

P.F. Chang's® cont... (Oct '12)

Main Menu (Cont):

	C	F	Cb
Seafood: *Per Whole Meal, Without Rice*			
Lemongrass Grilled Norw. Salmon	640	37	20
Crispy Honey Shrimp	660	38	53
Shrimp, with Candied Walnuts	1380	104	74
Sichuan Shrimp	360	16	32
Vegetarian Plates: *Without Rice*			
Coconut Curry Vegetables	1050	75	52
Ma Po Tofu	1030	70	44
Stir-Fried Eggplant	1010	88	50
Noodles Meins & Rice:			
PF Chang's Fried Rice, with Beef	1240	28	203
PF Chang's Lo Mein, with Pork	760	25	100
Singapore Street Noodles	700	17	105
Double Pan-Fried Noodles w/ Chkn	1030	48	108
Sides: *Per Small Dish*			
Shanghai Cucumbers	60	2	7
Sichuan-Style Asparagus	110	4	15
Spinach Stir-Fried with Garlic	110	8	8
Soups: Hot & Sour: 1 cup	70	2	9
1 bowl	380	11	48
Egg Drop : 1 cup	60	2.5	8
1 bowl	290	12	39
Desserts: *Per Whole Dish*			
Banana Spring Rolls	940	38	143
Great Wall of Chocolate Cake	1520	72	238
Mini Tiramisu	180	11	18

Pita Pit® ~ See CalorieKing.com

Pizza Hut® (Oct '12)

Fit' n Delicious: *Per ⅛ of 12" Pizza*

Chicken, Mushroom & Jalapeno	170	4.5	22
Chicken, Onion & Green Pepper	180	4.5	23
Green Pepper, Onion & Tomato	150	4	24
Ham, Onion & Mushroom	160	4.5	23
Ham, Pineapple & Tomato	160	4.5	24
Tomato, Mushroom & Jalapeno	150	4	23
Hand-Tossed Style: *Per ⅛ of 12" Pizza*			
Cheese Only	220	8	26
Dan's Original	260	12	26
Hawaiian Luau	240	9	27
Ham & Pineapple	200	6	27
Italian Sausage & Onion	240	10	27
Meat Lover's	300	16	26
Pepperoni	230	9	25
Pepperoni & Mushroom	210	8	26
Spicy Sicilian	240	11	26
Supreme	260	12	26
Triple Meat Italiano	260	12	26

Pizza Hut® cont... (Oct '12)

Pan: *Per ⅛ of 12" Pizza*	C	F	Cb
Cheese Only	240	10	27
Ham & Pineapple	230	4	28
Hawaiian Luau	260	12	28
Meat Lover's	330	18	27
Pepperoni & Mushroom	240	10	27
Supreme	290	14	27
Triple Meat Italiano	290	15	27
Veggie Lover's	230	9	28
Personal Pan: *Per 6" Pizza*			
Cheese Only	590	24	69
Ham & Pineapple	550	20	71
Meat Lover's	830	46	68
Supreme	720	36	69
Veggie Lover's	550	20	70
P'Zone: *Per ½ P'Zone*			
Classic	470	16	61
Meaty	550	23	61
Pepperoni	450	15	60
Thin 'n Crispy: *Per ⅛ of 12" Pizza*			
Cheese Only	190	8	22
Ham & Pineapple	180	6	23
Meat Lover's	280	16	22
Supreme	240	12	23
Veggie Lover's	180	6	23
Stuffed Crust: *Per ⅛ 14" Pizza*			
Cheese Only	340	14	39
Ham & Pineapple	330	12	41
Meat Lover's	480	26	39
Supreme	420	20	40
Veggie Lover's	330	12	41
Stuffed Pizza Rollers, *each*	220	10	24
Wings: *Per 2 Pieces, Without Dipping Sauce*			
Bone Out: Buffalo, all flav., 2.5 oz	190	9	18
Honey BBQ, 3 oz	220	8	27
Crispy Bone In:			
Buffalo, all flavors, 2.5 oz	230	15	16
Honey BBQ, 3 oz	260	14	24
Traditional: All American, 1.5 oz	80	5	0
Garlic Parmesan, 2 oz	180	16	1
Dipping Sauces: Marinara, 3 oz	60	0	12
Ranch, 1.5 oz	220	23	2
Pastas, Tuscani: *Per ½ Pan*			
Chicken Alfredo	580	32	49
Meaty Marinara	450	20	44
Desserts: Cinnamon Sticks (2)	160	4.5	26
Hershey's: Choc. Dunkers (2)	190	8	27
Chocolate Sauce, 1.5 oz	120	2.5	24
White Icing Dipping Cup, 2 oz	170	0	44

Pizza Ranch® (Oct '12)

Pizzas: Per 1/10 Slice of 12" Pizza

	C	F	Cb
Thin Crust: Bacon Cheeseburger	110	5	11
BLT	160	5	11
Bronco	110	5	11
Buffalo Chicken	110	5	9
California Chicken	110	5	10
Chicken Bacon Ranch	160	9	10
Chicken Broccoli Alfredo	100	4	10
Diced Chicken	80	2	10
Garlic Cheese; Italian Sausage	100	5	9
Pepperoni	90	3	10
Prairie (Veggie)	80	2	11
Roundup	100	4	11
Stampede	110	4	12
Sweet Swine	80	2	12
Texan (Taco)	150	5	18

Original Crust ~ Add 90 Cals and 18 g Carb to Thin Crust
Skillet Crust ~ Add 90 Cals & and 12g Carb to Thin Crust
For Complete Menu & Data ~ see CalorieKing.com

Pollo Tropical® ~ See CalorieKing.com

Popeye's® (Oct '12)

Chicken Pieces: Mild & Spicy With Skin

Breast, average	430	27	14
Leg, average	165	10	5
Thigh, average	270	20	8
Wing, average	210	14	8
Nuggets: 4 pieces, 1.75 oz	150	9	10
6 Pieces 2.65 oz	230	14	14
Tenders: Mild, 3 pieces, 4.45 oz	340	14	26
Spicy, 3 pieces, 4,45 oz	310	15	16
Louisiana Leaux:			
Baguette (1)	90	2	18
Green Beans: Regular, 3.5 oz	40	1.5	6
Large, 10 oz	120	4.5	18
Get Up & Geaux Kid's Meal	260	5	32
Naked BBQ Chicken Po'Boy	340	7	49
Naked Chicken Wrap	200	6	22
Sandwiches & Wraps: *Each*			
Chicken & Sausage Jambalaya	220	11	20
Chicken Po'Boy	660	34	61
Chicken Livers	1190	80	65
Loaded Chicken Wrap	310	13	33
Seafood: Catfish Fillets, 5 oz	460	29	27
Butterfly Shrimp (8)	290	17	21

Popeye's® ... cont (Oct '12)

Sides:

	C	F	Cb
Biscuit, 2 oz	260	15	26
Cajun Fries, regular, 3 oz	260	14	30
Cajun Rice, regular, 4.34 oz	170	5	25
Cole Slaw, regular, 4.87 oz	220	15	19
Corn on the Cob (1), 7.75 oz	190	2	37
Mashed Potatoes, regular, 5 oz	110	4	18
Onion Rings (12)	560	38	50
Red Beans & Rice, regular, 5.15 oz	230	14	23
Breakfast:			
Biscuits: Bacon	400	25	37
Chicken	490	26	47
Egg	510	29	41
Egg & Sausage	690	45	43
Sausage	540	36	41
Sausage & Gravy	510	33	42
Grits	370	5	80
Hashbrowns	360	20	41
Desserts:			
Hot Sweet Potato Pie 3.35 oz	350	19	41
Mardi Gras Cheesecake, 3 oz	310	19	32
Mississippi Mud Pie, 3 oz	280	7	51
Sliced Pecan Pie, 3.35 oz	410	21	52

Port of Subs® (Oct '12)

Figures Based on West Coast Outlets

	C	F	Cb

Cold Submarine S'wiches: Per 5" Sub with Cheese, Lettuce, Tomato Vinegar, Oil, Salt & Oregano

	C	F	Cb
#1 Ham, Salami, Capicolla & Pepperoni with Provolone	435	18	42
#2 Ham & Turkey, with Provolone	355	9	42
#3 Salami & Turkey, with Provolone	390	13	43
#4 Ham & Salami with Provolone	385	14	42
#5 Smkd Ham & Turkey, with Chedd.	370	10	43
#6 Vegetarian, with 3 Cheeses	450	21	45
#7 Roast Beef, with Provolone	365	10	42
#8 Turkey, with Provolone	360	8	44
#10 Rstd Chicken Brst, w/ Provolone	350	8	42
#11 Ham, with American Cheese	405	14	41
#12 Salami, with Provolone	395	16	42
#13 Peppered Pastrami Turkey Swiss	375	12	43
#15 Salami & Pepperoni, w/ Provolone	405	18	42
#16 BLT Sandwich	470	26	39
#17 Tuna, with Provolone	475	25	43
#18 Rst Beef & Turkey, w/ Provolone	360	9	43

Continued Next Page...

Updated Nutrition Data ~ www.CalorieKing.com
Persons with Diabetes ~ See Disclaimer (Page 22)

Port of Subs® ... cont (Oct '12)

Figures Based on West Coast Outlets **C** **F** **Cb**
Light Submarine S'wiches: Per 5" Sub,
(318 Calories or less) w/out Cheese, Oil or Mayo

	C	F	Cb
#2 Ham Turkey	305	5	47
#5 Smoked Ham & Turkey	318	6	43
#6 Vegetarian	248	5	42
#7 Roast Beef	314	6	42
#8 Turkey	310	5	44
#9 Peppered Pastrami	267	4	41
#10 Roasted Chicken Breast	300	4	42
#18 Roast Beef & Turkey	312	5	43

Wraps: With 12" Flour Tortilla, Cheese, Lettuce,
Tomato, Onion, Vinegar, Oil, Salt & Oregano

	C	F	Cb
#4 Ham, Salami, with Provolone	600	28	56
#8 Turkey, with Provolone	565	21	59
#11 Ham, with American Cheese	615	27	58

Fresh Salads: With Lettuce, Tomato & Onion, w/o Dressing

	C	F	Cb
Caesar: With Parmesan, 6 oz	35	0	11
Add Grilled Chicken, 10 oz	190	3	10
Chefs, 11 oz	300	18	10
Garden, 10 oz	70	2	11
Grilled Chicken, 10 oz	190	3	10
Tuna, 9 oz	250	18	9

Salad Dressings: Per 1.5 oz package

	C	F	Cb
Blue Cheese	220	23	2
Ranch	260	28	2
Fat Free Ranch	50	0	13

Sides: Per Regular, 8 oz

	C	F	Cb
Caesar Bow Tie Pasta Salad, 8 oz	355	18	37
Potato Salad	325	13	52

Desserts:

	C	F	Cb
Brownie, 4.5 oz	535	12	96
Chocolate Chunk Cookie, 4.5 oz	560	29	72

Pret A Manger® (Oct '12)

Baguettes: Per Pack **C** **F** **Cb**

	C	F	Cb
Balsamic Tuna, Tomato & Avocado	600	20	85
Chicken Mozzarella	590	18	82
Ham & Cheese	600	20	77

Slim: Brie, Basil & Tomato

	C	F	Cb
Slim: Brie, Basil & Tomato	345	14	41
Roasted Beef, Arugula & Parm.	290	9	28

Hot Food: Per Pack

	C	F	Cb
Toasties: Ham, Cheese & Mustard	540	26	44
Mozzarella & Pesto	400	16	48
Wraps: BBQ Pulled Pork	470	16	60
Buffalo Chicken	390	20	41

Sandwiches: Per Pack

	C	F	Cb
California Club	570	28	54
Chicken & Bacon	470	18	59
Tuna Salad	560	29	46
Slims: California Club	285	14	27
Chicken & Bacon	235	9	30
Chicken, Avocado & Balsamic	265	12	29

Pret A Manger® ... cont (Oct '12)

Wraps: Per Pack **C** **F** **Cb**

	C	F	Cb
Avocado Pine Nut	440	26	41
Crunchy Veggie	370	15	49
Roasted Turkey Caesar Salad	430	20	33
Roasted Turkey, Basil & Hummus	390	14	40
Spicy Shrimp & Cilantro	290	7	34

Soups: Per Medium Size Pack

	C	F	Cb
Broccoli & Cheddar	465	35	23
Carrot Ginger	165	7	27
Chicken Noodle	135	3	14
Chicken Tortilla	210	5	26
Chkn, Cilantro & White Bean Chili	465	21	36
Split Pea, with Ham	315	7	47

Salads: Per Pack, Without Dressing

	C	F	Cb
Chicken & Avocado	440	28	43
Chicken Caesar	420	16	23
Farmers Market	260	12	34
Lentil & Couscous Pot	100	4	14
Tuna Nicoise	290	15	13

Breakfast: Per Pack

	C	F	Cb
Baguettes: Cream Cheese	270	9	39
Egg & Bacon	370	17	37
Egg & Roasted Tomato	360	16	42
Oatmeal, regular, per pack	145	2	27

Bakery: Per Pack

	C	F	Cb
Cake: Carrot	370	26	29
Decadent Chocolate	300	16	34
Croissants: Plain	300	16	32
Almond	410	23	41
Pain au Chocolat	300	15	34
Muffins: Blueberry	450	24	56
Cranberry Orange	370	12	62

Beverages: Per Container

	C	F	Cb
Grapefruit Juice	100	0	23
Lemonade	110	0	29

Pretzelmaker® (Oct '12)

Pretzels: Per Serving **C** **F** **Cb**

	C	F	Cb
Bites: Plain, salted, large, 3.5 oz	250	1	52
Cinnamon Sugar, 3.8 oz	330	4	65
Pretzel Dogs: Mini (6)	300	19	23
Jalapeno	410	19	32
Pretzels: Caramel Crunch, 4.2 oz	300	4	58
Cinnamon Sugar, 3.88 oz	330	4	65
Garlic; Salted, average, 4.2 oz	310	4	60
Iced Cinnamon Swirl, 3.88 oz	330	4	65
Ranch, 4.2 oz	320	4.5	60
Unsalted, 4.2 oz	280	1	59

Continued Next Page...

Pretzelmaker® cont... (Oct '12)

Sauces: *Per Single Portion*

	C	F	Cb
Caramel	140	0	35
Cheddar Cheese	80	5	4
Cream Cheese	200	20	2
Honey Mustard	80	0	20
Icing	180	0	45
Ketchup	20	0	4
Mustard	10	0	1
Nacho Cheese	80	5	4
Pizza	20	0.5	6

Beverages: *Per 20 fl.oz Unless Indicated*

Blended Drinks:

	C	F	Cb
Cool Cappuccino	640	21	107
Lemon Twist	540	16	99
Mango Madness	520	16	89
Mocha Mania	620	20	106
Power Pomegranate	490	16	86
Strawberry Bananza	650	20	115
Lemonade, Original, 44 fl oz	380	0	91

Qdoba® (Oct '12)

Burritos:

	C	F	Cb

Each, with Flour Tortilla, Cilantro-Lime Rice, Black Beans, Salsa Verde, Sour Cream and Shredded Cheese

	C	F	Cb
Grilled Chicken	1100	39	126
Ground Beef	1150	45	127
Pulled Pork	1070	33	135

Signature Flavors: *With Flour Tortilla and Sauce*

		C	F	Cb
Ancho Chile BBQ, w/ Pulled Pork	555	14	78
Fajita Ranchera, w/ Gr. Chicken	535	18	58
Grilled Veggie	360	10	57
Queso, with Grilled Chicken	585	25	55

Grilled Quesadillas: *Each, With Flour Tortilla, Cheeses, Sour Cream and Guacamole*

	C	F	Cb
Grilled Chicken	1090	65	62
Shredded Beef	1090	62	63

3-Cheese Nachos: *Per Serving, With 3-Cheese Queso, Salsa Roja And Tortilla Chips*

	C	F	Cb
Grilled Chicken	960	52	86
Ground Beef	1010	58	87
Pulled Pork	930	46	95

Qdoba® cont... (Oct '12)

Tacos: *Each, With Lettuce, Cheese & Sour Cream*

	C	F	Cb
Crispy: Grilled Chicken	200	12	9
Ground Beef	215	15	10
Pulled Pork	185	10	12
Shredded Beef	195	12	11

Taco Salads: *With Lettuce, Black Bean & Corn Salsa, Fat Free Picante Ranch & Crunchy Flour Tortilla Bowl*

	C	F	Cb
Grilled Chicken	695	33	65
Ground Beef	745	39	66

Chips & Dip: *Includes Tortilla Chips*

	C	F	Cb
3- Cheese Queso	750	42	81
Guacamole & Salsa Roja	765	40	92

Breakfast Items: *With Flour Tortilla*

Breakfast Burrito: *Chorizo, Egg & Potato:*

	C	F	Cb
With 3-Cheese Queso Sauce	840	40	74
With Cheese & Ranchera Sauce	980	50	74

Quizno's Subs® (Oct '12)

Subs: *Per Regular, with Standard Menu Toppings on White Italian Roll*

	C	F	Cb
All Natural Chicken:			
Baja Chicken	970	47	82
California Chicken Club	870	40	75
Chicken Carbonara	920	44	69
Mesquite Chicken	850	38	72
Deli Style:			
Classic Italian	850	45	72
Honey Bacon Club	770	33	81
Meatball	950	56	77
The Traditional	720	32	72
Turkey Bacon Guacamole	850	42	77
Ultimate Turkey Club	730	31	71
Savory Steak:			
Double Cheese Prime Rib	810	38	75
French Dip	880	48	74
Peppercorn Prime Rib	810	42	72
Prime Rib Philly	890	45	80

Sliders: *Per Slider with Base Toppings, without Cheese or Dressings*

	C	F	Cb
Beef, Bacon & Cheddar	260	11	25
BLT Classic	220	9	24
Meatball	360	21	28
Smokey Chipotle Turkey	250	12	24
Turkey Club	250	10	25

Grilled Flatbreads: *Per Small*

	C	F	Cb
Basil Pesto Chicken	380	16	33
Chicken Bacon Ranch	460	23	34
Greek Chicken	430	21	34
Little Italy	480	28	33
Sonoma Turkey	360	15	35

Continued Next Page...

Updated Nutrition Data ~ www.CalorieKing.com
Persons with Diabetes ~ See Disclaimer (Page 22)

Quizno's Subs® cont... (Oct '12)

Wraps: Includes Dressing	C	F	Cb
Cobb	930	60	66
Honey Mustard Chicken	1030	64	80

Fresh Farmer Market Salads: Per Large, with Dressing			
Honey Mustard Chicken	720	56	27
Peppercorn Caesar, with Chicken	740	62	15

Savory Soups: Per Small Bowl, with 2 Crackers			
Broccoli Cheese	180	9	17
Chicken Noodle	140	4.5	19

Desserts: Chocolate Brownie	400	20	54
Cinnamon Sugar Cookie	510	22	73
Ultimate Choc. Chunk Cookie	500	24	68
Marshmallow Treat	340	8	66

Rally's/Checkers® (Oct '12)

Burgers/Sandwiches:	C	F	Cb
Bacon Dble Cheeseburger, w/ Chse	650	42	32
Big Buford	570	36	31
Cheese Double Cheese	510	31	31
Chili Cheeseburger	320	15	30
Rallyburger	390	22	32

Classic Wings: Extra Hot, 5 pieces	355	21	2
Honey BBQ, 5 pieces	390	17	18
Parmesan Garlic, 5 pieces	480	35	1

Fries:			
Chili Cheese, 7.75 oz	550	34	48
French: Medium, 4.25 oz	420	27	40
Large, 6 oz	590	38	57

Ranch 1® (Oct '12)

Sandwiches:	C	F	Cb
Chicken & Cheese	390	12	40
Chicken Philly, 9.25 oz	410	13	40
Original: Crispy Chicken, 11.5 oz	640	31	60
Crispy Spicy Chicken, 11.5 oz	470	9	68
Grilled Spicy Chicken, 10.25 oz	360	7	46

Bowls:			
Chicken Fajita, 10 oz	540	24	53
Chicken Platter, with Rice, 11.85 oz	270	6	28
Popcorn Chicken: Small, 5.5 oz	310	10	30
Large, 7.5 oz	420	14	40
Kids, 2 oz	120	4	11

Salads: Completed			
Grilled Chicken Caesar, 13.25 oz	430	30	14
Southwest Chicken, 17.5 oz	680	43	44

Fries: Medium, 5.75 oz	380	19	43
Large, 8 oz	530	27	58
Kids, 4.25 oz	280	15	31
Cheese: Medium, 7.3 oz	490	27	46
Large, 11 oz	760	44	66

Red Hot & Blue® (Oct '12)

Entrees: Per Serving	C	F	Cb
Delta Double: With Memphis Chkn	900	54	12
With Pulled Pork	793	60	9
Five Meat Treat	935	63	15
Ribs, Half Slab: Dry	935	72	14
Sweet	950	71	22

BBQ Sandwiches: Regular, Without Sides			
Beef Brisket	390	15	37
Carolina Chopped Pork	360	14	34
Pulled Pork	370	15	37

Salads: Without Dressing			
Grilled Chicken Caesar	770	46	47
RH & B Chopped Salad	850	42	55
Smokehouse Salad	670	36	36
Southern Fried Chicken	710	31	60

Soup, Memphis Corn Chowder, 1 bowl	270	12	23

Sides: BBQ Beans	255	2	48
Mashed Potatoes with Gravy	310	14	44
Potato Salad	405	28	33

Red Lobster® (Oct '12)

Lunch Menu: Without Condiments, Dipping Sauces Or Optional Side Dishes.

Seaside Starters:	C	F	Cb
Chilled Jumbo Shrimp Cocktail	120	0.5	4
Crispy Calamari & Vegetables	1520	97	115
Grilled Shrimp Bruschetta	650	26	58
Lobster Pizza	720	30	69
Pan Seared Crab Cakes	280	14	13
Parrot Isle Jumbo Coconut Shrimp	530	36	34
Shrimp Nachos	1090	64	94

Classics:			
Cajun Chicken Linguini Alfredo	780	39	56
Crunchy Popcorn Shrimp	280	14	26
Garlic Shrimp Scampi	130	8	0
Sailor's Platter	330	10	8
Seafood Stuffed Fish	160	5	6

Lighthouse/Fresh Fish Menu: Includes Broccoli			
Rainbow Trout, half portion	220	10	6
Salmon, half portion	270	9	6
Tilapia, half portion	210	3	9

Signature Combinations:			
Admiral's Feast	1280	73	92
Broiled Seafood Platter	300	10	9
Seaside Shrimp Trio	1060	54	78
Ultimate Feast	600	28	25

Continued Next Page...

Red Lobster® cont... (Oct '12)

Dinner Menu: Without Condiments, Dipping Sauces Or Optional Side Dishes.

Starters:	C	F	Cb
Crispy Calamari & Vegetables	1520	97	115
Golden Onion Rings	1430	100	121
Grilled Shrimp Bruschetta	650	26	58
Mozzarella Cheesesticks	680	39	49
Parrot Isle Jumbo Coconut Shrimp	530	36	34
Shrimp Nachos	1090	64	94
Soups: Per Cup			
Lobster Bisque	210	14	12
New England Clam Chowder	230	17	13
Seafood Gumbo	230	8	25
Lobster & Crab Entrees:			
Crab Linquine Alfrado, full serve	1120	50	95
Live Maine Lobster, steamed, 1.25 lb	230	1.5	0
Lobster & Shrimp Pasta, full serve	1020	50	86
Rock Lobster Tail	170	1	1
Snow Crab Legs Meat, 3.5 oz	180	2	0
Shrimp Entrees:			
Walt's Favorite Shrimp	550	30	39
Crunchy Popcorn Shrimp	560	27	51
Side Dishes: Baked Potato	220	1	47
Coleslaw	200	15	13
Creamy Lobster Mashed Potatoes	370	22	30
Fresh Broccoli	45	0.5	6
Fries	330	17	40
Home-Style Mashed Potatoes	210	10	27
Wild Rice Pilaf	180	3	34
Salads: Includes Dressing			
Caesar Salad: With Chicken	670	52	14
With Shrimp	620	51	14
Dipping Sauces: Per 1.5 oz			
Cocktail Sauce	40	0	9
Honey Mustard	280	26	12
Tartar Sauce	190	19	6
100% Pure Melted Butter	350	38	2
Desserts:			
Carrot Cake	600	36	63
Chocolate Wave	1490	81	172
Key Lime Pie	580	22	88
New York-Style Cheesecake			
with Strawberries	520	36	39
Warm Apple Crostada	670	32	85
Warm Chocolate Chip Lava Cookie	1070	51	142

For Complete Nutritional Data ~ see CalorieKing.com

Red Robin® (Oct '12)

Nutritional Information varies between restaurants. Please refer to Red Robin's website for further information

Appetizers: Per Whole Dish, with Standard Components	C	F	Cb
Garden Fresh Hummus Plate	775	41	82
Guacamole, Salsa & Chips	555	31	63
Jump Starters:			
Cheese Sticks, with Marinara Sce	605	33	49
Jalepeno Coins, fried, w/o Sauce	490	31	47
Onion Rings, without Sauce	520	28	62
Sweet Potato Fries, w/o Sauce	855	44	105
RR's Buzzard Wings,			
w/ Celery & Bleu Cheese Dress.	1395	114	5
Three For All, with condiments	1630	104	150
Towering Onion Rings,			
w/ Ranch Dressing & Mayo	1935	131	169
Triple S Riblets, w/ Fries & Sauce	995	49	82
Entrees: With Standard Components			
Arctic Cod Fish & Chips	1120	67	84
Clucks & Fries: Regular Style	1025	75	40
Buffalo Style	1270	103	40
Clucks & Shrimp Combo	1040	69	67
Ensenada Chicken Platter, 2 pieces	440	17	11
Prime Rib Dip	1020	58	73
Red's Nantucket Seafood Scatter	1245	75	97
Shrimp & Cod Duo	1425	83	134
Triple S Riblets & Clucks Combo	1255	69	80
Triple S Riblets, w/ Mac & Cheese	1905	116	119
Gourmet Burgers: With Standard Components			
A.1. Peppercorn	1070	61	73
All American Patty Melt	1355	100	66
Bleu Ribbon	1040	58	74
Burnin' Love	830	43	61
Guacamole Bacon	935	56	55
Prime Chophouse	1005	54	74
Royal Red Robin	1195	84	53
Sauteed 'Shroom	850	48	57
The Banzai	960	55	72
Whiskey River BBQ, with Beef	1145	70	77
Sandwiches: Per Sandwich			
Baja Turkey Club	735	47	29
Chicken: Bruschetta	615	27	45
California	745	37	53
Crispy	910	54	71
Simply Grilled	410	7	51
Teriyaki	795	39	66

Continued Next Page... ...

Red Robin® cont... (Oct '12)

Wraps: With Standard Components

	C	F	Cb
Caesar's Chicken	790	43	54
Whiskey River BBQ Chicken	1065	62	71

Soups:

	C	F	Cb
Chicken Tortilla:			
1 Cup	280	11	29
1 Bowl	560	21	61
Clam Chowder:			
1 Cup	350	21	25
1 Bowl	695	43	50
Roasted Vegetables:			
1 Cup	120	3	17
1 Bowl	250	7	36

Salads: Without Dressings or Bread

	C	F	Cb
Apple Harvest Chicken	410	19	25
Avo Cobb-O	550	30	17
Crispy Chicken Tender	875	53	41
Simply Grilled Chicken	370	14	20
Southwest Grilled Chicken, w/ Strips	710	35	46
Whiskey River BBQ Chicken, w Strips	715	31	63

Desserts:

	C	F	Cb
Gooey Chocolate Brownie Cake	820	31	133
Mountain High Mudd Pie	1370	61	187
Sundaes: Birthday	375	19	49
Hot Fudge	785	36	110
Nestle Tollhouse Cookie	700	33	99

Roly Poly® (Oct '12)

Wraps:

Per 6" White Tortilla Unless Indicated

Ham & Smoked Pork:

	C	F	Cb
Italian Classic	335	12	32
Key West Cuban Mix	330	9	44
Peachtree Melt	310	11	27
Pork Melt	310	11	26
Porky's Nightmare	320	12	28
Chicken: Basil Cashew Chicken	300	10	30
Catalina Chicken	315	11	28
Chicken Caesar	310	11	30
Chicken Fajita	315	9	28
Cobb Salad	255	12	27
Oriental Chicken	270	4	29
Santa Fe Chicken	305	11	28
Tuna: Classic Tuna Melt	340	17	26
Popeyes Tuna on Wheat	305	11	31
Texas Tuna Melt	310	11	30
Thai Hot Tuna	340	11	30
Turkey: California	330	12	31
Tuscan	220	2	31

Round Table Pizza® (Oct '12)

Appetizers:

	C	F	Cb
Buffalo Wings, 6 pieces	420	30	6
Garlic Bread, 6 pieces	420	21	54
With Cheese, 6 pieces	600	36	54
Garlic Parmesan Twists, 3 pieces	510	15	78
Honey BBQ Wings, 6 pieces	480	27	12

Pizzas: Per ½ of Large 14" Pizza

Original Crust: Cheese

	C	F	Cb
Cheese	230	9	25
Chicken & Garlic Gourmet	250	11	25
Chicken Smokehouse	270	12	26
Gourmet Veggie	240	10	27
Guinevere's Garden Delight	220	8	26
Hawaiian	220	8	27
Italian Garlic Supreme	270	14	25
King Arthur Supreme	270	13	26
Maui Zaui, with Polynesian Sce	260	10	29
Montague's All Meat Marvel	290	15	25
Pepperoni	240	11	24
Smokehouse Combo	290	14	26

Pan Crust: Cheese

	C	F	Cb
Cheese	300	11	38
Chicken & Garlic Gourmet	340	13	39
Chicken Smokehouse	360	14	40
Gourmet Veggie	320	12	41
Guinevere's Garden Delight	300	10	39
Hawaiian	300	10	40
Italian Garlic Supreme	360	16	39
King Arthur Supreme	340	14	39
Maui Zaui w/ Polynesian Sauce	340	12	43
Montague's All Meat Marvel	360	15	38
Pepperoni	320	13	38

Skinny Crust: Cheese

	C	F	Cb
Cheese	190	9	18
Chicken & Garlic Gourmet	220	11	18
Chicken Smokehouse	240	12	19
Gourmet Veggie	200	10	20
Guinevere's Garden Delight	180	8	19
Hawaiian	190	8	20
Italian Garlic Supreme	240	14	18
King Arthur Supreme	240	13	19
Maui Zaui w/ Polynesian Sauce	220	10	22
Montague's All Meat Marvel	260	15	18
Pepperoni	210	11	18

Sandwiches:

	C	F	Cb
Chicken Club	800	43	59
Ham Club	740	40	60
RT Veggie	630	32	65
Turkey Club	720	38	59
Turkey Sante-Fe	730	40	57

For Complete Nutritional Data ~ see CalorieKing.com

Rubio's Mexican Grill® (Oct '12)

Burritos: Each, with Flour Tortilla, **C** **F** **Cb**
without Chips

	C	F	Cb
Baja: Grilled Chicken	630	28	55
Steak	650	32	55
Bean & Cheese	760	37	78
Beer-Battered Fish	810	48	70
Grilled: Mesquite Shrimp	730	34	75
Ono	700	31	76
Veggie	770	35	83
Burrito Especial: Chicken	820	31	102
Steak	840	34	102
Health Mex,			
Chicken, w/ whole grain tortilla	500	9	74
Nachos: Regular	1270	78	112
With Chicken	1340	78	114
Quesadillas: Three Cheese	1120	70	87
Three Cheese Chicken	1200	70	89

Tacos: Each, Corn Tortilla

	C	F	Cb
Grilled Gourmet: Chicken	320	17	24
Steak	330	19	24
Street: Carnitas	100	4	8
Grilled Chicken	90	2.5	9
From The Sea: Blackened Ono	230	10	26
Chili-Lime Wild Salmon	230	9	25
Fish: Original	300	17	27
Especial	360	22	29
Gr. Gourmet Garlic Herb Shrimp	340	19	23
Salsa Verde Pan-Seared Shrimp	260	13	22
Smoky Red Chile Hand-Battered,			
Shrimp Taco	310	15	31

Two Taco Plate: With Corn Tortilla, Pinto Beans & Rice

	C	F	Cb
Blackened/Grilled Ono, average	700	21	97
Garlic Herb Shrimp Grilled Gourmet	900	41	93

Salads: Includes Dressing/Sauce

	C	F	Cb
Chicken Balsamic & Roasted Vege	310	11	29
Chicken Chipotle Ranch	450	31	22
Chicken Chopped	460	24	36
Chicken Grilled Grande Bowl	630	27	62

Salsas: Per 1 oz

	C	F	Cb
Picante	20	1	2
Other Varieties	5	0	1
Dessert, Churro, 1.5 oz	170	8	22

Ruby Tuesday® (Oct '12)

Shareables: Per Serve, w/out Sauce **C** **F** **Cb**

	C	F	Cb
Asian Dumplings	115	5	12
Fried Mozzarella	100	4	10
Jumbo Lump Crab Cake	70	4	4
Southwestern Spring Rolls	160	8	18
Spinach Artichoke Dip	310	19	27

Burgers: Without Sides

	C	F	Cb
Handcrafted: Alpine Swiss	995	65	55
Avocado Turkey Burger	910	54	59
Boston Blue	1145	72	77
Buffalo Chicken Burger	755	39	69
Chicken BLT	765	38	69
Triple Prime: Burger	875	56	54
Bacon Cheddar	1095	75	54
Cheddar	1035	70	54
Ruby's Classic	855	55	52
Smokehouse	1155	73	77
Turkey Burger	740	41	58

Fit & Trim Choices: Includes Menu Set Sides

	C	F	Cb
BBQ Grilled Chicken	345	9	23
Chicken Bella	455	22	15
Creole Catch	335	15	9
Grilled Salmon	410	24	10
Top Sirloin	425	25	12

Fork-Tender Ribs: Without Sides

	C	F	Cb
Asian Sesame Glazed, Half	515	30	17
Classic BBQ, Half	500	24	29
Memphis Dry Rub, Half	460	29	6

Premium Seafood: Without Sides

	C	F	Cb
Asian Glazed Salmon	455	27	15
Crab Cake Dinner	270	17	14
Creole Catch	240	10	0
Herb-Crusted Tilapia	400	24	11
Jamaican Jerk Shrimp on Rice Pilaf	540	7	89
Jumbo Skewered Shrimp	240	19	0
Salmon Florentine	460	29	7
Tilapia Trio on Rice Pilaf	985	48	66

Smart Eating,

	C	F	Cb
Grilled Chicken Wrap, w/o sides	495	17	47

Steakhouse Steaks: Without Sides

	C	F	Cb
Rib Eye	910	71	7
Top Sirloin	335	19	3
Triple Pime Meatloaf	560	34	37

Continued Next Page...

Ruby Tuesday® cont... (Oct '12)

Pasta Classics: Without Sides

	C	F	Cb
Chicken & Broccoli	1475	92	93
Chicken & Mushroom Alfredo	1195	64	87
Lobster Carbonara	1405	95	80
Parmesan Chicken	1345	74	110
Spaghetti Squash Marinara	260	11	32

Dressing: Per 1 oz

	C	F	Cb
Balsamic Vinaigrette	40	2	5
Blue Cheese	180	19	1
Honey Mustard	90	8	5
Italian	130	14	1
Ranch	90	9	1
Signature Parmesan	150	16	1
Thousand Island	80	7	5

Fresh, Fresh Sides:

	C	F	Cb
Baked Potato: Plain	260	2	52
Loaded Baked Potato	570	28	54
Creamy Mashed Cauliflower	135	8	14
French Fries	395	18	55
Garlic Cheese Biscuit	110	5	12
Onion Rings	340	19	37
Rice Pilaf	160	3	30
Sauteed Baby Portob. Mushrooms	140	10	6
White Cheddar Mashed Potatoes	290	17	29

Kid's Menu: Includes Set Menu Sides

	C	F	Cb
Chicken Breast	290	12	22
Chicken Tenders	465	22	31
Chop Steak	495	34	22
Fried Shrimp	475	25	45
Grilled Cheese	655	28	78

Desserts: Blondie for One

	C	F	Cb
Desserts: Blondie for One	540	23	77
Cakes: Double Chocolate	795	31	119
Italian Cream Cake	990	56	110
Cookies: Chocolate Chip	180	9	24
White Choc. Macadamia Nut	200	12	23
Cupcakes: Carrot Cake (1)	325	16	45
Red Velvet (1)	285	11	45
Tiramisu	535	28	65

For Complete Menu ~ see CalorieKing.com

Runza® (Oct '12)

Burgers:

	C	F	Cb
¼ lb Bacon Cheeseburger	510	31	26
¼ lb French Onion	490	29	25
¼ lb Legend Supreme	520	32	26
¼ lb Swiss Mushroom	480	29	24
Runza Way: ¼ lb Cheeseburger	410	22	27
½ lb Double Cheeseburger	670	39	29
¼ lb Hamburger	360	18	25
Junior: Cheeseburger	250	13	18
Cheeseburger Runza	270	13	21
Swiss Cheese Mushroom	300	17	18

Sandwiches:

	C	F	Cb
BBQ Chicken, grilled	390	9	46
Buffalo Chicken, grilled	350	10	36
Cheese Runza	580	24	69
Deluxe Chicken, grilled	360	11	37
Runzas: Original	530	20	67
Swiss Cheese Mushroom	630	28	68
Mini Runzas: Original	270	10	34
Cheeze	290	12	35
Onion Rings: Medium	320	19	35
Large	550	31	58
French Onion Dip, 2 oz	100	7	4

Salads:

	C	F	Cb
Asian Griled Chicken w/ dressing	400	6	58
Southwest Chicken Salad w/ Salsa	320	15	29
Sweet Berry Chicken w/o dressing	360	19	18
Dressings: Honey Mustard	310	28	14
Ranch	260	27	4

Soups: Per Bowl

	C	F	Cb
Chicken Noodle	290	8	33
Homemade Chili	320	17	22
Tomato Florentine	110	1	21
Vegetable Beef	110	3.5	13
Vegetable Cheese	190	11	14

Kids Meals: Includes Small Fries, Without Drink

	C	F	Cb
Junior: Cheeseburger, plain	250	13	18
Cheeseburger, Runza Way	270	13	21
Hamburger, plain, small	480	20	45
Swiss Cheese Mushroom	300	17	18

Desserts,

	C	F	Cb
Ice Cream, all flavors, 1 dish	230	7	34
Shakes: Cappuccino, reg., 16 oz	490	12	82
Vanilla, regular, 16 oz	430	12	66
Slushie, Pepsi	160	0	40

Ryan's Grill Buffet & Bakery® (Oct '12)
Entrees: Without Sides

	C	F	Cb
Beef: BBQ'd, 4 oz	140	5	16
Country Fried Steak, w/ gravy, 2.6 oz	220	13	16
Meatloaf, 3 oz	180	11	7
Perfect Pot Roast, 4.95 oz	160	7	9
Roasted, carved, 3 oz	230	15	0
Salisbury Steak, 3.53 oz	150	9	8
Chicken:			
Breasts: Country BBQ, 5.8 oz	310	16	6
Rotisserie, 5.3 oz	310	17	1
Traditional, Baked, 5.3 oz	310	17	0.5
Chicken & Dumplings, 4.95 oz	160	5	17
New Orleans Bourbon Street, 3 oz	180	8	9
Orange Chicken, 3 oz	340	22	26
Fish/Seafood: Baked Fish, 2 oz	90	4.5	0
Butter Crumb Alaskan Pollock, 1.75 oz	110	5	2
Butterfly Shrimp (6), 2.3 oz	210	9	24
Carved Salmon Filet, 3 oz	190	11	0
Clam Strips, 3 oz	320	20	28
Fried: Fish, 3 pieces, 3 oz	240	12	27
Shrimp (22), 3 oz	240	12	24
Wood Seared Salmon, 1 pce, 3 oz	220	16	0
Pasta/Spaghetti: *Per 4.95 oz Serving*			
Country Pasta Gratine	160	4	24
Creamy Penne Carbonara	260	17	17
Fire Grilled Chicken Alfredo	220	14	14
Grilled Italian Sausage Penne	180	11	14
Pork:			
Carved: Grilled Loin, 3 oz	140	10	0
Ham, 3 oz	100	5	0
Honey Glazed Baked, 1 sl, 3 oz	120	5	1
Ribs, BBQ/County-Style (3), 3.5 oz	420	27	15
Steak: Grilled, 2 oz	140	9	0
BBQ, grilled, 2 oz	150	9	3
Salads: *Without Dressing*			
Asian Chopped, 3.55 oz	90	4	13
Caesar, 1 cup, 2.5 oz	70	6	4
Greek, 2.65 oz	120	8	10
Seafood, 4.15 oz	310	26	15
Sides:			
Baked Potato, plain, 4.25 oz	150	0	36
BBQ Baked Beans, 3 oz	130	3	26
Cauliflower Au Gratin, 3 oz	50	2	8
French Fries, 2 oz	170	9	23
Fried Okra, 3 oz	220	12	28
Mashed Potatoes, 4 oz	70	0.5	13
Desserts: Cheesecake, plain, 1 sl.	230	12	28
Key Lime Pie, scratch, 1 sl., 2.5 oz	220	9	31
Lemon Meringue Pie, 2.25 oz	130	4.5	34

7-Eleven® (Oct '12)
7-Select Burritos:

	C	F	Cb
Bean and Cheese, 5 oz	320	10	47
Beef & Bean, 5 oz	360	16	44
Beef, Bean & Green Chile, 5 oz	360	15	44
Red Hot Beef, 5 oz	340	15	41
Bacon & Cheese Potato Stix, 3 oz	220	15	16
Bites: *Without Bun or Toppings*			
Big Bite Hot Dog, 2 oz	180	17	1
Breakfast Bite Sausage, 3 oz	250	21	2
Cheeseburger Bite Link, 4.2 oz	440	38	2
Qtr Pound Big Bite Hot Dog, 4 oz	360	34	2
Breakfast Sandwiches:			
Biscuits: Egg, Cheese & Ssg, 5.5 oz	460	32	31
Sausage, 3.3 oz	330	22	28
Croissant, Egg, Cheese & Ssg, 4.8 oz	410	30	20
Engl. Muffin, Egg, Chse & Ssg, 5 oz	390	25	24
Other Selections:			
Chicken Tender S'wich, 5.9 oz	350	8	45
Chicken Tenders (1), 3.3 oz	160	5	11
Maple Pancake Sausage (1), 2.6 oz	270	19	19
Pepperoni Pizza, 1 slice, 3.9 oz	300	14	30
Rollers: Buffalo Chicken (1), 3 oz	190	7	16
Corn Dog (1), 3.4 oz	320	21	23
Taquitos: *Per 1.3 oz Taquito*			
Bacon, Egg, Cheese & Potato	190	8	23
Jalapeno Cream Cheese	245	12	29
Monterey Jack & Chicken	280	14	30
Steak & Cheese	210	11	22
Wings: *Without Dipping Sauce*			
Boneless: Asian Habanero, 1 piece,	60	1	8
Buffalo, 1 piece, 1.1 oz	60	1.5	6
Bone In, Spicy Wing Zings, 1 wing	80	4.5	3
Sides: Hash Browns (1), 2 oz	100	5	12
Off the Shelf:			
Cupcakes: Choc. Crème Filled (1)	200	6	35
Orange Creme Filled (1), 2 oz	200	6	35
Cream Filled Cookie (1), av. all	150	6	22
Donuts: Choc. Covered (1), 1.9 oz	250	15	29
Minis: Chocolate (4)	310	19	34
Crunch (6), 3.5 oz	410	19	56
Powdered (6), 3 oz	370	18	48
Honey Buns: Glazed (1), 5 oz	620	35	70
Iced (1), 6 oz	820	58	68
Mini Muffins: Blueberry (1), 1 oz	70	4	7
Chocolate Chip (1)	80	4.5	8
Slurpees: *Average all flavors:*			
12 oz cup	95	0	26
22 oz cup	175	0	44
28 oz cup	220	0	56
Sugar Free, 12 oz cup	30	0	9

Saladworks® (Oct'12)

Salads: Without Dressing	C	F	Cb
Autumn Harvest	300	12	40
Bently	245	10	11
Buffalo Bleu	250	7.5	24
Chicken Caesar	285	4	19
Cobb	270	16	13
Fire Roasted Cabo Jack	390	19	31
Greek	185	10	18
Nuevo Nicoise	230	4	31
Sophie's Salad	310	14	35
Tivoli	430	19	31
Focaccia Fusion: Without Spread			
BLT	345	13	32
Chicken Monterey	385	12	35
Fajitalicious	380	12	33
Turkey Ranch	365	10	33
Dressings: Per 1 oz Ladle			
Balsamic: Regular	170	18	4
Fat Free	20	0	5
Classic French	130	12	6
Green Goddess	150	15	3
Oriental Sesame	90	4.5	12
Parmesan Caesar	150	17	1
Rustic Thousand Island	140	13	5

Extra Menu Items ~ See CalorieKing.com

Sandella's® (Oct'12)

	C	F	Cb
Grilled Flatbread: With Standard Toppings			
Brazilian Bacon	560	17	79
Brazilian Chicken	510	10	73
Pesto Chicken	610	28	56
Spinach & Bacon	660	39	52
Paninis: With Standard Toppings			
Chicken Delicato; Turkey Reuben, av.	490	16	53
Spinach, Ham & Swiss	550	20	61
Tuscan Chicken	540	21	55
Quesadillas: With Standard Toppings			
California; Chicken Fajita, average	505	23	53
Mediterranean	400	16	53
Salads: Includes ½ Flatbread & Dressing			
Fiesta	360	8	54
Greek	310	15	37
Rice Bowls: Includes Flatbread & Standard Toppings			
Black Bean & Rice	840	20	130
Chicken Fajita	750	20	104
Wraps: With Standard Toppings			
California Turke	410	10	55
Chicken Fajita	520	20	53
Pesto Turkey	460	15	54
Sweet & Spicy Chicken	400	7	64

Sarku Japan® (Oct'12)

D'Lite Meals:	C	F	Cb
Rice & Chicken Tempua, 15 oz	970	58	81
Rice & Shrimp Tempura, 11 oz	540	21	70
Vegetarian, 14 oz	360	0.5	79
Vegetarian Soba Noodle, 14 oz	710	24	106
Combos:			
Tempura: Chicken, 23 oz	1270	78	102
Chicken & Shrimp, 20 oz	980	53	95
Teriyaki: Beef, 19 oz	570	10	85
Beef & Shimp, 21 oz	630	11	85
Chicken, 22 oz	640	13	90
Chicken & Shrimp, 24 oz	700	14	90
Shrimp, 19 oz	500	2.5	83
Sauce, Teriyaki, 1.5 oz	45	0	9
Sides: Maki Roll, 2 oz	140	11	9
Rice: Steamed, 9 oz	290	0	64
Fried, 9 oz	330	4.5	62
Tempura Chicken, 1 piece, 2 oz	230	19	8
Tempura Shrimp, 1 piece, 0.8 oz	90	7	4

Schlotzsky's® (Oct'12)

	C	F	Cb
Oven-Toasted Sandwiches: Per Medium Size			
Angus: Beef & Provolone	750	29	80
Corned Beef	520	9	72
Corned Beef Reuben	880	37	79
Pastrami Reuben	880	37	79
Pastrami & Swiss	820	31	77
BLT	530	18	72
Chicken & Pesto	570	13	75
Chicken Breast	495	5	78
Chipotle Chicken	540	10	75
Homestyle Tuna	620	21	77
Santa Fe Chicken	655	21	72
Smoked Turkey Breast	485	7	76
Smoked Turkey Reuben	855	35	83
Turkey & Guacamole	520	10	77
Turkey Bacon Club	760	29	77
Original Style: The Original	775	34	76
Cheese	785	37	75
Deluxe	975	47	79
Ham & Cheese	725	26	79
Turkey	805	33	78
Wraps: Per Medium Size			
Chicken & Pesto	525	19	53
Homestyle Tuna	575	27	57
Santa Fe Chicken	610	25	54

Continued Next Page...

Schlotzsky's® cont... (Oct '12)

8" Pizzas: Per Pizza

	C	F	Cb
BBQ Chicken & Jalapeno	665	16	96
Chipotle Chicken	770	31	75
Combination Special	660	27	77
Double Cheese	595	22	74
Fresh Veggie	600	22	77
Grilled Chicken & Pesto	670	23	74
Pepperoni & Double Cheese	730	34	74
Smoked Turkey & Jalapeno	640	21	78

Salads: Without Dressing or Flatbread

	C	F	Cb
Cranberry, Apple, Pecan & Chicken	655	27	66
Hearts of Romaine, Chicken Caesar	415	18	26
Flat Bread, entree size, 4 slices	215	5	35
Garden	40	1	9
Potato	240	13	29
Turkey Avocado Cobb	600	32	40
Turkey Chef	415	24	16

Dressings: Per 3 oz

	C	F	Cb
Chunky Blue Cheese	455	49	3
Ranch, freshly prepared	325	33	5
Red Wine Vinaigrette	425	43	9
Robusto Italian	285	28	3
Tuscan Caesar	425	45	2

Soup: Per Bowl

	C	F	Cb
Broccoli Cheese	275	22	19
Chicken Tortilla	215	8	22
Timberline Chili	415	14	47
Tomato Basil	305	8	46

Chips:

	C	F	Cb
Baked: Regular; BBQ, average	140	3	25
Other varieties, average	220	12	25

Kid's Meals: Without Cookie or Drink

	C	F	Cb
Cheese Pizza	530	17	76
Cheese Sandwich	385	14	48
Ham & Cheese Sandwich	415	15	49
Pepperoni Pizza	580	22	76
Turkey Sandwich	335	6	50

Desserts:

	C	F	Cb
Brownie (1)	370	19	40
Carrot Cake, 1 slice	715	42	80
Creamy Cheesecake, 1 slice	540	33	50

Cookies: Per Cookie

	C	F	Cb
Choc./Fudge Choc. Chip, av.	160	7	23
Oatmeal Raisin; Sugar, average	150	6	24
Macadamia Nut	170	9	22

Second Cup® ~ see CalorieKing.com

Shakey's® (Oct '12)

Pizzas: Per Slice, ½ Large Pizza

	C	F	Cb
Cheese: Pan Crust	185	6	26
Thin Crust	150	5.5	18
Firehouse: Pan Crust	255	12	27
Thin Crust	220	12	19
Garden Veggie: Pan Crust	185	5.5	27
Thin Crust	150	5	19
Margherita: Pan Crust	175	5	26
Thin Crust	135	4.5	18
Rustic Garlic Chicken: Pan Crust	190	5.5	26
Thin Crust	155	5.5	18
Shakey's Special: Pan Crust	210	6.5	31
Thin Crust	195	10	18
Texas BBQ Chicken: Pan Crust	205	5	29
Thin Crust	170	5	21
Ultimate Meat: Pan Crust	280	14	26
Thin Crust	245	13	18
Additional Toppings: Beef	35	3	0
Cheese	15	1	0.5
Chicken	15	0.5	0
Pepperoni	25	2.5	0
Sausage	45	4	0.5

Shareables: Per Serving, Unless Indicated

	C	F	Cb
Chicken Strips (5)	620	31	48
Mojo Potatoes (5)	215	11	25
Mojo Supreme, serves 4-6	1950	120	160
Shakey's Spicy Wings (6)	495	29	27

Shakey's Famous Chicken: Per Piece

	C	F	Cb
Fried Chicken: Breast	475	26	16
Leg	170	19	6
Thigh	350	24	10
Wing	130	9	3.5

Shari's® (Oct '12)

Breakfast:

	C	F	Cb
Favorites:			
Farmhouse Biscuit Breakfast	1160	72	94
The Breakfast Sampler, with Butter Syrup	1460	84	133
Traditional Eggs Benedict, with Hashbrowns	810	46	61
Fruit Crepes: Apples	740	39	84
Burst O Berry	680	39	71
Omelettes: BMP	930	77	8
Denver; Spring Spinach, average	655	52	11
Fajita Chicken	700	52	13
Sauteed Shrimp & Cheese	590	39	8
Pancakes: B'milk, w/ Butter & Syrup	780	15	152
Shari's Potato Pancakes	570	17	96

Continued Next Page...

Shari's® cont... (Oct '12)

Breakfast (Cont):

	C	**F**	**Cb**
Specialties:			
Biscuits & Country Gravy: W/ Bacon	820	50	68
With Sausage	970	66	68
Classic Quiche: BMP	810	50	68
Lorraine; Three Cheese & Ham, av.	815	50	69
Vegetables	780	46	72
Meat Lover's Skillet, w/o side choices	1140	91	34
Western Scramble	1020	78	32

Lunch:

NW Flame-Grilled Burgers: *Without Sides*			
Blue Mountain Bleu Cheese	890	56	47
Double R Ranch Bacon Chseburger	1200	70	51
Garlic-Mushroom Swiss	1050	75	49
Old-Fashioned: Classic Hamburger	600	29	47
Classic Cheeseburger	680	35	46
The Ranch Hand BBQ Bacon	1080	67	65
Flatbread Paninis: *Without Sides*			
All American	760	37	60
Classic Reuben	870	39	67
Quiche Platters: *Without Sides*			
BMP; Ham & Three Cheese, av.	565	38	39
Lorraine	590	40	39
Salads: *Entrée Size*			
American Chopped, w/o Dressing	640	31	43
Asian, w/ Orange Chicken & Dress.	1020	55	107
Classic Grilled Chicken Caesar,			
without Dressing	710	46	41
Sandwiches: *Per Whole Sandwich, Without Side Choices*			
Favorites: Applewood BLT	420	22	37
Bistro Deli, with Ham	350	6	46
Cranberry Pecan Chicken Salad	690	36	64
Handcrafted: Baja Chipotle Chicken	840	48	59
Cuban, on Ciabatta	620	30	45
Prime Rib Dip	820	51	47

Dinner:

Down-Home BBQ Favorite,			
Baby Back Ribs, as served	1470	63	123
Flame Grilled Beef: *With Toast & Onion Rings*			
Center Cut New York Strip Steak	970	64	39
T-Bone Steak, 16 oz	1130	67	41
USDA Top Sirloin	600	32	40
Flame Grilled Chicken: *As Served*			
Chicken Chimichurri	1100	67	87
Chicken Mozzarella Bruschetta	740	40	54
Chicken Penne Alfredo	1080	55	94
Homestyle Classic,			
Pot Roast & Veggies, as served	1300	75	60

Shari's® cont... (Oct '12)

Dinner (Cont):

	C	**F**	**Cb**
Seafood Favorites: *As Served*			
Alask. Cod & Shrimp Combo Platter	1540	89	148
Hand Cut Alaskan Cod & Chips	1220	77	111
Desserts:			
Classic Pies: *Per Slice, as Served*			
Banana Cream Dream	600	36	56
Chocolate Cream Supreme	590	33	67
Gourmet Pies: *Per Slice, As Served*			
Creamy Caramel Pecan Crunch	710	45	71
Peanut Butter Chocolate Silk	660	45	60
S'mores Galore	570	31	68
Velvet Chocolate Silk	640	46	55

Sheetz® (Oct '12)

Breakfast:

	C	**F**	**Cb**
Plain Bagel, W/out Add Ons Or Dressing Unless Indicated			
Shmagelz: Bacon & Egg	530	27	53
Egg & American Cheese	440	19	50
Egg, Ham & Provolone	525	21	55
Shmiscuitz: Bacon & Egg	540	35	39
Egg & American Cheese	450	27	36
Egg, Ham & Swiss Cheese	550	30	41
Egg, Sausage & Amer. Cheese	625	44	36
Shmuffins: Bacon & Egg	410	25	29
Egg & American Cheese	320	17	26
Egg & Ham	310	11	30
Egg, Sausage & Cheddar Cheese	495	34	26
Egg & Steak	395	16	27
Cold Subz: Per 6" White Sub, w/0 Add Ons or Dressing			
American Cheese	350	11	45
BLT	445	19	48
Chicken Salad	490	23	54
Roast Beef	280	4	46
Turkey	295	4	47
Hot Subz: Per 6" White Sub, W/out Add Ons or Dressing			
Chicken	360	6	45
Meatball	370	13	48
Pepperoni	440	20	45
Hot Dogz, with Chili & Onions	310	19	27
Nachoz, Bueno/Grande,			
with Nacho Cheese	515	23	65
Saladz: Without Dressing			
Chef, with Shredded Cheese	250	12	13
Crispy Chicken, w/ Shredded Chse	370	16	31
Garden, with Shredded Cheese	130	8	8
Steak	210	8	8
Taco, with Shredded Cheese	355	18	39

Continued Next Page...

Sheetz® cont... (Oct '12)

Add Ons:	C	F	Cb
Bacon	150	12	2
Black Olives	15	1	0.5
Cheeses: American; Cheddar; Swiss	110	9	0
Hot Pepper Provolone	100	8	1
Parmesan	5	0.5	0.5
Green/Jalapeno Peppers	5	0	0.5
Shredded Lettuce; Diced Onions, av.	5	0	1
Tomatoes, sliced	5	0.5	1
Dressings/Sauces:			
Honey Mustard	10	0	4
Italian Romano	60	6	2
Marinara	10	0.5	1
Mayo; Ranch, average	145	16	1
Sidez:			
Chili, Mac & Cheese, 6.7 oz	130	6	14
Cole Slaw, 5 oz	200	9	28
Fryz: Bag, 3.2 oz	160	6	23
Cup, 5 oz	260	10	36
Cheese, 14.4 oz	670	32	81
Smokehouse, 15.38 oz	985	53	103
Beverage, Hot Chocolate, medium	290	1	56

Sizzler® (Oct '12)

Burgers/Sandwiches:	C	F	Cb
Burgers: Mega Bacon Cheeseburger	1010	61	48
Sizzler Burger: ⅓ lb	620	30	47
½ lb	760	40	47
Sandwiches: Grilled Chicken Club	645	28	48
Malibu Chicken	705	37	59

Hot Entrees: *Without Sides, Dipping Sauces & Condiments, Unless Indicated*

	C	F	Cb
Chicken: Grilled Fettuccini Alfredo	1000	56	62
Hibachi Chicken (1)	180	4	7
Lemon-Herb Chicken (1)	170	6	0
Malibu Chicken (1)	360	25	11
Pork Chop, with Apple Sauce	420	27	15
Ribs: Half Rack	625	39	37
Full Rack	1155	79	51
Seafood:			
Grilled Salmon, with Rice Pilaf	530	20	40
Grilled Shrimp: Fettuccine Alfredo	985	55	64
Skewers (2), with Rice Pilaf	455	16	42
Steaks: Bacon Wrapped Sirloin	555	35	5
Classic, 8 oz	395	21	1
Chopped Steak, 8 oz	520	30	17
Petite (6 oz)	295	16	1
Rib Eye, 14 oz	1055	66	1
Steak Combos: Classic Trio	860	47	36
Steak & Lobster Tail	410	17	2

Sizzler® cont... (Oct '12)

Prepared Salads: *Per 4 oz Serving, Without Dressing*

	C	F	Cb
Seafood, 4 oz	160	11	11
Sicilian Pasta, 2 oz	65	4	6
Three Bean, 1 oz	25	1	5
Waldorf, 4 oz	130	8	16
Salad Dressings: *Per 2 Tbsp, 1 oz*			
Honey Mustard	110	8	9
Italian, Low Fat	40	3	3
Ranch	115	12	1
Signature Blue Cheese	105	11	1
Thousand Island	100	9	5
Sides:			
Baked Potato, plain	265	4	51
Broccoli, 5 oz	45	0	7
French Fries, 5 oz	285	13	42
Rice Pilaf, 5 oz	225	4	39

For Complete Menu & Data ~ see CalorieKing.com

Skyline Chili® (Oct '12)

Burritos:	C	F	Cb
Chili Burrito Deluxe	640	33	44
Vegetarian Black Bean Deluxe	700	32	73

Ways: *Per Regular Serving*

Spaghietti, Chili & Cheddar Cheese:

	C	F	Cb
3 Way	780	41	52
4 Way Onion	800	41	58
4 Way Bean	850	42	65
5 Way	870	42	70
Bowls: Coney	780	61	8
Loaded Chili	510	31	23
Vegetarian Black Beans & Rice	370	14	47
Chili Spaghetti, regular	440	13	51
Potatoes: 3-Way Potato	600	25	63
Cheddar Potato	700	42	61
Sour Cream Potato	520	28	61

Salads: *Without Dressing Unless Indicated*

	C	F	Cb
Buffalo Chicken	190	8	10
Garden, with Croutons	140	8	13
Greek, regular size, with dressing	380	37	7
Wraps:			
Buffalo Chicken, w/ Ranch Dress.	680	39	56
Classic Chkn w/ Chili Ranch Dress.	650	36	56
Greek Chicken, w/ Greek Dressing	670	38	58
Sides: Chicken, 2.5 oz	70	1	1
Crackers, 1 bowl	60	1.5	11
Fries: Chili Cheese	750	40	66
French	390	13	63

Smoothie King® (Oct '12)

Fruit Smoothies: Per 20 fl.oz Cup **C** **F** **Cb**
Figures Include Turbinado. Without Turbinado,
deduct 100 calories and 23 carbs.

	C	F	Cb
Get Energy: Acai Adventure	455	5	92
Green Tea Tango	260	3	46
Power Punch	430	1	101
Shape Up, High Protein Smoothies:			
Almond Mocha	365	9	42
Banana	320	9	32
Chocolate	365	9	42
Snack Right: Banana Berry Treat	365	0	86
Berry Punch	360	0	91
Fruit Fusion	355	1	76
Grape Expectations	400	0	95
Stay Healthy: Blueberry Heaven	340	1	73
Hearty Apple	405	1	86
Mangosteen Madness	385	0	94
Orange KA-BAM	465	0	117
Trim Down: Blackberry Dream	300	1	72
MangoFest	285	0	72
Passion Passport	395	0	96
Slim-N-Trim: Chocolate	295	2	57
Orange Vanilla	215	1	46
Strawberry	375	1	84
Strawberry Kiwi Breeze	375	0	90
The Shredder: Chocolate	310	3	36
Strawberry	355	1	56
Vanilla	285	2	30

32 fl.oz Cup: Multiply 20 fl.oz figures by 1.5
40 fl.oz Cup: Multiply 20 fl.oz figures by 2
Kids Kup Smoothies: Per 12 fl.oz Cup

	C	F	Cb
Berry Interesting	275	0	69
Choc-A-Laka	245	3	44
Gimme-Grape	265	0	64
Smarti Tarti	200	0	49

Snappy Tomato (Oct '12)

Pizza: Per Slice , ⅛ of Large Pizza **C** **F** **Cb**

	C	F	Cb
Buffalo Grilled Chicken	250	5	32
Cheese	220	7	30
Hawaiian	370	18	33
Meat Topper	430	23	31
Pepperoni	340	17	31
Ranch	370	21	31
Snapperoni	390	22	31
Snappy Ultimate	460	26	33
Supreme	340	17	32
Veggie	240	8	33

Snappetizers, Snappy Wings (3),
	C	F	Cb
Plain, without sauce, 2.6 oz	160	11	0

Sonic Drive-In® (Oct '12)

Burgers: With Standard Toppings **C** **F** **Cb**

	C	F	Cb
Green Chile Cheeseburger	710	43	44
Jr.	340	17	34
Jr. Deluxe	380	23	32
Veggie with Mustard	450	14	64
Sonic: W/ Mayonnaise	740	48	44
With Mustard	640	37	43
Bacon Cheeseburger, w/ Mayo	870	59	45
Cheeseburger, with Mayonnaise	800	54	44
Super Sonic:			
Bacon Dble Cheeseburger, w/ Mayo	1280	92	44
Dble Cheeseburger, w/ Mayo	1220	87	45
Coneys:			
All Beef Chili Cheese	410	26	30
Footlong, ¼ pound	830	54	54
Toaster Sandwiches: Chicken Club	810	46	63
Bacon Cheeseburger	840	49	59
Wraps: Crispy Chicken	490	23	49
Grilled Chicken	390	14	39
Chicken: Chicken Strips (5)	490	27	26
Jumbo Popcorn Chicken:			
Small, without Sauce, 4 oz	380	22	27
Large, without Sauce, 6 oz	560	32	41
Sides: Per Medium Serving			
French Fries: Plain, 4 oz	360	17	49
With Cheese, 5.5 oz	490	26	53
With Chili & Cheese, 7.25 oz	560	31	57
Mozzarella Sticks, w/o sauce, 5 oz	440	22	40
Onion Rings, 5.5 oz	440	21	55
Tater Tots: Plain, 5 oz	360	19	43
With Cheese, medium, 6 oz	450	28	43
With Chili & Cheese, med., 8.2 oz	540	33	48
Breakfast:			
Burritos: Bacon, Egg & Cheese	430	25	36
Sausage, Egg & Cheese	450	28	36
Steak & Egg	550	31	41
SuperSonic	540	33	46
French Toast Sticks: With Syrup (4)	570	25	76
Without Syrup (4)	480	25	54
Sandwiches:			
Breakfast Bagel: With Bacon	550	22	68
With Sausage	630	32	68
CroisSonic, Sausage, Egg & Cheese	600	49	28
Ultimate Meat & Cheese Burrito	820	60	43

Continued Next Page...

Fast - Foods & *Restaurants*

Sonic Drive-In® cont... (Oct '12)

Desserts:	C	F	Cb
Banana Split	490	18	76
Single Topping Sundaes:			
Chocolate	500	22	69
Hot Fudge	520	27	63
Pineapple	440	22	55
Sonic Blasts: M&M's, small, 14 oz	910	49	106
Oreo; Snickers, small, 14 oz, av.	900	48	103
Beverages: Per Regular Size, 14 oz			
Floats/Blended:			
Diet Coke; Diet Dr Pepper	260	14	28
Coca-Cola	330	14	49
Malts: Chocolate	630	32	79
Strawberry	520	26	63
Vanilla	550	32	60
Shakes: Banana	620	31	80
Chocolate	620	31	77
Pineapple; Strawberry, average	570	31	67

For Complete Nutritional Data ~ see CalorieKing.com

Souplantation® (Oct '12)

Soups: Per Cup	C	F	Cb
Regular:			
Chesapeake Corn Chowder	290	17	30
Classical Minestrone	120	2	20
Cream of Mushroom	290	24	15
New Orelans Jambalaya	210	11	18
Vegetarian Harvest	200	10	23
Breads: Sourdough	150	0.5	27
Buttermilk Cornbread, 1 piece	140	2	27
Focaccia, Garlic Asiago	160	8	19
Pasta: Per 1 Cup			
Arizona Marinara	360	11	47
Brocc. Cheese Baked Potato Topper	120	7	10
Carbonara Pasta, with Bacon	290	10	43
Creamy Bruschetta	360	16	43
Chicken Tetrazzini	480	23	47
Creamy Cilantro Lime Pesto	360	20	37
Curried Pineapple & Ginger	200	2	40
Fettuccine Alfredo	390	18	44
Fire-Roasted Tomato Basil Alfredo	370	14	44
Garden Vegetable, with Meatballs	310	10	44
Vegetarian Marinara, with Basil	260	4	44
Prepared Salads: Per ½ Cup			
BBQ Potato	170	9	21
Carrot Raisin	90	3	17
Dijon Potato, with Garlic Dill Vinegar	150	12	9
Greek Couscous, w/ Feta & Pinenuts	210	10	25
Thai Noodle, w/ Chkn & P'nut Sce	190	10	19

Souplantation® cont... (Oct '12)

Bakery:	C	F	Cb
Chocolate Brownie	180	8	26
Muffins: Chocolate Chip	170	8	22
French Quarter Praline	250	10	35
Fruit Medley Bran	130	0.5	29
Desserts: Per ½ Cup			
Apple Medley	70	0	18
Banana Royale	80	0	20
Caramel Apple Cobbler	360	12	68
Rice Pudding	110	2	20

For Complete Nutritional Data ~ see CalorieKing.com

Southern Tsunami® (Oct '12)

Rolls: With White Rice	C	F	Cb
Hybrid: Berry, 6 oz	230	5	44
Blueberry: Salmon, 8 oz	350	15	45
Shrimp, 8 oz	330	12	45
Done Deal, 7 oz	370	17	39
Happy Mango, 8 oz	440	21	53
Jalapeno, 8 oz	310	7	48
Mango Shrimp, 6 oz	370	19	41
Red Rock Fujisan, 7 oz	400	15	42
Spicy Mango Roll, 8 oz	400	17	46
Ultimate Chili Combo, 6 oz	290	9	41
Chef Samplers: A, 9.5 oz	410	2	65
B, 7.5 oz	360	6	57
Plus Rolls: Per Two 3 oz Servings, 6 oz			
California	230	4	44
Cream Cheese Plus: Salmon	290	11	39
Shrimp	260	8	39
Tuna	280	8	39
Eel	300	9	46
Seaside Plus: Eel	380	15	47
Salmon	290	7	45
Shrimp	230	1	45
Steelhead	270	7	39
Tuna	280	1	45
Spicy Plus: Salmon	280	9	39
Shrimp	240	5	39
Steelhead	270	7	39
Tuna	270	5	39
Vegetable	230	4	46

Continued Next Page... ...

Southern Tsunami® cont... (Oct '12)

Rolls (Cont):

Hybrid Rolls: *With Brown Rice*

	C	F	Cb
Berry, 6 oz	200	6	44
Blueberry: Salmon, 8 oz	320	15	34
Steelhead, 8 oz	310	14	34
Crunchy: Dragon, Hot, 6 oz	270	10	30
Tempura, 6 oz	260	7	37
Jalapeno, 8 oz	250	7	39
Mango Shrimp, 6 oz	350	19	33
Red Rock Fujisan, 7 oz	370	16	31
Ultimate Chili Combo, 6 oz	250	10	30
Wraps: Avocado Salad Roll, 4.6 oz	130	5	21
Berry, 4.6 oz	180	8	25
California, 6.6 oz	270	17	28
Smoked Salmon Salad, 4.6 oz	210	10	21

Salads: Without Dressing

	C	F	Cb
Edamame, 4 oz	120	7	9
Seared Tuna, 9 oz	210	8	18

Dressings/Sauces: Eel Sauce, 1 T.

	C	F	Cb
Eel Sauce, 1 T.	35	0	8
Ginger Dressing, 2 Tbsp	50	2	8
Peanut Sauce, 2 Tbsp	30	1	6
Sweet Chili, 3 fl.oz	300	0	72
Wasabe Dressing, 2 Tbsp	30	2	2

Starbucks® (Oct '12)

Brewed Coffee: *Figures based on 16 fl.oz Grande Without Whipped Cream*

	C	F	Cb
Caffe Misto (Au Lait): W/ Whole Milk	130	7	10
With Nonfat Milk	70	0	10
With Soy Milk	100	3	13

Hot Espresso Beverages:

	C	F	Cb
Caffe Latte: With Whole Milk	220	11	18
With Nonfat Milk	130	0	19
With Soy Milk	170	4.5	23
Cappuccino: With Whole Milk	140	7	12
With Nonfat Milk	80	0	12
With Soy Milk	120	3.5	16
Caramel Macchiato: W/ Whole Milk	270	11	34
With Nonfat Milk	190	1	35
Cinn. Dolce Latte: With Whole Milk	300	10	40
With Nonfat Milk	210	0	42
Espresso: 1 doppio, 2 fl.oz	10	0	2
1 solo, 1 fl.oz	5	0	1
Espresso Con Panna, 1 Solo, 1 fl.oz	30	2.5	2

Starbucks® cont... (Oct '12)

Chocolate: W/out Wh. Cream

	C	F	Cb
Hot Chocolate:			
With Whole Milk	330	13	47
With Soy	290	7	51
White Hot Chocolate:			
With Whole Milk	450	17	62
With 2% Milk	420	12	62
With Nonfat Milk	360	6	62
With Soy Milk	410	11	66

Iced Espresso: Per 16 fl.oz Grande, Without Whipped Cream

	C	F	Cb
Caffe Latte:			
With Whole Milk	150	7	13
With Nonfat Milk	90	0	13
With Soy Milk	130	3.5	17
White Choc. Mocha:			
With Whole Milk	360	11	55
With Nonfat Milk	310	6	56
With Soy Milk	340	8	58

Frappuccino Blended Coffee: Cold, per16 fl.oz Grande With Whole Milk, Without Whipped Cream

	C	F	Cb
Caffe Vanilla	310	3	68
Caramel	280	3.5	64
Cinnamon Dolce	240	3	51
Coffee	240	3	50
Double Chocolaty Chip	290	8	53
Espresso	230	2.5	50
Java Chip	340	7	67
Mocha	290	4	61
White Chocolate Mocha	330	5	66

Frappuccino Blended Creme: Cold, per 16 fl.oz Grande, With Whole Milk And Whipped Cream

	C	F	Cb
Cinnamon Dolce Creme	350	16	49
Tazo Green Tea Creme	430	16	68
Vanilla Bean Creme	400	16	59
White Chocolate Creme	420	18	59

Smoothies: Per16 fl.oz Grande, With 2% Milk, Without Whipped Cream

	C	F	Cb
Orange Mango	270	1.5	53
Strawberry	300	2	60

Tazo Teas: Per 16 fl.oz Grande, With Whole Milk

	C	F	Cb
Hot Tea Latte: Awake	210	7	31
Chai	270	7	45
Earl Grey	200	7	29
Green Tea	390	13	57
Iced Tea Latte: Awake	120	2	24
Chai	260	7	44
Green Tea	320	9	51

Kid's Drinks & Others:

	C	F	Cb
Apple Juice, Cold, 12 fl.oz	190	0	49
Apple Juice, Steamed, 8 fl.oz	110	0	28

Continued Next Page.. ...

Fast - Foods & Restaurants

Starbucks® cont... (Oct '12)

Drink Extras:	C	F	Cb
Caramel Drizzle, 1 teaspoon	15	0.5	2
Flavored Syrup: 1 Pump	20	0	5
Sugar-Free, 1 Pump	0	0	0
Mocha Syrup, 1 Pump	25	0.5	6
Sweetened Whipped Cream:			
Grande/Venti, cold drinks, average	115	11	3
Grande/Venti, hot drinks	70	7	2
Breakfast Specialities:			
Bacon, Gouda & Egg Frittata, on Artisan Roll	350	18	30
Egg White, Spinach, Feta Wrap	290	10	33
Egg White/Turkey Bacon & Cheese on Muffin	320	7	43
Oatmeal: 1¼ oz, without sugar	140	2.5	25
With brown sugar, ½ oz	190	2.5	38
Bistro Boxes:			
Cheese & Fruit, 5.3 oz	480	28	39
Chicken & Hummus, 6.3 oz	260	7	25
Chipotle Chicken Wrap	290	12	26
Salumi & Cheese	360	17	34
Tuna Salad, 5.9 oz	380	21	25
Sandwiches & Paninis:			
Ham & Swiss Panini	360	9	43
Rstd Tomato & Mozz. Panini	390	18	44
Rstd Vegetable Panini	350	12	48
Tarragon Chicken Salad Sandwich	420	13	46
Turkey & Swiss Sandwich	390	13	36
8-Grain Roll, Plain	350	8	67
Bagels: Everything with Cheese	280	2	56
Multigrain	300	3	60
Plain	280	1	59
Bars & Brownies:			
Blueberry Oat Bar	370	14	47
Double Chocolate Brownie	410	24	46
Marshmallow Dream Bar	210	4	43
Cakes: Per Slice			
Banana Nut Loaf, 4.25 oz	490	19	75
Pumpkin Bread, 4.25 oz	390	14	61
Pound: Iced Lemon, 4.5 oz	490	23	67
Marble, 3.75 oz	350	13	54
Starbuck's Classic Coffee, 4 oz	440	19	63
Reduced Fat Cakes:			
Banana Chocolate Chip Coffee	400	8	80
Cinnamon Swirl	340	9	62
Very Berry Coffee	350	10	59
Cookies: Chocolate Chunk	380	17	51
Outrageous Oatmeal	370	14	56
Croissants: Butter	310	18	32
Chocolate	300	17	34
Doughnuts, Old-Fashioned Glazed	420	21	57

Starbucks® cont... (Oct '12)

Muffins:	C	F	Cb
Apple Bran	350	9	64
Bountiful Blueberry	370	14	55
Zucchini Walnut	490	28	52
Sweet Rolls & Danish:			
Apple Fritter	420	20	59
Cheese Danish	420	25	39
Morning Bun	350	16	45
Parfaits: Greek Yogurt Honey, 6 oz	300	12	44
Peach Raspberry, 8.1 oz	300	4	57
Strawberry & Blueb. Yogurt, 8.1 oz	300	3.5	60
Petites: Cake Pops, average, 1.5 oz	165	9	23
Cherry Pie, 1.7 oz	170	7	24
Red Velvet Whoopie Pie, 1.4 oz	190	11	21

Ice Cream ~ See Page 107
Bottled Drinks ~ See Page 37
Coffee Mix (VIA) ~ See Page 35

Steak Escape® (Oct '12)

Burgers: With Set Menu Board Toppings, Without Condiments	C	F	Cb
Single	590	32	48
Double	860	50	52
Double Philly	700	35	43
Double Char	870	50	49

Sandwiches: With Set Menu Board Toppings, Without Condiments

	C	F	Cb
6": Classic Italian	600	33	46
Turkey Club	360	9	42
Wild West BBQ	460	13	49
12": Buffalo Chicken	1080	44	126
Fire Escape	880	26	90
Triple Cheesesteak	1220	57	89

Wraps: With Set Menu Board Toppings, Without Condidments

	C	F	Cb
French Onion	630	28	56
Ragin Cajun	470	17	50
Teriyaki Chicken	520	18	55

Salads: Without Dressing

	C	F	Cb
Grilled: Chicken; Steak, average	425	25	15
Ham	360	22	17

Sides:

	C	F	Cb
Fresh Cut Fries: Small	510	26	61
Regular	700	36	84
Cheddar & Bacon, regular	910	52	91
Ranch & Bacon, regular	1160	82	86
Killer Potatoes: Chicken	470	15	54
Ham; Turkey, average	420	12	56
Loaded: Bacon & Ranch	670	46	51
Cheddar & Bacon	430	17	56

For Complete Nutritional Data ~ see CalorieKing.com

Updated Nutrition Data ~ www.CalorieKing.com
Persons with Diabetes ~ See Disclaimer (Page 22)

Steak 'n Shake® (Oct '12)

The Original Steakburgers:	C	F	Cb
Single	280	11	30
Double 'n Cheese	440	25	31
Triple	510	30	30
Bacon 'n Cheese Double	480	28	31
Cheesy Cheddar	480	27	32
Guacamole	700	48	47
Spicy Chipotle	640	41	42
Chili Bowls: 3-Way (1)	830	36	94
5-Way (1)	1170	63	99
Deluxe (1)	1220	74	81
Sandwiches:			
Guacamole Grilled Chicken	580	31	59
Spicy Chicken	490	21	51
Turkey Club	420	16	45
Signature Steak Franks: Regular	380	27	22
Cheesy Cheddar	490	36	24
Chicago Style	420	27	30
Chili Cheese	620	44	31
Salads: Without Dressing			
Apple Pecan Grilled Chicken	330	8	39
Fried Chicken	470	26	34
Southwest Grilled Chicken	490	26	46
Fries: French, regular	440	21	60
Large	640	30	87
Cheese: Regular	610	34	67
Large	810	43	94
Breakfast:			
Bagels Sandwich: With Bacon	450	16	51
With Sausage	570	29	50
Biscuits: Bacon, Egg & Cheese	520	35	32
Egg & Cheese	450	30	31
Sausage & Egg	600	44	31
Sausage, Egg & Cheese	650	48	31
With Sausage Gravy: Half order	540	37	43
Full Order	1070	74	86
Hash Browns: Shredded	290	23	19
Side order, 5 pieces	260	17	23
Perfect Start Oatmeal	340	11	57
Skillets: Country	1230	93	63
Portobello & Swiss	1040	87	27
Hand Dipped Shakes: Per Regular			
Banana; Mocha	610	20	100
Butterfinger	830	29	135
Chocolate; Vanilla, average	620	20	101
Cookies 'n Cream	760	25	124

Subway® (Oct '12)

6" Sandwiches (6g Fat or Less): C F Cb
Figures based on 9-grain wheat bread, lettuce, tomatoes, onions, green peppers and cucumbers. Oil or mayo not included.

	C	F	Cb
Black Forest Ham	290	4.5	46
Oven Roasted Chicken	320	5	47
Roast Beef	320	5	45
Subway Club	310	4.5	46
Sweet Onion Chicken Teriyaki	380	5	59
Turkey Breast	280	3.5	46
Turkey Breast & Black Forest Ham	280	4	46
Veggie Delite	230	2.5	44

6" Sandwiches: Figures based on 9-grain wheat bread, lettuce, tomatoes, onion, green peppers, cucumbers and cheese. Oil or mayo not included.

	C	F	Cb
Big Philly Cheesesteak	500	17	51
BLT	320	9	43
Buffalo Chkn w/ Reg. Ranch Drssng	420	16	46
Chicken & Bacon Ranch Melt	570	28	47
Cold Cut Combo	370	13	46
Italian B.M.T.	410	16	46
Meatball Marinara	480	18	59
Spicy Italian	480	24	46
Steak & Cheese	380	10	48
Subway Melt	370	11	47
Tuna	470	24	44

Kids Meal Sandwiches: Figures based on 9-grain wheat bread, lettuce, tomatoes, onions, green peppers and cucumbers. Oil or mayo not included.

	C	F	Cb
Black Forest Ham	180	2.5	30
Roast Beef	200	3	30
Turkey Breast	180	2	30
Veggie Delite	150	1.5	29

Condiments & Sauces: For 6" Sandwiches

	C	F	Cb
Chipotle Southwest, ¾ oz	100	10	1
Honey Mustard, Fat-Free, ¾ oz	30	0	7
Mayonnaise: 1 Tbsp, ½ oz	110	12	0
Light, 1 Tbsp, ½ oz	50	5	0.5
Mustard, Yellow or Deli Brown, 2 tsp	5	0	0.5
Olive Oil Blend, 1 tsp	45	5	0
Ranch Dressing, ¾ oz	110	11	1
Sweet Onion, Fat-Free, ¾ oz	40	0	9

Extras: For 6" Sandwiches

	C	F	Cb
Bacon Strips (2)	45	3.5	0
Cheese: American, 2 triangles, ¼ oz	40	3.5	1
Cheddar, 2 triangles, ¼ oz	60	5	0
Swiss, 2 triangles, ¼ oz	55	4.5	0
Chicken Strips, 2.5 oz	80	1.5	0

Continued Next Page....

Subway® cont... (Oct '12)

Breakfast:

Egg Muffin Melts with Egg White: *Figures based on light wheat English muffin, cheese & egg white*

	C	F	Cb
Egg White & Cheese, with Ham	170	4	24
Breakfast B.M.T. Melt	220	8	25
Bacon, Egg White and Cheese	180	5	24
Mega Melt	300	17	24
Sausage, Egg White & Cheese	270	15	24
Steak, Egg White & Cheese	180	4	25
Sunrise Subway Melt	210	6	26

Egg Muffin Melts: *Figures based on light wheat English muffin, cheese & regular egg.*

Breakfast B.M.T.	240	10	25
Bacon, Egg & Cheese	200	7	24
Egg & Cheese	170	6	24
Egg & Cheese, with Ham	190	6	24
Steak, Egg & Cheese	200	6	25
Sunrise Melt	230	8	26

6" Breakfast Omelet Sandwiches: *Figures based on 9-grain bread, cheese & regular egg*

Bacon, Egg & Cheese	410	16	45
Egg & Cheese	360	12	44
Egg & Cheese with Ham	390	13	45
Steak, Egg & Cheese	430	15	47
Sunrise Melt	470	17	48

Regular Egg On Mornin' Flatbreads: *Figures based on flatbread, cheese and regular egg.*

Egg & Cheese	190	7	21
Breakfast B.M.T.	250	12	22
Bacon, Egg & Cheese	210	9	21
Steak, Egg & Cheese	210	8	22
Sunrise Melt	240	10	23

Breakfast Sides,

Hash Browns, 4 pieces	210	10	28

Salads (6g Fat or Less): *Figures based on lettuce, tomatoes, onions, green peppers, olives & cucumbers. Dressing or croutons not included.*

Black Forest Ham	110	3	11
Grilled Chicken & Baby Spinach	130	2.5	10
Oven Roasted Chicken Breast	130	2.5	9
Roast Beef; Subway Club, av.	140	3.5	10
Sweet Onion Chicken Teriyaki	200	3	24
Turkey Breast/Ham, average	110	2.5	11
Veggie Delite	50	1	9

Salad Dressing:

Chipotle Southwest	260	27	2
Fat Free Italian, 2 oz	35	0	7
Honey Mustard	80	1	18
Oil and Vinegar	190	21	0
Ranch, 2 oz	290	30	3
Sweet Onion	100	0	24

Subway® cont... (Oct '12)

Soups: *Per 10 oz Bowl*

	C	F	Cb
Chili Con Carne	280	8	35
Chipotle Chicken Corn Chowder	130	2.5	22
Creamy Potato with Bacon	250	14	26
Minestrone	90	1	15
New England Style Clam Chowder	150	5	20
Roasted Chicken Noodle	110	2	15
Spanish Style Chicken & Rice w/ Pork	110	2.5	16
Tomato Garden Vegetable w/ Rotini	90	0	20
Vegetable Beef	100	2	15

Chips: Lay's Classic, 1.5 oz 230 15 23

Baked Lay's, 1.1 oz	130	2	33

Cookies & Desserts:

Apple Slices, 1 package, 2.5 oz	35	0	9
Chocolate Chip Cookie, 1.5 oz	220	10	30
Oatmeal Raisin Cookie, 1.5 oz	200	8	30
Raspberry Cheesecake, 1.6 oz	200	9	29
Yogurt Parfait, with granola	160	2	30

Sweet Tomatoes®

Same Menu & Data as Souplantation ~ See Page 242

Swiss Chalet® (Oct '12)

Starters:

	C	F	Cb
Garlic Loaf, without Cheese, 8.46 oz	700	40	73
Chalet Chicken Wings (8), with sauce	550	34	23
Cheese Perogies (7)	420	10	69
Caesar Salad without Dressing	90	3	13

From The Grill: *Without Sides*

Burgers: Classic Hamburger	710	39	43
Classic Bacon & Cheese	890	54	46
Veggie	470	13	57
BBQ Ribs: Half Rack	650	42	6
Full Rack	1300	85	11

Rotisserie Chicken: *Meat Only*

Double Leg, with Skin	490	31	0
Half Chicken, with Skin	530	27	0
Quarter Chicken:			
Dark meat, without Skin	160	8	0
Dark meat, with Skin	240	16	0
White meat, without Skin	220	6	0
White meat, with Skin	290	11	0
Chicken Pot Pie, 1 pie	560	32	39

Sandwiches: *Without Sides*

Classic Hot Chicken, white meat	520	11	51
Flatbread: Hickory Chicken	700	32	70
Southwest Chicken	710	37	64

Stir-Frys:

Chicken: With Rice	900	36	103
Without Rice	620	32	47
Vegetable, with Rice	690	28	103

Continued Next Page...

Fast - Foods & Restaurants

Swiss Chalet® cont...(Oct '12)

Wrap,

	C	F	Cb
Rotisserie Chicken Club	710	32	57

Entree Salads: Without Dressing

	C	F	Cb
Spinach Chicken Salad	410	25	28
Sweet Heat Salad with Chicken	340	9	30
West Coast Salad with Chicken	460	21	21

Dressings/Sauces:

	C	F	Cb
Caesar Dressing, 1 oz	180	18	2
Chalet Dressing, 1 Tbsp, 1 oz	160	14	6
Chalet Dipping Sauce, 3.5 oz	25	0.5	5
Greek Dressing, 1 oz	140	14	2

Sides:

	C	F	Cb
Gravy, 4 oz	45	1.5	7
Mashed Potatoes, 5 oz	150	4	27
Sauteed Mushrooms, 6 oz	140	1	30
Seasoned Rice, 6 oz	240	3.5	48

Desserts/Pies: Apple Pie

	C	F	Cb
Desserts/Pies: Apple Pie	440	19	65
Coconut Cream Pie	540	33	57
Lemon Meringue Pie	400	11	73
Old Fashioned Carrot Cake	260	16	24
Pecan Pie	590	29	79

Taco Bell® (Oct '12)

Burritos:

	C	F	Cb
½ lb Cheesy Potato	540	26	59
½ lb Combo	460	18	53
7-Layer	510	19	68
Beefy 5-Layer	550	22	68
Cantina, Chicken	760	27	96
Chili Cheese	380	17	41
Grilled Chicken	420	18	48
Supreme: Beef	420	16	52
Chicken; Steak, average	390	13	52

XXL Grilled Stuft:

	C	F	Cb
Beef	880	42	94
Chicken; Steak, average	825	36	91

Chalupas:

	C	F	Cb
Supreme: Beef	370	21	31
Chicken	340	18	29
Steak	340	18	29
Fresco: Bean Burrito	350	9	57
Crunchy Taco	170	7	20
Soft Tacos: Chkn; Grilled Steak, av.	150	4	19
Fresco	170	7	20
Supreme, Chicken; Steak, av.	340	9	50

Gorditas:

	C	F	Cb
Cheesy Crunch	490	29	39
Supreme: Beef	300	14	31
Chicken	270	10	29
Steak	270	11	29

Nachos: Regular

	C	F	Cb
Nachos: Regular	320	19	33
BellGrande	760	39	82
Cheesy	270	15	30

Taco Bell® cont...(Oct '12)

Tacos:

	C	F	Cb
Crunchy: Regular	170	10	12
Supreme	200	12	15
Double Decker: Regular	320	14	37
Supreme	350	16	40
Soft: Beef	200	9	19
Beef Supreme	230	11	22
Chicken	170	6	18
Crispy Potato	270	13	31
Fresco Chicken	150	3.5	18
Grilled Steak	250	14	19

Specialities:

	C	F	Cb
Cantina Bowl, Chicken	560	22	64
Cheese Roll-Up	190	9	18
Chilli Cheese Burrito	380	17	41
Crunchwrap Supreme	540	21	71
Enchiritos: Beef	360	17	34
Chicken	340	14	32
Steak	330	14	32
MexiMelt	270	14	21
Mexican Pizza, 7.5 oz	540	31	47
Quesadillas: Cheese	480	27	40
Steak	520	28	41
Tostada	250	10	30

Taco Salads:

	C	F	Cb
Express with Chips	580	29	59
Fiesta: Beef	780	42	74
Chicken	720	35	70
Steak	720	36	70

Volcano Menu:

	C	F	Cb
Burrito	780	41	80
Nachos	970	58	92
Taco	230	16	14
Sides: Cheesy Fiesta Potato	290	17	32
Cinnamon Twists	170	7	26
Mexican Rice	120	3.5	20
Pintos 'n Cheese	180	7	20

Condiments & Sauces:

	C	F	Cb
Avocado Ranch Dressing, ½ oz	80	8	1
Creamy Jalapeno Sauce, ½ oz	70	7	1
Green Tomatillo Sauce, 1 oz	10	0	2
Guacamole, ¾ oz	35	3	2
Pepper Jack Sauce, ½ oz	70	7	1
Pizza Sauce, 1 oz	10	0	2
Salsa: Original, ¾ oz	5	0	1
Fire Roasted; Verde, ¼ oz	5	0	1
Sour Cream, Reduced Fat, ¾ oz	30	2	2

Fast - Foods & *Restaurants*

Taco Bell® cont... (Oct '12)

Beverages: Per 16 fl.oz

	C	F	Cb
Classic Limeade Sparkler	150	0	39
Dr Pepper	200	0	54
Frutista Freeze: Mango Strawberry	250	0	62
Strawberry	280	0	70
Lipton Raspberry Iced Tea	160	0	42
MUG Root Beer	200	0	52
Mountain Dew Baja Blast	220	0	58
Tropicana Pink Lemonade	200	0	54

Note: Nutritional data in New York outlets may vary slightly.
Please check Taco Bell website

Taco Cabana® (Oct '12)

Cabana Burritos: Includes Flour
Burrito & Menu Set Toppings

	C	F	Cb
Beef	950	42	96
Chicken	900	37	99
Steak Fajita	910	39	96

Flameante Chicken: Includes Rice, Beans, Lettuce,
Pico de Gallo & 2 Flour Tortillas

¼ Chicken Dark Dinner	950	41	87
¼ Chicken White Dinner	800	23	87
½ Chicken Dinner	1620	63	146

Sizzling Fajitas: Includes All Standard
Toppings & 2 Flour Tortillas

Chicken	740	20	98
Steak	760	24	98

Tacos:

Crispy: Ground Beef	180	10	11
Stewed Chicken	160	7	13
Soft: Bean & Cheese	300	14	32
Beef	230	9	22
Black Bean	200	4	34
Carne Guisada	190	6	21
Chicken, stewed	210	7	23

Sides & Add-Ons: Per Serving

Black Beans, 4 oz	80	0	14
Borracho Beans	140	3	20
Guacamole, 3 oz	110	9	7
Queso, 3 oz	200	15	5
Refried Beans	250	13	24
Rice	120	1	25
Salsa: Fuego; Roja, 1 oz	5	0	1
Verde, 1 oz	10	0	1
Sour Cream: 3 oz	160	14	3
For Chicken Enchilada	170	6	20
Tortillas: 6" Corn	70	1	15
6" Flour	120	3	19

Taco Del Mar® (Oct '12)

Baja Bowls: As Served

	C	F	Cb
Mondo: Carne Asada Steak	490	15	62
Chicken; Shredded Beef	520	17	62
Fish	570	34	46
Ground Beef	570	23	62
Pork	500	15	61
Vegan	360	8	64

Burritos: As Served
Mondito: Per 9.6 oz Unless Indicated

Carne Asada Steak	440	13	65
Chicken; Shredded Beef	460	14	65
Fish, 10.7 oz	510	23	61
Ground Beef	480	17	65
Pork	450	13	65
Vegan, 9.3 oz	380	9	66

Mondo: Per 18.45 oz Unless Indicated

Carne Asada Steak	820	23	118
Chicken; Shredded Beef	860	25	118
Fish, 19 oz	900	42	102
Ground Beef	900	32	118
Pork	840	24	117
Vegan, 18 oz	700	16	120

Platters: As Served
Enchilada: Per 2 Enchiladas

Carne Asada Steak	780	28	104
Cheese	870	38	104
Chicken; Shredded Beef, average	820	30	104
Ground Beef	860	36	105
Pork	800	28	103

Enchilada/Taco: Per 1 Enchilada &1 Taco

Carne Asada Steak	820	30	109
Chicken; Shredded Beef	850	32	108
Ground Beef	900	38	109
Pork	830	30	108

Quesadillas: As Served

Carne Asada Steak	1170	49	135
Chicken; Shredded Beef	1200	51	135
Ground Beef	1250	57	136
Pork	1180	50	134

Nachos: As Served

6 Layer Cheese	1050	62	96
Super: Carne Asada Steak	1140	65	98
Chicken; Shredded Beef, av.	1170	67	97
Ground Beef	1220	74	98
Pork	1150	66	97

Salads: As Served

Cabo: Chicken; Shredded Beef	420	19	36
Fish	450	22	47
Pork	400	18	36
Taco: Carne Asada Steak	610	29	57
Ground Beef	690	37	60

Note: Nutritional Information varies from
state to state. Please refer to Taco Del Mar Website

Updated Nutrition Data ~ www.CalorieKing.com
Persons with Diabetes ~ See Disclaimer (Page 22)

Taco John's® (Oct '12)

Burritos:	C	F	Cb
Bean Burrito	370	11	53
Beef Grilled Burrito	590	32	53
Beefy Burrito	440	21	42
Chicken & Potato Burrito	480	21	56
Chicken Grilled Burrito	590	30	50
Combination Burrito	410	16	47
Crunchy Chicken & Potato Burrito	580	27	67
Meat & Potato Burrito	520	25	57
Super Burrito	450	20	50
Tacos: Soft Shell, Chicken	190	6	21
Taco Bravo	330	13	38
Taco Burger	280	12	29
Specialties:			
Taco Salad w/o dressing	540	33	40
Chicken Taco Salad w/o dressing	500	27	39
Crunchy Chicken Taco Salad w/o dress.	630	36	53
Super Nachos: Small	420	25	37
Regular	790	47	72
Super Potato Oles: Small	650	40	59
Regular	1090	67	98
Quesadilla Melt: Cheesy	450	24	40
Fajita Beef	550	29	46
Fajita Chicken	520	25	45
Crunchy Chicken without sauce	370	18	29
Snacks: Chips & Queso	430	25	43
Cini-Sopapilla Bites	200	8	34
Sides: Potato Oles: Small	480	27	52
Medium	670	38	73
Large	860	49	94
Refried Beans: With Cheese	320	7	46
Without Cheese	260	2.5	45
Mexican Rice	250	6	45
Condiments:			
Bacon Ranch, 1.5 oz	120	9	10
House Dressing, 1.5 oz	70	7	2
Nacho Cheese, 3 oz	110	9	5
Salsa, 2 oz	10	0	2
Sour Cream, 2 oz	120	10	3
Desserts:			
Apple Grande	260	11	39
Choco Taco	390	21	48
Churro	200	9	29

Taco Mayo® (Oct '12)

Burritos:	C	F	Cb
Bean	495	16	71
Beef	490	23	41
Super: Beef	540	23	57
Chicken	405	16	39
Melts: Tamale	615	34	50
Tostada	525	32	35
Quesadillas: Chicken	675	37	46
Fajita Chicken	700	39	47
Fajita Steak	725	40	47
Tacos: Crispy Taco, Beef	160	9	10
Soft Taco: Beef	230	11	17
Chicken	185	6	16
Salads: Acapulco: Chicken	680	50	35
Steak	705	51	35
SalsaLita Steak	305	8	33
Taco Steak	445	25	30
Sides: Mexicali Rice	160	1	36
Refried Beans	295	9	43
Potato Locos, Small	380	24	36

Taco Time® (Oct '12)

Burritos:	C	F	Cb
Beef, Bean & Cheese	490	17	55
Chicken B.L.T.	690	39	43
Big Juan: Chicken	580	16	70
Ground Beef	630	23	73
Casita: Chicken	490	17	42
Ground Beef	540	24	46
Crisp Burrito: Chicken	380	17	33
Ground Beef	430	21	36
Pinto Bean	360	14	47
Soft Burrito: Ground Beef	430	16	43
Pinto Bean	370	10	54
Veggie	520	17	73
Tacos:			
Soft Tacos: Per 7 oz Unless Indicated			
Chicken	360	9	40
Ground Beef	420	16	43
Super Soft Wheat Taco: Beef	590	23	63
Chicken	530	16	59
Other Favorites: Cheddar Melt	250	12	25
Nachos Grande	930	43	96
Tostada: Bean	230	13	21
Chicken	320	13	22
Ground Beef	380	20	25
Breakfast:			
Burritos: Egg & Bacon, 7.5 oz	510	24	49
Egg & Cheese, 5.75 oz	370	16	40
Ultimate, 11 oz	860	58	52
Omelets: Cheese, 8 oz	490	36	6
Country, 13.25 oz	720	54	20
Nacho, 15.5 oz	740	48	26

Continued Next Page...

Taco Time® cont... (Oct '12)

Fries:	C	F	Cb
Cheddar Fries, medium, 7 oz	500	35	39
Mexi Fries, medium, 6 oz	390	26	38
Stuffed Fries, medium, 7 oz	460	28	42
Sides: Chips, Taco, oz	150	3.5	27
Mexi-Rice, 3.5 oz	80	0.5	17
Refritos, with Chips, 6 oz	230	7	29
Salads:			
Regular: Chicken Taco, 9.5 oz	310	13	22
Ground Beef Taco, 9 oz	370	20	24
Tostada Delight: Chicken, 9 oz	450	19	35
Ground Beef, 9 oz	490	26	36
Desserts: Churro: Plain	210	16	17
With Cinnamon & Sugar	250	16	27
Crustos	290	6	58
Empanada, Apple	230	7	40

Target Food Court (Oct '12)

Entrees: Per Order	C	F	Cb
Beef Hot Dog	340	20	27
Chicken Tenders	270	10	18
Kids: Chicken Nuggets	180	7	12
Macaroni & Cheese	300	9	45
Personal Pan Pizza: Per Order			
Cheese	590	24	69
Italian Sausage	750	39	69
Pepperoni	610	26	67
Sandwiches: Ham & Swiss, 6.1 oz	370	10	40
Turkey & Havarti	720	40	47
Turkey & Provolone	330	12	36
Toasted Flatbreads:			
Chicken Marinara	180	8	15
Chicken Spinach Artichoke	160	7	17
Salads: California Chicken	550	30	31
Chicken Caesar, 13 oz	550	36	20
Harvest Chicken	550	29	39
Soups: Chicken Noodle	90	2	11
Tomato Basil	180	11	15
Snacks: Apples & Caramel	100	1	23
French Fries	230	9	33
Popcorn	300	16	33
Yogurt Parfait	320	5	59
Treats: Brownie	410	18	57
Chocolate Chip Cookies	510	26	68
Churro	180	5	32
Pretzels: Bavarian, with Butter	490	6	93
And Cinnamon Sugar	520	6	102
Smoothies: Mango; Strawb., av.	230	0	57
Strawberry	240	0	60
ICEE's: Coca Cola, 20 oz	180	0	45
Dr Pepper, 20 oz	330	0	75
Pepsi, 32 oz	240	0	61

TCBY® (Oct '12)

Soft Serve Froz. Yogurt: Per 4 fl.oz	C	F	Cb
Cheesecake	110	2	23
Golden Vanilla	120	2	23
Peanut Butter	130	2	26
No Sugar Added, Fat Free,			
average all flavors	80	0	22
(Note: Carb figure includes Sugar Alcohols)			
Sorbet,			
average all flavors, 4 fl.oz	100	0	25
Hand-Scooped Frozen Yogurt:			
Butter Pecan: Kid's, 4 fl.oz	150	7	17
Small, 6.4 fl.oz	240	11	27
Regular, 12.8 fl.oz	480	22	54
Choc. Chunk Cookie Dough:			
Kid's, 4 fl.oz	150	6	23
Small, 6.4 fl.oz	240	10	37
Regular,12.8 fl.oz	480	19	74
Peaches & Cream:			
Kid's,4 fl.oz	110	2.5	18
Small, 6.4 fl.oz	175	4	29
Regular, 12.8 fl.oz	350	8	58
Peanut Butter Delight: Kid's 4 fl.oz	170	8	21
Small, 6.4 fl.oz	270	13	34
Regular, 12.8 fl.oz	540	26	68
Vanilla Bean: Kid's,4 fl.oz	110	3	18
Small, 6.4 fl.oz	175	5	29
Regular, 12.8 fl.oz	350	10	58
Cakes: Per 1/10 Cake			
Choc. & Van. Yogurt Dble Crunch	350	18	43
White Choc. Mousse Yog. w/ Choc.	310	14	42
Pies: Per 1/10 Pie			
Chocolate Decadence	330	13	49
Cookies & Creme	320	15	42

TGI Friday's® (Oct '12)

Appetiers: As Served, Per Serve	C	F	Cb
Crispy Green Bean Fries	900	65	69
Fried Mozzarella	770	46	54
Pan Seared Potstickers	780	65	80
Sesame Jack Chicken Strips	1100	35	162
To Share: Per Whole Dish, As Served			
Classic Mediterranean Hummus	1010	42	133
Jack Daniels Sampler	1840	64	234
Loaded Potato Skins	2030	131	161
Spinach Florentine Flatbread	440	27	31
Tostada Nachos	1410	97	57
Tuscan Spinach Dip	1110	73	86

Continued Next Page...

Fast - Foods & Restaurants

TGI Friday's® cont... (Oct '12)

Black Angus Burgers: With Fries

	C	F	Cb
Cheeseburger	1110	72	73
Jack Daniel's Burger	1360	74	127
Kansas City BBQ Burger	1510	85	137
NY Cheddar & Bacon Burger	1410	89	99
Sedona Black Bean Burger	1160	72	101
Turkey Burger	890	46	91

Sandwiches: Without Sides Unless Indicated

California Club	870	52	53
Caribb. Chicken w/ sweet pot. fries	1210	49	151
Jack Daniel's Chicken	1140	58	106
Triple Stack Reuben	920	52	69

Black Angus Steaks: Without Sides

Flat Iron	380	27	2
Sirloin: Petite	370	24	3
With Half Rack Ribs	850	44	40
Sirloin: 10 oz	600	45	3
With Grilled Shrimp Scampi	900	70	6

Chicken & Pasta: As Served

Chicken Fingers	1000	67	66
Dragonfire Chicken	670	15	99
Pasta: Bruschetta Chicken	920	42	90
Cajun Shrimp & Chicken	1010	47	84
Chicken Piccata	1200	69	98

Jack Daniels Grill: Without Sides Unless Indicated

Chicken	620	8	79
Chicken & Shrimp	570	11	77
Flat Iron Steak	590	16	80
Ribs & Shrimp with fries & slaw	1770	81	174
Sirloin & Shrimp	1010	41	102

Salads: Includes Dressing

Balsamic-Glazed Chicken Caesar	500	28	46
Chipotle Yucatan Chicken	860	60	46
Pecan-Crusted Chicken	1100	71	51
Strawberry Fields, with Grilled Balsamic Chicken	600	46	39
Dressing: Balsamic Vinaigrette	300	31	7
Bleu Cheese	320	34	2
Honey Mustard	310	29	12
Ranch	210	22	2

Sides: Ginger-Lime Slaw

	120	10	5
Mashed Potatoes	210	10	21
Parmesan Steak Fries	660	49	47
Seasoned Fries	290	23	19

TGI Friday's® cont... (Oct '12)

Soups: Per 10 oz Bowl

	C	F	Cb
French Onion	280	16	21
Soup Of The Day: Chicken Noodle	230	9	24
Broccoli Cheese	300	25	11
New England Clam Chowder	500	30	45
Tomato Basil	300	24	20
Tortilla	250	12	22

Desserts:

Brownie Obsession, ½ serve	620	30	80
Ice Cream Strawberry Shortcake, ½ serve	550	23	67
Oreo Madness	700	61	91
Vanilla Bean Cheesecake	970	61	91

Signature Slushes: Per 22 oz Tumbler

Blue Rasperry	310	0	75
Mango Peach Lemonade	150	0	41
Red Bull Passion	220	0	54
Ruby Red Bull	200	0	51

Thundercloud Subs® (Oct '12)

Subs: Small, w/ Standard Toppings

	C	F	Cb
Classic: BLT	405	17	40
Smoked Chicken	295	4	40
Turkey	280	4	41
Hot Subs: Meatball	650	32	56
Hot Pastrami	430	13	41
Signature Subs: Club	480	19	43
California Club	510	23	45
NY Italian	570	30	42
Office Favorite	850	40	81
Texas Tuna	700	45	44
Veggie Delite, with Hummus	360	10	53

Tim Hortons® (Oct '12)

Breakfast:

	C	F	Cb
Sandwiches: Regular Size			
Bagel BELT with Cheese	460	16	59
Bacon, Egg & Cheese	440	25	35
Breakfast Sausage & Biscuit	420	27	32
Egg & Cheese	390	21	35
English Muffins: Bacon, Egg & Chse	330	15	33
Sausage, Egg & Cheese	450	27	33
Wraps: Bacon	270	16	18
Egg & Cheese	220	12	17
Sausage	390	28	18
Hashbrowns, 1.75 oz	100	5	12

Continued Next Page...

251

Tim Horton's® cont... (Oct '12)

Sandwiches: Regular, on White Bun **C** **F** **Cb**
with Standard Ingredients

	C	F	Cb
BLT	420	18	47
Chicken Salad	350	9	48
Ham & Swiss	400	12	48
Toasted Chicken Club	390	7	52
Turkey Bacon Club	380	7	55

Wrap Snackers:

BBQ Chicken, 3.5 oz	180	6	19
Chicken Ranch, 3.5 oz	190	8	17

Soups: Per Small 10 oz Bowl

Beef Barley w/ Portobello Mshrm	110	2	18
Chicken Noodle	110	2.5	19
Cream of Broccoli	160	10	15
Hearty Potato Bacon	230	13	23
Split Pea with Ham	160	2.5	28
Turkey & Wild Rice	120	1.5	24

Baked Goods: Each

Cookies: Chocolate Chunk	230	9	35
Oatmeal Raisin Spice	220	8	35
Peanut Butter	280	16	27
Triple Chocolate	250	13	31

Donuts:

Cake: Chocolate Glazed	260	10	39
Old Fashioned Plain	260	19	20
Sour Cream Plain	270	17	27
Filled: Blueberry	230	8	36
Boston Cream	250	9	37
Canadian Maple	260	9	41
Strawberry	230	8	36
Honey Cruller	320	19	37
Yeast, Apple Fritter	300	11	49

Timbits, Low-Fat:

Cake, Glazed: Chocolate	70	2.5	10
Sour Cream	90	4.5	12
Old Fashion, Plain	70	5	5
Filled, all varieties	60	2	10
Yeast: Apple Fritter	50	1.5	9
Honey Dip	60	2	9

Desserts: Per 6 oz Container

Low Fat Yogurt: Creamy Vanilla	160	2.5	32
Strawberry	150	2.5	28

Beverages:

Cafe Mocha, 10 fl.oz	170	6	27
Coffee w/med. sugar/cream, 10 fl.oz	75	3.5	9
Hot Chocolate, 10 fl.oz	240	6	45

Iced Cappuccinos: *Per Small, 12 fl.oz*

Original: With milk	180	1.5	39
With cream	300	15	41

T.J. Cinnamons® (Oct '12)

Bakery: **C** **F** **Cb**

	C	F	Cb
Cinnamon Roll, Original, 5.25 oz	505	10	73
Cinnamon Twist (1), 2.5 oz	260	14	33
Sticky Bun Smear w/ Pecans, 1.25 oz	180	12	18
T.J. Cream Cheese Icing, 1 oz	115	5	18

Beverages: Per 12 fl.oz Serving

Mocha Chill, w/o Whipped Cream	265	4	46

Togo's Eatery® (Oct '12)

Sandwiches: **C** **F** **Cb**

Cold: Per Regular White Bread With Standard
Toppings, Without Dressing

	C	F	Cb
Albacore Tuna	550	17	73
Roast Beef & Avocado	570	13	69
The Italian	780	34	71
Turkey & Avocado	530	15	74
Turkey, Bacon Club	530	16	67
Turkey, Ham & Cheese	540	13	67
Vegetarian: Avocado & Cucumber	450	11	75
Egg Salad & Cheese	640	28	70
Hummus	650	27	85
Hot: BBQ Beef	670	19	85
Chicken	480	4	71
French Dip	690	17	66
Pastrami	770	37	66
Roast Beef	580	9	66

Toasted Sandwiches: *Per Regular Size With Menu*
Board Featured Bread

Clubhouse	660	23	80
Pepper Jack Pastrami	980	57	68
Uncle Toby's Italian	880	47	73

Salad Wraps: Includes Whole Wheat Wrap, Standard
Toppings & Dressings

Asian Chicken with Asian Dressing	670	32	74
BBQ Chicken Ranch w/ Buttmlk Ranch	640	30	72
Chicken Caesar w/ Caesar Drssng	550	20	67
Santa Fe Chicken with Spicy Pepitas	800	44	75

Salads: Per Full Salad, Without Dressing

BBQ Chicken Ranch	390	20	32
Chicken Caesar	210	6	17
Farmer's Market			
Santa Fe Chicken	370	16	33

Tropical Smoothie Cafe® (Oct '12)

Breakfast:

	C	F	Cb
Wraps: Early Bird, regular size	850	51	54
All American, regular size	620	26	53

Toasted Sandwiches: *Without Chips or Fruit*

	C	F	Cb
Cranb. Walnut Ckn Salad, on Wheat	635	36	59
Turkey Bacon, w/ Ranch, on Ciabatta	520	15	52
Turkey Guacamole, on Wheat	500	10	66
Ultimate Club, w/ Chipotle Mayo on Ciabata	605	25	52

Toasted Wraps: *On Garlic Herb Tortilla, Without Chips Or Fruit*

	C	F	Cb
Hummus Veggie	615	25	78
Jamaican Jerk Chicken, with Sauce	670	18	86
King Caesar, with Caesar Dressing	625	29	56
Totally Turkey, w/ Ranch Dressing	575	20	56

Fresh Salads: *Includes Standard Dressing*

	C	F	Cb
Chicken Caesar	325	21	10
Southwest Chicken, w/ SW Ranch	540	29	44
Thai Chicken	375	11	43

Simply Indulgent Smoothies: *With Turbinado*

	C	F	Cb
Beach Bum	510	5	123
Chocolate Chiller	530	7	118
Peanut Butter Cup	655	21	117
Tropi-Colada	460	1	129

Low Fat Smoothies: *With Turbinado*

	C	F	Cb
Blimey I imey	475	0.5	124
Blue Lagoon	305	1	79
Hawaiian Breeze	370	0.5	93
Rockin Raspberry	380	0.5	99
Strawberry Beach	440	0.5	113
Sunrise Sunset	425	0.5	109

Supercharged: *With Turbinado*

	C	F	Cb
Health Nut	490	5.5	97
Lean Machine	425	0	111
Muscle Blaster	430	3	89
Peanut Paradise	650	19	99

With Splenda, deduct 200 calories & 50g carbs

Tubby's® (Oct '12)

Subs: *Per Regular, w/o Condiments*

	C	F	Cb
Deli-Subs: Classic Italian	610	14	75
Ham & Cheese	500	10	76
Turkey Breast & Cheese	500	9	74
Grilled Burger Subs: Big Tub	650	25	78
Burger Special	760	33	78
Cheeseburger Italiano	740	33	76
Pizza Burger	630	25	75

Tubby's® Cont... (Oct '12)

Subs (Cont): *Per Regular Size*

Grilled Chicken Subs:

	C	F	Cb
Chicken	440	4.5	72
Chicken & Broccoli	520	10	75
Chicken & Cheddar	510	10	73
Chicken Fajita	520	10	75

Grilled Steak Subs:

	C	F	Cb
Portobella Mushroom Steak	835	26	52
Pepper Steak & Cheese	570	15	76
Steak & Cheese	560	15	74
Steak Special	590	16	76

Specialty Items: BLT

	C	F	Cb
BLT	540	20	71
Cold Veggie	470	9	79
Italian Sausage	630	26	77
Tuna	530	9	74
Veggie Stir Fry, hot	470	9	79

Uno Chicago Grill® (Oct '12)

Appetizers: *Per Whole Dish*

	C	F	Cb
Crispy Cheese Dippers, 11.4 oz	850	47	80
Pizza Skins, 25 .4 oz	2070	140	147
Shrimp & Crab Fondue, 16.4 oz	1120	81	64

Burgers: *Without Sides*

	C	F	Cb
BBQ, with Bacon & Cheddar (1)	1020	71	33
Buffalo Cheddar (1)	890	62	29
Uno (1)	780	53	28

Entrees:

Chicken: *Per Whole Dish, Without Sides Or Breadstick*

	C	F	Cb
Baked Stuffed Chicken, 11.8 oz	360	14	10
Chicken Milanese, 22.5 oz	850	56	46
Chicken Thumb Platter, 10.5 oz	480	17	34

Steak & Seafood: *Per Whole Dish w/o Sides Or Breadstick*

	C	F	Cb
Baked Haddock, 11.85 oz	580	35	12
Grilled Shrimp & Sirloin, 15 oz	660	29	8
Lemon Basil Salmon, 8.65 oz	490	34	0
The Chop House Classic, 8.2 oz	410	14	0

Thin Crust Pizza: *Per ⅓ Pizza*

	C	F	Cb
Mediterranean, Traditional Crust	310	15	33
Pepperoni, Flatbread Base	330	15	32
Roasted Eggplant, Spinach & Feta, Traditional Crust	295	11	38
Sides: French Fries, 7.6 oz	450	33	36
Red Bliss Mashed Potatoes	270	14	34
Roasted Seasonal Veges, 7.2 oz	80	4.5	10
Steamed Seasonal Veges, 6.25 oz	100	7	9

Villa Fresh Italian® (Oct '12)

Pizzas: Per Slice

	C	F	Cb
Neapolitan: Cheese, ⅙ pizza	405	13	49
Bacon & Tomato, ⅙ pizza	500	20	50
Deluxe, ⅙ pizza	505	21	52
Stuffed: Baked Ziti, ⅛ pizza	815	28	100
Meat, ⅛ pizza	840	41	74
Spinach and Mshrm, ⅛ pizza	730	33	77
Stromboli: *Per Stromboli*			
Chicken Broccoli	615	19	73
Pepperoni	805	40	71
Sausage	735	33	73
Pasta & Italian Specialties:			
Baked Spaghetti Bolognese, 15.8 oz	590	22	69
Baked Ziti, 15 oz	595	25	66
Chicken Alfredo, 16 oz	580	11	80
Meat Lasagna, 13.5 oz	695	21	94
Pasta Primavera, 10 oz	300	10	37
Spinach Lasagna, 19 oz	995	45	106
Spaghetti, 12 oz	755	34	94
Vegetables,			
Sauteed, Fresh, 5.45 oz	215	20	7.5

Vocelli Pizza® (Oct '12)

Pizzas: Per ⅛ of Medium Pizza

	C	F	Cb
Gourmet: Buffalo Chicken	240	9	27
Chicken Alfredo Spinaci	230	8	27
Philly Steak	270	12	27
Pasta: Chicken Alfredo, 18 oz	1080	55	100
Chicken Parmesan, 20 oz	1030	35	132
Chicken Pesto, 18 oz	1110	59	99
Hot Subs:			
Chicken Florentine, 8.5 oz	480	21	40
Chicken Pesto, 7.5 oz	410	17	34
Chicken Parm. on Ciabatta, 7 oz	440	18	45
Salads: *Per Regular Size, Without Dressing*			
Antipasta, 16 oz	270	16	17
Chicken Caesar, 8 oz	125	3	5
Mediterranean, 16 oz	270	18	17
Tuscan Chicken	290	13	12
Appetizers:			
Bruschetta, 1 slice, 4.65 oz	230	11	25
Buffalo Wings, bone in, 9 oz	720	54	2
BBQ Wings, bone in, 9 oz	760	53	14
Garlic Bread, 1.75 oz	230	11	27
Dessert: Cannoli (1), with cream	150	7	17
Tiramisu, 4 oz	340	21	34

Wahoo's Fish Taco® (Oct '12)

Bowls: With White Rice & Black Beans

	C	F	Cb
#7 Blackened/Charbroiled Chkn, av.	860	15	127
# 8 Charbroiled/Teriyaki Fish, av.	930	22	126
#9 Veggie	760	11	141
#10 Carnitas/Kahlua Pig, average	1025	25	131
Classic Burrito, A la Carte:			
Carne Asada	480	19	53
Carnitas	605	22	54
Charbroiled/Blackened:			
Fish, average	545	23	53
Chicken, average	495	18	52
Mushroom	405	16	55
Shrimp	400	16	53
Veggie, w/ White Rice & Black Beans	635	19	98
Tacos, A la Carte:			
Blackened Chicken	185	5	22
Carne Asada	180	5	22
Carnitas	235	8	23
Veggie w/ White Rice & Black Beans	215	4	36
Side Kicks: Brown Rice	350	7	64
White Beans	285	3	54
Salads: *Chips Not Included*			
Blackened Chicken	415	22	14
Charbroiled Chicken	415	21	14
Charbroiled Fish	485	29	14

For Complete Nutritional Data ~ see CalorieKing.com

WAWA® (Oct '12)

Breakfast:

	C	F	Cb
Bagels: Plain	290	1	60
Plain, with Butter	490	23	60
Cinnamon Raisin	290	1	63
Cinnamon, with Cream Cheese	410	13	65
Everything	310	6	56
Bowls: *Per Bowl, Without Syrup*			
Creamed Chipped Beef On White	290	10	40
Pancake: Without Syrup	330	10	56
With Bacon	370	12	57
With Sausage	490	24	57
With Turkey Sausage	420	16	57
Scrambled Egg: With Bacon	370	25	9
With Sausage	500	38	9
Ciabatta Melts: *On Shorti Roll, Without Extras*			
Scrambled Eggs: With Bacon	530	20	58
With Beef Cheesesteak	620	23	60
With Ham & Swiss	670	27	62
Italian Style	640	26	60
Sizzlis: *Without Hashbrowns*			
Bagels: Bacon, Egg & Cheese	370	15	42
Pork Roll, Egg & Cheese	420	19	42

Continued Next Page...

254

WAWA® cont... (Oct '12)

Lunch:

Bagel Sandwiches: *With Plain Bagel, w/o Toppings*

	C	F	Cb
BLT	390	8	62
Chicken Salad	630	29	66
Egg Salad	650	35	66

Cold Hoagies: *On Shorti Roll, Without Toppings*

	C	F	Cb
Egg Salad	560	36	46
Tuna Salad	620	38	48
Turkey	320	5	46

Soups: *Per Medium Serving*

Broccoli Cheddar	340	26	17
Maryland Crab	120	1	20
Minestrone	140	3.5	23

Sides: *Per Medium Serving*

Chili	250	8	32
Macaroni & Beef	350	11	43
Macaroni & Cheese	500	25	49
Mashed Potatoes	530	33	52
Meatballs in a Cup	360	25	20
Steak, Ale & Cheddar	480	29	32
Stuffing	400	23	42

Dinner:

Breaded Chicken Strips: 230, the

3 piece	240	13	16
5 piece	400	22	27

Hot Dogs: *Without Toppings, Mustard or Sauce*

¼ Pound	400	27	21
Big Bacon Cheese Dog	640	40	41

Hot Hoagies: *On Shorti Roll, Without Toppings*

Beef Cheesesteak	340	9	42
Chicken Cheesesteak	340	7	42
Meatballs	560	28	60

Soups: *Per Medium Serving*

Baked Potato w/ Cheddar & Bacon	450	32	28
Italian Wedding	130	4.5	16

Quesadillas: Beef

Quesadillas: Beef	550	30	36
Cheese	520	32	36
Chicken	550	28	35

Bakery:

Croissant, Plain	280	14	35
Muffins: Banana Walnut	670	34	83
Blueberry	610	30	78
Chocolate Chip	680	34	86
Corn	640	29	87

Beverages: *Per 24 oz*

Hot Cappuccino: Original	370	13	63
English Toffee	340	9	63
Smoothie, Strawberry Banana	690	0	180

Wendy's® (Oct '12)

Old Fashioned Hamburgers: With Standard Toppings

	C	F	Cb
Dave's ¼ lb Single	580	33	42
Dave's ½ lb Double	800	48	42
Dave's ¾ lb Triple	1060	67	42
Baconator: Single	660	40	40
Double	970	63	40
Son of Baconator	700	43	40
Bacon Deluxe Double	890	56	42
Double Stack	400	21	26
Jr. Bacon Cheeseburger	400	24	25
Jr. Cheeseburger	290	13	26
Jr. Cheeseburger Deluxe	350	19	27
The "W"	580	33	40

Sandwiches: With Standard Toppings

Asiago Ranch Club: With Spicy Chkn	710	37	57
With Homestyle Chicken	730	38	59
Crispy Chicken	380	20	37
Homestyle Chicken Fillet	560	23	57
Spicy Chicken Fillet	530	22	55
Ultimate Chicken Grill	390	10	43

Go Wraps: Homestyle Chicken

Go Wraps: Homestyle Chicken	350	17	32
Grilled Chicken	260	10	25
Spicy Chicken	340	16	31

Natural Cut Fries: Value

Natural Cut Fries: Value	230	11	30
Small, 4 oz	320	16	42
Medium, 5 oz	420	21	55
Large, 6½ oz	530	25	68

Crispy Chicken Nuggets: 5 pieces

Crispy Chicken Nuggets: 5 pieces	220	14	13
10 pieces	450	29	26

Sauces: Barbecue Nugget

Sauces: Barbecue Nugget	45	0	11
Heartland Ranch Dipping	120	12	3

Garden Sensations' Salads: Full, Without Toppings or Dressing

Apple Pecan Chicken	350	11	30
Baja	540	32	34
BLT Cobb	390	20	9
Spicy Chicken Caesar	470	25	26

Dressings: Classic Ranch, 1 pkt

Dressings: Classic Ranch, 1 pkt	100	10	2
Italian Vinaigrette, 1 pkt	70	6	4
Thousand Island, 1 pkt	160	15	5

Sides:

Chili, Large, 16 oz	310	9	31
Hot Stuffed Baked Potatoes: Plain	270	0	61
Sour Cream & Chives	320	3.5	63
Frosty, Chocolate/Vanilla, small	290	8	48

Frosty Shakes: Per Large 24 oz, With Whipped Cream

Caramel	1000	19	195
Chocolate	880	17	165
Strawberry	810	16	153
Vanilla Bean	870	16	169

For Complete Nutritional Data ~ see CalorieKing.com

255

Whataburger® (Oct '12)

Burgers

	C	F	Cb
All Time Favorites:			
A.1. Thick & Hearty Burger	1050	64	65
BBQ Cheddar Burger	1060	63	67
Chop House Cheddar Burger	1160	75	59
Green Chili Double	1010	62	68
Honey BBQ Chicken Strip S'wich	1070	56	97
Whataburger Patty Melt	1100	75	54
Justaburger	290	15	25
Whataburger: Original	640	32	61
Bacon & Cheese	800	44	61
Double Meat	880	51	61
Triple Meat	1130	70	61
Jr.	300	15	28
Jalapeno & Cheese	730	39	61
Chicken:			
Whatachick'n: Burger	570	27	64
Bites: 6 pieces, without sauce	390	19	31
9 pieces, without sauce	540	27	42
Strips, 3 pieces, without sauce	610	34	42
French Fries: Small, 3 oz	260	13	41
Medium, 4.5 oz	390	20	47
Large, 6 oz	520	27	63
Onion Rings: Medium, 4.25 oz	400	25	37
Large, 6½ oz	590	38	56
Salad, Garden, without dressing	170	9	15
Breakfast:			
Cinnamon Roll	390	9	71
Biscuits: Plain	300	17	32
With Bacon	350	20	32
With Gravy	510	30	48
With Jelly	340	17	41
With Sausage	540	37	32
Honey Butter Chicken	590	36	50
Biscuit Sandwiches:			
With Bacon	500	32	34
With Sausage	690	49	34

Whataburger® cont... (Oct '12)

Breakfast (Cont):	C	F	Cb
On A Bun: With Bacon	320	18	26
With Sausage	510	35	26
Platters: With Bacon	640	41	34
With Sausage	830	59	34
Taquitos: With Bacon & Egg	380	20	28
With Bacon, Egg & Cheese	420	24	28
With Cheese	370	20	28
Desserts:			
Chocolate Chunk Cookie	230	11	31
Hot Apple Pie, 3 oz	270	14	34
Beverages:			
Malts: Chocolate, 20 oz	670	16	123
Vanilla, 20 oz	590	17	99
Shake, Chocolate, 20 oz	630	16	111

White Castle® (Oct '12)

Burgers:	C	F	Cb
Cheeseburger: Single	170	9	15
Double	300	17	20
Sliders: Original	140	6	13
Double	240	12	21
Chicken Ring with Cheese	380	30	16
Chicken Breast with Cheese	390	28	20
Fish with Cheese	340	24	18
Surf & Turf with Cheese, 6 oz	540	38	27
Sides:			
Chicken Rings: 6 rings, 5 oz	530	47	12
9 rings, 7½ oz	790	71	18
Clam Strips, regular, 4.5 oz	210	17	5
Fish Nibblers, regular, 5 oz	320	16	28
French Fries, 5.6 oz	350	23	33
Mozzarella Cheese Sticks, 3 sticks	440	33	22
Onion Chips, 6 oz	670	50	46
Onion Rings, Homestyle, 5 oz	480	33	40
Sauces & Condiments: Per Packet			
Ketchup, 1 pkt	10	0	2
Mayonnaise, 1 pkt	60	7	0
Ranch Dressing, 1 oz	150	17	1
Sauces: BBQ, 1 pkt	10	0	3
Seafood, 1 oz	30	0	7
White Castle Zesty Zing, 1 oz	120	11	4

Updated Nutrition Data ~ www.CalorieKing.com
Persons with Diabetes ~ See Disclaimer (Page 22)

Wienerschnitzel® (Oct '12)

Hot Dogs:	C	F	Cb
Original: *On Standard Bun*			
Chili	300	14	31
Chili Cheese	350	18	31
Deluxe	280	13	30
Kraut	260	12	28
Plain	270	13	28
Stadium	280	13	30
Original: *On Pretzel Bun*			
Chili	430	16	57
Kraut; Mustard; Plain	400	15	54
Stadium	410	15	56
Angus All Beef: *On Pretzel Bun*			
Chicago	570	26	67
Chili Cheese	600	32	57
Bacon Wrapped: On Standard Bun			
Original	370	23	27
Street Style	400	26	29
Corn Dogs: Regular	250	17	15
Mini (6 pack)	320	22	12
Junkyard Dog, Orig., on Seeded Bun	490	26	45
Sides: Chili Cheese Fries	540	38	39
Fries: Regular	300	22	25
Large	430	31	35
Jalapeno Poppers (3)	210	11	21
Breakfast:			
Biscuits: Egg, Bacon, Cheese	440	25	36
Egg, Sausage, Cheese	540	34	40
Burritos: Egg, Bacon, Cheese	490	25	39
Egg, Sausage, Cheese	590	34	43
French Toast Sticks	490	29	49
Syrup, 1 oz	120	0	31
Desserts:			
Cones: Plain, 5 oz.	250	9	41
Chocolate Dipped, 5 oz.	450	27	50
Floats: Mountain Dew; Root Beer, av.	440	12	85
Tropicana Strawberry Lemonade	450	12	82
Freezees: Butterfinger	620	24	100
Oreo; M&M	630	25	99
Reese's Peanut Butter Cup	630	26	97
Sundaes: Caramel; Hot Fudge av.	400	16	63
Chocolate	390	14	64
Pineapple; Strawberry	370	14	59
Shakes, average all flavors	650	23	110
Drinks: 16 fl.oz, without ice			
Lipton Raspberry Iced Tea	180	0	45
Mountain Dew	230	0	61
Mug Root Beer	210	0	57

Winchell's® (Oct '12)

Donuts: Per Donut	C	F	Cb
Buttermilk Bars: Choc Iced; Glazed	420	19	61
Jelly Filled:			
Apple with Cinnamon Crumb	370	15	53
Raspberry with Glaze	390	13	61
Strawberry with Sugar	380	13	60
Old Fashioned, Glazed; Maple Iced	410	17	60
Raised Ring: Choc. Iced	270	10	41
Sugared	230	9	34

WingStreet (Oct '12)

Chicken:	C	F	Cb
Crispy Bone In Wings: *Per 2 Pieces*			
All American, 2 oz	200	14	8
Buffalo, Mild/Med./Hot, 2.75 oz	230	15	16
Garlic Parmesan, 2.5 oz	300	25	9
Honey BBQ, 3 oz	260	14	24
Bone Out Wings: *Per 2 Pieces*			
All American, 2 oz	150	8	11
Buffalo, Mild/Medium, 2.5 oz	190	9	18
Garlic Parmesan, 2.5 oz	260	19	11
Honey BBQ, 3 oz	220	8	27
Traditional Wings: *Per 2 Pieces*			
All American, 1.25 oz	80	5	0
Buffalo, Medium/Hot, 2 oz	110	6	8
Garlic Parmesan, 2 oz	180	16	1
Spicy Asian, 2.3 oz	130	5	13

Woody's Bar-B-Q® (Oct '12)

Starters:	C	F	Cb
Breaded Wings (10)	700	47	13
Beef Chili Cheese Fries	805	38	63
Dinner Entrees: Without Sides			
½ Chicken	840	56	0
Baby Back Ribs, ½ Rack	260	20	1
Beef Prime Rib	760	62	1
Sandwiches: Per Regular, Without Sides			
Beef	390	14	28
Pork	490	26	29
Wraps: Without Sides			
Beef BBQ	380	13	31
Pork	440	21	31
Dogs: Chili Cheese	630	48	26
Slaw	580	44	32

For Complete Nutritional Data ~ see CalorieKing.com

Fast - Foods & Restaurants

Yoshinoya® (Oct '12)

Bowls: With Sauce	C	F	Cb
Beef Bowl: Regular	730	27	91
Large	1040	38	131
With Vegetables: Regular	650	20	95
Large	960	29	141
Beef & Chicken Combo:			
Large, with skin	1190	36	151
Large, without skin	1150	33	151
Teriyaki Chicken Bowl:			
Regular, with skin	790	18	190
Large, with skin	1140	25	165
Vegetable Bowl, regular	440	3	97
BBQ Style Plates:			
Beef Plate: W/ Fried Rice & Ndles	850	35	98
With Fried Rice	830	38	89
With Steamed Rice	800	31	100
With Fried and Steamed Rice	810	34	95
Beef & Chicken Plates:			
With Fried Rice & Noodles	950	38	101
With Fried Rice	920	40	92
With Noodles	970	36	109
Chicken Plates: W/ Fried Rice & Ndles	700	23	79
With Fried Rice	720	24	84
With Steamed Rice	690	17	94
With Fried and Steamed Rice	710	21	89
Kids, Chicken	360	7	53
Desserts: Cheese Cake, 3.5 oz	330	19	35
Chocolate Cheesecake, 3.5 oz	370	22	37

Z Pizza® (Oct '12)

Pizzas: Small, Per Slice	C	F	Cb
Creations: Berkeley Vegan	180	8	19
California	150	6	19
Casablanca	190	9	18
Greek	150	6	17
Italian; Mexican; Napoli, av.	180	8	18
Provence	160	7	20
Santa Fe	180	7	20
Thai	170	6	19
Tuscan	160	7	18
ZBQ	170	5	21
Rusticas: Per Slice			
Chicken Sausage	105	3	11
Curry Chicken & Yam	135	4	17
Mediterranean	145	8	12
Moroccan	120	6	13
Pear & Gorgonzola	135	5	13
Calzones: Meat Calzone	760	36	75
Veggie Calzone	600	22	80
Salads: Small, Without Dressing			
Arugula	450	37	23
Caesar Side	200	17	8
California	90	5	13
Pear and Gorgonzola	530	44	25

Zaxby's® (Oct '12)

Zappetizers: With Sauce	C	F	Cb
Fried White Cheddar Bites w/ sce	820	52	62
Onion Rings, 5 oz	780	56	59
Spicy Fried Mushroom, 5.7 oz	620	46	43
Tater Chips, 5.2 oz	940	68	72
Meal Dealz: With Sauce, without Drink			
Big Zax Snak	950	52	82
Buffalo Wings, without sauce	900	56	51
Chicken Finger Nibbler	1330	71	137
Most Popular: As Served			
Chicken Finger Plate: Regular	1260	72	99
Large	1775	105	129
Wings & Things	1490	92	85
Sandwich Baskets: Includes Fries			
Cajun Club	1140	58	98
Club	1250	73	99
Wings & Fingerz: With Sauce			
Buffalo Fingerz: 5 pieces	630	42	15
10 pieces	1050	65	27
Buffalo Wings: 5 pieces	540	40	3
10 pieces	880	60	4
Chicken Fingerz: 5 pieces	610	39	19
10 pieces	1230	80	36
Zax Kidz: Without Drink			
Kiddie Cheese	490	29	49
Kiddie Finger	570	36	40
Kiddie Nibbler	610	33	61
Zalads: With Texas Toast, Without Dressing			
Blue, with Blackened Chicken	605	29	34
Caesar Zalad:			
With Fried Chicken	730	39	39
With Grilled Chicken	570	26	29
House Zalad: With Fried Chicken	765	42	44
With Grilled Chicken	605	29	34
Salad Dressings:			
Blue Cheese, 1 packet, 1.25 oz	180	19	2
Honey French, 1.25 oz	150	12	9
Honey Mustard, 1.25 oz	150	13	6
Lite Ranch, 1.25 oz	90	8	3
Mediterranean, 1.25 oz	140	14	4
Ranch, 1.25 oz	160	16	2
Thousand Island	230	24	3
Sides: Celery Basket, with sauce	370	40	6.5
Cole Slaw, 2.2 oz	140	11	12
Crinkle Fries, regular, 5 oz	360	16	48
Texas Toast, basket, 3 wedges, 4.3 oz	440	20	60

Zero Sub's® ~ see CalorieKing.com

Updated Nutrition Data ~ www.CalorieKing.com
Persons with Diabetes ~ See Disclaimer (Page 22)

Notes on Cholesterol

- **Cholesterol is a white waxy substance produced** mainly by our liver. It is also found in animal food products. Plant foods have no cholesterol.

- **Cholesterol is essential to life.** It is a structural part of every body cell wall and is the building block for vitamin D, sex hormones, and bile acids which help in the digestion of dietary fats.

- **The body makes sufficient cholesterol** for its needs and does not rely on cholesterol in the diet. Dietary fats have a major influence on blood cholesterol levels - more so than dietary cholesterol.

- **A high blood cholesterol level increases** the risk of atherosclerosis - the thickening of arteries that can reduce or block blood flow to the heart, brain, eyes, kidneys, sex organs and other body parts.

  This in turn increases the risk of heart attack, stroke, blindness, kidney failure, impotence and other blood circulatory problems.

  Other risk factors which increase the risk of atherosclerosis include high blood pressure, smoking, obesity and uncontrolled diabetes.

BLOOD CHOLESTEROL

CHECK YOUR RISK!

Total Cholesterol Level (mg/dl)		Risk of Heart Attack
▼		▼
240 and above	~	High Risk
200 - 239	~	Borderline/High
Below 200	~	Desirable

♥ **Know your cholesterol level,** particularly if there is a family history of heart disease or stroke. If level is high, see your doctor.

♥ **All adults should have** their cholesterol, HDL and triglycerides tested at least every 5 years.

HEART ATTACK WARNING SIGNALS

Many victims die before reaching the hospital by ignoring warning signals and delaying medical help.
Symptoms vary and commonly include:

- **Chest pain,** vice-like squeezing or burning sensation in center of the chest or between the shoulder blades, or in the mid-back. Pain may even feel like severe indigestion.

- **Pain** may be felt in the arms, shoulders, neck or jaw.

- **Shortness of breath** often occurs with or before chest discomfort.

- **Other signs,** with or without pain, include a cold sweat, nausea or light-headedness.

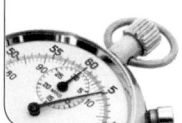

If you experience any of the above symptoms call IMMEDIATELY for medical help. Every minute counts.

Call 9-1-1 or your emergency number

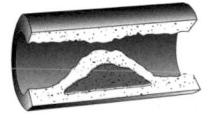

▲ Atherosclerosis can clog arteries and impede blood flow to the heart or other body organs.

▼ A thrombus (blood clot) can form on unstable, festering athero-sclerotic plaque and rapidly block blood flow. A heart attack or stroke can result.

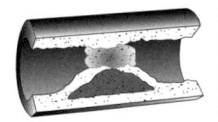

Fats & Cholesterol Guide

The amount and type of dietary fat has the greatest influence on blood cholesterol levels.

Fats in food are a mixture of 3 basic types: saturated, monounsaturated, and polyunsaturated. Animal fats are mainly saturated while plant oils and fish oils are mainly mono- and polyunsaturated.

Saturated fats have subgroups known as long-chain, medium-chain, and short-chain fats. Most of the long chain fats raise blood cholesterol, and increase the risk of blood clots and thrombosis leading to artery blockage.

Long-chain saturated fats are found mainly in full-cream milk, cheese, butter, cream, fatty meats and sausages, and processed foods.

Monounsaturated fats tend to more selectively lower 'bad' LDL cholesterol and maintain the protective 'good' HDL cholesterol in the bloodstream – but only if they replace saturated fats in the diet.

Foods rich in monounsaturates include canola and olive oils, canola margarine, peanuts, and avocados.

Polyunsaturated fats consist of two main classes. **Omega-6** polyunsaturates tend to lower blood cholesterol. Rich sources include safflower, sunflower and corn oils.

Omega-3 polyunsaturated fats can lower blood cholesterol; significantly lower blood triglycerides; and reduce the rise of thrombosis, heart arrythmmia, and artery spasm.

Best practical omega-3 sources include canola oil and margarine, soybean oil and fish.

A balanced intake of the two omega classes is important for optimal health. For most Americans, slightly increasing omega-3 intake would help attain a more ideal balance.

Trans fats from hydrogenated vegetable oils and shortenings should also be avoided. They are common in commercial baked and fried food products such as cakes, muffins, pastries, doughnuts, fried snacks and french fries.

> Note: All fats are high in calories and need to be limited for weight control.

DIETARY FATS COMPARISON

- ■ Saturated Fat
- ▨ Monounsaturated Fat
- Polyunsaturated Fats:
  - ☐ Linoleic (Omega-6)
  - ■ Alpha-Linolenic (Omega-3)

OILS	PERCENTAGE CONTENT			
CANOLA OIL	7	63	20	10
LINSEED/FLAX OIL	9	19	17	55
SAFFLOWER OIL	9	14	77	
GRAPESEED OIL	10	22	68	
SUNFLOWER OIL	11	23	66	
CORN OIL	14	32	52	2
OLIVE OIL	14	76	10	
SOYBEAN OIL	15	23	54	8
PEANUT OIL	19	45	34	2
COTTONSEED OIL	26	16	58	
PALM OIL	51	39	10	

SPREADS & FATS
Saturated Fat includes 'Trans Fats'   ☐ WATER CONTENT

LIGHT MARGARINE	14	14	21	51	
CANOLA MARGARINE	18	45	12	6	19
POLYUNSATURATED MARG	24	20	36	20	
BUTTER	57	18	2	24	
LARD	41	47	12		
BEEF FAT	44	37	4	15	

GOOD SOURCES OF OMEGA-3 FATS

Plant Sources	Omega-3 Fats (Grams)
Canola Oil, 1 Tbsp, ½ fl.oz	1.5g
Flaxseed Oil, 1 Tbsp	8g
Soybean Oil, 1 Tbsp	1.2g
Canola Margarine, 1 Tbsp, ½ oz	1g
Soybeans, cooked, ½ cup, 4 oz	0.5g
Walnuts, ½ oz	0.5g

FISH - Per 4 oz Serving

High Content: Salmon (Chinook), Tuna, **3g**
Trout (Lake), Sardines, Herring, Mackerel **3g**

Medium Content:
    Salmon, (Pink/Red/Coho), 4 oz **2g**

Fair Content: Per 4 oz Serving
Bass, Catfish, Cod, Grouper, Hake,
Halibut, Kingfish, Perch, Pollock, Shark, } **0.5-1g**
Trout (Rainbow), Tuna, Crab,
Oysters, Blue Mussels, Shrimp, Squid

How Much Is Needed?

As little as 1-2 grams daily of omega-3 fats may benefit general health. High doses of fish-oil supplements should only be taken as directed by your doctor.

Dietary Cholesterol

Cholesterol in food varies in its effect on blood cholesterol level (BCL) from person to person. Much depends on the amount and type of fat and fiber eaten at the same meal.

Any elevating effect of dietary cholesterol on BCL is more likely to occur when the diet is high in saturated fat. Little elevation, if any, generally occurs when dietary fats are balanced in favor of monounsaturated and polyunsaturated fats (including omega-3 fats).

For example, while fish does contain cholesterol, the omega-3 fats can prevent any increase in BCL. Conversely, a meal containing no cholesterol but rich in saturated fat may result in a significant increase in BCL.

Consequently, the need to be overly concerned about dietary cholesterol is being de-emphasized in favor of the approach of limiting total fat, saturated fat, and trans fat in particular – and substituting unsaturated fats.

The liver usually cuts back its own cholesterol production in response to cholesterol in the diet. Many people can consume normal amounts of high-cholesterol foods without concern.

However, it is difficult to identify just who is at risk - the so-called 'hyper-responders'. Because over 50% of Americans have a BCL above ideal levels, the **American Heart Association** advises all Americans to be prudent and limit their cholesterol intake to less than 300mg daily, as well as to adopt a heart-healthy diet.

This limitation still allows the inclusion of most foods that are regularly eaten – even the overly maligned egg.

> Eggs contain a modest 5 grams of fat per large egg. Barely 2 grams is saturated, the rest being monounsaturated or polyunsaturated.
>
> By comparison, a cup of whole milk has 8g fat of which almost 5g is saturated.

CHOLESTEROL COUNTER

Cholesterol is found only in foods of animal origin. Plant foods contain no cholesterol.

	Cholesterol mg
Meat - Average all types:	
Lean Meat, cooked, 120g	100
Fatty Meat, cooked, 120g	100
Fat, thick strip, 60g	40

Note: While lean meat and fat have similar amounts of cholesterol, choose lean meat to limit fat intake.

Chicken/Turkey, average, 120g	100
Organ Meats: Liver, fried, 4 oz	500
Brains, beef, pan fried, 3 oz	1700
Sausages: Frankfurter, 40g	25
Salami, 2 slices, 55g	40
Bacon: 3 slices, cooked, 30g	20
Fish: Fish fillets, average, ckd, 120g	70
Tuna/Salmon, canned, 100g	50
Scallops, 9 medium, 3 oz	30
Prawns, raw, 100g	110
Oysters, raw, 6 medium, 85g	45
Crayfish, Crab, cooked, 100g	70
Eggs (Chicken), 1 large	210
1 medium	180
Egg White, *Scramblers*	0
Milk/Yoghurt: Whole, 1 cup, 250ml	30
Light/low-fat Milk (1%), 1 cup	10
Skim/Non-fat, 1 cup	10
Soy Milk, Tofu, Tempeh	0
Cheese: Natural/Hard/Cream, 30g	30
Cottage, low-fat, 2 Tbsp, 40g	5
Cream Cheese, 30g	25
Fats: Butter, 1 Tbsp, 20g	45
Margarine, Oils (vegetable)	0
Mayonnaise, 1 Tbsp	10
Cream: Heavy, whipping, 2 Tbsp, 40g	40
Light/Sour, 2 Tbsp	10
Ice Cream: Full-fat (10–11%), 100ml/50g	20
Low-fat (less than 4%), 50g	5
Fruit, Vegetables, Avocados	0
Nuts, Seeds, Grains	0
Coffee, Tea, Beer, Wine	0

For Comprehensive Food Listings ~ see CalorieKing.com

Blood Cholesterol ~ Diet Hints

DIETARY HINTS TO LOWER BLOOD CHOLESTEROL

1. Maintain a healthy weight.
If overweight, lose weight with a sensible, low-fat meal plan and daily exercise.

2. Reduce saturated fat intake by:
(a) eating less dairy fat. Choose low-fat or fat-reduced varieties of milk, yogurt, soy drinks, cheese, and ice cream.

(b) replacing saturated fats with fats and oils rich in monounsaturated and polyunsaturated fats. Choose vegetable oils such as canola, olive, sunflower and soybean. Avoid solid frying fats.

Note: *Promise Active* and *Benecol* spreads contain plant stanol esters which can lower total and LDL cholesterol.

(c) eating less fat from meat and poultry. Choose lean cuts of meat and skinless chicken. Go easy on lunch meats, salami and fatty sausages. Enjoy fish.

(d) eating less saturated and trans fats from baked and fried fast-foods. Avoid deep-fried foods. Avoid donuts, cakes, pastries and cookies unless made with healthier fats and oils.

3. Increase your soluble fiber intake.
Foods rich in soluble fiber include beans, lentils, chick peas, hummus, nuts, seeds, psyllium-seed husks and psyllium-fiber supplements. Oat bran, rice bran and barley are also good sources, as are fruit, vegetables and avocados.
(*See Fiber Guide - Page 264-269*).

4. Eat more soy bean products such as: soy drinks, tofu, tempeh (cultured soy beans), soy flour, soy vegetarian foods and edamame (fresh green soybeans).

Soy protein in place of animal protein can significantly decrease high blood cholesterol levels as well as 'bad' LDL cholesterol and blood triglycerides while 'good' HDL cholesterol is maintained. For best results, eat at least 25g of soy protein per day (from 3-4 servings).

5. Eat more fruit, vegetables, and whole grains in place of high-fat foods. Aim for 2 fruits and 5 servings of vegetables per day. They also contain valuable antioxidants. The fat of avocados (and most nuts) is mainly unsaturated and can lower blood cholesterol levels.

6. Limit cholesterol to 300mg per day.
(Extra Notes ~ See Previous Page)

7. Avoid brewed unfiltered coffee (espresso; plunger-style). Several cups per day may raise blood cholesterol. Filtered coffee is fine.

8. Spread your food intake over the day.
Have 5-6 small meals per day rather than just 2-3 large meals. Nibbling, versus gorging, favors lower blood cholesterol.

ALCOHOL – WINE

Alcohol is a mixed bag. Moderate amounts of 1-2 drinks daily appear to reduce the risk of heart attack and ischemic stroke in older persons.

However, larger amounts increase the risk of high blood pressure, obesity, heart failure and hemorrhagic stroke, and can aggravate hypertriglyceridemia: as well as many other health hazards. (*See Alcohol Guide – Page 23*)

The speculative benefits of moderate alcohol intake have been overstated in the media. The overriding harmful effects of excess alcohol do not allow its recommendation for any aspects of health promotion.

Fruit, Vegetables & Tea Also Protect:
Red wine and red grapes (more so than white) contain antioxidants which may help protect cholesterol in the blood from becoming oxidized.

Many fruits, vegetables, grains, nuts and tea also contain protective antioxidants.

How Fats Affect Blood Flow

Fats in the diet affect more than blood cholesterol levels. They can also strongly influence blood clot formation and thrombosis, as well as blood flow and ultimate oxygen delivery to body parts and organs.

While advanced atherosclerosis can impede blood flow to the heart and other organs, it is thrombosis (complete blockage by blood clots) or arterial spasm which commonly results in a heart attack or stroke.

Plant and fish oils rich in omega-3 fats lessen the risk of blood clots, thrombus formation, and artery spasm by reducing platelet stickiness and adhesion to artery walls. This reduces the risk of atherosclerotic plaque becoming unstable and reactive.

Omega-3 fats also improve blood flow by reducing blood viscosity and increasing the flexibility of red blood cells (RBC) that need to flex and twist on themselves in order to squeeze through tiny narrow capillaries often half their diameter.

A diet high in saturated fats has the opposite effect by stiffening RBC membranes and increasing blood viscosity, thereby hindering blood flow. The stiffening of the RBC membrane also reduces its ability to release vital oxygen to body cells and take up carbon dioxide.

Stiff red blood cells may also form aggregates that resemble coin stacks. In narrow blood vessels, this further impedes blood flow and impairs oxygen release through the much-lessened surface area of red blood cell membranes exposed to blood. (Smoking, lack of exercise, and stress can have similar adverse effects on thrombosis, red blood cell flexibility, and blood flow.).

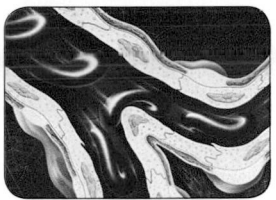

▲ **Picture of Healthy Blood Flow**

Flexible red blood cells twist and slide through tiny capillaries - often half the diameter of red blood cells.

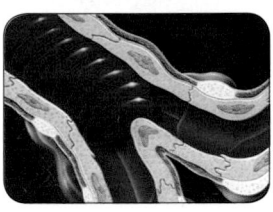

▲ **A Not-So-Healthy Picture!**

Red blood cells have lost their flexibility and ability to twist and slip through capillaries. They are stacked up, thereby impeding blood flow.

A diet high in saturated fats can contribute to this picture - as can smoking, lack of exercise, and stress.

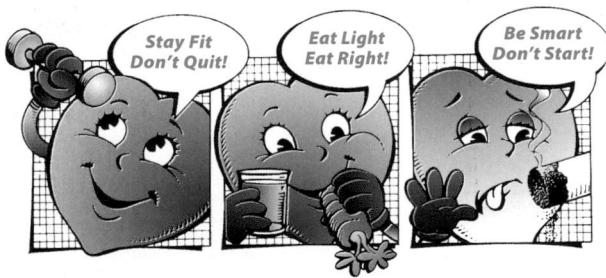

Fiber Guide

Introduction `Fiber`

Fiber is the general term for those parts of plant food that we cannot digest (although bacteria in the large bowel partly digests fiber through fermentation). It is not found in foods of animal origin (meats, dairy products).

Fiber promotes intestinal health, bowel regularity, can benefit diabetes and blood cholesterol levels, and may help prevent colon cancer. High-fiber foods also assist weight control.

Most Americans don't eat enough fiber – less than 20 grams/day - instead of a healthier 25 to 35 grams/day.

Types of Fiber

Plant foods contain a mixture of different fibers in varying proportions. Insoluble and soluble fiber categories are based on their solubility in water. All types of fiber are beneficial to the body.

◆ **Insoluble fibers** (cellulose, hemi-celluloses, lignin) make up the structural parts of plant cell walls.

Best **food sources** are wheat bran, corn bran, rice bran, wholegrain cereals and breads, beans and peas, nuts, seeds, and the skins of fruits and vegetables.

These fibers absorb many times their own weight in water. They create a soft bulk and hasten the passage of waste products through the intestines.

They promote bowel regularity, and aid in the prevention and treatment of uncomplicated forms of **constipation, diverticulosis and hemorrhoids.**

The risk of colon cancer may also be reduced by fiber's diluting effect on potentially harmful substances.

◆ **Soluble fibers** (pectin, gums, mucilages) are found mainly within plant cells, soy milk (whole bean) and products.

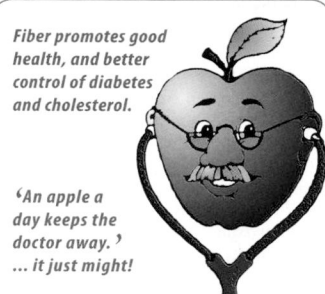

Fiber promotes good health, and better control of diabetes and cholesterol.

'*An apple a day keeps the doctor away.*'
... it just might!

Types of Fiber (Cont)

Best Sources of Soluble Fiber: Fruits and vegetables, oat bran, barley, beans and peas, prunes, psyllium and flax seed.

These fibers form a gel which slows both stomach emptying and the absorption of sugars from the intestines. **This helps to control blood sugar levels.**

Weight control is also aided by the slower emptying of the stomach and the feeling of **fullness provided by soluble fiber.**

Some soluble fibers can lower **blood cholesterol** by binding bile acids and excreting them. More body cholesterol must then be broken down to supply bile acids for emulsification of dietary fats. **Rice bran, while not high in soluble fiber, can also lower blood cholesterol.**

◆ **Resistant starch** is that part of starchy foods (approx. 10%) which is tightly bound by fiber and resists normal digestion. Friendly bacteria in the large bowel ferment and change the resistant starch into short-chain fatty acids, which are important to bowel health and may protect against colon cancer.

Starchy foods include bread, cereals, rice, pasta, potatoes and legumes.

Fiber & Weight Control

Fiber can assist weight control in several ways. Fiber rich foods such as fresh fruit and vegetables, potatoes and wholegrain bread contain few calories for their large volume (due to their low-fat, high-water content).

Their bulk fills the stomach and satisfies the appetite much sooner than fiber-depleted foods. The extra chewing time also contributes to satiety, and gives the stomach time to register a feeling of fullness. Excessive calories are less likely to be consumed.

Fiber-depleted foods and drinks are more concentrated in calories; e.g. fats, sugar, candy, soft drinks, fruit juices, alcohol. They require little or no chewing. Large amounts with excessive calories can be consumed before the appetite is satisfied.

Example: Whereas one fresh apple might satisfy the appetite, an apple juice drink with the equivalent sugars and calories of 2-3 apples only minimally satisfies the appetite. (See illustration below.)

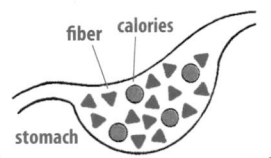

High-fiber foods fill the stomach. Fewer calories are consumed.

Low-fiber foods are more concentrated in calories. More food must be eaten to fill the stomach.

EFFECTS OF REMOVING FIBER FROM FOOD

2-3 pieces of fresh fruit produces 1 glass of fruit juice. The removal of fiber concentrates the sugar and calories.

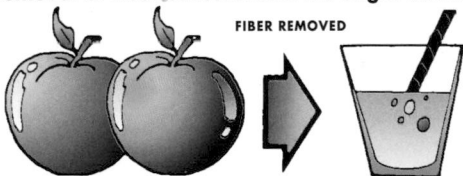

FIBER REMOVED

Fresh Fruit		Fruit Juice
High Fiber	←	Negligible Fiber
Low Calorie Density	←	High Calorie Density
Long Eating Time	←	No Eating Time (Drink)
Satisfies Hunger	←	Does Not Satisfy Hunger
Sugar Slowly Absorbed	←	Sugar More Quickly Absorbed
Less Insulin Required	←	More Insulin Required

Fiber Guide ~ Constipation

Constipation

Constipation can reasonably be defined as a failure to have a bowel movement at least every second day – and just as importantly, without straining or pain.

Typically, constipated stools are too hard, too narrow and too small.

The **main cause** is simply a lack of dietary fiber. Other contributing factors include insufficient fluids, too little exercise, emotional stress, gastrointestinal disease, lack of proper dentition to chew high-fiber foods, and some medications (e.g. some antacids, antidepressants, pain medications).

Note: Check with your doctor to rule out any underlying medical problem – especially if you have a change in bowel habits in middle-age or later years.

DESIRABLE FIBER INTAKE

Adults: 25-35gm per day
Children (under 18): Age + 5gm
Example: 6-year old (6 + 5)= 11gm

SAMPLE FOOD QUANTITIES
For 35 Grams of Fiber/Day

	Fiber
Breakfast Cereal (higher-fiber)	5g
plus 4 slices wholegrain Bread	6g
plus 3 servings fresh Fruit	9g
plus 1 medium Potato (w. skin)	
or 1 cup Brown Rice	4g
or ½ cup wholegrain Pasta	
plus 3-4 servings Veggies/Salad	6g
plus 1 cup Bean Soup	
or ¼ cup Baked/Soy Beans	
or ½ cup Corn/Peas/Lentils	5g
or 1¼ oz Almonds (natural)	
or 3 medium Figs	

HINTS TO INCREASE FIBER AND AVOID CONSTIPATION

1 **Breakfast is an important** contributor to daily fiber intake. Eat high-fiber breakfast cereals (bran-based cereals, oatmeal etc.). Add 1-2 tablespoons of unprocessed bran.

Dried fruits, chopped nuts, soy grits, and seeds are also excellent additions to cereals.

Note: A gradual increase in fiber will prevent bloating, gas or pain. People intolerant to bran may benefit from psyllium-based fiber supplements and cereals.

2 **Drink adequate water daily.** Fiber works by absorbing many times its own weight in water.

3 **Eat wholegrain breads,** or fiber-enriched breads. They have over double the fiber of regular white bread.

4 **Enjoy fruit as fresh fruit** with skin rather than as fruit juice. Enjoy wholegrain pasta, barley, brown rice, nuts and seeds.

5 **Eat more vegetables,** salads and legumes – especially cooked beans, lentils, potatoes with skins, avocado, broccoli, brussels sprouts, cabbage, carrots, celery, and peas.

6 **Add bran** (barley/rice/wheat) or soy grits to soups, casseroles, yogurt, desserts, cookies, cakes. Also use whole-meal flour or soy flour in place of white flour. Use nuts, seeds, and ground linseed.

7 **Snack** on fresh or dried fruits, carrot or celery sticks, popcorn, nuts or seeds, wholegrain crackers, high-fiber bars (low-fat). Limit amounts if overweight.

8 **Exercise regularly** to strengthen abdominal muscles and stimulate the gut. Keep up water intake, especially in warm weather.

9 **Avoid** indiscriminate and regular use of harsh laxatives. They can overstimulate the intestinal muscles and may make normal bowel activity impossible. It may take several weeks to restore normal bowel function.

Breakfast Cereals   Fiber

General Mills:

	Fiber
Basic 4, 1 cup, 2 oz	3
Cheerios (Honey Nut; Multigrain), 1 c., 1 oz	2
Fiber One, ½ cup, 1.1 oz	14
Multi-Bran Chex, 1 cup, 2 oz	7
Oatmeal Crisp Almond, 1 cup, 2 oz	4
Raisin Nut Bran, 1¼ cup, 2 oz	6
Total, average all types, ¾ cup, 1 oz	3
Wheat Chex, 1 cup, 2 oz	6
Wheaties ¾ cup, 1 oz	3

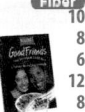

Health Valley:

	Fiber
Amaranth Flakes, ¾ cup, 1 oz	3
Crunches & Flakes, ¾ cup, 1.9 oz	4
Fiber 7 Flakes, ¾ cup, 1 oz	7
Golden Flax, ¾ cup, 1.9 oz	6
Granola (Low-Fat),⅔ cup, 2 oz	6
Healthy Fiber Flakes, ¾ cup, 1.1 oz	4
Oat Bran Flakes, all types, ¾ cup, 1 oz	2
Oat Bran O's, ¾ cup, 1 oz	3
Real Oat Bran, ½ cup, 1.7 oz	5

Kellogg's:

	Fiber
All-Bran, ½ cup, 1.1 oz	10
All-Bran w. Extra Fiber, ½ cup, 1 oz	13
All-Bran Bran Buds, ⅓ cup, 1 oz	13
Corn Flakes, Fruit Loops, Smacks 1 cup, 1 oz	1
Cocoa/Rice Krispies Treats, 1¼ cup, 1 oz	0
Complete: Wheat Flakes, ¾ c., 1 oz	5
Oat Bran Flakes, ¾ cup, 1.1 oz	4
Corn Pops, 1 cup, 1.1 oz	0
Cracklin' Oat Bran, ¾ cup, 1.7oz	6
FiberPlus Antioxidants:	
Berry Yogurt Crunch, 1 c., 1.9 oz	10
Cinnamon Oat Crunch ¾ c., 1.1 oz	9
Frosted Mini Wheats, 24 bisc., 2 oz	5
Granola w. Raisins, ⅔ cup, 2.1 oz	3
Raisin Bran, 1 cup, 2.1 oz	7
Smart Start, Strong Heart,	
Cinnamon Raisin, 1 cup, 1.8 oz	4
Special K, 1 cup, 1.1 oz	0.5

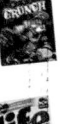

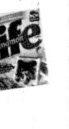

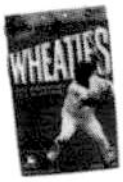

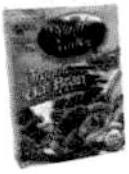

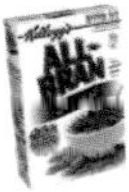

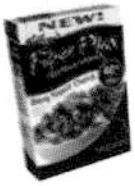

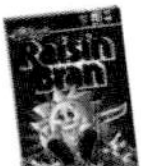

Fiber ~ Fiber (grams)

Breakfast Cereals (Cont)   Fiber

	Fiber
Kashi: GoLEAN Cereal, 1 cup, 1.8 oz	10
GoLEAN Crunch!, 1 cup, 1.9 oz	8
GoLEAN Bars, avg. (1)	6
Good Friends: Original, 1 cup, 1.9 oz	12
Cinna-Raisin Crunch, 1 cup, 1.8 oz	8
Heart to Heart, ¾ cup, 1.2 oz	5
7 Whole Grain Pilaf, ½ cup, cooked, 5 oz	7
7 Whole Grain Puffs, 1 cup, 0.7 oz	1
Quaker: Cap'n Crunch, ¾ cup, 1 oz	1
100% Natural Granola,	
avg., ½ cup, 1.8 oz	3
Crunchy Corn Bran, 1 cup, 1 oz	5
Life Cereal, ¾ cup, 1.1 oz	2
Oat Bran, ½ cup, 1.4 oz	6
Oatmeal, average, 1 packet	3
Post: 100% Bran, ⅓ cup, 1 oz	9
Alpha Bits, 1 cup, 1 oz	2
Blueberry Morning, 1 cup, 1.9 oz	5
Cocoa/Fruity Pebbles, 1 cup, 1 oz	0
Cranberry Almond Crunch, 1 cup, 1.8 oz	3
Fruit & Bran, 1 cup, 1.9 oz	6
Grape-Nuts, ½ cup, 2 oz	7
Great Grains, ⅔ cup, 1.9 oz	5
Honey Bunches of Oats, ¾ cup, 1.1 oz	2
Shredded Wheat & Bran, ½ cup, 2 oz	8

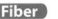

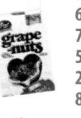

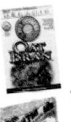

Brans & Supplements, Metamucil

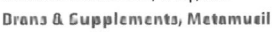

	Fiber
Oat Bran: 1 Tbsp (level)	1
⅓ cup, (5½ Tbsp.)	5
Rice Bran, raw. ¼ cup, 1 oz	6
Wheat Bran (unprocessed):	
Raw, 1 Tbsp	1.5
2 Tbsp (level), ¼ oz	3
¼ cup, (4 Tbsp.), ½ oz	3
Wheat Germ: Raw, ¼ cup, 1 oz	4
Psyllium Seed Husks, 2 Tbsp	8
Fibersure: 1 heaping tsp	5
Metamucil: Orange, 1 rnd Tbsp, 11g	3
Fiber Wafers (2)	6

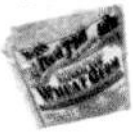

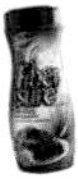

Hot Cereals, Oatmeal

	Fiber
Bulgur (cracked Wheat), ckd, 1 cup	8
Corn/Hominy Grits, dry, 3 Tbsp, 1 oz	0.5
Cream of Wheat, cooked, ¾ cup	1
Oatmeal (uncooked ⅓ cup), ckd, ⅔ cup	3

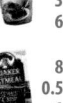

Fiber Counter

Breads & Crackers | Fiber

Bread: White, 1 slice, 1 oz — 0.6
Whole-wheat, 1 slice, 1 oz — 1.5
Wholegrain, 1 slice, 1 oz — 2
Rye, Pumpernickel, 1 slice — 1.5
Bagel/Roll/Bun, 1 medium, 2 oz — 1.5
Pita, whole wheat, 6½" pocket — 4.5
Crackers: Graham, average, 2 — 0.4
Saltine, 4 crackers — 0.4
Crispbreads (Rye), average, 2 — 4
Matzo 1 board, 1 oz — 1
Rice Cakes, average, 1 cake — 0.3
Tortilla: Regular, 6" — 0.5
Whole-wheat, 6" — 1.3

Barley, Pasta, Rice & Flours

Barley, pearled, raw, ¼ cup, 1.7 oz — 8
Rice: White, cooked, 1 cup — 0.6
Brown, cooked, 1 cup — 3.5
Rice-A-Roni, average, 1 cup, prepared — 1.5
Spaghetti/Noodles: Cooked, 1 cup — 2
Whole-wheat, cooked, 1 cup — 4
Flour: Wheat, All-purpose, 1 cup, 4½ oz — 3.5
Whole-Wheat, 1 cup, 4½ oz — 15
Cornmeal, stone ground, 1 cup, 4½ oz — 13
Carob Flour, 1 cup, 3½ oz — 41
Rye Flour, 1 cup, 3½ oz — 15
Soy Flour: Defatted, 1 cup, 3½ oz — 17
Full-fat, raw, 1 cup, 3 oz — 8
Soy Meal, defatted, 1 cup, 4½ oz — 14

Frozen Entrees & Dinners

Average All Brands: Per Serving
Beans/Chili base, average — 6-10
Potato/Pasta base, average — 4-6
Vegetable base, average — 3
Meat/Chicken base, average — 2-3
Pizzas, ¼ large, average — 3
Vegetarian Soy Burgers, 1 pattie — 4

Soups

Chicken Noodle, 1 cup — 0.5
Tomato Soup, average, 1 cup — 0.5
Vegetable Soup, average, 1 cup — 3
Health Valley: Per 1 Cup Serving
Black Bean; Minestrone — 8
Tomato — 1
5-Bean Vegetable; Lentil & Carrots — 10
Mushroom Barley; Vegetable — 4
Split Pea — 8

Fast Foods & Restaurants | Fiber

Hamburgers: Small, average — 1.5
Large/Whopper, average — 2.5
Hot Dog, Regular — 1.5
French Fries: Small serving, 2½ oz — 2.5
Regular/Medium, 3½ oz — 3.5
Chicken Nuggets, 6 pack — 0.5
Chicken Sandwich, average — 2
Taco, average — 4
Sundaes, Shakes, Soft Drinks — 0
Arby's: Baked Potato w. Broc. & Cheese — 8
Roast Beef Sandwich, regular — 2
Denny's: Grilled Chicken Salad, no bread — 4
Classic Burger, no fries — 2
Club Sandwich, no fries — 4
Grilled Chicken Sandwich, no fries — 4
Domino's (12"): Classic/Thin, 1 slice — 1
Deep Dish, 1 slice — 3
Feast Pizza, Classic/Thin, 1 slice — 2
McDonald's: Big Mac — 3
Hamburger; Quarter Pounder — 2
Egg McMuffin — 1
Grilled Chicken Caesar Salad — 3
Pizza Hut: Per 1 Slice, Medium
Pan Pizza: Cheese, Pepperoni — 1
Supreme — 2
Thin 'n Crispy, Supreme — 2
Hand-Tossed, average all varieties — 2
Subway: Sandwich, white roll, av. — 2
w. Honey Wheat Roll, average — 3.2
Salads, average — 4

Cakes, Cookies, Snack Bars

Apple/Fruit Pie, 1 serving, 4 oz — 2
Cake: w. plain flour, 1 serving, 3.4 oz — 1.5
w. whole-wheat flour, 1 serving — 3
Carrot Cake, 4 oz — 3
Cookies, oatmeal, (3 small/1 large) — 1
Donuts, Medium, 1 oz — 0.7
Fruit Cake, 1 serving, 1½ oz — 2
Fig Bars, 1 cookie, ½ oz — 0.7
Muffins, Oat Bran (2 small, 1 large), 4 oz — 5
Granola Bars, average, 1 bar — 2
Atkins Advantage Bars, average — 7
Clif Bars, 2.5 oz — 5
Curves, Chocolate Peanut Bar, 25g — 5
Fi-Bar Chewy & Nutty 1 bar — 1
Fiber One (Gen. Mills), 1.4 oz bar — 9
FiberPlus, all bars, 1.2 oz — 9
Health Valley: Fruit/Granola Bars — 3
Cereal Bars — 3
Luna Bars, avg., 1.7 oz — 1
Special K, Protein Meal Bar, 1.6 oz — 3

268

Chocolate, Chips, Popcorn

	Fiber
Cheese Balls/Curls/Twists	1
Chocolate, Hard Candy, 1 oz	0
Chocolate with nuts/fruit, 2 oz bar	1.5
Mars Bar, 1.8 oz	1
Potato Chips, corn chips, 1 oz	1
Popcorn, 3 cups	3
Pretzels, Twists (6)	1

Nuts, Seeds

	Fiber
Almonds: Natural, 25 nuts, 1 oz	3.5
Blanched (skins removed), 1 oz	3
Cashews, Filberts, Pecans, 1 oz	1.7
Peanuts, Mixed Nuts, Coconut, 1 oz	2.5
Peanut Butter, 2 Tbsp, 1 oz	2
Pistachio Nuts, dried, shelled, 1 oz	3
Walnuts, Black/English, dried, 1 oz	2
Seeds: Amaranth, 2½ Tbsp, 1 oz	3.5
Flax Seeds, 3 Tbsp, 1 oz	7
Psyllium Seed Husks, 5 Tbsp, 1 oz	20
Quinoa Seeds, 3 Tbsp, 1 oz	1.7
Sesame Seeds, whole, 1 oz	3.4
Sesame Butter/Tahini, 2 Tbsp, 1.1 oz	1.4
Sunflower kernels, ¼ cup, 1 oz	3.8
Teff Seeds, 1 oz	3.8

Fruit – Fresh

	Fiber
Apples: 1 medium, 5½ oz (whole)	
with skin + core	3.7
with skin, no core	3.2
without skin, no core	1.7
Apricots, 2 medium, 4 oz	1.5
Avocado, average, ½ medium	6.7
Banana, 1 medium, 6 oz (w. skin)	3
Blueberries, raw, ½ cup, 2½ oz	1.7
Cherries, sweet, raw, 8 fruits, 1.6 oz	1
Grapefruit, average, ½ fruit, 10 oz	1.4
Grapes, 1 medium bunch, seedless, 7 oz	2
Kiwifruit, 1 medium, 2.7 oz	2.3
Mango, 1 medium, 11 oz (whole)	1.6
Melons, Cantaloupe, 4 oz (edible)	1
Nectarine, 1 medium, 4 oz	1.9
Olives, average all types, 7 jumbo, 2 oz	1.5
Oranges, 1 medium (7-8 oz w. skin)	
5½ oz (peeled)	3.8
Passionfruit, 2 medium, 2½ oz	5
Peaches, 1 large, 6 oz	2
Pears, raw, 1 medium, 6 oz	4.5
Pineapple, 1 slice, 3 oz	1.2
Plums, 2 medium, 6 oz	1.8
Strawberries, 6 medium/3 large, 2 oz	1
Watermelon, 4 oz (edible)	0.5

Fruit – Dried, Juice

	Fiber
Dried Fruit: Apricots, 8 halves, 1 oz	2.2
Dates (3 med); Raisins (2 Tbsp), 1 oz	1.5
Figs, 3 medium, 1½ oz	5
Prunes, 4 medium, 1 oz	2
Fruit Juice: Orange/Apple etc, 1 glass	<0.5
Prune Juice, 5 oz	1.4
Carrot Juice, 8 oz	1.8

Vegetables

	Fiber
Asparagus, 4 medium spears	1.3
Bean Sprouts, ½ cup, 2 oz	1
Beans: Snap/Green, ½ cup, 2 oz	2
Baked Beans in Tom Sce, ½ c, 4½ oz	5
Dried Beans, ckd, average, ½ cup	7
Beets, ckd, slices, ½ cup, 3 oz	1.7
Broccoli, cooked, ½ cup, 3 oz	2.4
Brussels Sprouts, ckd, ½ cup, 3 oz	3.5
Cabbage: White, ckd, ½ cup, 2½ oz	1
Red, ckd, ½ cup, 2½ oz	2
Carrots, 1 medium (7½"), ½ cup, 3 oz	2.5
Cauliflower, cooked, 3 flowerets, 2 oz	1.5
Celery, raw, diced, 1 cup, 3½ oz	1.6
Chick Peas (Garbanzos), ckd, ½ c., 3 oz	6.5
Corn: Kernels, cooked, ½ cup, 2½ oz	2.5
Corn on the Cob, 1 ear, 5 oz	4
Cucumber/Lettuce/Mushrooms, 2 oz	0.5
Eggplant, raw, sliced, ½ cup , 1½ oz	2
Lentils, cooked, ½ cup, 3½ oz	8
Mixed Vegetables, frozen, cooked, ½ cup	3
Onions, Raw, 1 medium, 4 oz	1.5
Spring Onions, chop., ¼ cup, 1 oz	0.7
Peas: Green, Raw, 2½ oz	3.7
Cowpeas (Black-eyed), ckd, ½ cup	10
Split Peas, ckd, ½ cup, 3½ oz	8
Peppers, sweet, raw, 1 large, 6 oz	3
Potatoes: 1 medium, with skin, 5 oz	4
without skin	2.5
½ cup mashed, 3½ oz	1.5
French Fries, small, 2.6 oz	3
Spinach, cooked, ½ cup, 3 oz	2.2
Squash: Summer, cooked, ½ cup, 3 oz	2.5
Winter, cooked, ½ cup, 3½ oz	2.4
Tomatoes: 1 medium, 4½ oz	1.5
Tomato Sauce, 1 cup	0.3
Soybean Products: Miso, ½ c., 5 oz	7.4
Tempeh, cooked, 1 piece, 3 oz	2
Tofu, ½ cup, 4.4 oz	0.4

Salads

	Fiber
Side Salad, average	1
Bean Salad, ½ cup	5
Coleslaw, ½ cup	1
Potato Salad, ½ cup	2

Protein Guide

General Notes

- **Protein has many important body functions.** It builds and repairs muscle, and is the basis of our body's organs, hormones, enzymes, and antibodies to fight infection.

- **Protein is also an emergency fuel** in the absence of sufficient carbohydrate and fats. For this reason, weight loss should be gradual so as to preserve protein levels in muscle, the heart and other body organs.

- **It is easy to obtain sufficient protein,** even if vegetarian. **Plant proteins are not inferior to animal proteins.** In fact, eating more soy and other plant proteins, and less animal protein, may help to build stronger bones and prevent osteoporosis, and may help to control blood cholesterol levels.

- **When changing to a vegetarian diet,** include soybeans, and other beans, soy milk drinks (calcium-enriched), lentils, tofu, tempeh, nuts and wholegrain breads and cereals. Milk, yogurt, cheese and eggs can enhance nutrient intake.

Protein & Muscle

- Although muscles are built of protein, protein is not a special fuel for working muscle cells – carbohydrates and fats are.

- In fact, a diet high in protein (and fat) and low in carbohydrate can significantly reduce the performance of endurance sports athletes. **Carbohydrates** are the best fuel for muscles exercised for long periods.

- Any **extra protein** required by athletes and body-builders can easily be obtained from the extra food eaten to satisfy hunger and energy needs.

- Remember, **excessive protein** intake will not build bigger muscles. Any excess is converted and stored as fat. Excess protein can also strain the kidneys, which excrete the waste products of protein metabolism.

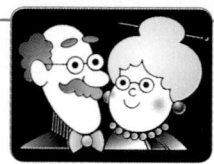

Elderly people (and dieters) must eat sufficient food to ensure adequate protein intake.

Inadequate protein leads to a drop in immune response with greater susceptibility to illness and infections. Muscle strength and muscle mass also drop.

Protein needs are easily met with sensible eating. Athletes who eat enough food for their energy needs can obtain sufficient protein.

RECOMMENDED DAILY PROTEIN INTAKE
~ HEALTHY RANGE ~
(Lower figure is RDA)

		PROTEIN
Children:	1-3 yrs	13g-26g
	4-8 yrs	19g-38g
	9-13 yrs	34g-64g
Males:	14-18 yrs	52g-120g
	19+	56g-120g
Females:	14+	46g-110g
Pregnancy:		71g-120g
Breastfeeding:		71g-120g

Note: On lower-calorie diets, aim for higher amounts of protein within the Healthy Range.

Pro ~ Protein (grams)

Meat

	Pro
Steak: *Average all cuts, lean (no fat)*	
Small (4 oz raw/3 oz cooked)	23
Medium (6 oz raw/4¼ oz cooked)	34
Large (10 oz raw/7¼ oz cooked)	57
Roast Beef, lean, 2 slices, 3 oz	24
Ground Beef patty, lean, cooked, 3 oz	21
Lamb chop, broiled, 3 oz	22
Liver, cooked, 3 oz	23
Veal cutlet, 1 medium	23
Pork, cooked, lean, 3 oz	24
Bacon, 3 medium slices	6
Ham, roasted, 2 pieces, 3 oz	18
Ham, luncheon, 2 slices, 1½ oz	7
Pastrami *(Oscar Mayer)*, 3 sl., 1¾ oz	10
Sausages: Bologna, 2 sl., 2 oz	7
Braunschweiger, 2 sl., 2 oz	8
Pork link, thick, 2 oz	6
Frankfurter, 1⅓ oz	5
Salami, hard, 3 slices, 1 oz	7
Vegetarian *(Boca Burger)*, 1 pattie	13

Chicken/Turkey: *Without Skin*

	Pro
Chicken, cooked; Breast, Roasted, 4 oz	36
Leg/Thigh,Roasted, 2 oz	14
½ Whole Chicken	60
Drumstick, Rstd, 1 med., 3 oz	13
Turkey: Light meat, cooked, 3 oz	28
Dark meat, lean, 3 oz	24

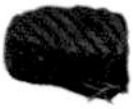

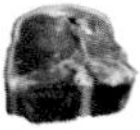

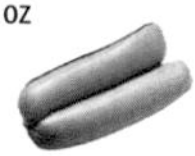

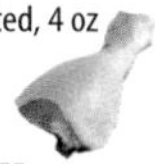

Fish

	Pro
Fresh Fish: *Per 4 oz, cooked*	
Cod, Flounder/Sole, Pollock	28
Catfish, Haddock, Halibut, M/Mahi	28
Ocean Perch, Swordf., Orange Roughy	28
Canned Fish: Tuna, Light, 3 oz	25
White, 3 oz	23
Salmon, pink, 3 oz	17
Salmon, red, 3 oz	17
Sardines, 3 whole (3"), 1¼ oz	9
Anchovies, 1 can, 1½ oz	13
Shellfish: Crabmeat, 3 oz	17.5
Clams, raw, 4 large/9 sml, 3 oz	11
Crayfish, cooked, 3 oz	20
Lobster, cooked, 3 oz	17
Oysters, raw, 6 medium, 3 oz	7
Scallops, 2 lge/5 small, 1 oz	5
Shrimp, raw, 6 large, 1½ oz	8.5
Fish Products: Fish Sticks, 4 sticks	10
Fish Portions, in batter, 4 oz	13
Gefilte Fish, 1 medium ball, 2 oz	8

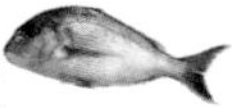

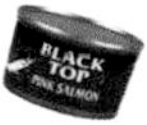

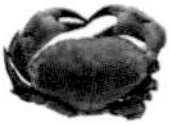

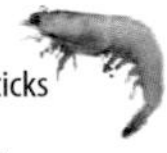

Eggs

	Pro
1 Large Egg, whole	6
Egg Yolk	3
Egg White	3
Omelet: Plain, 2 eggs	13
Ham & cheese	17
Egg Substitutes, (liquid):	
Egg Beaters, 1/4 cup, 2 oz	4.5
Better 'n Eggs/Scramblers, ¼ cup, 2 oz	6

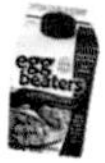

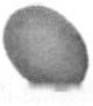

Milk, Yogurt, Ice Cream

	Pro
Milk: Whole: 2%, 1 cup	8
Low-Fat (1%); Fat-Free, 1 cup	8.5
Chocolate Milk, 1 cup	8
Thick Shake: Chocolate, 10 oz	9
Vanilla, 10 oz	11
Soymilk, (fortified), average, 1 cup	7
Soy Dream, Enriched, shelf-stable, 1 cup	7
Yogurt: Plain, 6 oz	10
Fruit flavors: 6 oz	8
8 oz	11
Ice Cream: Rich, ½ cup	2
Regular, Vanilla, ½ cup	2.5
Sherbet, ½ cup	1
Custard, baked, ½ cup	7

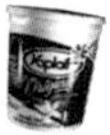

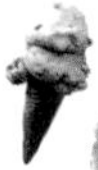

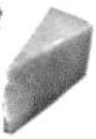

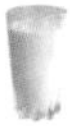

Cheese

	Pro
Hard Cheeses, average, 1 oz	7
Cottage Cheese, ½ cup	13
Cream Cheese, avg., 1 oz	2
Ricotta, part skim, ½ cup	14

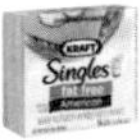

Bread, Bagels, Biscuits

	Pro
Bread, w. enriched flour: 1 slice, 1 oz	2
4 thin slices, 4 oz	8
4 thick slices, 6 oz	1.2
Bagel, plain 2 oz	6
Biscuits, 1 oz	2
Pita Bread, 1 pita, 1½ oz	4
Pumpernickel, 1 slice, 1 oz	3

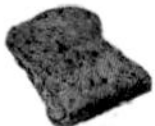

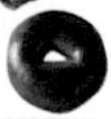

Infant/Baby Foods

	Pro
Infant Formula Milk:	
Enfamil/Gerber/Similac:	
Regular/Low Iron , 5 fl.oz	2.2
With Iron, 5 fl.oz	2.2
Isomil/Nursoy/ProSobee	3
Baby Cereals: *Average all brands*	
Dry, 4 Tbsp, ½ oz	1
Jars, w. fruit, 4½ oz	1

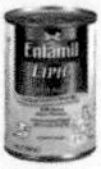

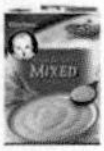

Protein Counter

Breakfast Cereals	Pro
Hot Cereals ~ *Cooked:*	
Bulgur, cooked, 1 cup, 5 oz	9
Oatmeal: Reg., non-fortified, 1 cup	6
Instant, fortified, avg., 1 pkt	4
Quaker, all flavors, ½ cup	5
Corn/Hominy Grits: 1 cup	3
Quaker: Reg., 3 Tbsp, 1 oz	2
Instant White, 1 packet	2
Cream of Wheat, 1 cup	4
Brands ~ *Ready-To-Eat*	
Arrowhead: Average all varieties, 1 oz	3
General Mills: Basic 4, 1 cup, 2 oz	4
Cheerios, Original, 1 cup, 1 oz	3
Cocoa Puffs, 1 cup, 1 oz	1
Kix, 1⅓ cups, 1 oz	2
Multi-Bran Chex, 1 cup, 2 oz	4
Country Corn Flakes, 1 cup, 1.2 oz	2
Total Raisin Bran, 1 cup, 2 oz	3
Wheaties ¾ cup, 1 oz	3
Health Valley: Oat Bran O's, ¾ cup, 1 oz	3
Amaranth Flakes, ¾ cup, 1 oz	3
Bran Flakes w. Raisins, ¾ cup, 1.1 oz	5
Low-Fat Granola, ⅔ cup, 2 oz	5
Real Oat Bran Alm. Crunch, ½ cup, 1.7 oz	6
Golden Flax, ¾ cup, 1.9 oz	6
Kashi: Friends, 1 cup, 1.9 oz	5
GoLean Crunch!, 1 cup, 1.9 oz	9
7 Whole Grain Flakes, 1 c., 1.8 oz	6
Kellogg's: All-Bran: ½ cup, 1 oz	4
Complete Oat Flakes, ¾ c., 1.1 oz	3
Cocoa Krispies, ¾ cup, 1 oz	1
Corn Flakes, 1 cup, 1 oz	2
Low-fat Granola w. Raisins ⅔ c., 2.1 oz	4
Product 19, 1 cup, 1 oz	2
Raisin Bran, 1 cup, 2 oz	7
Rice Krispies, 1¼ cup, 1.2 oz	2
Smart-Start Healthy Heart, 1 c., 1.8 oz	6
Special K: Regular, 1 c., 1.1 oz	6
Protein Plus, ¾ cup, 1 oz	10
Post: Raisin Bran, ⅔ cup, 2 oz	4
Grape Nuts, ½ cup, 2 oz	6
Quaker: Crunchy Corn Bran, 1 cup, 1 oz	2
100% Natural Granola, ½ cup, 1.7 oz	5
Life, ¾ cup, 1.1 oz	3
Cap'n Crunch, ¾ cup, 1 oz	1
Oat Bran, ½ cup, 1.4 oz	7

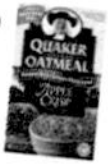

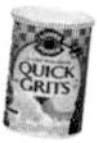

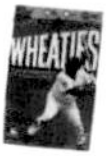

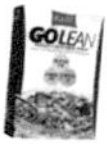

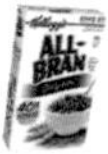

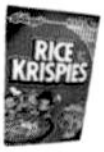

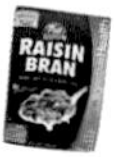

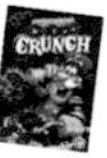

Brans & Wheatgerm	Pro
Oat Bran, raw, 1 Tbsp	2
Rice Bran, raw, 2 Tbsp	1
Wheat Bran, unprocessed, 2 T.	1
Wheat Germ, 2 Tbsp, ½ oz	4
Grains & Flours, Yeast	
Amaranth, ½ cup, 3.4 oz	14
Barley, ½ cup, 3.2 oz	12
Buckwheat Flour, Whole-groat, 1 cup	15
Carob Flour, 1 cup, 3.6 oz	5
Corn Flour, 1 cup, 4 oz	11
Corn Meal, 1 cup, 4½ oz	8
Flour: White, 1 cup, 5.6 oz	9
Wholegrain, 1 cup, 4¼ oz	16
Millet, wholegrain, 1 cup, 3½ oz	12
Rye Flour: Dark, 1 cup, 4½ oz	18
Light, 1 cup, 3½ oz	9
Soy Flour, full fat, 1 cup, 3 oz	29
Yeast: Brewers, 2 Tbsp, ½ oz	8
Nutritional Yeast Flakes *(Red Star),* 1 heaping Tbsp, ½ oz	8
Rice, Spaghetti, Macaroni	
Rice: Brown/White, average 1 cup cooked, 6½ oz	5
Spaghetti/Macaroni/Noodles (enriched):	
Cooked, 1 cup, 4½ oz	7
Canned: in Tomato Sce, ½ cup	2
with Meatballs, 1 cup, 8 oz	10
Macaroni & Cheese, 1 cup, 9 oz	8
Soups	
With Noodles/Vegetables, 1 cup	3
With Meat/Beans/Peas, 1 cup	8
Fruit	
Fresh/Canned:	
Average, all types 1 medium/2 small fruit	1
Avocado, ½ medium	2
Dried Fruit: Apricots, 8 halves, 1 oz	1
Dates, 6 dates, 2 oz	1.5
Figs, 4 medium figs, 2 oz	2
Prunes, 5 medium, 1½ oz	1
Raisins, 1 oz	1
Fruit Juice: Average, 1 cup	0.5
Prune Juice, 6 fl.oz	1
Tomato Juice, 1 cup, 8 fl.oz	1.5

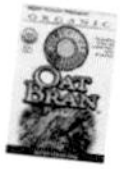

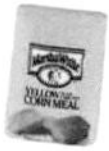
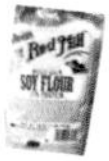

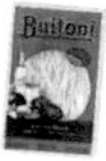

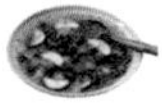
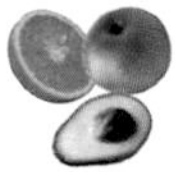
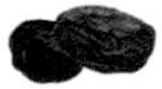
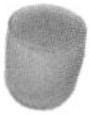

Vegetables | Pro

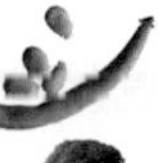

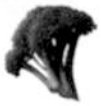

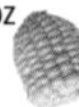

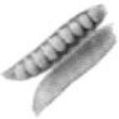

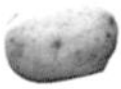

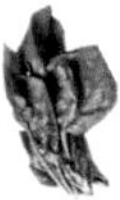

	Pro
Beans: Snap/green, ½ cup, 2 oz	1
Dried: Average all types, cooked, ½ cup	7
Baked Beans, ½ cup 4½ oz	5
Bean Sprouts, mung, 1 c., 4 oz	3
Broccoli, 3 raw, ½ cup, 1½ oz	1.5
Cabbage; Cauliflower, raw, 1 c. 3 oz	1.5
Corn: raw, ½ cup kernels, 3 oz	2.5
1 ear trimmed to 3½"	2
Lentils, cooked, ½ cup, 3½ oz	9
Mushrooms, raw, ½ c., sliced	1
Peas: Green, raw, ½ c., 2½ oz	4
Split Peas, cooked, 1 cup, 7 oz	16
Potatoes: *Cooked:*	
1 medium, with skin, 5 oz	3.3
without skin, 4 oz	2.3
French Fries, small, 2.6 oz	2
Potato Salad, ½ cup, 4 oz	3.5
Pumpkin, ½ cup mashed, 4.3 oz	1
Seaweed, kelp, 1 oz	<1
Spinach, cooked, ½ cup, 3 oz	2.7
Squash, ckd, all types, ½ cup	1
Tomatoes, 1 medium, 4½ oz	1
Vegetables, mixed, ckd, 1 cup	2.5
Soybeans, cooked, ½ cup, 3 oz	14

Tofu, Tempeh, Miso

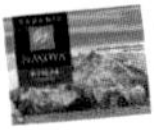

Tofu, raw, firm, ½ cup, 4½ oz	10
Tempeh, ½ cup, 3 oz	16
Miso, ½ cup, 5 oz	16
Miso Soup, 1 cup	3
Soybean Protein *(TVP)*, 1 oz	18

Cakes, Pastries, Pies

(Made with enriched flour)

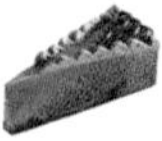

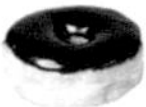

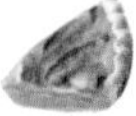

Carrot w. cream cheese frosting, 4 oz	4
Cheesecake, 1 piece, 4 oz	6
Chocolate, 1 piece, 2 oz	2
Fruitcake, 1 piece, 3 oz	4
Plain, 1 piece, 3 oz	4
Croissant, plain, 2 oz	5
Danish Pastry, 1 pastry, 2¼ oz	4
Donuts, average, 2 oz	4
Muffins, average, 1 med., 1½ oz	3
Pancakes, 4" diam., two, 2 oz	4
Pies: Fruit, 1 piece, 5½ oz	4
Pecan, 1 piece, 5 oz	7
Puddings, average, ½ cup, 4½ oz	4
Waffles, 1 large, 2½ oz	7

Peanut Butter | Pro

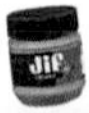

	Pro
Regular: 2 Tbsp, 1.1 oz	8
Peter Pan Plus, 2 Tbsp, 1.1 oz	8

Sugar, Honey, Jam

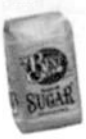

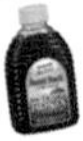

Sugar: White	0
Brown, 1 Tbsp	0
Molasses: Light/Med., 1 Tbsp	0
Blackstrap, 1 Tbsp, ¾ oz	0
Corn Syrup, 1 Tbsp, ¾ oz	0
Honey, Jams, Jelly	0

Candy, Chocolate, Carob

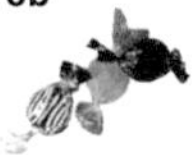

Candy, sugar-based	0
Chocolate: Plain, 2 oz bar	4
with nuts, 2 oz bar	6
Carob, plain, 2 oz	6

Cookies, Crackers, Chips

Cookies, average, 4 cookies	2
Crackers, Graham, 2½" sq., (2)	1
Rice Cakes, average, one	1
Corn/Potato Chips, 1 oz	2

Nuts:

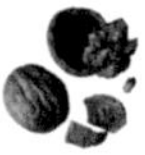

Almonds, shelled, 20-25 nuts	6
Brazil Nuts, 7-8 medium nuts, 1 oz	4
Cashews, 12-16 nuts, 1 oz	5
Macadamias, 1 oz	2
Peanuts, dry rsted, 40 nuts, 1 oz	6
Pecans, 24 halves, 1 oz	2
Walnuts, 15 halves, 1 oz	4

Seeds:

Sesame Seeds, dry, 1 Tbsp	2
Pumpkin Kernels, dry, hulled, 1 oz	7
Sunflower Seeds, dried, hulled, 1 oz	6
Tahini, 1 Tbsp, ½ oz	2.5

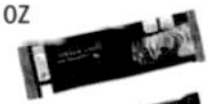

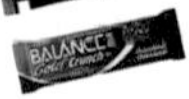

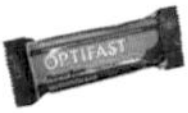

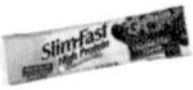

Granola & Food/Protein Bars

Granola Bars, avg., 1 bar, 2 oz	2
Anytime Health,	
Meal Bars, 80g	20
Snack Bars, 50g	12
Balance Bars, Orig. 1.76 oz	14
Bariatrix, Proti-Bars (1), 1.4 oz	15
Dr Soy, Protein Bars, 1.76 oz	11
GeniSoy, Protein Bar, 1.6 oz	14
Jenny Craig, Bars, 1.8 oz	4
Met-Rx, "Big 100", 3.5 oz	27
Myoplex, Carb Sense Bar, 2.5 oz	26
Optifast, Peanut Butter, 1.59 oz	8
PowerBar: Harvest/Performance	10
Slim-Fast, High Protein Meal, 1.7 oz	15
Optima Meal, 2 oz bar	8
Special K: Protein Meal, 1.6 oz	10
Protein Snack, 0.9 oz	4

Protein Counter

High Protein Drinks	Pro
Anytime, Health:	
Whey Protein Isolate,	
All flavors, 1 oz	25
Atkins, Shakes, 11 fl.oz can	18
Boost, High Protein, 8 oz	10
Carnation, Instant Breakfast, 10 oz	13
Curves, Protein Drink, 2 scoops, dry	15
dotFIT: FirstString, 4 scoops, 5.2 oz	42
Meal Replacement,	
Chocolate, 2 scoops, 2.2 oz	20
WheySmooth, Choc., 2 scoops, 2.2 oz	40
Ensure, Plus, 8 oz can	13
Gatorade: Nutrition Shake, 11 oz	20
Protein Recovery Shake, 11 oz	20
GeniSoy, Shake, 1 scoop, 1.2 oz	14
Kashi GoLean, Shake, 2 sc., 2.1 oz	21
Met-Rx, RTD 40	40
Myoplex, Original Nutrition Shake, 1 pkt	42
Optifast 800, made up, 8 fl oz	14
Resource (Novartis), Standard, 8 fl.oz	15
Slim-Fast Shakes: Meal, 11 oz can	10
High Protein, 11 oz can	15
Optima, 11 oz can	10
Special K20, Protein Water, 16 fl.oz	5
Walgreens, Slim For Less, 11 oz can	10
Weider, Mass 1000, 4 scoops, 7 oz	34

Coffee, Tea, Soda	
Coffee, Coffee Substitutes, 1 cup, 8 fl.oz	0
Coffee w. 2 oz milk, 1 cup, 8 fl.oz	2
Caffe latte, large, 16 fl.oz	12
Cappuccino, large, 16 fl.oz	8
Frappuccino, avg., 16 fl.oz	6
Hot Chocolate, with milk, 1 cup, 8 fl.oz	8
Soft Drinks/Soda	0
Tea, all types	0

Beer, Wine, Spirits	
Beer, 12 fl.oz	1
Wines, red/white, 1 glass	0
Spirits/Liquor	0

Fast-Foods/Burgers	
Pancakes, Average all outlets, 3	8
Shakes, Chocolate, 16 fl.oz	12
Sundaes, Average all outlets	7
Arby's: Roast Beef Sandwich, regular	20
Chicken Club Salad	32
Roast Beef Sandwich, Super	21
Burger King: Whopper S/wich	29
Bacon Double Cheeseburger	32
BK Big Fish Sandwich	24

Fast Foods/Burgers (Cont)	Pro
Carl's Jr:	
Famous Star Hamburger w/ Cheese	27
Charbroiled Chicken Club Sandwich	39
Super Star Hamburger w/ Cheese	47
Domino's Pizza: Deep Dish (12")	
Beef, 2 slices	10
Cheese, 2 slices	12
Pepperoni, Sausage, 1 sl.	10
KFC: Original, Breast	42
Crispy Strips, 3 strips	33
Snacker, Regular	15
McDonald's: Big Mac	25
Cheeseburger	15
Chicken McNuggets (6)	14
Crispy Chicken Classic Burger	28
Filet-O-Fish	15
Hamburger	12
Quarter Pounder w. Cheese	29
French Fries: Small, 2.5 oz	3
Large, 5.4 oz	6
Salads w. Chicken, average	30
Triple Shake, average, 16 fl.oz	16
Breakfast: Egg McMuffin	18
Bacon, Egg & Cheese McGriddles	15
Sausage Burrito	12
Sausage McMuffin w. Egg	21
Pizza Hut: Per Medium, 1 slice, ⅛ Pizza	
Thin 'n Crispy, Supreme	10
Pan Pizzas, average	11
Hand Tossed, Pepperoni	10
Fit n' Delicious, Ham/Pineapple/Tomato	7
Subway: 6" Subs	
Roast Beef	26
Meatball Marinara	24
Roast Chicken Breast	23
Subway Club	26
Sweet Onion Chicken Teriyaki	26
Taco Bell: Bean Burrito	12
Chicken Quesadilla	28
Chicken/Steak Enchirito	21
Gordita Baja Beef	13
Steak Burrito Supreme	18
Taco Supreme	11
Wendy's: ¼ lb Single Burger	27
Chicken Club	37
Jr Hamburger	13

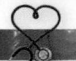

High Blood Pressure

High Blood Pressure

Many American adults have hypertension (high blood pressure), and are unaware of it. It is generally symptomless, so **have your blood pressure checked annually** – particularly if it runs in the family.

Untreated hypertension overworks the heart, damages arteries and promotes atherosclerosis. This in turn greatly increases the risk of heart disease, stroke, blindness, kidney disease and impotence. The earlier hypertension is detected, the sooner it can be brought under control.

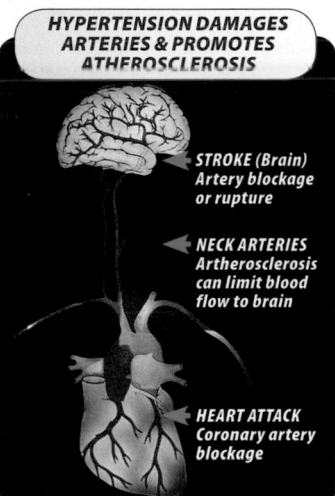

HYPERTENSION DAMAGES ARTERIES & PROMOTES ATHEROSCLEROSIS

STROKE (Brain) Artery blockage or rupture

NECK ARTERIES Artherosclerosis can limit blood flow to brain

HEART ATTACK Coronary artery blockage

BLOOD PRESSURE CLASSIFICATION

For Adults Age 18 & Older ~ Not Acutely ill or on Medication (American Heart Association)

	DIASTOLIC		SYSTOLIC
Normal ➤	Below 80	and	Below 120
Prehypertension ➤	80-89	or	120-139
Hypertension:			
Stage 1 ➤	90-99	or	140-159
Stage 2 ➤	100 or more	or	160 or more

Treating Hypertension

Prehypertension (in the chart above) means you don't have high blood pressure now but are likely to develop it in the future.

You can take steps to lessen the risk by adopting healthy lifestyle habits such as:
- reducing sodium intake
- eating adequate fruit and vegetables
- losing weight if overweight
- limiting alcohol to 2 drinks or less daily
- quitting smoking
- exercising regularly, managing stress.

Stage 1 hypertension can often be treated with the above lifestyle changes.

Stage 2 hypertension usually requires drug therapy. However, salt restriction, abstaining from alcohol, and the above lifestyle changes will improve the success of drug therapy, and enable smaller drug doses to be prescribed.

STROKE KNOW THE WARNING SIGNS

Stroke is a medical emergency! If you notice one or more of these signs, call 9-1-1 or your doctor immediately.

These signs may be signalling a possible stroke or transient ischemic attack:

- **Sudden weakness** or numbness in your face, arm, or leg on one side of your body
- **Sudden confusion,** trouble speaking or understanding
- **Sudden trouble seeing,** in one or both eyes
- **Sudden trouble walking,** dizziness, loss of balance or coordination
- **Sudden severe headache** - 'a bolt out of the blue' – with no apparent cause

Salt & Sodium Guide

Salt & Sodium

- **Sodium is a mineral element** most commonly found in salt (sodium chloride). It also occurs naturally in much smaller amounts in animal and plant foods, and water – normally sufficient for our needs without having to add salt to our diet.

- **Sodium is required** for nerve and muscle function, as well as to balance the amount of fluid in our tissues and blood. Sodium acts like a sponge to attract and hold fluids in body tissues.

- **Excess sodium** can cause water retention, and increase the risk of developing hyper-tension. Very high salt intake may also increase the risk of stomach cancer.

- **Too little sodium** may cause low blood pressure (hypotension), and decrease blood flow to the heart, brain and kidneys – especially during exercise. (A certain blood volume is required to sustain the blood pressure needed for adequate blood flow in the capillaries).

Salt-Sensitive Persons

- **Normally, our kidneys** excrete excess dietary sodium. The thirst we feel after a salty meal is the body calling for water to dilute the sodium, and enable the kidneys to flush out excess sodium.

- **However, 'salt - sensitive'** persons (up to 70% of adults) tend to retain excess sodium (above approximately 3000mg daily) instead of excreting it. Such persons are more likely to develop hypertension and would benefit most from sodium restriction. Assume you are susceptible if there is a family history of hypertension.

- Although not everyone will benefit, **all Americans are being asked to moderate their salt and sodium intake** as a public health measure – particularly because so many do not know whether or not they have hypertension, and also because we do not know just who is salt-sensitive.

FINDING HIDDEN SODIUM

On average, **less than one third of our sodium intake comes from the salt shaker.**
The rest is hidden in processed foods that have salt added during manufacture.

Sodium compounds added to food or medicinals can also contribute significant sodium.

Sodium bicarbonate in particular is widely used in antacid tablets (such as *Alka Seltzer*) and powders. Sodium bicarbonate contains 27% sodium by weight. Each gram contributes 270mg sodium. Large amounts of sodium can be unwittingly consumed – up to 600mg per tablet. (See Antacids ~ Page 280)

Example: 2 *Alka-Seltzer* Tablets = 1000mg sodium

Other sodium compounds include monosodium glutamate (MSG), sodium ascorbate, sodium nitrite, and sodium citrate.

POTASSIUM BALANCES SODIUM

Potassium helps to balance sodium by helping the kidneys to excrete excess sodium.
Fruit and vegetables are rich sources of potassium – another reason to ensure you have your 5-7 servings every day.
Nuts also provide potassium as well as magnesium and other heart-healthy nutrients and anti-oxidants. Eat them unsalted.
Note: This info is only for people with normal kidney function. Also not for persons on potassium-sparing diuretics.

ALCOHOL DANGER
Excessive alcohol intake contributes to hypertension. Susceptible persons should limit alcohol intake to 1-2 drinks per day.

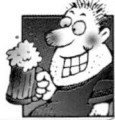

Salt Sodium Guide

Sodium accounts for only 40% of the weight of salt (sodium chloride). Examples:
1 gram (1000mg) Salt has 400mg Sodium
1 teaspoon (5g) Salt has 2000mg Sodium

HINTS TO REDUCE SODIUM

- **Cut down use of the salt shaker.** Start with an easy 50% cut in sodium by using Lite Salt (*Morton*) or *Cardia* Salt. Then gradually cut back until you can leave the salt shaker off the table. Sea salt is still high in sodium.

- **Use fresh herbs,** and salt-free seasonings to add flavor to food.

- **Choose low-sodium,** sodium-free, and reduced-sodium products in place of regular, salted products.

- **Check food labels for sodium levels.** FDA Guidelines for sodium descriptors are:
  - **Reduced Sodium:** At least 25% less sodium than the original product
  - **Low Sodium:** 140 mg or less/serving
  - **Very Low Sodium:** 35mg or less/serving
  - **Sodium Free:** Less than 5mg/serving
  - **No Salt Added:** Made without the salt normally added, but still contains the sodium that is a natural part of the food

- **Use reduced-sodium breads,** butter and margarine. Regular varieties are considered high in sodium in view of their significant contribution to our diet.

- **Go easy on salty condiments and sauces** such as ketchup, mustard, soy sauce, spaghetti sauces, and salad dressings. Use low-sodium varieties.

- **Limit pizzas and salty fast-foods.** Check the *CalorieKing.com* food database.

- **Avoid salty snack foods** such as potato chips, corn chips, salted nuts, pretzels and cheesy-flavored snacks. **Choose unsalted** popcorn, nuts or seeds. Eat more fruit.

- **Don't salt children's food** to your taste.

- **Avoid antacids with** sodium bicarbonate (such as *Alka-Seltzer*). They are high in sodium. Look for low-sodium alternatives.

FOODS HIGH IN SODIUM

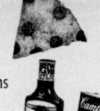
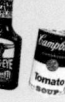
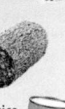

- Cheese, Butter, Margarine
- Pickles, Sauerkraut, Olives
- Condiments, Sauces
- Salad Dressings
- Canned vegetables/salads/beans
- Deli Salads (with dressing)
- Frozen/Packaged Meals/Entrees
- Soups: Canned/dry; bouillon cubes
- Meats: Ham, bacon, sausage, luncheon meats, smoked meats
- Canned Fish (in brine/salt)
- Sea Salt, Garlic/Celery Salt
- Snack Foods (potato chips, pretzels)
- Tomato Juice (Canned), V8 Vegetable Juice
- Fast Foods: Pizza, Burgers, Chicken
- *Alka-Seltzer* Antacid
- Bread (regular)

MODERATE SODIUM

- Meat, Fish, Poultry - Unprocessed
- Milk, Yogurt, Soy Drinks, Eggs
- Peanut Butter
- Breakfast Cereals (less than 200mg/serving)
- Chocolate Candy, Fruit/Nut Bars
- *Reduced Sodium & Low Sodium* Products

FOODS LOW IN SODIUM

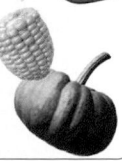

- Products labelled *Very Low Sodium*, or *Sodium Free*
- Bread (No Salt Added)
- Fresh fruits and vegetables
- Canned and Dried Fruits
- Potatoes, Rice, Pasta
- Dried Beans & Lentils, Tofu
- Nuts & Seeds (unsalted)
- Corn & Popcorn (unsalted)
- Pepper, Spices, Herbs
- Jam, Honey, Syrup
- Candy, Gum
- Hard & Jelly Candy
- Coffee, Tea, Alcohol
- Fresh Fruit Juices, Water

Sodium Counter

The American Heart Association recommends a sodium intake of **less than 1500mg/day**

Sodium ~ Sodium (mg)

Milk & Dairy Products

	Sodium
Milk: Whole/lowfat/skim, average 1 cup, 8 fl.oz	120
Whole, low sodium, 1 cup	5
Choc Milk, 1 cup	130
Soy Milk, 8 fl.oz	30
Buttermilk, cultured, 8 fl.oz	250
Dry/Powder, skim, ¼ cup, 1 oz	110
Yogurt, with fruit average, 8 oz	130
Cheese: Bleu, 1 oz	330
Parmesan, 1 oz	450
Kraft Cheddar, 2% milk, 1 oz	230
Philadelphia Cream Cheese, 1 oz	90
Process Cheese., average,1 oz	430
Swiss, 1 oz	40
Cottage Cheese, ½ cup, 4 oz	450
Ricotta Cheese, ½ cup, 4 oz	150

Ice Cream, Frozen Yogurt

Icecream, average, ½ cup	50
Frozen Yogurt, ½ cup	50

Fats/Oils

Butter/Margarine:	
Regular, 2 Tbsp, 1 oz	230
Unsalted, reg., 2 Tbsp, 1 oz	5
Mayonnaise, avg., 2 Tbsp, 1 oz	160
Oils/Lard/Drippings	0
Cream, average, 1 Tbsp	5
Coffee-Mate: Powdered, 1 tsp	2
Liquid, 1 Tbsp	5

Eggs

Whole, 1 large	70
Omelet, 2 egg, plain	220
w. cheese	400
Egg Beaters: Original, ¼ cup	115
Flavors, average, ¼ cup	230

Meats

Meat, average all types, cooked (Beef/Lamb/Veal/Pork), 4 oz	80
Corned Beef, cooked, 3 oz	800
Bacon, cooked, 2 sl., ½ oz	270
Ham, 3 oz	1100

Chicken & Turkey

Chicken/Turkey, cooked, unsalted, 4 oz	80
Stuffing Mixes, average., ½ cup	500

KFC ~ See Page 281 (Fast-Foods)

Sausages & Meats

	Sodium
Bologna, 1 oz	280
Frankfurter, 2 oz	640
Ham, chopped, ¾ oz slice	290
Liverwurst (Braunschweiger), 1 oz	320
Pepperoni, 5 slices, 1 oz	570
Salami, cooked, 1 oz	350
dry/hard, 1 oz	600
Sausage, 1 oz link	220
Pork, 2 oz patty	260
Spam: Classic, 2 oz	790
25% Less Sodium, 2 oz	580
Turkey Roll, 1 oz	160

Fish: Fresh Fish, average, plain	
Cooked, 4 oz (no bone)	60
Broiled w. butter, 4 oz	150
Breaded & fried, 4 oz	320
Fish fillets, batter-dipped 3 oz	350
Fish sticks, 1 oz stick	160
Gefilte Fish (w. broth), 1 pce, 1½ oz	220
Herring, pickled, 2 pces, 1 oz	260
Lobster, meat only, 4 oz	180
Oysters, fresh, 6 med., 3 oz	95
Salmon: Canned, 3 oz	460
No Salt Added, 3 oz	65
Smoked fish, average, 3 oz	650
Tuna: Canned, regular, 3 oz	330
No Added Salt, 3 oz	40
Spicy Flavored, 5 oz can	550

Entrees & Meals

Frozen Meals, average	600-900
Lean Cuisine, average	700
Stouffer's, average	580
Dinners, average	900-1200
Side Dishes, average	400-600
Pizza, frozen, ¼ large, 6 oz	800-1200
Microwave Cup Meals	900-1200
Cup O'Noodles, average	1500

Pizza ~ See Page 281 (Pizza Hut)

More Sodium Counts:
www.CalorieKing.com

Sodium Counter

Soups

	Sodium
Condensed, average, 1 cup, 8 oz	800-1000
Low Sodium, average	70
Chicken Noodle, average, 1 cup	900
Bouillon Cube, average	950
Ramen Noodle Soup, av., 3 oz pkg	1500
Soup Cups, average	850
Soup Mixes, average, 1 cup	900

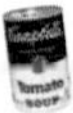

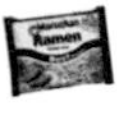

Condiments, Sauces, Dressings

A-1 Sauce, 1 Tbsp	280
Barbecue Sauce, 1 Tbsp	130
Bragg's Liquid Aminos, 1 tsp	220
Chili Sauce, 1 Tbsp	230
Ketchup: Tomato, 1 Tbsp	180
Low Sodium, 1 Tbsp	20
Mayonnaise, 1 Tbsp	80
Mustard, 1 tsp	70
Pizza Sauce, ½ cup	700
Salad Dressings, 2 Tbsp, 1 oz	160-400
Spaghetti Sauce, ½ cup	500
Soy Sauce, 1 Tbsp	900
Lite *(Kikkoman),* 1 Tbsp	600
Sweet & Sour, ½ cup	250
Tabasco, 1 tsp	25
Vinegar, Lemon Juice	0
Worcestershire, 1 Tbsp	200
Tomato: Sauce, 1 cup	1200
Paste/Puree (salted), ½ cup	1000
No Salt Added, ½ cup	25

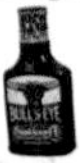

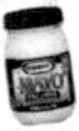

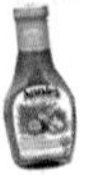

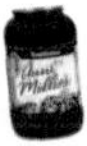

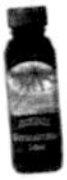

Salt & Salt Substitutes

Table Salt: 1 teaspoon, 6g	2400
Single Serve package, 1 g	400
Cardia Salt, 1 teaspoon	1080
Lite Salt *(Morton),* 1 teaspoon, 6g	1200
***Morton/No Salt* Substitute,** 1 tsp	5
Garlic/Onion/Seasoned Salt, 1 tsp, 4g	1350
Garlic/Seasoned Salt 1 teaspoon, 4g	1300
Sea Salt, 1 teaspoon, 5g	2250

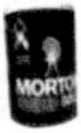

Seasonings, Herbs & Spices

Baking Powder, 1 tsp, 3g	340
Baking Soda (Sodium bicarb), 1 tsp, 3g	810
Accent (Flavor Enhancer), 1 tsp	600
Chili Powder, 1 tsp, 3g	25
Curry Powder	0
Lemon Pepper *(Lawry's),* 1 tsp	340
Meat Tenderizer, 1 tsp, 5g	1750
MSG (Monosodium glutamate), 5g	500
Mrs Dash Blends/Marinades	
Old Bay, Seasoning (Less Sodium), 1 teaspoon, 2.4g	380
Pepper, Mustard (dry), 1 tsp	1
Yeast, Nutritional, 1 Tbsp	10

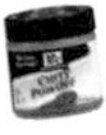

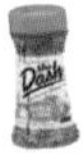

Breakfast Cereals

	Sodium
Kellogg's:	
All-Bran, ½ cup, 1 oz	80
Special K, 1 cup, 1.1 oz	220
Corn Flakes, 1 cup, 1 oz	200
Just Right, ¾ cup, 1 oz	240
Mini Wheats Frosted, 24 bisc., 1.8 oz	5
Health Valley Cereals, 1 serving	5
Quaker: Cap'n Crunch, ¾ cup, 1 oz	200
Crunchy Corn Bran, ¾ cup, 1 oz	230
100% Natural Granola, ½ cup, 1 oz	15
Puffed Rice/Wheat, 2 cups, 1 oz	1
General Mills: Total, ¾ cup, 1 oz	190
Oatmeal: Regular, ¾ cup	1
Instant *(Quaker),* ⅔ cup (1 pkt)	270

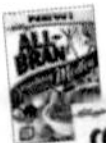

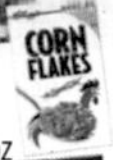

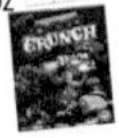

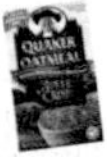

Breads, Bagels, Crackers

Bread: Thin Slice, average 1 oz	140
Thick Slice, 1½ oz	210
Low Sodium, 1 oz	10
Bagels: Plain, medium, 2 oz	200
Large, take-out, average, 4 oz	550
Sara Lee, 3.4 oz	500
Biscuits, average, 1 oz	180
Bun/Roll: 1 medium, 1½ oz	200
Large, 4 oz	560
Crackers: Saltine, 2 crackers	70
Low Salt *(Premium),* 2	25
Graham, 2 regular	50
Croissant, Plain, average, 2 oz	280
Rice Cakes, average	25
Ritz Crackers, Low-Sodium, 1 oz	60
Ry-Krisp Crispbread, Sesame, 2	100

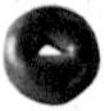

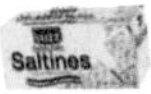

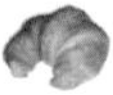

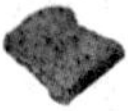

Cookies, Cakes, Desserts

Cookies: Average, 2-3 cookies, 1 oz	100
Average, 2½ oz	180
Baked Custard, ½ cup	100
Brownie, 1½ oz	130
Carrot Cake, 8 oz	650
Cheesecake, 7 oz	350
Cinnamon Sweet Roll, 2 oz	250
Danish, Apple/Fruit	250
Donut, average	150
Muffins: 1 medium, 2 oz	150
1 extra large, 4 oz	300
Pancakes, (4"), x 3	360
Fruit Pies, average, 7 oz	600
Pudding: Average, ½ cup	160
Jell-O (Mix), Instant, ½ cup	400
Waffles: Home-made, 7", 2½ oz	350
Frozen: Average, 1¼ oz	260
Aunt Jemima, avg, 2½ oz	565

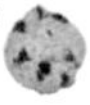

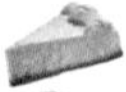

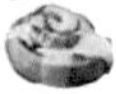

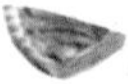

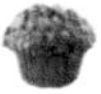

Sodium Counter

Fruit & Juices

	Sodium
Fresh Fruit, average all types, 1 serving	1
Dried/Canned Fruit, ½ cup	1
Fruit Juice: Fresh, sqz'd, 6 fl.oz	1
Commercial, aver., 6 fl.oz	20
Tomato Juice (Campbell's), 6 fl.oz	570
Low Sodium (No Salt Added)	20
V8 Vegetable (Campbell's): 5.5 fl.oz can	290
12 fl.oz bottle	630
Low Sodium, 5.5 fl.oz can	95

Vegetables

Fresh/Frozen (No Salt Added): Per ½ Cup

	Sodium
Asparagus, Bean Sprouts, Corn	3
Beets, Carrots, Celery, ½ cup	40
Broccoli, Cabbage, Cauliflower	10
Cucumber, Green Beans, Mushroom, Okra	3
Onions, Peas, Potato, Pumpkin, Squash	3
Peppers, Hot Chili, raw, each	3
Spinach, Turnips, ½ cup, ckd	40
Tomato, 1 medium, 5 oz	10
Canned: Asparagus, 4 spears	300
Beans, baked in tomato sauce	450
Beets, ½ cup, 3 oz	240
Corn Kernels, ½ cup, 3 oz	190
Creamed, ½ cup, 4½ oz	330
Mushrooms w. butter sce, 2oz	550
Peas, ½ cup, 3 oz	250
Sauerkraut, ½ cup, 4 oz	750

Pickles, Olives

	Sodium
Olives, pickled: Green, 1 large	90
Ripe/black, 1 large	40
Pickles: Bread & Butter, 4 sl., 1 oz	200
Dill, 1 pickle, 2½ oz	900
Sweet, 1 gherkin, ½ oz	130

Soybean Products

	Sodium
Miso (Soy Paste), ¼ c., 2½ oz	2500
Soybean Protein Isolate, 1 oz	280
Tempeh, Natural, ½ cup, 3 oz	5
Tofu, average, ½ cup, 4 oz	5

Jam, Honey, Syrups

	Sodium
Jam/Jelly, 1 Tbsp	2
Honey/Maple Syrup, 1 Tbsp	1
Log Cabin Syrup, 1 fl.oz	35
Lite, 1 fl.oz	90

Peanut Butter

	Sodium
Peanut Butter: Regular, 2 Tbsp, ½ oz	190
Low Sodium (Jif), 2 Tbsp	65
Unsalted (Trader Joe's), 2 Tbsp	5

Snacks, Nuts

	Sodium
Cheese Balls/Curls, 1 oz	280
Cheetos, 1 oz	290
Corn/Tortilla Chips, average, 1 oz	220
Fritos, Lightly Salted, 1 oz	80
Granola bars, average, 1 bar	80
Nuts: Plain, unsalted, 1 oz	1
Lightly salted, 1 oz	80
Salted or Honey Roasted, 1 oz	160
Popcorn: Plain (unsalted), 1 cup	1
Flavored, average, 1 cup	60
Salt added, 1 cup	180
Potato Chips: Plain, 1 oz	160
Lay's, Lightly Salted, 1 oz	90
Flavored, average, 1 oz	250
Pretzels: Regular, 3, 1 oz	450
Soft, salted, large	1000

Candy, Chocolate

	Sodium
Chocolate, milk, 1 oz	30
Fudge, chocolate, 1 oz	55
Candy Bars, average, 1½ oz	60
Hard Candy, Jelly Beans, 1 oz	10
Licorice, 1 oz	30

Beverages, Alcohol

	Sodium
Coffee, Tea, 1 cup	1
Cocoa, dry, plain, 1 Tbsp	0
Mix, average, 1 envelope	120
Quik (Nestle), 2 tsp	35
Soft Drinks, average, 8 fl.oz	20
Mineral Water, Perrier, 8 fl.oz	5
Gatorade Thirst Quencher, 8 fl.oz	110
Red Bull, 8½ fl.oz can	200
Water, Average, 1 cup, 8 fl.oz	5
Alcohol: Beer, average, 12 fl.oz	15
Wines, average, 4 fl.oz	10
Spirits (distilled), 1½ fl.oz	1

Antacids ~ Alka-Seltzer

	Sodium
Alka-Seltzer (Per Tablet):	
Original; Heartburn	570
Extra Strength	590
Lemon Lime	500
Gold	310
Alka-Mints, chewable	0
Bromo Seltzer, ¾ capful	760
Picot, 1 packet, 5g	670
Rolaids, All types	0
Tums, Regular/Extra Strength	0

Cold & Flu ~ Alka-Seltzer Plus

Effervescents, average, 1 tablet	480
Fast Crystal Packs; Liquid Gels	

Sodium Counter

Fast-Foods & Restaurants | Sodium

Burger King:

Burgers: A1 Steakhouse XT — 1930
Cheeseburger — 740
Double Bacon Cheeseburger — 1180
Hamburger — 520
Whoppers: Original — 1020
With Cheese — 1450
Whopper Jr. with Cheese — 750
Chicken, Original — 1390
Sides: French Fries, medium, salted — 670
Onion Rings, medium — 630
Breakfast: Ham, Egg & Cheese Croissanwich — 1110

Denny's:

Better Burgers: Classic Cheeseburger — 1410
Western — 1820
Sandwiches: Club — 1530
Spicy Buffalo Chicken Melt — 3820
Steak & Seafood: Lemon Pepper Tilapia — 1520
T-Bone & Breaded Shrimp — 1490
Soups, Salads & Sides: Chicken Noodle, 12 oz — 1300
Clam Chowder, 12 oz — 1820
Breakfast: Buttermilk Pancakes (3) — 1770
Ham & Cheddar Omelette — 1330
Southwestern Sizzlin Skillet — 2140
Sides: Coleslaw, 3 oz — 520
Everything H. Browns w/ Onions, Cheese & Gravy — 3820
Garlic Bread, 2 pieces — 350
Hash Browns, 5 oz — 650
Vegetable Rice Pilaf, 5 oz — 820
Desserts: Carrot Cake, 8 oz — 660
Hershey's Chocolate Cake, 5 oz — 400

Jack In The Box:

Burgers: Bacon Untimate Cheeseburger — 1840
Hamburger — 570
Jumbo Jack with Cheese — 1250
Sandwiches: Homestyle Ranch Chicken Club — 1940
Turkey, Bacon & Cheddar — 2130

KFC:

Chicken Breast: Original — 710
Extra Crunchy — 1010
Grilled — 460
Popcorn Chicken: Individual, 4 oz — 1160
Value Box — 1900
Strips, Crispy, 3 pieces — 1280
Wings, Boneless Honey BBQ, 3 wings — 1020
Sandwiches: Grilled Filet — 850
Grilled Twister — 1300
Snackers, average all varieties — 700
Sides: Macaroni & Cheese — 880
Mashed Potatoes with Gravy — 530
Potato Wedges — 740

Fast-Foods & Restaurants | Sodium

McDonalds:

Burgers. Angus Bacon & Cheese — 2070
Big Mac — 1040
Cheeseburger — 750
Double — 1150
Hamburger — 520
McChicken — 830
Quarter Pounder with Cheese — 1190
McNuggets: 6 pieces — 600
BBQ Sauce, 1 package, 1 oz — 260
Sandwich: Prem. Grilled Chicken Ranch BLT — 1440
French Fries: Small, 2.5 oz — 160
Medium, 4.1 oz — 270
Large, 5.4 oz — 350
Ketchup, 1 package, 10g — 110
Breakfast: Egg McMuffin — 820
Big Breakfast, reg. size Biscuit — 1560
Hash Browns, 2 oz — 310
Hotcakes, with Syrup & Whipped Margarine — 665
McSkillet Burrito, with Sausage — 1390
Happy Meal: Cheeseburger/Fries/Choc. Milk — 1060
Desserts/Shakes: Hot Fudge Sundae — 180
Chocolate Triple Thick Shake, 16 fl.oz — 250

Pizza Hut:

Pan Pizza, 12": *Per ½ Pizza, 4 Slices*
Meat Lovers — 3300
Cheese; Ham & Pineapple; Veggie, average — 2100
Pepperoni; Hawaiian Luau; Dan's Original, av — 2400
Supreme; Triple Meat; Spicy Sicilian, average — 2800
Thin 'N Crispy ~ *Add an extra 100mg to above figures*

Subway:

6" Lowfat Sandwich: *W/o Condiments/Dressings/Cheese*
Roast Beef/Chicken, average — 800
Subway Club; Turkey; Ham — 1150
Sweet Onion Chicken Teriyaki — 1000
Veggie Delite — 400
6" Sandwiches: *Without Condiments*
BLT; Tuna, average — 950
Philly Chsestk; Meatball Mar.; Subway Melt — 1550
Italian B.M.T.; Spicy Italian, average — 1800
12" Footlong ~ *Double above figures*

Taco Bell: *Per Single Item*
Burritos: ½ lb Combo — 1640
Supreme: Beef; Chicken; Steak, average — 1400
Chapulas; Gorditas: Average — 750
Nachos: Regular — 520
BellGrande — 1300
Specialties: Cheese Quesadillas — 1120
Tacos: Chicken, Soft — 660
Crunchy; Supreme, average — 340

Other Restaurants ~ www.CalorieKing.com

Index C - E

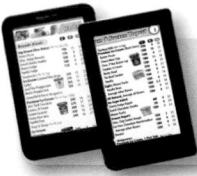
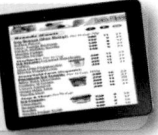

Index E - J

Index O - S

FAST-FOODS INDEX
~ PAGE 175 ~

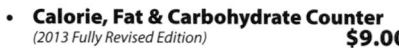
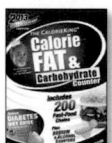 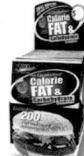 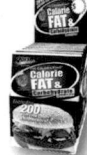
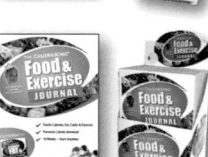
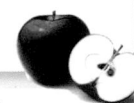
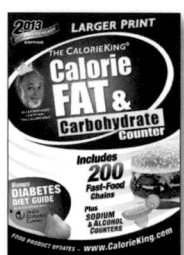
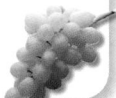

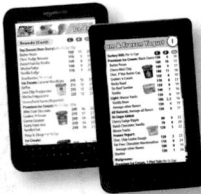
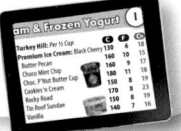